Laser Therapy

Clinical Practice and Scientific Background

A guide for research scientists, doctors, dentists, veterinarians and other interested parties within the medical field.

By
Jan Tunér and Lars Hode

Prima Books AB
2002

Prima Books AB
Spjutvägen 11
772 32 Grängesberg
Sweden
Fax +46 240 23037
www.prima-books.com

Printed by UP Print, Tallinn, Estonia
Illustrations and book design by Anders Nobel

ISBN 91-631-1344-9

Preface

Over 30 years have passed since the first reports appeared on the biological effects of non-thermal laser light. Medical treatment with therapeutic laser light has thus passed through its infancy, childhood, and early maturity, and is now on the cusp of middle age. Maturity has made its mark. The debate that initially raged over whether or not therapeutic lasers should even be used has gradually subsided. Research efforts have matured both qualitatively and quantitatively. The question is no longer whether or not therapeutic lasers have biological effects, but rather how they work and how best to use them.

Today we can safely say that therapeutic lasers have an important biological effect, and a very positive one at that. What is not yet clear are the optimal doses, intensities and treatment intervals and many details in the complicated chain of mechanisms. Extrapolating from cell and animal research to clinical treatment of humans is no easy task. There is also a degree of uncertainty regarding the optimal wavelengths for various indications. The effects of varying pulse frequency remain uncertain.

Despite the questions that remain, we believe that therapeutic lasers have a tremendous and as yet untapped potential in the field of healthcare. It is now clear that therapeutic lasers have no undesirable side effects in the hands of a reasonably qualified therapist. The method is sterile, painless, and often less expensive than methods already in use. Certain indications, such as paraesthesia and mucositis are unique for laser therapy, insofar as there are no effective conventional treatment methods. Therapeutic lasers are effective against herpes and zoster and without the strong side effects of pharmacological treatment. The pharmacological side effects in rheumatic therapy are severe and lead to additional therapy and costs whereas laser therapy has no such side effects. These are just a few examples of the advantages of laser therapy.

We have done our best to address both clinicians and researchers in this book. Such an approach has its pitfalls. The clinician will undoubtedly want more practical advice, the researcher more scientific details. To the clinician, we would emphasise that other, more "hands-on" publications are available. But clinical success is not achieved through picture books and simplifications alone. A deeper knowledge of laser medicine will yield better clinical results as well as and greater pleasure in working. We would encourage researchers to see this book as a sort of "smörgåsbord", a good place to sample various topics and, using the bibliography, find the original studies and explore them more deeply. To make the book somewhat easier to read, we have put some of the more complex topics in a separate chapter.

The scientific literature on therapeutic lasers encompasses some 2,500 titles, including congressional reports and abstracts. Of these, we have catalogued 1,500 and read 1,200 in the original. Most studies of the latter category are included in the book's bibliography, and mini-abstracts have been written for some 400. The majority of these mini-abstracts concern studies that showed positive effects of laser therapy. Many negative studies are listed, but we have chosen to emphasise the positive. We do so not with the goal of sweeping negative findings under the rug, but in order to confirm that there really are scientific grounds for every statement in this book. Much can be learned from the negative studies, as well; all parameters cannot possibly be rosy. But the negative studies need close analysis, too, and in one section of the book we have carefully dissected a number of the better-known, putatively negative studies.

The previous edition of this book was written and published in 1999. Although only three years have passed, an important development has been seen. A lot of sound scientific work has been published. We have tried to include the most relevant new studies, emphasising the clinical side. New powerful and comparatively inexpensive semiconductor lasers have emerged. These new lasers have shown that dosages and power densities can be increased at an advantage, in relation to those recommended in the previous book.

This book is the third English title by these authors. The previous books were "Laser Therapy in Dentistry and Medicine" and "Low Level Laser Therapy - clinical practice and scientific background". Although a casual reader would recognise much of the material in the old books, the present book is different in many ways. New research has been added, new chapters written, old chapters re-edited and updated. This upgrading is important in a scientific field like laser therapy, where new and important knowledge has been added during recent years.

It is our hope that this book will be of use to all those who have an interest in the therapeutic use of lasers. We are eager to continue the dialogue that we have with our readers and are grateful to receive suggestions and criticism, both positive and negative.

Jan Tunér
D.D.S

Lars Hode
Dr.Sci

Terminology in this book

The therapeutical lasers used today are mainly below 500 mW. However, many lasers generally used for surgery can be defocused and arranged to give energy densities of the same values as the former. Thus, a therapeutic laser could be defined as a laser using energy densities below the threshold where irreversible changes in cells occur.

Regarding the therapy, we have chosen to use the term **laser therapy** (instead of Low Level Laser Therapy), mostly out of a desire to dispense with a lot of unnecessary words. This is the dominant term in use today, but there is still a lack of consensus.

Regarding the laser instrument, we have chosen to use the term therapeutic laser rather than "low-level laser", since high-level lasers are also used for laser therapy. Another reason is that many of the traditional laser types today are not really Low Level any more and the trend is towards higher output power.

The term "soft laser" was originally used to differentiate therapeutic lasers from "hard lasers", i.e. surgical lasers. Several different designations then emerged, such as "MID laser" and "medical laser". "Biostimulating laser" is another term, with the disadvantage that one can also give inhibiting doses. The term "bioregulating laser" has thus been proposed. One of the most frequent terms, "low-power laser", is also misleading, since high-power lasers, too, are used for laser therapy.

An unsuitable name is "low-energy laser". The energy transferred to tissue is the product of laser output power and treatment time, which is why a "low-energy laser", over a long period of time, can actually emit a large amount of energy.

Other suggested names are "low-reactive-level laser", "low-intensity-level laser", "photobiostimulation laser" and "photobiomodulation laser".

Thus, it is obvious that the question of nomenclature is far from solved. This is because there is a lack of full agreement internationally, and the names proposed thus far have been rather unwieldy. Feel free to forget them, but remember laser therapy until agreement is reached on something else.

Suggested key words in computer search: laser therapy, low level laser therapy, biostimulation, bioregulation, low power laser, soft laser, therapeutic laser, medical laser, MID laser, low energy laser, low reactive-level laser, low intensity laser, low intensity-level laser, photobiostimulation, photobiomodulation, LILT, LELT and LPLT.

Contents

Chapter 1 Some basic laser physics 1

1.1 Electromagnetic radiation 2

1.1.1 Wavelength and frequency 2

1.1.2 Photon energy 2

1.1.3 The electromagnetic spectrum 2

1.1.4 The optical field 3

1.1.5 Radiation risks 3

1.1.6 Can electromagnetic radiation cause cancer? 4

1.1.7 Protective mechanisms 5

1.2 Various sources of radiation 5

1.2.1 Natural sources of radiation 5

1.2.2 Man-made sources of radiation 5

1.2.3 The light-emitting diode (LED) 6

1.2.4 The laser 8

1.2.5 Laser design 8

1.2.6 The properties of laser light 12

1.2.7 Coherence 12

1.2.8 Polarisation 15

1.2.9 Output power 16

1.2.10 Continuous and pulsed lasers 16

1.2.11 The pulse peak power 17

1.2.12 Average power output 17

1.2.13 Power density 17

1.2.14 Collimation 19

1.2.15 Risk of eye injury 19

1.2.16 Decisive factors in the risk of eye injury 22

1.3 Laser types in medicine and surgery 26

1.4 The surgical lasers 27

1.4.1 The Carbon dioxide laser (CO_2-laser) 28

1.4.1.1 Carbon dioxide lasers in surgery 29

1.4.1.2 Carbon dioxide lasers in dental applications 31

1.4.2 The Nd:YAG laser 33

1.4.2.1 Nd:YAG lasers in surgery 33

1.4.2.2 Nd:YAG lasers in dentistry 33

1.4.3 Ho:YAG lasers 35

1.4.4 Er:YAG lasers 35

1.4.5 Argon laser 37

1.4.6 Copper vapour laser 37

1.4.7 KTP/532-laser (frequency doubled Nd:YAG laser) 37
1.4.8 Ruby laser 38
1.4.9 Alexandrite 39
1.4.10 High power semiconductor lasers 39
1.4.11 Dye laser 39
1.4.12 Excimer laser 39
1.5 Therapeutic lasers 40
1.5.1 The Helium-Neon laser (HeNe) 40
1.5.2 Indium-Gallium-Aluminium-Phosphide lasers (InGaAlP) 41
1.5.3 Gallium-Aluminium-Arsenide lasers (GaAlAs) 41
1.5.4 The Gallium-Arsenide laser (GaAs) 42
1.5.5 The defocused strong lasers 43
1.5.6 Some "exotic lasers" 44
1.5.7 The krypton laser 44
1.5.8 The nitrogen laser 44
Chapter 2 Therapeutic instruments 45
2.1 A customer's guide 46
2.1.1 History 46
2.1.2 What will tomorrows lasers look like 47
2.1.3 Hand held lasers and automatic devices 48
2.1.4 Which type of laser is best suited to which task? 49
2.1.4.1 HeNe laser and InGaAlP laser 49
2.1.4.2 GaAs laser 50
2.1.4.3 GaAlAs lasers 50
2.1.4.4 Combination probes 51
2.1.4.5 Therapeutic CO_2-lasers 52
2.1.5 Which laser should I buy? 52
2.1.6 Stronger = better? 53
2.1.7 How much should a laser cost? 55
2.1.8 Is a therapeutic laser really worth the money? 56
2.1.9 Do you need to update your laser? 56
2.2 Ten points to consider when choosing an instrument 56
2.3 How do I maintain my laser? 59
Chapter 3 Biostimulation 61
3.1 History 62
3.2 A few words on mechanisms 65
3.2.1 Photoreceptors 67
3.3 What parameters to use 68
3.3.1 Laser parameters 68

3.3.1.1	*Which wavelength?*	*68*
3.3.1.2	*Output power*	*69*
3.3.1.3	*Average output power*	*69*
3.3.1.4	*Power density*	*69*
3.3.1.5	*Energy density*	*70*
3.3.1.6	*Treatment dose*	*70*
3.3.1.7	*Calculation of doses*	*71*
3.3.1.8	*Dose ranges*	*72*
3.3.1.9	*Calculation of treatment time for a desired dose*	*75*
3.3.1.10	*"Ready reckoner"*	*75*
3.3.1.11	*Dose per point*	*77*
3.3.1.12	*Pulsed or continuous light*	*77*
3.3.1.13	*Pulse frequency*	*78*
3.3.2	Patient parameters	79
3.3.2.1	*Treatment area*	*79*
3.3.2.2	*Treatment intervals*	*80*
3.3.2.3	*Pre- or postoperative treatment?*	*82*
3.3.3	Treatment method parameters	83
3.3.3.1	*Local treatment*	*83*
3.3.3.1.1	*Shallow problems*	*83*
3.3.3.1.2	*Deeper problems*	*83*
3.3.3.1.3	*Treating inside the body*	*84*
3.3.3.2	*Systemic treatments*	*84*
3.3.3.2.1	*Acupuncture.*	*84*
3.3.3.2.2	*Trigger points*	*87*
3.3.3.2.3	*Spinal processes*	*88*
3.3.3.2.4	*Dermatome*	*88*
3.3.3.2.5	*Blood irradiation*	*88*
3.3.3.2.6	*Lymph nodes*	*91*
3.3.4	Combination treatment	91
3.3.5	Interaction with medication	91
3.4	**Other considerations**	**92**
3.4.1	What about collimation?	92
3.4.2	Depth of penetration, greatest active depth	92
3.4.2.1	*Factors that reduce penetration*	*94*
3.4.2.2	*Tissue compression*	*95*
3.4.2.3	*How deep does the light penetrate?*	*95*
3.4.3	The importance of the tissue and cell condition	95
3.4.4	In vitro/in vivo	97
3.5	**Laser Therapy with high output lasers**	**98**

3.5.1 Laser therapy with carbon dioxide lasers ... 98
3.5.2 Laser therapy with Nd:YAG lasers ... 100
3.5.3 Laser therapy with ruby lasers ... 101
3.6 Risks and side effects ... 101
3.6.1 The importance of a correct diagnose ... 102
3.6.2 Cancer ... 102
3.6.3 Cytogenetic effects? ... 102
3.6.4 A false picture of health ... 103
3.6.5 Tiredness ... 103
3.6.6 Pain reaction ... 103
3.6.7 Do high doses of laser therapy damage tissue? ... 103
3.6.8 Protection against radiation injury ... 104
3.7 How to measure effects of laser therapy ... 105
3.7.1 Thermography ... 105
3.7.2 Magnetic resonance imaging ... 106
3.7.3 High resolution digitised ultrasound B-scan ... 106
3.7.4 Tensile strength ... 106
3.7.5 Other objective methods ... 106
3.8 "Is laser therapy effective?" ... 107
3.8.1 Does laser therapy really work? ... 107
3.8.2 Why the controversy? ... 108
3.8.3 Does it have to be a laser? ... 109
3.8.4 FDA (Food and Drug Administration) ... 110
3.8.5 "There is no documentation on that!" ... 111
3.8.6 Confused? ... 112
3.8.7 Experience and attitudes ... 113
3.8.8 The funding of research ... 114
Chapter 4 Medical indications ... 115
4.1 Who and what can be treated? ... 116
4.1.1 Allergy, acne systica gravis and eczema ... 116
4.1.2 Arteriosclerosis ... 117
4.1.3 Asthma ... 117
4.1.4 Arthritis ... 118
4.1.5 Blood pressure ... 125
4.1.6 Bone regeneration ... 126
4.1.7 Cancer ... 130
4.1.8 Cardiac conditions ... 134
4.1.9 Carpal tunnel syndrome ... 135
4.1.10 Cerebral palsy ... 136
4.1.11 Crural and venous ulcers ... 137

4.1.12 Depression, psychosomatic problems 139
4.1.13 Diabetes 140
4.1.14 Duodenal/gastric ulcer 141
4.1.15 Epicondylitis 141
4.1.16 Fibrositis/fibromyalgia 143
4.1.17 Gynaecologic indications 145
4.1.18 Headache/Migraine 146
4.1.19 Haemorrhoids 147
4.1.20 Herpes simplex 147
4.1.21 Immune system modulation 149
4.1.22 Inner ear conditions 151
4.1.23 Laryngitis 151
4.1.24 Lichen 151
4.1.25 Low back pain 152
4.1.26 Microcirculation 152
4.1.27 Morbus Sluder 155
4.1.28 Mucositis 155
4.1.29 Muscle regeneration 155
4.1.30 Nerve conduction 156
4.1.31 Nerve regeneration and function 157
4.1.32 Oedema 162
4.1.33 Ophthalmic problems 164
4.1.34 Pain 166
4.1.35 Plantar fasciitis 170
4.1.36 Salivary glands 171
4.1.37 Sinuitis 172
4.1.38 Spinal cord injuries 173
4.1.39 Sports injuries 174
4.1.40 Strain injuries 175
4.1.41 Tendinitis/bursitis 176
4.1.42 Tinnitus, vertigo, Ménière´s disease 178
4.1.43 Tonsillitis 183
4.1.44 Trigeminal neuralgia 184
4.1.45 Thrombophlebitis 185
4.1.46 Tuberculosis 185
4.1.47 Urology 185
4.1.48 Warts 188
4.1.49 Whiplash-associated disorders 188
4.1.50 Wound healing 189
4.1.51 Zoster 196
4.2 Anecdotal indications 198

4.2.1 Obesity ... 198
4.2.2 Wrinkles ... 198
4.2.3 Cellulites ... 199
4.2.4 Hair loss ... 199
4.2.5 Problems with orgasm ... 199

Chapter 5 Dental laser therapy ... 201

5.1 What is "a god dentist" ... 202

5.2 On which patients can laser therapy be used? ... 203

5.3 Dental indications ... 203

5.3.1 Alveolitis ... 204
5.3.2 Anaesthetics ... 204
5.3.3 Aphthae (canker sores) ... 205
5.3.4 Bleeding ... 206
5.3.5 Caries ... 207
5.3.6 Dentitio dificilis ... 209
5.3.7 Endodontics ... 210
5.3.8 Extraction ... 211
5.3.9 Gingivitis ... 213
5.3.10 Herpes zoster ... 215
5.3.11 Hypersensitive dentine ... 215
5.3.12 Implantology ... 218
5.3.13 Jaw fractures ... 219
5.3.14 Leukoplakia ... 219
5.3.15 Lingua geographica (glossitis) ... 219
5.3.16 Lip wounds ... 220
5.3.17 Mucositis ... 220
5.3.18 Nausea ... 220
5.3.19 Nerve injury ... 220
5.3.20 Oedema ... 221
5.3.21 Oral surgery ... 221
5.3.22 Orthodontics ... 222
5.3.23 Pain ... 224
5.3.24 Mild dental pain ... 224
5.3.25 Paediatric dental treatment ... 224
5.3.26 Periodontics ... 225
5.3.27 Prosthetics ... 228
5.3.28 Secondary dentine formation ... 229
5.3.29 Temporo-mandibular disorders (TMD) ... 230

5.4 Other dental laser applications ... 234

5.4.1 Dental photo dynamic therapy ... 234

5.4.2 Composite curing 235
5.4.3 Tooth bleaching 235
5.4.4 Dental casts 235
5.4.5 Caries detection 235
5.5 Case reports 235

Chapter 6 Dental research 239

Argentina 240
Córdoba University, Faculty of Dentistry, Córdoba 240
Australia 240
University of Queensland, Dental School 240
Royal Perth Hospital, Plastic Surgery and Maxillofacial Unit, Perth 241
Austria 241
Universitätsklinik für Kiefer- und Gesichtschirurgie, Vienna 241
Belgium 241
University of Ghent, Department of Orthodontics. 241
Brazil 241
UNESP, Faculdade de Odontologia, São José dos Campos, S.P. 241
Bauru School of Dentistry. University of São Paulo 242
University of São Paulo, Dentistry School 242
University of São Carlos, Sao Carlos, Sao Paulo 242
Universidade de Castelo Branco, São Paulo 243
Universidade de Castelo Branco, São Paulo 243
Universidade Federal de Pernambuco, School of Dentistry 244
Bulgaria 244
University of Medicine, Plovdiv, Department of Therapeutic Stomatology 244
Canada 244
McGill University, Faculty of Dentistry, Division of Oral and Maxillofacial Surgery, Montreal 244
Université Laval, Faculty of Dentistry, Quebec 244
China 245
West China University of Medical Sciences, Chengdu 245
Fourth Military Medical University, Xian 245
Nanfang Hospital, Stomatological Department, Guangzhou. 245
Croatia 245
Medicinski fakultet Rijeka, Katedra za stomatologiju, Rijeka 245
Cuba 246
University of Havana. DIEES-IMRE, La Habana 246
Czech Republic 246
Institute of Dental Research, Prague 246
Charles University, Prague 246
Denmark 246
Aarhus Universitet. Royal Dental College, Aarhus 246
Royal Dental College, Department of Oral and Maxillofacial Surgery, Copenhagen 247
Odense University Hospital, Odense 247
Egypt 247
Alexandria University, Faculty of Dentistry and Medicine 247
Finland 247
University of Helsinki, Department of Oral Surgery, Helsinki 247

France 247
Institut Pasteur de Lyon, Faculté d'Odontologie, Lyon 247
Faculté d'Odontologie de Marseille, Laboratoire de Biologie 248
Hôpital de la Pitié, Service d'anatomie pathologique, Paris 248
Faculté de Chirurgie Dentaire, Paris 248
Department of Radiotherapy, Cancer Centre, Marseilles 249
CHU, Service de Stomatologie, Dijon 249
Germany 249
Johannes Gutenberg-University, Mainz. 249
Universität Hannover, Institut für Biophysik, Hannover 249
University of Heidelberg, Dental School, Department of Conservative and Preventive Dentistry 249
Great Britain 250
Dental Hospital, Department of Maxillofacial Surgery, Cardiff 250
University Dental School, Department of Oral and Maxillofacial Surgery, Manchester 250
The Royal London School of Medicine and Dentistry, London 250
Institute of Dental Surgery, Department of Microbiology, London 251
University of London, Department of Microbiology. 251
University of Glasgow, Division of Neuroscience 251
Indonesia 252
Fakultas Kedokteran Gigi Universitas Airlangga, Laboratorium periodontia 252
Israel 252
Italy 252
Ospedale A. Cardarelli. Div di Odontostomatologia e Traumatiolgia Maxillo-Facciale, Naples 252
Università di Torino. Instituto Policattedra di Clinica Odontostomato-logica 253
University of Modena, Department of Dentistry and Oral Surgery, Modena 254
Università degli Studi di Firenze, Instituto di Odonto-gnato-stomatologia, Florence. 254
Università degli studi di Bologna, Instituti policattedra di clinica odontostomatologica, Bologna. 254
Japan 255
Niigata University, School of Dentistry 255
Iwate Medical University, School of Dentistry, Department of Oral Pathology, Morioka 255
Keio University, Department of Dentistry and Oral Surgery, Tokyo 255
Nihon University, School of Dentistry, Department of Endodontics, Tokyo 256
Showa University, School of Dentistry, Department of Endodontics, Tokyo 257
Tokyo Dental College, Department of Orthodontics. 258
Hiroo Metropolitan General Hospital, Tokyo 258
Ohu University, Graduate School of Dentistry, Ohu 258
Nihon University School of Dentistry, Matsudo, Chiba 259
Aichi-Gakuin University, Nagoya 259
Kyushu University, Faculty of Dentistry, Department of Preventive Dentistry, Fukuoka 260
Korea 262
Seoul National University, College of Dentistry, Department of Oral Diagnostics 262
Wonkwang University, School of Dentistry, Department of Oral Diagnostics and Oral Medicine 263
Dankook University, Department of Dentistry, Choongnam 263
Pusan National University, College of Dentistry, Department of Oral Medicine 263
Chonbuk National University, School of Dentistry, Department of Oral Medicine 264
Kuwait 264
Ministry of Public Health, Dental Centre, Department of Crown and Bridge 264
The Netherlands 264
University of Amsterdam, Academic Centre for Dentistry, Department of Masticatory Function 264
University of Nijmegen, Department of Orthodontics and Oral Pathology 265
Norway 265

University of Oslo, Faculty of Dentistry, Department of Oral Surgery and Oral Medicine 265
Poland 266
Medical Academy of Bialystok, Department of Conservative Dentistry 266
Medical University of Lodz, Institute of Dentistry, Lodz. 266
Portugal 267
Romania 267
University of Medicine and Pharmacy, School of Dentistry, Department of Oral Rehabilitation. 267
Disciplina de Propedeutica Stomatologica, Universitatea "Ovidius" Constanta. 267
Russia 267
Moscow Institute of Medicine and Stomatology 267
Voronezh State Medical Academy, Voronezh 268
State Research Centre for Laser Medicine, Moscow 269
Singapore 271
National University of Singapore, Faculty of Dentistry 271
South Africa 271
University of Pretoria, Faculty of Dentistry, Centre for Stomatological Research. 271
Spain 271
Faculty of Odontology, Department of Oral Medicine and Maxillo-facial Surgery, Madrid 271
Hospital Provincial de Madrid 271
Universidad de Oviedo, Escuela de Estomatología 272
Universidad Nacional, Faculdad de Odontología, Córdoba. 272
Universitat Rovira i Virgili, Facultad de Medicina i Ciencia de la Salut, Reus. 272
Sweden 272
Karolinska Institutet, Department of Periodontology, Stockholm 272
Switzerland 272
Université de Genève, Geneva 272
La Carita Hospital, Locarno 273
Taiwan 273
Pharmaceutical Industry Technology and Development Center, Taipei Hsien. 273
Thailand 273
Khon Kean University, Bangkok 273
Turkey 273
Istanbul School of Dentistry, Istanbul 273
Gazi University, Faculty of Dentistry, Ankara 273
Marmara University, Department of Oral and Maxillofacial Surgery 274
United Arab Emirates 274
Clinic for Laser & Physiotherapy, Dubai 274
USA 274
Baylor College of Medicine, Texas Children's Hospital, Department of Pathology. 274
University of Illinois, School of Dentistry, Department of Material Science 274
University of California, School of Dentistry, San Francisco 274
Center for Dental AIDS Research, Waukegan, Ill. 274
University of Connecticut, School of Dental Medicine, Farmington 275
University of Nebraska, College of Dentistry, Lincoln, Nebraska 275
Department of Periodontics, Maxwell AFB, Alabama 275
University of Maryland, Department of Oral-Maxillofacial Surgery, Baltimore, MD. 275
Uzbekistan 275
First State Medical Institute, Tashkent 275

Chapter 7 Veterinary use 277

Chapter 8 Contraindications 285

8.1 Pacemaker 286

8.2 Pregnancy 286

8.3 Epilepsy 286

8.4 Thyroid gland 286

8.5 Children 287

8.6 Cancer 288

8.7 Radiation therapy patients 288

8.8 Diabetes 289

Chapter 9 Laser therapy on the Internet 291

9.1 Laser therapy on the Internet 292

9.2 Internet discussion groups 292

9.2.1 Tinnitus 292

9.2.2 Wavelength 292

9.2.3 Coherence 294

9.2.4 Polarisation 294

9.2.5 Laser power 295

9.2.6 Light emitting diodes (LED) 298

9.2.7 Pulse frequencies 301

9.2.8 FDA approval 302

9.2.9 Miscellaneous 310

Chapter 10 The difficult dose and intensity 311

10.1 Basics about energy 312

10.2 Output power 313

10.3 Power density 314

10.4 The laser beam 316

10.5 The laser probe 318

10.6 Pulsed lasers 319

10.7 Energy density 319

10.8 Treatment dose 320

10.9 The dose does not depend on the intensity 325

10.10 Dose per point 328

10.11 More about treatment technique 329

Chapter 11 The Mechanisms 333

11.1 Are the biostimulative effects laser specific? 334

11.1.1 Is it possible to prove that laser therapy doesn't work? 334

11.1.2 Comparisons between coherent and non-coherent light 335

11.1.2.1 Hode's hamburger ... 338
11.1.2.2 Hode's big burger ... 340
11.1.3 Abrahamsson's apple ... 341
11.1.4 Moonlight ... 342
11.1.5 How deep does light penetrate into tissue? ... 343
11.1.6 Bright Light Phototherapy ... 345
11.1.7 Similarities and differences ... 348
11.2 Possible primary mechanisms ... 348
11.2.1 What characterises the light in a laser speckle? ... 350
11.2.2 Porphyrins and polarised light ... 350
11.2.3 Cell cultures and tissue have different optical properties ... 351
11.2.4 Is laser therapy an effect of heat development in the tissue? ... 352
11.2.5 Fluorescence - luminescence ... 353
11.2.6 Multi-photon effects ... 354
11.2.7 Lasing effects in tissue ... 354
11.2.8 Non linear optical effects ... 355
11.2.9 Opto-acoustic waves ... 356
11.3 Secondary mechanisms ... 356
11.3.1 Effects on pain ... 356
11.3.2 Effects on blood circulation ... 358
11.3.3 Stimulatory and regulatory mechanisms ... 358
11.3.4 Effects on the immune system ... 359
11.3.5 Other interesting possibilities ... 360
11.4 Summary of mechanisms ... 361
11.5 Diagnostics with Therapy Lasers ... 363
11.6 Photodynamic Therapy - PDT, ... 363
11.7 Other medical uses of lasers ... 363
Chapter 12 A guide for scientific work ... 365
12.1 Methodology of a trial ... 368
12.2 Parameters ... 369
Technical parameters ... 369
Treatment parameters ... 369
Medical parameters ... 370
12.2.1 Closer description of the technical parameters ... 370
1) Name of instrument (producer) ... 370
2) Laser type and wavelength ... 370
3) Laser beam characteristics ... 371
4) Number of sources ... 371
5) Beam delivery system ... 371
6) Pulsed or continuous emission ... 371

7) Output power 372
8) Power density at probe aperture 372
9) Calibration of the instrument 373
12.2.2 Closer description of the treatment parameters 373
1) Treatment area 373
2) Dose: Energy density 373
3) Dose per treatment and total dose 374
4) Intensity: Power density 374
5) Treatment method 374
6) Treatment distance (spot size), type of movement, scanning 374
7) Sites of treatment 375
8) Number of treatment sessions 375
9) Frequency of treatment sessions 375
12.2.3 Closer description of the medical parameters 376
1) Description of the problem to be treated 376
2) Patients (number, age, sex) 376
3) Exclusion criteria 376
4) Inclusion criteria 376
5) Condition of patient 376
6) Pre-, parallel- or post-medication 376
7) Treated with other methods before 377
8) Drop-out rate 377
9) Follow up 377
10) Outcome measures 377
11) Statistical Analysis 377
12) Economy 377
Conclusion 377

Chapter 13 The laser therapy literature 379

13.1 The positive double blind studies 380

13.2 The negative double blind studies 388

13.3 Are all the negative studies really negative? 391

13.3.1 "I heard it through the grapevine" 391
13.3.2 Positive from negative 392
13.3.3 Negative from negative 392
13.3.4 Dose development 392
13.3.5 Pitfalls 393

13.4 The Cochrane analyses – can they be improved? 412

13.5 Poor documentation – compared to what? 418

13.6 The Russian experience 418

13.7 The work of Tiina Karu 421

13.8 English language books on laser therapy: 430

13.9 Books in other languages, with ISBN. 431
13.10 Laser journals 433

Chapter 14 References - Abbreviations 435

14.1 Numeric references referred to in the book. 436
14.2 Alphabetical register of references 499
14.3 Abbreviations 559

Alphabetic index 561

List of figures

Figure 1.1	Wavelength distribution of light from various sources	7
Figure 1.2	Star wars	9
Figure 1.3	Principle design of a laser	10
Figure 1.4	Photographed laser speckles	14
Figure 1.5	Laser speckles	14
Figure 1.6	Coherent and non-coherent light	15
Figure 1.7	Different types of pulsing	18
Figure 1.8	Laser and light-bulb	21
Figure 1.9	Laser and eye-risk	23
Figure 1.10	Portable CO_2-laser	29
Figure 1.11	Hyperplasia removed with Er:YAG laser	36
Figure 1.12	Absorption coefficient for melanin and hemoglobin	38
Figure 2.1	Small rechargeable 300 mW GaAlAs laser	46
Figure 2.2	Courtesy: Glen Calderhead	47
Figure 2.3	Typical scanner	48
Figure 2.4	Therapeutic laser, including three different laser types	49
Figure 2.5	Therapeutic CO_2-laser, 10-15 W to tissue	52
Figure 2.6	900 mW GaAlAs (810 nm) probe	54
Figure 3.1	The Swedish daily Svenska Dagbladet, October 31st, 1963	62
Figure 3.2	"The historic mice" I. Courtesy: Andrew Mester	64
Figure 3.3	"The historic mice" II. Courtesy: Andrew Mester	64
Figure 3.4	Apple ready reckoner	76
Figure 3.5	Cumulative dose	81
Figure 3.6	Shorter treatment intervals	81
Figure 3.7	Methods of blood irradiation. Modified from Gasparyan	90
Figure 3.8	Depth of penetration, direct contact	93
Figure 3.9	Depth of penetration, distance	94
Figure 4.1	Oropharyngeal carcinoma	131
Figure 4.2	Typical mucositis	133
Figure 4.3	Typical labial HSV-1	148
Figure 4.4	Facial paresis	161
Figure 4.5	Stye day one and two, following HeNe laser therapy.	165
Figure 4.6	Sinuitis maxillaris before and after GaAlAs laser therapy.	172
Figure 4.7	Skin wound	189
Figure 5.1	Aphthae	206
Figure 5.2	Endodontics	210
Figure 5.3	Extraction	212
Figure 5.4	Hypersensitve dentine	216
Figure 5.5	Angular chielitis	220
Figure 5.6	Location of the P 6 point	220
Figure 5.7	Evaluation of microcirculation in tender points	230

Figure 7.1	Laser probe for veterinary use	281
Figure 10.1	Typical diode collimator	314
Figure 10.2	Laser with focusing lens	315
Figure 10.3	Even beam distribution	316
Figure 10.4	Gaussian beam distribution	316
Figure 10.5	Measured power distribution in typical probe apertures	317
Figure 10.6	Arndt-Schulz law	320
Figure 10.7	Laser on skin	323
Figure 10.8	Lasers on skin	324
Figure 10.9	Lasers on skin, short - long wavelength	325
Figure 10.10	Treatment of an open leg ulcer	326
Figure 10.11	Treatment outside of an open leg ulcer	327
Figure 10.12	Apple	328
Figure 10.13	Distributed light	329
Figure 10.14	Treatment technique	330
Figure 11.1	Hode's hamburger	338
Figure 11.2	Set-up for Hode's hamburger experiment	339
Figure 11.3	Extended set-up	340
Figure 11.4	Different light sources have different spectra	340
Figure 11.5	Enlarged real laser speckles	342
Figure 11.6	Transilluminated hand	343
Figure 11.7	The mechanism of laser therapy	362

List of tables

Table 1.1 The electromagnetic spectrum ... 3
Table 1.2 Different lasers, their wavelengths and use ... 26
Table 1.3 Typical surgical lasers and their wavelengths ... 27
Table 1.4 Typical therapeutic lasers and their wavelengths ... 40
Table 3.1 Dose to skin surface ... 71
Table 3.2 Output power dependent on pulse frequency ... 72
Table 3.3 Dose ranges for different lasers and indications ... 73
Table 3.4 Treatment time with a GaAs-laser ... 76
Table 3.5 Treatment time with a GaAlAs laser ... 77
Table 3.6 Pulse frequency - laser acupuncture ... 78
Table 4.1 Arthritis ... 119
Table 4.2 Tendinitis/Bursitis different characteristics ... 177
Table 11.1 Absorption ... 344
Table 11.2 BLT literature ... 347
Table 11.3 Examples of different dose levels in vitro ... 349
Table 13.1 Waylonis G W et al ... 394
Table 13.2 Jensen H et al ... 395
Table 13.3 Basford J R et al ... 396
Table 13.4 Taube S et al ... 397
Table 13.5 Lundeberg T, Haker E, Thomas M ... 398
Table 13.6 Masse J-F et al ... 399
Table 13.7 Smith R J et al ... 400
Table 13.8 Klein R G et al ... 401
Table 13.9 Seichert N et al ... 402
Table 13.10 Mulcahy D et al ... 403
Table 13.11 de Bie et al ... 408
Table 13.12 Laser therapy - ultrasound ... 418
Table 13.13 Indication Russian/Ukranian language literature ... 420

Chapter 1
Some basic laser physics

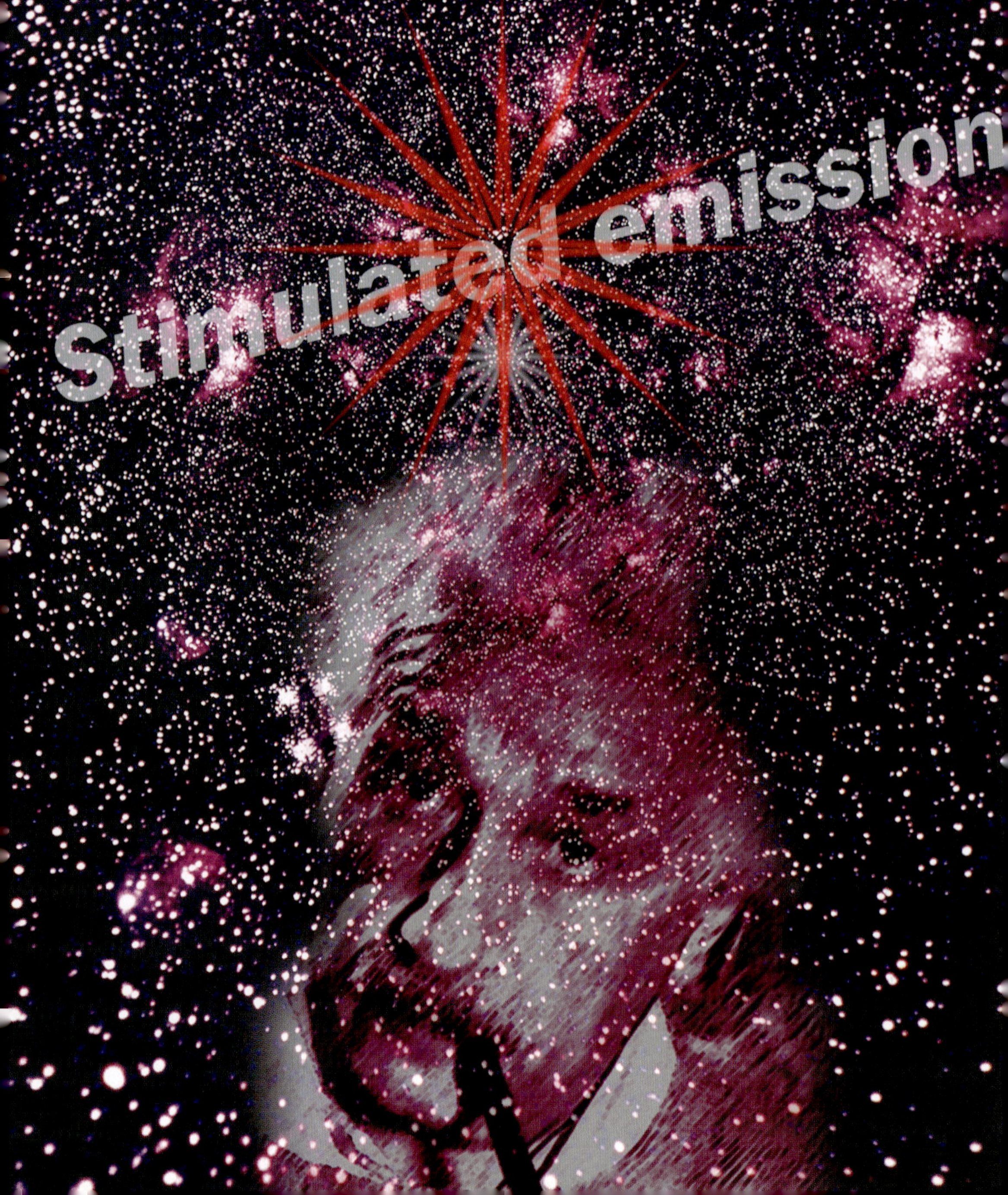

1.1 Electromagnetic radiation

This book is not intended to be a textbook of physics. The aim of this chapter is first and foremost to explain to the reader why some lasers can be harmful to the eyes. We will also describe briefly the various types of laser which are used within medicine and some of their characteristics.

The radiation emitted by the sun, light bulbs, fires, radio transmitters, etc., is called electromagnetic radiation. This is a form of energy consisting of photons - packets of energy - that travel at the speed of light, i.e. approximately 300,000 kilometres per second in a vacuum. Photons can be seen as wave particles or wave packets. Each photon is thus a small packet of energy in the form of a wave element, in which the wave (in the same way as water waves or sound waves) has a defined wavelength and a frequency related to that wavelength.

1.1.1 Wavelength and frequency

The relationship between wavelength (λ) and frequency (ν) is:

$$\lambda \times \nu = c$$

where c = the speed of light in the medium of interest. (In media other than a vacuum the formula will be: $\lambda \times \nu = c/n$ where n is the index of refraction.)

Within the part of the electromagnetic spectrum that we call the radio frequency field, frequency is often used instead of wavelength (e.g. for FM radio stations – 87-108 MHz). In the other parts of the we would have to use unmanageably high numbers and therefore use the wavelength in all but a few cases. We will from now on use wavelength, rater than frequency, because “frequency” often arises in discussions about pulsed radiation and is used to denote pulse frequency (number of pulses per second).

1.1.2 Photon energy

Photons of different wavelengths have different energy levels. Photon energy (E) is proportional to frequency (λ) and can be expressed as

$$E = h \times \nu = h \times c/\lambda$$

where h is equal to Planck’s constant. If we use wavelength instead of frequency, photon energy would be inversely proportional to the photon’s wavelength. Photons with a long wavelength therefore have a low energy, while photons with a short wavelength have a high energy.

1.1.3 The electromagnetic spectrum

Electromagnetic radiation spans an enormous range of wavelengths, often referred to as the wavelength spectrum, and the different parts of this spectrum have been given different names. The table on next page shows each part in terms of its name, range of wavelength, a description of its use, and an example of the source of the radiation. The electromagnetic spectrum, subranges, wavelengths, use and typical sources

Name	Wavelengths	Used for	Source
Radio waves	1000 -1 m	Radio, TV, telecommunications, cellular telephones	Radio transmitters, electric cables
Microwaves	1000 -1 mm	Radar, telecom, microwave ovens, speed measuring	Klystrons, magnetrons, masers
Infrared (IR)	1000 - 0.8 µm	Radiation heaters, infrared heating, remote control	Hot objects, IR lamps, fires, LEDs, lasers
Visible light	800 –400 nm	Illumination, photography, imaging, holography	Light-bulbs, flash lamps, candles, LEDs, lasers
Ultraviolet (UV)	400 -1 nm	Solarium, curing of plastics, sterilisation	UV lamps, lasers, accelerators
X-rays	1000 -1 pm	X-raying, radiation treatment of tumours	X-ray tubes, accelerators
Gamma Rays	1000 -1 fm	Radiation treatment of cancer, sterilisation of food	Radioactive isotopes, particle accelerators

Table 1.1 The electromagnetic spectrum

1.1.4 The optical field

The spectrum of electromagnetic radiation that follows the laws of optics includes wavelengths between approximately 1 nm and 1000 µm and is usually referred to as "optical radiation", even though most of it lies outside the visible spectrum (wavelengths of about 400-800 nm). Both infrared (IR) and ultraviolet (UV) radiation exhibit many similarities to visible light and are therefore regarded as part of the optical field. When using the term "light" from now on, we will be referring to infrared and ultraviolet radiation as well as visible light.

1.1.5 Radiation risks

Special considerations relating to the eyes will not be discussed in this section; See chapter 1.2.15 "Risk of eye injury" on page 19.

Because different wavelengths have different energy levels, the risks of exposure to various kinds of electromagnetic radiation are also of varying magnitude. High-energy photons (gamma rays, X-rays and ultraviolet light) can "break" (ionise) atoms and break up chemical bonds in molecules which they encounter, while low-energy photons (radio waves and microwaves, infrared and visible light) do not cause ionisation but only excitation and heating. Photons in the optical field, either as visible light, ultraviolet or infrared, can be reflected, transmitted (that is, go right through) or absorbed when they come in contact with matter. Tissue is generally more transparent to wavelengths near infrared (800 - 1200 nm) than to visible light. When a photon is absorbed, it sheds all of its energy into the matter and is annihilated. The energy shed is transformed into another type of energy, most often thermal. Consequently, if high-power radiation (many watts = many photons per second) encounters an object, a great deal of heat can result (for example, a stone in the sun becomes hot). By concentrating a beam on a small area, e.g. by focusing it, a high power density is achieved in that small area and the heat built up during the absorption of the radiation can be so great that the beam burns, melts or vaporises the material in the area encountered. This technique is used in surgical lasers. In this way, all radiation (if sufficiently intense) can injure an individual or an object.

However, those types of radiation involving photons in which the energy level is so high that they can ionise are dangerous even at low intensities, because ionisation is by nature damaging. This type of radiation is usually called ionising radiation.

In principle, all ionising radiation is carcinogenic, since cell damage may result from exposure to it. All electromagnetic radiation with a wavelength shorter than 320 nm (UVB radiation, UVC radiation, X-rays, and gamma radiation) is ionising, and thus in principle dangerous to us even in relatively low quantities. In the range from 320 nm to 400 nm (the UVA band), long-term exposure - to sunlight or in a solarium, for example - has been shown to cause damage, though only rarely cancer.

As far as the visible band (400-800 nm) goes, there are people who are oversensitive to light (photo allergy), and who can only tolerate red light (light with wavelengths over 600 nm) and therefore cannot go out in daylight. Since therapeutic lasers always have wavelengths above 630 nm, such photo allergy sufferers tolerate laser therapy but cannot be exposed to the light of a candle.

1.1.6 Can electromagnetic radiation cause cancer?

Electromagnetic radiation can injure living organisms if it

1) is of sufficient intensity to burn (many watts) and/or
2) contains high-energy photons (short wavelength).

N.B. Whether the photons come from a “natural” or from an artificial light source is of no significance - one photon with a certain energy is exactly the same as another one with the same energy!

There is a fairly clear wavelength limit at which photon energy becomes so high that the photons can ionise matter that they meet. This limit is 320 nm, (for physicists: this corresponds to 3.91 eV) so that photons with a shorter wavelength than this are capable of ionising molecules or atoms in tissue and hence can cause cancer (they are carcinogenic).

An example of a source of radiation which produces carcinogenic ultraviolet radiation is the quartz lamp. The casing of such a lamp is not made of glass but of quartz. This material, unlike glass, allows ultraviolet radiation to pass through it and tolerates much higher temperatures. Quartz lamps produce much of their radiation in the wavelength field around 250 nm. Ultraviolet radiation with such a short wavelength is very aggressive and is used, for example, to kill bacteria and other microorganisms. Because the radiation from quartz lamps is carcinogenic, these lamps were banned in most countries about 40 years ago. A laser with the same wavelength and the same strength is just as dangerous - no more, no less. (See chapter 3.6 “Risks and side effects” on page 101.) The risk factor depends on both the dose (input energy, measured in joules per cm^2 of skin) and the power density (intensity) of the radiation.

1.1.7 Protective mechanisms

Human beings have always been subjected to solar radiation. The sun emits all of the types of radiation shown in the table on the previous page, though only radio waves, microwaves, infrared radiation (thermal radiation), visible light, and the longwave part of ultraviolet radiation are not absorbed by the atmosphere and therefore reach the surface of the earth. Of those types of radiation that reach the ground, only a small part of the ultraviolet radiation (known as UVB) is dangerous to human beings. We have as a consequence developed protective mechanisms against it. Special cells (melanocytes) in the outer skin produce melanin, which absorbs UV radiation and prevents it from reaching the deeper and more sensitive tissues.

1.2 Various sources of radiation

1.2.1 Natural sources of radiation

The sun is our main natural source of radiation and energy. Like the light used for general illumination, it has a very wide spectrum (i.e. it is composed of photons with considerably varying wavelengths). On the earth’s surface, solar radiation has its highest intensity at 440 nm, blue light, above and below which it decreases. The sun, then, is actually blue, though any self-respecting child will draw it in yellow. It looks yellow to us because our eyes are most sensitive to yellow - 550 nm. Below 440 nm, the intensity of solar radiation drops, falling to zero at 290 nm (with the ozone layer in its present state). The carcinogenic part of solar radiation lies between 290 and 320 nm, and is known as UVB radiation. There is no upper limit to the sun’s long wave radiation, but at very long wavelengths - radio waves - the intensity is low. (See Figure 1.1 “Wavelength distribution of light from various sources” on page 7.)

1.2.2 Man-made sources of radiation

All conventional light sources are more or less broadband. The most narrow-banded are low-pressure gas discharge lights, such as neon lights (red) or sodium lights (yellow). These often feature a dominant wavelength, meaning that most photons have this wavelength or a wavelength close to it. These light sources have a function in some ways reminiscent of a laser's.

Of all the hundreds of types of lamps, we have chosen to study only two types in more detail: the light emitting diode and the laser. They are both used in therapeutic instruments and it is important to know the difference between them.

1.2.3 The light-emitting diode (LED)

Another light source, which is relatively narrow-banded, is the light-emitting diode. This is a small, inexpensive semiconductor lamp, which should not be confused with a laser. Typical LEDs produce red, yellow, green, blue or even white light (three LEDs in one case). There are LEDs which emit infrared radiation, generally with wavelengths around 950 nm (entirely invisible). These are often used in television remote control units.

According to the European Standard IEC 601, an LED is: "*Any semiconductor p-n junction device which can be made to produce electromagnetic radiation by radiative recombination in the semiconductor in the wavelength range from 180 nm to 1 mm, produced primarily by the process of spontaneous emission.*"

The diagram shows the wavelength distribution of light from various sources, including sunlight, filament lamps, fluorescent lamps, and several different lasers. Note that the spectrum of a laser is shown as a narrow vertical line; the laser emits light of only "one" wavelength. This line has nothing to do with the fact that laser light is sometimes collimated to a narrow beam!

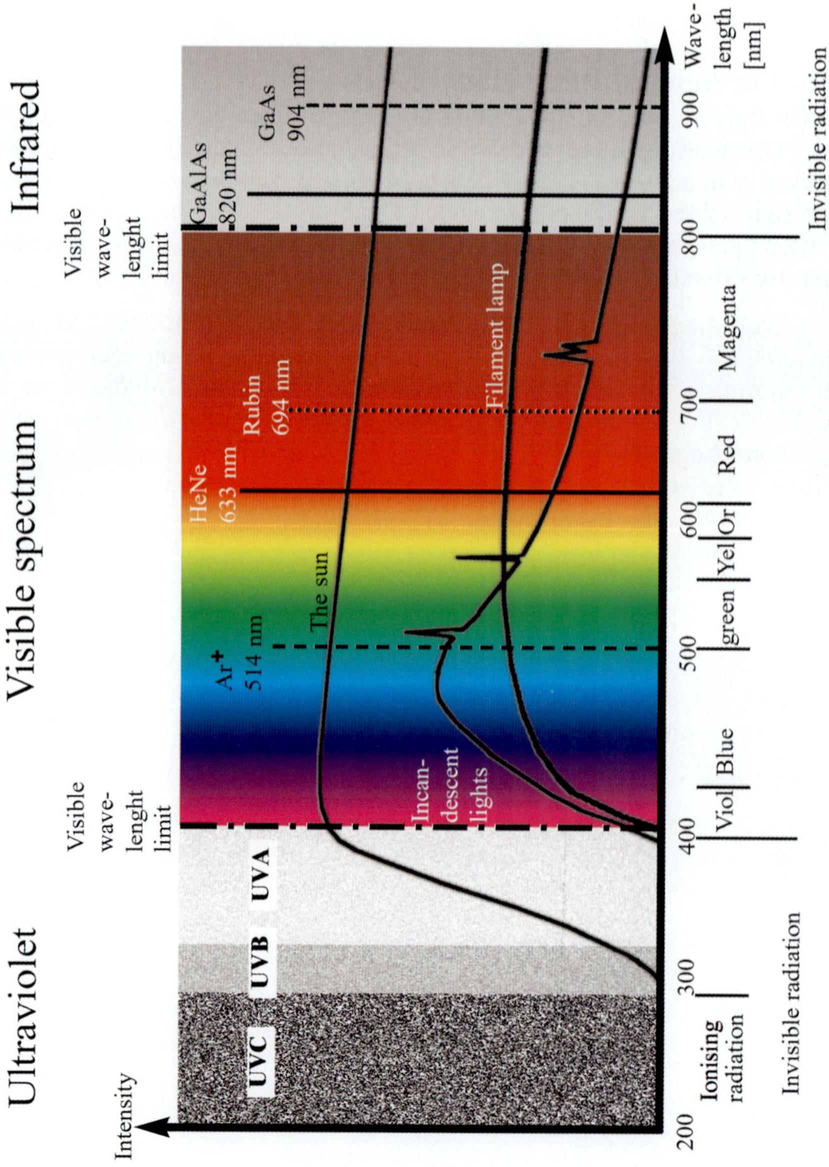

Figure 1.1 Wavelength distribution of light from various sources

1.2.4 The laser

The laser is the latest and most advanced of our light sources. The word LASER is an acronym for **L**ight **A**mplification by **S**timulated **E**mission of **R**adiation.

As a point of interest, the first name suggested for the laser was "Light Oscillation by Stimulated Emission of Radiation" - but this resulted in the unfortunate acronym LOSER.

Credit for the development of laser theory is generally given to Albert Einstein. In his theory "Zur Quantum Theories der Strahlung", published in 1916, he first used the name stimulated emission. Other and more important steps have been taken by Arthur Shawlow, Charles Townes and Theodor Maiman. Maiman presented the first working laser, a ruby laser, at a press conference on 7th July 1960.

Strictly speaking, a laser is a light amplifier if the radiation produced is within the visible range or a radiation amplifier if the radiation produced is within the infrared or ultraviolet radiation ranges. A predecessor of the laser was the MASER (Microwave Amplification by Stimulated Emission of Radiation). It works on the same principle as the laser, but within the microwave range.

According to the European Standard IEC 601, the definition of a laser is: "*Any device which can be made to produce or amplify electromagnetic radiation in the wavelength range from 180 nm to 1 mm primarily by the process of controlled stimulated emission*".

1.2.5 Laser design

A laser, whether large or small, always includes the following parts:

Energy source	(power supply)
Lasing (amplifying) medium	(solid, liquid or gas)
Resonating cavity[1]	(mirrors)

How energy is supplied to the lasing medium depends on the structure of the medium. The energy source may be an electrical current, optical radiation from a flash lamp or another (pumping) laser, radio waves or microwaves, or a chemical reaction.

1. There exists lasers without resonating cavity but we will not go into that as it would lead away to far.

"Star wars" chemical laser"

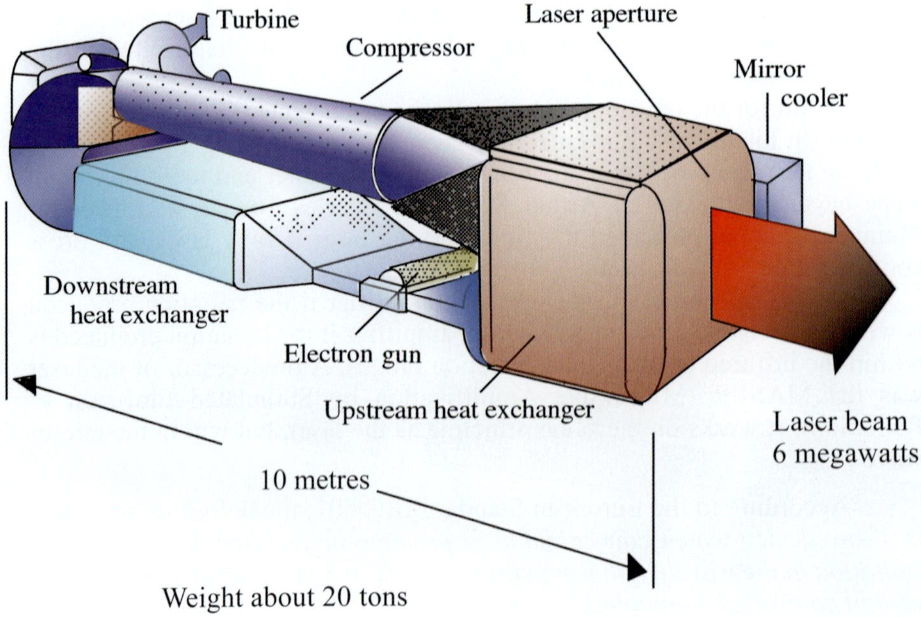

GaAs laser diode

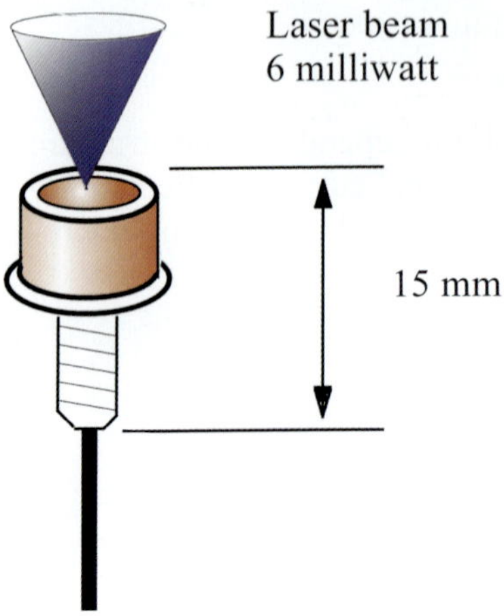

A laser can be seen as a tool: Tools have different shapes and sizes and different use

Two different lasers are shown here: Weight 20 tons and 2 grams, respectively. One for destruction (but was never built) and one for healing.

Figure 1.2 Star wars

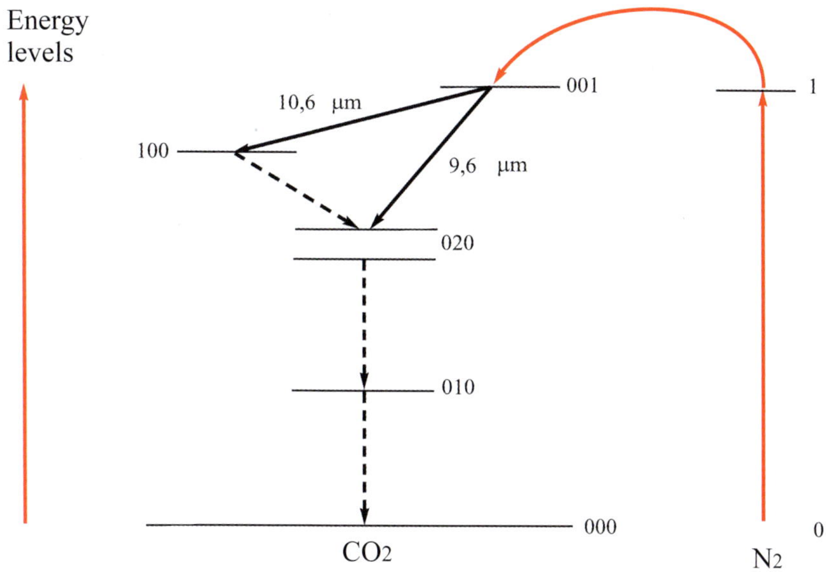

Energy diagram for CO_2 laser

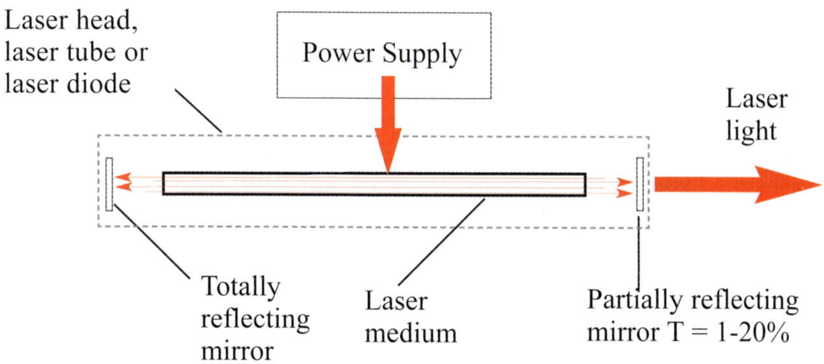

Figure 1.3 Principle design of a laser

The lasing medium must be able to store the energy supplied, which it does by a process called population inversion. This stored energy can then be emitted in an organised fashion, known as stimulated emission of radiation. When a photon with the right photon energy enters the electromagnetic field of the excited atom with energy stored in this way, some of the energy is emitted by the creation of an identical photon. The first photon is not absorbed. Hence, both the new and the old photon can then stimulate other atoms in the lasing medium to emit their stored energy. It is like a chain reaction, causing an "avalanche" of light in which all the photons have exactly the same photon energy.

Hence, the radiation from a laser always has a certain fixed wavelength, which is determined by the structure of the lasing medium and does not, like the radiation from other light sources, consist of a wide range of wavelengths. There are currently thousands of different types of laser, and these produce light, UV, or IR radiation of various wavelengths. Usually a laser has one characteristic wavelength, though it is sometimes possible to choose within a range of wavelengths. This is most common among semiconductor lasers. There are a few lasers designed in such a fashion that the wavelength can be changed, even during operation - tuneable lasers..

> Summary: Stimulated emission only occurs when the incident photon has exactly the same energy as the released photon; the first photon causes release of the second photon simultaneously, i.e. the second photon must follow the oscillations of the first photon, so that the two photons oscillate in phase. This phase-locked, wavelength specific, photon chain reaction results in the monochromatic (one wavelength), coherent (fixed phase relation) characteristics of laser light.

Further, the lasing medium is generally elongated in shape, often in the form of a channel (gas lasers) or a narrow rod (solid state lasers) or doped channel (semiconductor lasers), and is fitted with mirrors at its ends. These mirrors form the resonating cavity. The light produced in the lasing medium is reflected back into the lasing medium several times and stimulates new light production. The resonating cavity is of two-fold importance: it increases the lasing medium's amplification and makes the light more coherent. (See chapter 1.2.7 "Coherence" on page 12.) The elongation and mirror arrangement also make it possible for the light to emerge as a parallel beam (that may be focused to an extremely small point). To extract the light from the laser, one mirror is made somewhat transparent - most often 1-20% transparency, so that between 99% and 80% of the light is reflected back. Hence, the light intensity inside a laser is always higher than the output power.

Other optical components may be arranged between the mirrors, permitting wavelength selection, polarisation of the laser light, or Q-switching (a pulsing method making it possible to achieve very intense and very short pulses). By inserting a non linear crystal, optical overtones (e.g. double frequency) can be generated - one example of this is the KTP laser. (See chapter 1.4.7 "KTP/532-laser (frequency doubled Nd:YAG laser)" on page 37.)

1.2.6 The properties of laser light

Laser light has two essential characteristics which differentiate it from "normal" light:

(1) its very narrow bandwidth
(2) its high level of coherence

Coherence means that the photons are well ordered - they are connected and build light waves that remain synchronised with one another over long distances, (See Figure 1.6 "Coherent and non-coherent light" on page 15.) A narrow bandwidth is necessary for a high degree of coherence. These two characteristics are typical of all laser light and are important with regard to laser therapy. Neither of them, however, has any major significance in the use of lasers as surgical instruments. Two other characteristics that many people believe are typical of lasers are:

(3) parallel beams
(4) high intensity

These characteristics can often be brought about in a laser by altering the size and geometric design of the lasing medium and resonating cavity as mentioned above, but they are easy to change. Laser light does not need to be parallel or particularly strong. These two characteristics are, however, most important with respect to lasers as surgical instruments. They are also the properties of laser light that make it harmful to the eye under certain circumstances. Narrow and parallel beams can allow the entire volume of light to pass through the pupil of an unprotected eye - it is thus not difficult to imagine how an intense laser light source can be dangerous to our light-sensitive eyes. (See Figure 1.9 "Laser and eye-risk" on page 23.)

1.2.7 Coherence

Coherence generally means order, or synchronicity. When a troop of soldiers is marching, it moves coherently, but if the soldiers are free to leave, they start to move incoherently. The same is true of the sound emanating from a flute (a flute is a typical "sound laser" - it has a resonance cavity, and its sound is monochromatic and coherent).

Soldiers marching (moving coherently) over a bridge will influence the mechanical structure other than they would if they were walking or running (moving incoherently) over the same bridge.

The tone of a flute may cause a crystal glass to break due to interference and resonance, but a wide-band, incoherent sound of the same intensity cannot break the glass. Interference is the effect of adding two or more waves. This addition may result in either amplification (constructive interference) or attenuation (destructive interference) of the resulting amplitude. Amplification is what makes extra high peaks when water waves meet, or what makes one pitch sound particularly strong when we sing at various pitches in the bathroom.

When a rough surface is illuminated with visible laser light, a kind of grainy quality can be observed in the light. These grainy elements, or granules, are called laser speckles, (See Figure 1.5 “Laser speckles” on page 14.) and occur as a result of interference between different light beams. This is because light with a sufficiently high coherence length can be “combined” in the same way that waves of water combine when they meet. (More about speckles and their medical importance in chapter 11.1.3.)

Waves of coherent light stay in phase in long trains of waves. The length of these trains of waves, the coherence length, may vary from one light source to another. An ordinary light bulb has a low coherence length, a matter of thousandths of a millimetre. A HeNe laser, on the other hand, may have a very high coherence length - decimetres or even several metres. A semiconductor laser usually has a coherence length of no more than a millimetre or so.

N.B. In a laser beam, the different parts of the wave field can have a fixed phase relation but are usually not “in phase”. (See Figure 1.6 “Coherent and non-coherent light” on page 15.)

The concept of coherence consists of both spatial and temporal coherence and it is mainly the former that is of interest here. However, the two are related to each other through the relation: $\Delta\omega \times \Delta t \geq 2\pi$ where $\Delta\omega$ represents the frequency interval within which the radiation is emitted and where Δt is close to the coherence time - higher Δt means a higher degree of temporal coherence.

Literature:

Nicola [511] developed a technique of causing highly reproducible inflammatory lesions on the skin of rats. HeNe light at 1 J/cm^2 produced an acceleration of the healing process. Incoherent light of the same wavelength and dose was less favourable.

In a study by Rosner [493] the effect of HeNe laser in the regeneration process of crushed optical nerves was estimated. While HeNe laser postponed the degenerative process, non-coherent infrared light was ineffective or affected the injured nerves adversely.

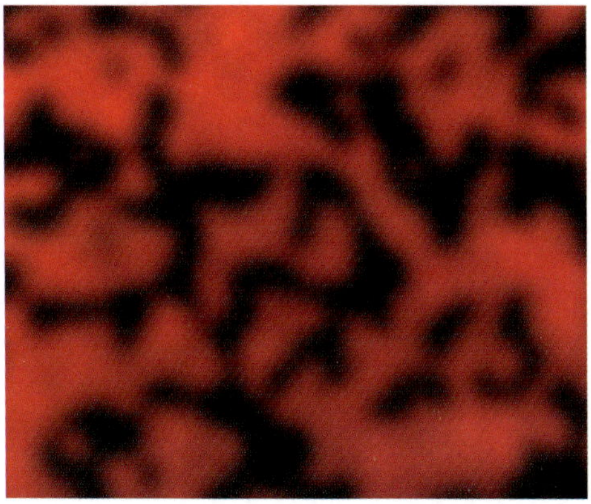

Figure 1.4 Photographed laser speckles

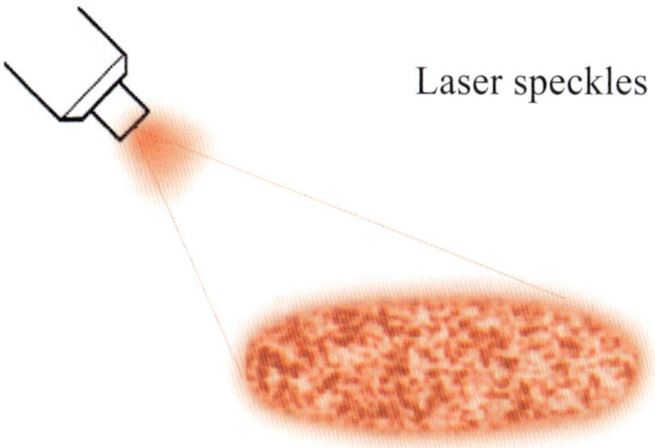

If a rough surface is illuminated by visable laser light, the laser light shows a speckled structure due to interference. This phenomenon is called laser speckles and occurs in the eye of the viewer.

Figure 1.5 Laser speckles

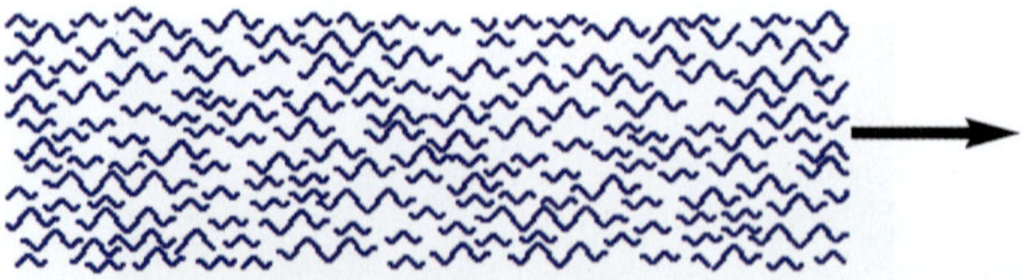

A paralell beam of light with short coherence length. This is often called "incoherent" or non-coherent light - lamp light.

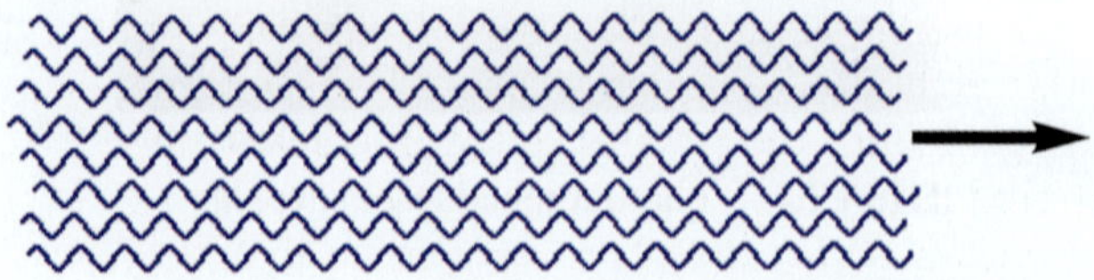

A paralell beam of light with long coherence length. This is often called "coherent" light - laser light.
N.B. Coherence has nothing to do with paralellity and the waves do not have to be in phase.

Figure 1.6 Coherent and non-coherent light

1.2.8 Polarisation

Light - whether from a laser or another source - can be non-polarised or polarised. It can also be more or less polarised (partially polarised). There are two types of polarisation: linear and circular, which can be described using the following analogy. We can take a long rope and tie one end round a tree, then stretch the rope so that it does not touch the ground. We then create wave motion by moving the rope up and down - the waves move vertically in accordance with the up and down movement. The wave is vertically linearly polarised. If we instead move the rope from side to side, the wave is horizontally linearly polarised. Finally, if we rotate the rope, a corkscrew-like wave motion results. This is circular polarisation, and we can differentiate between right and left rotational circular polarisation. (Both linear and circular polarisation are special cases of the more general elliptical polarisation, which - as well as the circular polarisation - can be left or right handed rotational).

Polarised light can be achieved by filtering with "polarisation" filters. Special prisms or other optical components (e.g. a Brewster window) can also be used. Most lasers and other light sources are not equipped with polarising means and consequently emit non-polarised light. (For more information about the importance of polarisation, read chapter 11.1).

1.2.9 Output power

Power is measured in watts (W). The strength or power output of a laser is thus measured in watts or milliwatts (mW = a thousandth of a watt). Higher output power is of some consequence in that at a higher power output one achieves a higher power density, which is often desirable. Also, a higher output power means that a certain desired dose (input energy, measured in joules per cm^2 of skin) is more quickly reached because energy is the same as power multiplied by time.

When you buy an ordinary lamp, it is always its power consumption, i.e. its input power, that is specified, and almost never its output power (radiance). Hence a 60 W lamp consumes 60 watts and yields, typically, 1 - 2 watts of visible light power. The remaining 98 – 99% of the input power is converted to heat in the glass casing and metal socket and to directly emitted, invisible infrared radiation. The power specified for a laser is always its output power. Hence a 60 W laser consumes more than 60 watts but yields 60 watts of (visible or invisible) radiation power.

1.2.10 Continuous and pulsed lasers

A light source usually emits light at a constant intensity. This is known as continuous wave (cw) emission. However, it is also possible to make lasers and other lamps with varying intensity, known as amplitude modulated emission. The variability of modulated light may be small (low degree of modulation) or large (high degree of modulation). In the extreme case (100% modulation), the intensity periodically reaches zero. If the light intensity only varies between a maximum and zero, the modulation is known as square-wave amplitude modulation, and the light source is said to be pulsed – the same as switching it on and off. (See Figure 1.7 “Different types of pulsing” on page 18.)

A pulsed light source can be pulsed either electrically, by switching its electrical power on and off, or by interrupting the light, for example, by using a chopper (mechanical shutter, Kerr cell, Pockels cell, etc.). It may be pulsed at a high or a low frequency, i.e. with many or few pulses per second. If the lamp (or laser) emits visible light and is pulsed at a low frequency (up to about 30 pulses per second), we can see that the light is blinking.

If the lengths of the periods of light are equal to the lengths of the periods of zero intensity, the “duty cycle” is 50%, as light is emitted during 50% of the overall time.

Some lasers and other lamps can be pulsed like flash bulbs with extremely short and very intense light pulses and rather long intermission times (very low duty cycle). This type of rather extreme pulsing is usually called superpulsing. Examples of lasers that can be superpulsed are YAG lasers, CO_2-lasers and GaAs lasers.

Note 1. Pulse frequency has nothing to do with the frequency of the light itself - the carrier wave. (See chapter 1.1.1 “Wavelength and frequency” on page 2)

Note 2. “Frequency modulation” has nothing to do with this. It refers to the variation of the frequency of the carrier wave.

1.2.11 The pulse peak power

When a laser is pulsed, the laser light power varies between the pulse peak output power and zero. It is possible to design a laser to achieve extremely high pulse peak output power - even trillions of watts. However, the pulse duration is then correspondingly low. The peak pulse power value is of importance for the penetration of light into tissue. The power density during these very high power pulses is of course also very high, yielding an extremely high photon flux with an increased probability of multi-photon effects. (See chapter 3.4.2.3 “How deep does the light penetrate?” on page 95 and chapter 11.2.6 “Multi-photon effects” on page 354.)

1.2.12 Average power output

For pulsed lasers, the output power value to be used for dose calculation is the laser's average power. (See chapter 3.3.1.7 “Calculation of doses” on page 71.) When a laser is chopped, the pulsing can have different duty cycles. If the light is "on" for 30% of the time and "off" for 70% of the time, the duty cycle is 30%. Then the average power is 30% of the peak power (if the switching is momentary, i.e. a true square wave). The duty cycle of the GaAs-laser is extremely low - in the order of 0.001. (See Figure 1.7 “Different types of pulsing” on page 18.)

1.2.13 Power density

Power density is another way of saying "light intensity" or "light concentration", and is the light output power per unit area of the target being illuminated by the laser light. This is usually measured in watts per square centimetre (W/cm^2). High power density is achieved, for instance, at the focal point of a magnifying glass. If the magnifying glass is moved closer to the objective point, so that the light spot grows, the light is spread over a wider area and the power density is correspondingly lower. Spreading the light over a larger area leads to a directly proportional reduction of power density.

For example, a 10 mW laser with the light focused on an area of 1 mm^2 gives a power density of 1 W/cm^2. A surgical laser with 10 W output power focused on a spot with a diameter of 0.1 mm, gives a power density of more-than 100,000 W/cm^2. Power density is of significance both in laser surgery and laser therapy.

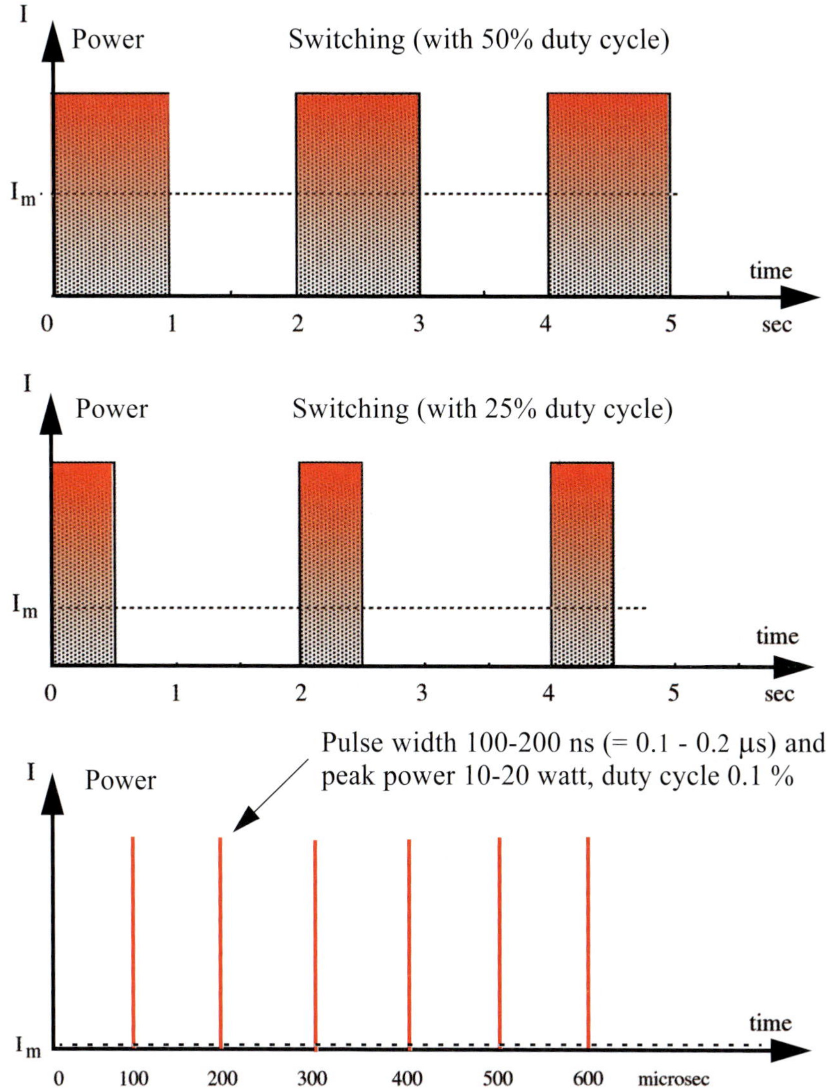

This diagram shows typical superpulsing: i.e. the ratio between the peak power and average power is very high.

Figure 1.7 Different types of pulsing

1.2.14 Collimation

It is a common misconception that light from a laser is always in the form of a parallel beam. The light from a gas laser is usually rather parallel (typically in the order of milli-radian), while the light from a diode laser (without collimating optics) is ordinarily much more divergent, with an angle of "spread" of around 30-90 degrees. This is mainly due to diffraction when the light is emitted from the resonator mirror on the semiconductor crystal. If a collimating lens or lens system is placed in front of the diode, the light's parallelity can be increased. This is called collimation. A collimated beam is quite parallel, and with such a beam, we can irradiate from a distance and still achieve high power density over a small area.

1.2.15 Risk of eye injury

Even in the infancy of laser technology there was an awareness of the increased risk of eye damage compared to conventional light sources. Hence, new rules were introduced to handle this hazard. Lasers were divided into five categories (Class 1, 2, 3A, 3B and 4) according to their potential to damage the eye. Classes 1-3A are considered safe, whereas Class 3B involves a certain risk and Class 4 a definite risk. Class 4, for example, comprises strong industrial and surgical lasers capable of burning and cutting. Note that this classification has nothing to do with the medical use, efficiency or quality of lasers but refers solely to the possible risk of eye injury.

In most countries only physicians and dentists are allowed to use Class 4 lasers (and veterinarians, in the treatment of animals). The practical job can then usually be delegated to nurses or other staff members.

To date, only a handful of accidents involving lasers have been reported and the only severe accidents concern contact with high voltage power supplies. Reports on eye injuries are very rare, and, when they do occur, injuries involve either the use of very strong industrial lasers where protective measures have been ignored or laboratories where people, over time, have become careless. Furthermore, in several cases the person in question has not even been aware of an eye injury, although there has been a visible scar on the retina. In the book "Therapeutic lasers", professor David Baxter writes: "In the only reported case of eye injury during therapeutic laser treatment, a chartered physiotherapist using a treatment unit on loan from a supplier suffered 60% corneal abrasion from the protective wings on the side of the goggles provided with the apparatus".

Another aspect is that, in the treatment of diabetic retinopathy, a strong argon or diode laser beam is directed right into the eye, and often some hundreds of laser pulses are fired. Still, the patient is not aware of any injury and reports that his vision is fine. In the treatment of cataract, a strong Nd:YAG laser is directed and fired right into the eye. Vision corrections are performed with an Excimer laser, evaporating parts of the cornea. CO_2-lasers, too, are used in eye surgery. All these lasers are strong and capable of burning tissue!

So, even though there are lasers capable of causing eye damage, the risk should not be exaggerated. Too often the fear of laser light is a greater risk than the laser itself! For example: a car driver being blinded by a laser pointer can lose control of his vehicle out of fear because he realises that he has been hit by a laser (and he "knows" this is very dangerous). But if he is blinded by a sunbeam, he will not be frightened, just blinded for a spell. Usually a sunbeam blinds a person much more than a laser pointer, because the laser pointer can only hit one eye at a time and for a much shorter time due to the narrowness of the beam.

A lot has been written about the laser as a military weapon to make soldiers blind. Well, that is not possible. At close range and with large lasers, it would be possible to inflict eye injury if an invisible beam were to be used. But in reality, no laser makes a person blind. Pilots could be disturbed by visible laser light but not made blind. Also, the user of the laser weapon would reveal his position and turn himself into a target. Still, the common military use of lasers is as distance measuring devices, beam-riding missiles and target designators – a laser points at a target and a "smart" bomb or missile sees the laser spot and flies to it. Amendations have been proposed to the Geneva Convention to forbid the use of laser as a weapon, but we think it would be much more sensible to suggest that guns be forbidden, as a bullet can do much more harm than a beam of light.

There are light sources which are more hazardous to the eyes than the corresponding lasers. One such device usually called IPL (Intense Pulsed Light) using a powerful flash lamp with a band-pass filter. It emits light pulses in the wavelength region 600 to 900 nm and with pulse energies around 50 joules per cm^2 aperture area. The aperture is usually rectangular and in the order of one by three cm. Like ruby and alexandrite lasers, this instrument is used in hair removal – the light is absorbed in dark hairs and then converted to heat, which burns the surrounding follicle to destruction or injury. This is called photo epilation. If this aperture is directed towards an unprotected eye, this can cause a much more severe injury than staring into the beam of e.g. an uncollimated ruby laser with fibre-optic transmission made for hair removal. But as these flash lamp devices are not lasers, there are no restrictions in their use!

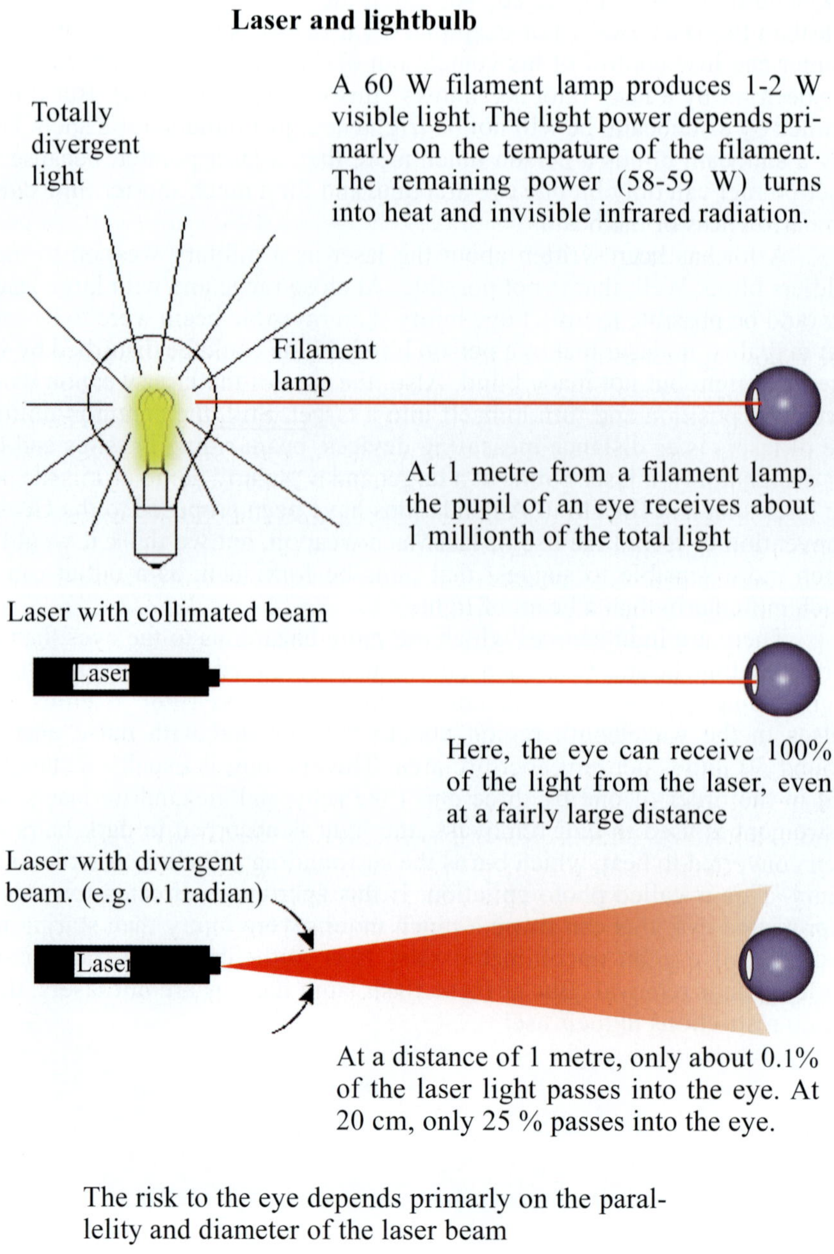

Figure 1.8 Laser and light-bulb

In 1998 there was an outbreak of laser hysteria in the Danish press. A train engineer was reported to have suffered a 20% loss of vision after having been irradiated by two young boys, using a laser pointer. In addition, a car driver was reported to have been injured in a similar fashion. This is, of course, pure nonsense. Laser pointers do not injure the eye! They are far too low-powered and the blink reflex will automatically reduce the exposure time.

The restrictions in the use of class 3B lasers as therapeutic instruments have been lifted in Europe since no reports of eye damages from these lasers have ever been reported.

1.2.16 Decisive factors in the risk of eye injury

The following factors are of importance in the eye risk of various lasers. (See Figure 1.9 “Laser and eye-risk” on page 23.)

- The divergence of the light beam: A parallel light beam of small diameter is by far the most dangerous. It can enter the pupil in its entirety and be focused by the eye’s lens to a spot with a diameter of hundredths of a millimetre. The entire light output is concentrated on this small area. With a 10 mW beam, the power density can be up to 12,000 W/cm^2.
- The output power of the laser: It is fairly obvious that a powerful laser (many watts) is more hazardous to stare into than a weak laser.
- The exposure time: The shorter the exposure time is, the stronger the light can be without risk of injuries. For visible light, the blink reflex affords a good protection.
- The wavelength of the light: Within the visible wavelength range, we respond to strong light with a quick blink reflex. This reduces the exposure time and thereby the light energy which enters the eye. Light sources which emit invisible radiation, whether an infrared laser or an infrared diode, always entail a higher risk than the equivalent source of visible lightRadiation at wavelengths over 1,400 nm is absorbed by the eye’s lens and thus rendered safe, provided the power of the beam is not too high. Radiation at wavelengths over 2,500 nm is absorbed by the cornea and is less dangerous. (See Figure 1.9 “Laser and eye-risk” on page 23.)

Desicive factors in the risk of eye injury

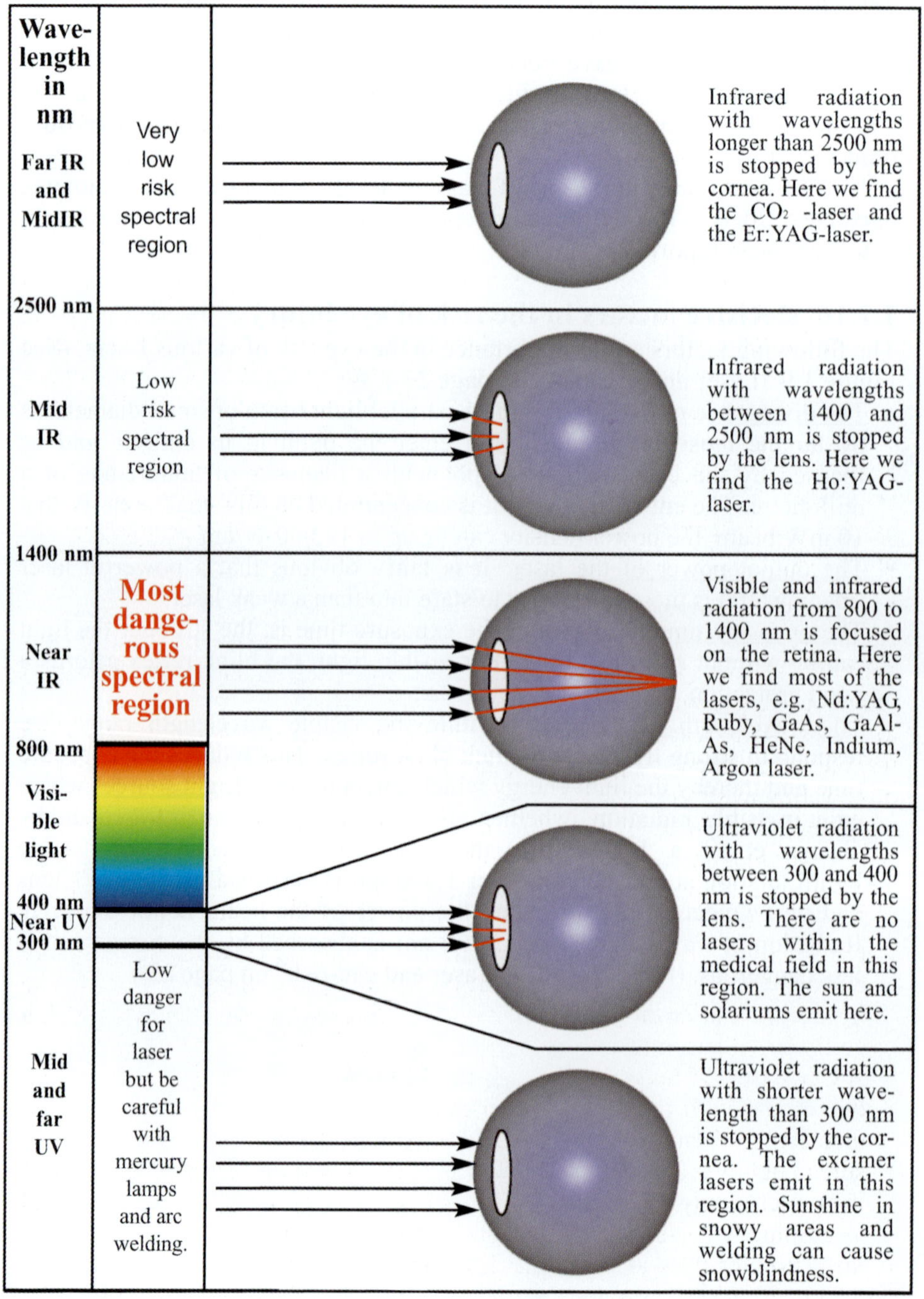

Figure 1.9 Laser and eye-risk

- The distribution of the light source: When looking at a light source, an image of the source is projected on the retina. If the light source is concentrated, as is often the case with lasers, the image will be projected as a point, provided it lies within our accommodation range, i.e. the area in which we can see clearly. A widely spread light source is projected onto the retina in a correspondingly wide image, with the light spread over a larger area, and with a lower power density as a consequence. For example: a clear light bulb (which is apprehended as a more concentrated light source) is worse to look at than a "pearl" light bulb. A laser system with several light sources spaced apart, such as a multiprobe with several laser diodes (the probe is the part of the laser you hold and apply to the area to be treated: a single probe means there is only one laser diode in the probe, as opposed to a multiprobe, which has several laser diodes) may be very powerful as a whole, yet constitutes a lesser hazard to the eye than it would if the entire power output was emitted by one laser diode, because the diodes' separate placement means that they are reproduced in different places on the retina.

We have often heard this kind of remark: "If it's a class 3B laser then it's fine, otherwise it is not effective!" This is, of course, entirely incorrect, and has led manufacturers to produce lasers that meet the 3B classification in order to sell higher volumes.

Let us look at two examples:
A GaAlAs laser with a wavelength of 830 nm, an output of 1 mW and a well-collimated beam (1 mrad divergence) is classified as laser class 3B as it is judged to be hazardous
to the eye. The reason for this is partly the collimated beam, and partly the wavelength, which is just outside the visible range and hence provokes no blink reflex in strong light.

- A HeNe laser with a wavelength of 633 nm, an output of 10 mW (10 times stronger than the laser in the previous example) and divergent beams (1 rad divergence, which corresponds to a cone of light with a top angle of about 57°, which is often the divergence of light from a fibre-optic cable) is classified as laser class 3A because, owing to its divergence, it cannot damage the eye (only a small portion of the light will hit the pupil). The light from a laser diode is usually rather divergent unless it is fitted with a collimating lens or lens system.
- A CO_2-laser (10 600 nm wavelength) of EDL (defocused) type, with 15 watt output and with the radiation uniformly spread out over a surface with a diameter of 5 cm, will be classified as a class 4 instrument. If instead it is spread out over a surface of 10 cm diameter, it will be classified as a class 1 instrument (only class 1 and 4 have this wavelength) and is hence regarded as absolutely eye-safe in spite of its high output power.

A laser pointer uses an InGaAlP laser with a wavelength usually between 650 and 670 nm (red light). The output power is in the order of 0.5 to 3 mW, focussed in a well-collimated beam. The spot size is usually 5 to 10 mm in diameter at a distance of 1 metre. If you look straight into the beam, the light looks very strong. However, these devices are completely harmless and no eye injury has been reported. But many people are afraid of them. As a comparison, an arrow or a dart can completely destroy an eye - a laser pointer is harmless.

As for therapeutic lasers, patients often ask: "Is it enough to shut your eyes if you receive laser treatment to the face, or must you have protective glasses?" Yes, it is enough to close your eyes! It is actually sufficient to shut your eyes even if a very powerful laser is being used. It is quite possible to treat a stye on the eyelid without risk, even if it is located right in front of the pupil [129]. The reason for this is that the eyelid spreads the light so that the lens cannot focus it. The light is spread over the entire retina and, with a 10 mW laser, we get a power density over the retina of 0.001 W/cm^2, which is about ten million times lower than if the eye were open and the beam parallel.

However, the use of protective glasses can be of benefit, particularly if powerful, collimated lasers in the infrared spectral region are used. In any case, protective glasses give the patient a sense of security. Furthermore, therapists never run the risk of a claim for damages from a patient if they make sure the patient always wears protective glasses during treatment. (Patients may well convince themselves that the laser has a negative effect on their eyes.)

Bear in mind, though, that protective glasses for HeNe or InGaAlP lasers are of no use whatsoever when using other laser types.

Warning: The use of normal sunglasses increases the risk of eye injury. The filtration mechanism of sunglasses is a wide band attenuation, giving a much lower absorption of a particular laser wavelength than real protection goggles give. In addition to this, the darkness of the glasses makes the pupil dilate and let in more light. They provide a false sense of security!

<ins>Summary:</ins> Although most lasers are harmless, some lasers certainly can cause eye injury. The most dangerous types combine power (> 100 mW) with a collimated beam and have a wavelength in the interval 700 nm – 1400 nm. So called laser pointers are harmless. A divergent beam can be quite strong and still carry a low risk; the more divergent, the less risk.

1.3 Laser types in medicine and surgery

In the table below, the names, wavelengths, working modes, and uses of the most common laser systems in medicine are listed. .

Laser name	Wavelength	Pulsed or cont.	Medical use
Crystalline laser medium:			
KTP/532	532 nm	p/c	leg vein treatment
Ruby	694 nm	p	tattoo and hair removal
Alexandrite	755 nm	p	bone cut, hair removal
Nd:YAG	1064 nm	p/c	coagulation of tumours
Ho:YAG	2130 nm	p	surgery, root canal, lithotripsia
Er:YAG	2940 nm	p	dental drill, laser peeling
Ti:sapphire	tuneable	p	two-photon PDT
Semiconductor lasers:			
InGaAlP	630-700 nm	c	biostimulation
GaAlAs	780-820-870 nm	c	biostimulation and surgery
GaAs	904, 905 nm	p	biostimulation
Liquid laser medium:			
Dye laser	tuneable	p/c	kidney stones
Rhodamine	560-650 nm	p/c	PDT, dermatology
Gas lasers:			
Excimer	193, 248, 308 nm	p	eye, vascular surgery
Argon	350-514 nm	c	dermatology, retinopathy
Copper	578 nm	p/c	dermatology
HeNe	633, 3390 nm	c	biostimulation
CO_2	1064 nm	p/c	dermatology, surgery

Table 1.2 Different lasers, their wavelengths and use

There are other types, but those mentioned above are the most common. The Dye laser is expensive to buy and to run and is gradually being replaced by other laser types. The semiconductor lasers can also be tuned, (± 10 nm) simply by varying the working temperature. The Ti:sapphire laser can produce extremely short pulses, down to the femto-second region.

1.4 The surgical lasers

The most typical surgical lasers and their wavelengths:

CO_2-laser	10,600 nm
Nd:YAG laser	1,064 nm
Ho:YAG	2,130 nm
Er:YAG	2,940 nm
Argon laser	514 nm
Copper vapour laser	578 nm
KTP laserfrequency-doubled Nd:YAG	532 nm
Ruby laser	694 nm
Alexandrite	755 nm
Stronger types of GaAlAs laser	typically 800-870 nm
Dye laser	400-900 nm
Ti:sapphire laser	700-900 nm
Excimer laser	193, 248, 308, 351 nm

Table 1.3 Typical surgical lasers and their wavelengths

In order for a laser to be suitable for use as a surgical laser, it must be powerful enough to heat up the tissue to temperatures over 50 °C. A surgical laser can either be used in continuous wave or pulsed mode. These lasers can be broadly divided into three groups, according to their output:

1. vaporising (superficial complaints, e.g. condyloma) 1-5 W.
2. light cutting (superficial incisions, e.g. plastic surgery) 5-20 W.
3. deep cutting (conisation, major surgical operations) 20-100 W.

The main aim of this book is not to instruct colleagues in the profession who work with or are thinking of working with surgical lasers - a great deal of literature on this subject already exists. Nevertheless, in this chapter we will be describing some of the surgical lasers on the market so that the reader can appreciate the difference between surgical and therapeutic lasers and thereby answer their patients' questions.

For those who already have a surgical laser, it is worth knowing that it can usually also be used in biostimulation - even powerful, destructive lasers do have laser therapy effects. It is well known that surgery with carbon dioxide lasers means less postoperative pain compared with conventional surgical techniques, and this may partly be due to its biostimulatory effect. Laser surgery, for instance, is followed by minimal scarring. This is suggested by Calderhead [304] to be an “alpha-phenomenon”, meaning that the lower laser light intensities in the periphery of the target area have biostimulative effects.

1.4.1 The Carbon dioxide laser (CO_2-laser)

As mentioned earlier, most types of laser are named after a combination of the components (or the main component) of the lasing medium. The main component of the CO_2-laser is thus carbon dioxide. This laser usually produces radiation with a wavelength of 10.6 micrometers (10600 manometers), which is high in the infrared band of the spectrum. The advantage of radiation with a long wavelength is that it is absorbed by water to a great extent, and by objects which contain water, such as tissue. This makes the CO_2-laser largely non-hazardous to the eye. See Figure 1.9 “Laser and eye-risk” on page 23, chapter 1.2.15 “Risk of eye injury” on page 19 and chapter 1.2.16 “Decisive factors in the risk of eye injury” on page 22. Ordinary spectacles or glass or plastic discs in a suitable frame are a sufficient protection for this wavelength.

Because of the high absorption rate in water and organic matter, the CO_2-laser beam has a shallow depth of penetration 99% is absorbed within 0.2 mm [296]. (See chapter 1.1.5 “Radiation risks” on page 3.) This also makes it very easy to evaporate and remove tissue without causing a deeper burn. Papilloma virus warts, for example, can be vaporised with only minor damage to the underlying tissue. The colour and melanin content of the tissue are not significant in relation to the rate of absorption.

A disadvantage associated with the long wavelength is that it is difficult to produce optical fibres with satisfactory transmission properties. There are fibres made from silver halide salts, which appear to be usable. Thin, flexible wave-guides in the form of small tubes of single-crystal sapphire can also be used to conduct the CO_2-laser beam. Up until now, the best way to get the light out from the laser tube has been to use mirror optics in articulated arms. However, this is relatively expensive and sensitive to knocks and bumps. The mirror setting requires a high level of precision, and the articulated arms are consequently sensitive to mechanical shocks.

Also, small plastic tubes, internally coated with dielectric layers, have been tested as wave-guides. Internally coated metal tubes are also being used in spite of some disadvantages. The most promising wave-guide technique may be small flexible glass tubes, internally coated with dielectric layers.

A CO_2-laser can be made very powerful - with an output of millions of watts - though such a laser would be as big as a house and very nearly require its own power station! Powerful lasers of this kind are used in industry to cut and process metal. Modern CO_2-lasers with an output under 200 W are often radio-wave excited with sealed gas systems, and do not require, as their predecessors did, any gas supply, gas refilling, or high voltage. Their lifetime is usually very long.

Today's surgical CO_2-lasers can also be superpulsed. This means that the laser light is emitted in a train of short but very intense pulses. In the case of tissue evaporation, this results in less burning under and around the vaporisation zone.

1.4.1.1 Carbon dioxide lasers in surgery

One of the advantages of the carbon dioxide laser is that the energy it produces is strongly absorbed by water and all organic matter. This means that layer after layer of tissue can be removed without nearby tissue being affected to any great extent. At the same time, the CO_2-laser coagulates blood in small vessels, making it possible to work in a controlled fashion.

Imagine the removal of pre-cancer cells on the uterus or a fungal infection from the floor of a patient's mouth, when the instruments you have to choose between are a scalpel and a carbon dioxide laser. It is not difficult to see the advantages of the laser. The scalpel causes profuse bleeding, making it difficult to see where the healthy tissue starts, and the practitioner is working with a knife close to well-vascularised tissue. With the laser we can vaporise fractions of a millimetre at a time and our vision is not impeded as there is generally no bleeding, and, furthermore, sutures are unnecessary. The same applies to an operation on a haemangioma on the lip. No bleeding, no sutures. The whole operation takes a couple of minutes and can be done on an outpatient basis. Subsequent check-ups are generally unnecessary. By focusing the beam, it can also be used like a scalpel, so it is possible to take a biopsy with a CO_2-laser.

Another interesting property of the CO_2-laser is that, when cutting, evaporating or coagulating the tissue, pain persists for only a few seconds after the burning has stopped. This is in contrast to when you burn yourself on a hot iron, your oven or hot water, leaving a pain for 20 to 30 minutes unless cold water or ice is applied to the site of the burn. The reason for this difference in pain perception is not known.

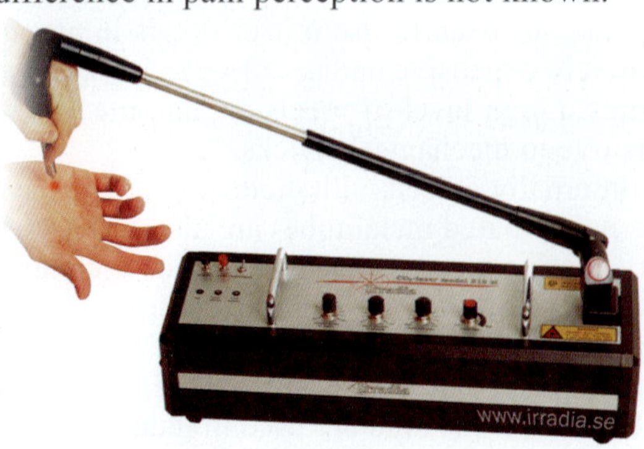

Figure 1.10 Portable CO_2-laser

The mucosa consists of 80-90% water, which argues for the use of carbon dioxide lasers. In the target area of a focused laser the temperature is between 150 and 300 degrees, depending on the laser output and the cross section of the beam, while from a distance of 0.5 mm from the "laser gun" the temperature drops to around 50 degrees. The power output used should be determined from case to case. The volume of liquid covering the mucous membrane must also be taken into consideration, as it affects the energy uptake of the tissue. Mucous membrane conditions such as lichen and leucoplakia can be removed by vaporising the tissue once a biopsy has been performed.

The healing process after an operation using a carbon dioxide laser is a little slower than after conventional surgery, but, on the other hand, the postoperative discomfort is considerably milder and the final cosmetic result much more acceptable (the latter is of course more important in cases of treatment of the face). The absence of bleeding may be the cause of the slower healing. The laser beam also kills off any residual infection in the operating area, which contributes to the healing process.

It is important to remove tissue with a certain extra margin, in order to remove clinically invisible change in the transitional zone between healthy and cancerous or infected tissue.

The disadvantages of carbon dioxide lasers used to be their size and price. Around 100 kg and US $30,000 - $40,000 has been a rough guide. The latest technical advances have led to lighter (around 15 - 20 kg) and cheaper (US$15,000 - US$25,000) lasers. They use sealed-off laser tubes without the need for gas refilling or high voltage. They may also be completely silent and may even be made battery powered and thereby mobile. Carbon dioxide lasers can be made very powerful, but for dermatological and ENT use, 1-10 W usually suffices.

In general surgery, the CO_2-laser has been used for a long time. One good indication for the laser is haemorrhoidectomy. Other good indications are fimosis and circumcision. The healing after excision of penis cancer has proved to be very good. In sleep apnea, CO_2-laser is used for uvulopalatoplasty in the treatment of snoring. The laser can also be used in laparoscopy. Typical benefits of laser surgery are less pronounced postoperative oedema and pain compared to conventional methods. Sutures are often not required.

Another use of CO_2-laser is so called transmyocardial revascularisation (TMR), in which a number of small holes are made through the heart muscle wall [572]. TMR is a modern therapeutic approach in the treatment of patients with severe chronic ischemic cardiac disease. Clinical data from 1800 worldwide TMR-treated patients show that TMR can improve cardiac status in cases without preoperative congestive heart failure. The mechanisms underlying beneficial TMR effects are not well understood, but there seems to be some evidence that biostimulation plays a role. Channels made by mechanical tools do not give the same favourable result. In a recent study the following result was presented: In a follow-up at 6 months, clinical data indicate that CO_2-laser TMR was able to improve clinical status in 50 of 61 laser-treated patients, whereas 5 did not show any benefit and 6 died. Histopathological investigations revealed tissue remodelling comparable with different stages of wound healing. The cicatricial tissue in the original laser-created channels displayed a stronger immunostaining for collagen type III than for type I. And the authors conclude: "Clinically, TMR improves cardiac function in some patients with severe ischemic cardiac disease, but pathophysiological data as well as morphological features from human myocardium could not explain this phenomenon. Therefore, TMR treatment should be used only as 'the last chance' in patients with severe angina pectoris. "

Another surgical use of CO_2-laser is as a drilling tool in laser-assisted hair transplantation [573]. These lasers deliver high bursts of energy of short duration and vaporise the hair transplantation recipient sites, which are consistent in depth and diameter.

Gynaecology was the first main field of use for the CO_2-laser. It can be used to evaporate genital condyloma, cervical neoplasia etc. In the case of conisation a rather strong CO_2-laser is needed, due to the deep incision needed in the blood rich tissue.

In dermatology, the CO_2-laser is very well suited for excision of superficial tumours, evaporation of angioma, verrucae, syringoma, tricho-epithelioma, adenoma sebaceum, steatocystoma, hidradenitis suppurativa, condyloma, neurofibromatosis, xanthelasma, rhinophyma, actinic cheilitis, venous lacuna, spider naevi, hematoma, telangiectasia, superficial basaloma, lentigo solaris, lentigo senilis etc.

A good field for the CO_2-laser is plastic surgery, such as eyelid operations (blepharoplasty). Even in tattoo treatment, this laser can be very useful. Our own experience is that the safest method is to evaporate very superficially over the tattoo and not to go down to the tattoo pigments, especially on shoulders and trunk, as the risk of keloid scarring is high in these areas. The CO_2-laser has also been used for so called laser peeling - a very superficial tissue ablation in the face - for the removal of wrinkles and acne scars. The mechanism is partly thermic by remodelling and contraction of the collagen, partly biostimulative.

An interesting application is to use a relatively low powered CO_2-laser to weld or solder tissue instead of suturing. Tissue welding gives less risk of scarring and can be done with high precision. Human albumin (HAS) can be used as a solder.

1.4.1.2 Carbon dioxide lasers in dental applications

In dentistry, the carbon dioxide laser has been used experimentally in cariotic tissue. If caries is removed with a carbon dioxide laser, a number of positive effects result. The residual infection in the dentinal tubuli is removed, the cavity bottom is almost vitrified, and a secondary dentine-stimulating effect can be achieved in the odontoblasts. Some promising experiments have been conducted relating to the treatment of pulp lesions, although the disadvantages currently outweigh the advantages. It is only possible to get at open caries, which must first be uncovered with a rotating instrument. The enamel contains only 10% water, so the temperature soon reaches destructive levels if hit by the carbon dioxide laser. Intraoral access has been improved by "wave conductors", bendable tubes, but access (and wave conductors) are still not good enough for the method to be used on a routine basis within cariology. A powerful suction system is needed to remove smoke and malodorous vapour.

Aphthae can be treated with small doses of carbon dioxide laser.

Dental necks can be successfully treated by CO_2-laser by closing the dentinal tubules [442].

Flap operation is an interesting indication for carbon dioxide lasers. All granulation on the inside of the flap can be removed, and the flap edge can be contoured. Rossman [236] and Israel [237] note in their studies that the normally unavoidable epithelium down-growth in the pocket is reduced after the flap is treated in this way.

Frenectomy is performed much more quickly with a carbon dioxide laser. No suturing is required, and the subsequent course of healing is very positive.

Gingivectomies have been described in the literature, but are not a recommended operation for the inexperienced laser operator, in view of the damage to the dental hard tissue and prosthetic replacements which can result. However, special tools which protect the tooth substance have been developed. The CO_2-laser can, on the other hand, be used in flap operations to remove granulation and to treat the exposed root surface. Necrotic cement can be removed and dentine tubuli can be sealed. It has been reported that by changing the structure of the root surface, the regeneration of fibroblasts is improved. A special form of gingivectomy is that performed on patients on Dilantine and related medicines. The strong hyperplasia is well suited to carbon dioxide lasers as the bleeding is minimal. A gingivectomy is first performed with a focused beam, and then the gingiva is contoured with a defocused beam.

Haemangiomas are also appropriately removed with laser once the size of the tumour has been carefully determined. Bear in mind that many haemangiomas are like the tip of the iceberg. The majority of laser-treated oral soft tissues are left to heal "per secundam", that is, by secondary intention without sutures.

Hyperplasia of various kinds is appropriately removed by incision. After anaesthetics, the tissue is stabilised with a pair of tweezers, and then an incision is made using single pulses.

Preprosthetic surgery can be performed with a carbon dioxide laser. Hypertrophic tubera and "flabby ridges" can be peeled off layer by layer. The patient can start using dentures much more quickly than after conventional surgery because the oedema is much smaller than if a scalpel were used. In crown and bridge therapy, the uncovering of the preparation margin is a good indication if access is acceptable. There is no retraction of the tissue as with electro-surgery.

Retention cysts such as ranula and mucocele can either be removed in their entirety or fenestrated by laser. By comparison with conventional surgery, a lower recurrence frequency has been reported when lasers are used.

Root canals can be sterilised by carbon dioxide laser [441]. The laser energy helps kill off the root canal's microflora, and partially seals the side canals and apex delta. A special adapter is needed to allow the laser beam to reach the apical region of the tooth. Studies are going on where a dentine-like material is pushed down to the apex region as a "plug", and then the laser is used to "solder" the plug to the tooth substance. Perforations of the root canal could also be sealed with this kind of plug. Laser can, in certain situations, replace retrograde root filling in apical surgery. The laser energy kills infections and seals the side canals.

1.4.2 The Nd:YAG laser

This type of laser produces light in a single crystal of Yttrium-Aluminium-Garnet doped with an additional substance. The most common such substance is elemental neodymium (Nd). The full name of this laser is thus Nd:YAG. Normally the laser is pumped by a very strong flash lamp.

Another new type of Nd:YAG-laser is the diode laser pumped YAG-laser. Here, powerful GaAlAs-lasers are used to pump optical energy to the Nd:YAG-laser rod instead of using a flash lamp. The output wavelength is then the typical 1064 nm. The advantage of this laser is its smaller size.

In spite of its high output power, the Nd:YAG laser also has biostimulating effects [152, 202, 218, 1062].

1.4.2.1 Nd:YAG lasers in surgery

The Nd:YAG laser has been used in general surgery for many years but is being replaced more and more by the CO_2-laser, which has better evaporation and cutting properties. However, the Nd:YAG laser is very good for coagulation and is a good tool for coagulating tumours. This is called hyperthermia and the effect on cancer is based on the fact that healthy tissue can be heated to a higher temperature than the tumour cells before being killed. Usually the laser beam is brought to the centre of the tumour by means of an optical fibre.

1.4.2.2 Nd:YAG lasers in dentistry

The output of the dental Nd:YAG laser is variable, and can be anything between 0 and 15 watts. Its pulsing can also be varied. Both these parameters should be adjusted to suit the type of treatment, even during the operation itself.

Only the treatment of soft tissue, aphthae and "drilling" have up to now been fully accepted by odontological experts, but many other interesting indications have been tested. The Nd:YAG laser for "drilling" was a pioneer in the area but has now been replaced by the Er:YAG laser, which is more suited for "drilling"and other dental procedures. Some of the possibilities of the dental YAG lasers are presented below.

Analgesia. It is possible to cut soft tissue and excavate caries without causing pain. The mechanism is unclear.

Anaesthesia of teeth. By irradiating a tooth for a few minutes with increasing intensity, local anaesthesia of the tooth can be brought about using energy densities ranging from 2 to 40 J/cm^2, preferably starting with short pulses, slightly below the pain threshold, and gradually increasing until anaesthesia is achieved. No lasting damage to the pulp as a result of this treatment has been observed. The anaesthesia is most easily achieved on young teeth. The more sclerotic the pulp space, the poorer the effect.

Caries. Superficial caries in the enamel can be treated as described above, that is, without removing tooth substance. A defect does remain, in the form of a small pit, but the surface is more resistant to caries than normal enamel. Profound caries can be removed painlessly with Nd:YAG laser. The sound is rather like the popping of popcorn, and the procedure takes longer than with the turbine. If can often be the case that the dentist must first uncover the caries area with a turbine. The psychological benefits tend to outweigh the practical drawbacks, although the absence of pain is always a significant benefit. Glass ionomer or composite materials are chosen as filling materials. The enamel is etched with the laser. Even if caries treatment with YAG laser is much more time-consuming, it is quite inspiring to be able to uncover a subgingival Class V filling without anaesthetics and without causing any bleeding, and then excavate the caries and etch the edge of the enamel - all with the same instrument. Often the excavation must be started with the turbine but the more profound parts of the decay can, to great advantage, be removed with the laser. The “feeling” of the manual probe will tell you when you have reached sound dentine. Postoperative problems are less frequent than in conventionally excavated and bonded restorations. Tooth structures are transparent to the Nd:YAG wavelenght. It is therefore necessary to use a black dye on the tooth prior to “drilling”. Thus, removing tooth structure is not the greatest advantage of Nd:YAG.

Fissure sealing. Laser-treated enamel is restructured and made more acid-resistant. This restructuring is possible through laser treatment of the fissure system. It is also thought that the bacteria in the bottom of the fissure can be killed and that it is possible to fuse the fissure. It is still possible to seal with resin, if so desired. The enamel can be etched by the laser but acid etch is considered to give better bonding.

Herpes simplex. As any other laser with proper dosage, Nd:YAG will successfully treat herpes simplex lesions. When treated with a higher intensity than in conventional laser therapy, the lesions will shrink within seconds and will then fall off after a few days.

Hypersensitive dentine. The sensitive root surface is “painted” with the laser, using water-cooling. Organic matrix is coagulated and the tubuli are closed.

Periodontics. Nd:YAG laser has been tested for a number of purposes within periodontics. A typical treatment could be as follows. The probe is moved down close to the bottom of the pocket and is then moved in a sweeping motion around the tooth. By this means, a large part of the bacterial flora in the pocket is eliminated. The laser probe is then moved in all directions over the root cement. The calculus is loosened up, and can be more easily removed, using conventional methods. The probe is then finally moved into the pocket epithelium. The granulation tissue is vaporised, and the result is pocket curettage. No anaesthetic is required. Different outputs and pulsation times are used for different operations. The optimal dosages and procedures for this kind of therapy still remain to be established.

Bi- and trifurcations are a challenging indication for Nd:YAG treatment. The flexible fibre will reach areas where the curette often fails.

Soft tissue treatment. It is possible to cut soft tissue without causing bleeding and without the need for anaesthetics. The uncovering of preparation margins is also possible, as are smaller operations, such as the removal of hyperplasia and minor frenectomies. The cutting output is, however, low and the operation takes longer than with carbon dioxide lasers. The tissue tends to stick to the probe. Unlike electrocautery, there will be no tissue retraction

Sterilisation of root canals. The biggest problem with the treatment of non-vital teeth is the apical infection. By moving the thin laser probe down into the apical area, and slowly moving it back, one can kill off bacteria in both the apex delta and the side canals. It has also been discussed whether it is possible, with an appropriate dosage, to seal the apex and side canals by melting the canal walls. It appears that the CO_2-laser is better suited to this indication, as studies have shown that the Nd:YAG laser can vitrify the canal walls, but that microscopic cracks occur.

Further literature: [926, 927]

1.4.3 Ho:YAG lasers

The Ho:YAG-laser (short for CTH:YAG-laser, with the dopant substances chromium, thulium and holmium in the YAG host), emits a wavelength of 2130 nm in the infrared part of the spectrum. This wavelength couples well into water and body fluids and can be transmitted through a silica fibre for easy and accurate beam delivery.

The Ho:YAG-laser is used for fragmentation of gall stones, kidney stones and stones in the urinary bladder. It has also been used successfully in the treatment of endometriosis. It can cut, evaporate and coagulate tissue. Further, it is used for shrinking of cartilage in e.g. knee joints and in the spinal cord.

It is not known if biostimulative effects occur when it is used. The Ho:YAG-laser is not dangerous to eyes unless directly focused on the eye.

1.4.4 Er:YAG lasers

The Er:YAG laser has elemental erbium as dopant. It works at a wavelength of 2940 nm and is, like the other members of the YAG family, pulsed. A great benefit of this wavelength is that it is not as harmful to the eyes (unless directly focused on the cornea) as the Nd:YAG laser. The main use of this laser type in surgery is for laser peeling. Compared with the CO_2-laser, it is less painful during treatment and the healing is somewhat faster. However, it has not quite as good an effect on wrinkles and acne scars as the CO_2-laser unless used for more than one session.

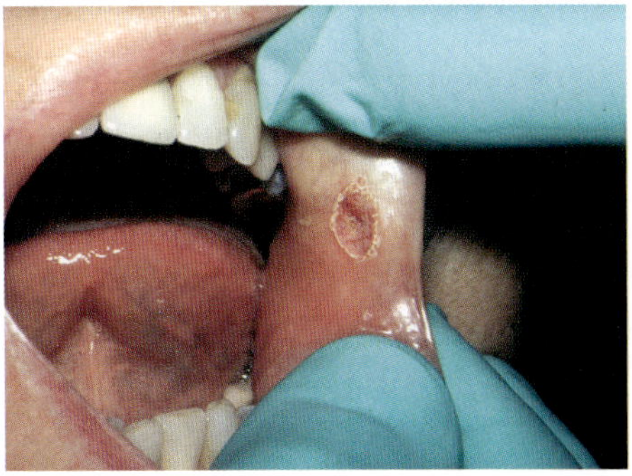

Figure 1.11 Hyperplasia removed with Er:YAG laser
Courtesy: Continuum Lasers

In dentistry, the Er:YAG is excellent for dental hard tissue and is therefore more suited for the treatment of caries than Nd:YAG-lasers. The wavelength 2940 nm is optimally absorbed by the water in the tooth substance and by the OH-ion in the hydroxy apatite. To avoid overheating, a jet of water accompanies the laser beam, in the same way as with a conventional drill. This water-cooling should reduce the laser's energi density considerably, but for various reasons the reduction is relatively small. The treatment is generally painless and the concept is obviously very interesting. Enamel, dentin, and composites can be removed with this laser, but not metals such as amalgam. Apart from working as a "drill" the Er:YAG laser can be used in minor surgical procedures such as frenectomies, tongue ties and pulpectomies, frequently without anaesthesia. It can also be used to treat aphthae and herpes simplex. Using thin fibres it is also possible to sterilise infected root canals and reduce bactererial growth in periodontal pockets. The Er:YAG "drill" is obviously slower than the traditional drill but has the advantage of requiring no anaesthesia (in most cases), so several quadrants can be treated during the same session. There is no temperature rise in the pulp; on the contrary the temperature is reduced by the water spray. With the Er:YAG laser, dentistry has taken a large leap from the old "extension for prevention" to "minimal invasive dentistry".

A newcomer in the Er:YAG family is the ErCr:YSGG laser (Erbium-Chromium:Yttrium-Scandium-Gallium-Garnet) with a wavelength of 2870 nm. The water is claimed not only to serve as a coolant but also to give a “hydrokinetic” action in order to make the “drill” more effective. However, it is not clear that it really gives a better drilling effect.

One of the difficult parts of the Erbium lasers is beam delivery. The first lasers used articulated arms with mirrors, a solution that is expensive and clumsy since the dentist has to move it at different angles. To make an optical fibre, the light conducting materials available were not transparent enough. Typically a one meter fibre reduced the output to 50% and a two meter fibre reduced it to 25%. Also, the fibres were easily burned at the input end. Today, there are flexible fibres of very pure quartz, transmitting more than 80% over a length of two meters.

Another method is to use a hollow wave guide with a dielectric surface material reflecting the beam. There are basically two problems with this solution, namely that the output power depends on the bending angles and that it easily breaks if bent too much.

Further literature: [201, 160, 1156, 1157, 1158].

1.4.5 Argon laser

Like the CO_2-laser, the argon laser (or rather, the argon ion laser) is a gas laser, usually emitting light with a wavelength of 514.5 nm (green light). It is much used in the treatment of diabetic retinopathy. However, other lasers, such as semiconductor laser types or KTP-lasers, are gradually replacing the argon laser. In the same way, the argon laser has been used in dermatology to coagulate haemangiomas but is now being replaced by the KTP/532-laser, the Dye laser or the Copper vapour laser. Argon laser at 488 nm has also been used to cure composite fillings and for tooth bleaching.

1.4.6 Copper vapour laser

This laser type is the strongest of the neutral metal vapour lasers. In its most typical form, it emits light at a wavelength of 578 nm (yellow). It is used in dermatology to coagulate haemangiomas and telangiectasis.

1.4.7 KTP/532-laser (frequency doubled Nd:YAG laser)

If a Nd:YAG laser is combined with a non-linear crystal (such as KDP, KTP, LiNbO3, etc.), light can be emitted at other wavelengths. One such combination is a Nd:YAG laser and a KTP crystal (Potassium Titanyl Phosphide), which is used for frequency doubling and hence also halves the wavelength to 532 nm (green light). Such instruments are often called KTP/532. A laser with this wavelength is a better alternative to the argon laser for treating haemangiomas, small telangiectasis, and red tattoos.

These lasers are normally pulsed (which the argon laser is not) with typical pulse lengths from microseconds to milliseconds. They can also be made to yield pulse trains.

Further, it has been observed that the KTP-laser radiation also has an effect on wrinkles, sometimes called “Non-Ablative Laser Treatment” of wrinkles. The energy density is set lower than the pain threshold, which makes the treatment painless. Practically no side effects have been noted. If the KTP-laser treatment is combined with a Ruby-laser treatment or Nd:YAG-laser treatment, even better results are obtained. The mechanism behind this is biostimulation.

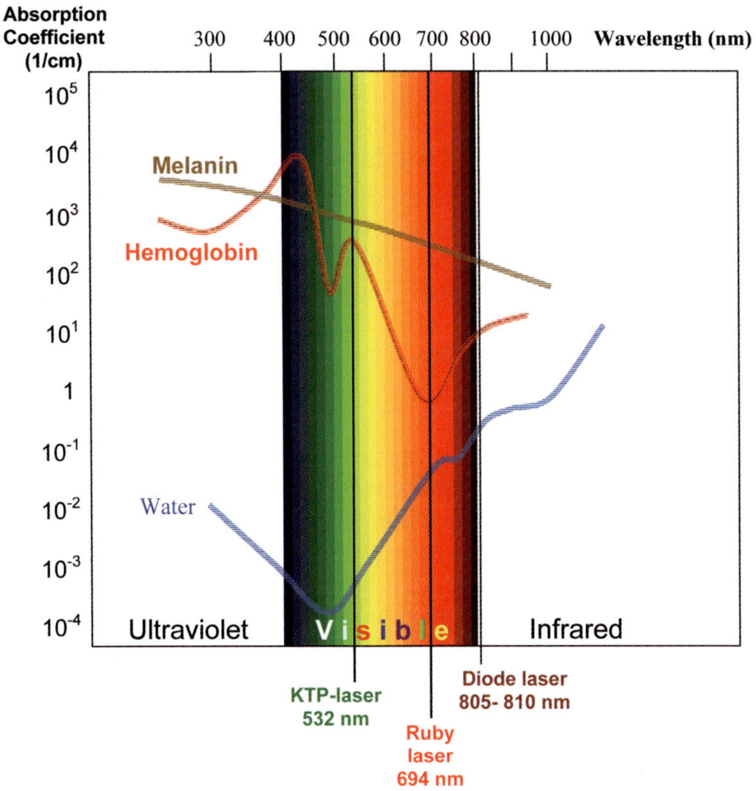

Figure 1.12 Absorption coefficient for melanin and hemoglobin

1.4.8 Ruby laser

This is the oldest of all lasers. The first working laser, presented at a press conference arranged at the Hughes Aircraft Laboratory in Los Angeles, on July 7, 1960, was a Ruby laser. This laser is a solid-state laser using a single, rod-shaped ruby crystal. It emits pulsed light at a wavelength of 694 nm (red light). This laser is currently used in dermatology to remove unwanted hair and to treat blue or green tattoos. In dentistry the ruby laser has been used to produce double-pulse holograms.

It is worth remembering that it was a Ruby laser that Endre Mester used when he discovered what he called biostimulation. The Ruby laser is still a useful instrument in the treatment of leg ulcers, decubitus, herpes labialis, herpes zoster, scars etc.

In the diagram above, it can be seen that the ruby laser has minimal absorbtion in blood and that KTP laser has hundred times higher absorbtion.

1.4.9 Alexandrite

This laser is also pulsed and can be made tuneable, usually within a range of 720-800 nm. Normally, it emits deep red visible light at a wavelength of 755 nm. It is primarily used to remove unwanted hair, as in cases of hirsutism. Q-switched, mode-locked versions are sometimes used to drill and cut bone.

1.4.10 High power semiconductor lasers

Today, semiconductor lasers of the GaAlAs type (with several stacked diode chips) can emit up to 200 W in continuous mode. Typical wavelengths range from 800-880 nm. This laser type can replace the Nd:YAG in surgery and coagulation. It has also been used with some success for hair removal. Its advantages are that it is small, relatively inexpensive, and relatively insensitive to mechanical shock and vibrations.

1.4.11 Dye laser

The active medium in a dye laser is a fluorescent organic dye dissolved in a liquid solvent, usually water. The input energy usually comes from another, external laser (such as an argon, nitrogen, or XeCl laser) or from a flash lamp. The main feature of the dye laser is its tuneable wavelength output and ability to produce ultra-short pulses. Dye lasers are used in dermatology to coagulate certain skin problems such as unwanted tattoos, haemangiomas, and telangiectasis. A version that can produce extreme pulsing can be connected to an optical fibre to blast kidney stones.

A method for detecting and destroying cancer tumours with dye lasers, is photodynamic therapy. It is often performed in two steps: detection and destruction. Detection is based on the following. HPD (hematoporphyrin derivate), a light sensitive flourescensing substance, at a dose of 10 mg/kg, or Photofrin, labelled with an antibody specific to the kind of tumour in question, is injected in the patient intravenously 24 hours prior to light irradiation. By irradiating the patient with green light and looking at the irradiated area through red bandpass filters, fluorescence can be seen. Fluorescence will occur at areas with higher concentrations of the dye, indicating the presence of a tumour. By irradiating the tumour area with light with a wavelength around 630 nm, the HPD will split, releasing toxic agents in the tumour area, possibly killing the tumour. The dye laser is often used as it is strong and can be tuned to the most efficient wavelength. It has been established [24], [25] that the depth of laser light penetration is sufficient to obtain a biological response (necrosis) as far down as 10 mm in the tissue

1.4.12 Excimer laser

The Excimer laser (193, 248, 308, 351 nm) is mainly used for vision correction. The most promising technique, the LASIK surgery is a procedure that corrects for near- or far-sightedness by evaporation of the surface of the cornea. The curvature of the cornea makes it work like a lens as a part of the eye's lens system, and by changing the curvature, the focus length and refraction quality of this system can be adjusted. The short wavelength of the Excimer laser enables it to be absorbed by the surface of the cornea, and the evaporation process can be very carefully controlled by means of a computer. Both nearsighted and farsighted persons can be helped, and the technique can also be used to adjust astigmatism. This method is very safe nowadays and the whole procedure is a matter of hours.

1.5 Therapeutic lasers

The most typical therapeutic lasers and their wavelengths:

HeNe laser	633 nm	Gas laser
InGaAlP lasers	633-700 nm	Semiconductor laser
GaAlAs lasers	780-890 nm	Semiconductor laser
GaAs laser	904 nm	Semiconductor laser
Defocused CO_2-laser	10,600 nm	Gas laser
Defocused Ruby laser	694 nm	Solid state laser
Defocused Nd:YAG laser	1,064 nm	Solid state laser

Table 1.4 Typical therapeutic lasers and their wavelengths

We recognise here three typical surgical laser types - the CO_2-laser, the Ruby laser and the Nd:YAG laser. The Ruby laser was actually the very first biostimulative laser, used by Endre Mester. As a matter of fact, the other surgical lasers could also be used as therapeutic instruments. When strong lasers are used for biostimulation, one only needs to make the beam wide enough not to burn. The patient will then feel only a mild heat. An alternative is to scan rapidly over the area to be treated with a narrow beam. In this case, it is important to have a safety mechanism to ensure that laser light cannot be emitted unless the scanning system is really working, to prevent the patient being burned if the scanning beam stops.

1.5.1 The Helium-Neon laser (HeNe)

This laser, the oldest in laser therapy use after ruby laser, consists of a large laser tube of glass containing a low-pressure gas mixture, which is connected to a high voltage source. It emits visible, red light with a wavelength of 633 nm. The laser generally works continuously, but can be pulsed by switching the electric power supply or by means of a beam chopper or similar unit. In that case, half the output is lost (if the duty cycle is 50%) compared to the continuous working mode. Typical output is 1-10 mW, sent directly (parallel beams) or via fibre optics to a treatment probe (usually divergent light). Instruments containing a HeNe laser are usually rather large and fragile because of the sensitive laser tube. There are laser tubes that are well protected by cushioning material, though the size problem still remains.

The HeNe laser is the most coherent of the different therapeutic types, having a coherence length of centimetres to metres. This is an important factor for the biological result. (See Table 3.3: "Dose ranges for different lasers and indications" on page 73 and Figure 11.4 "Different light sources have different spectra" on page 340.)

In a therapeutic instrument, the HeNe laser light is aimed at the area to be treated either directly, via scanning mirrors, or transfered via a fibre-optic light conductor. The light conductor can either be a mono-fibre or consist of a number of small, thin fibres (fibre bundle). Mono-fibres have much less power loss (typically 1-10%), but are more expensive. Fibre bundles often give a power loss between 20% and 50%, depending on quality. As can be seen, there are a number of practical disadvantages associated with HeNe laser equipment.

For treatment with skin contact, the depth of penetration of a useful level of light from a HeNe laser is 6-8 mm at 3.5 mW output and 8-10 mm for a laser with 7 mW output. (For a more detailed explanation, see chapter 3.4.2 "Depth of penetration, greatest active depth" on page 92.) The depth of penetration thus increases only minimally with increased output.

1.5.2 Indium-Gallium-Aluminium-Phosphide lasers (InGaAlP)

The InGaAlP is named GaAlInP laser in some of the literature. It belongs to a group of semiconductor lasers in which the crystal contains gallium, aluminium, indium, and phosphorus. They are related to the GaAlAs lasers and emit light in the wavelength range of 630-700 nm. Small lasers of this kind within the 650-700 nm wavelength range are often used as pointers in lectures. Developments in this field have taken the InGaAlP laser wavelength down towards and even below the HeNe laser's 633 nm, and the HeNe laser is gradually being replaced by the cheaper, smaller and more robust 633-700 nm InGaAlP laser. InGaAlP lasers make this wavelength available in a more practical form than the HeNe laser, with its expensive, large, and sensitive laser tube.

> One should bear in mind, though, that diode lasers emit light with a shorter coherence length than gas lasers, and we have noticed that the biological effects of light from these types of 633 nm lasers are less obvious than using He-Ne laser light. With higher output – e.g. 25-50 mW – similar results seem obtainable through using higher power densities and higher doses.

1.5.3 Gallium-Aluminium-Arsenide lasers (GaAlAs)

This type of laser comprises an entire family of semiconductor lasers. The wavelength can be selected within the 780-890 nm range, but in therapeutic use is usually between 800 and 830 nm, which is invisible, being just inside the infrared area. (However, if one looks straight into a GaAlAs laser probe without protection goggles, one can see a small red glowing point due to the remnant eye sensitivity at that wavelength). These lasers are continuous in their method of operation, but can be pulsed, in which case they are not superpulsed like the GaAs laser, but switched, which means that around half the power output (with a 50% duty cycle) is lost compared to when not pulsed. The depth of penetration of this type of laser is around 2-3 cm.

The GaAlAs laser has grown increasingly popular during the 1990s as it is very easy to run electrically. Small rechargeable lasers have been put on the market, not much larger than an electrical toothbrush. They can run on regular or rechargeable batteries. 30-100 mW laser diodes are now relatively cheap and the GaAlAs laser provides “a lot of mW for the money”. There are also GaAlAs lasers on the market with an output of more than 1000 mW. A warning should be issued about these lasers - the dangers of eye injury are very real at such high outputs, particularly if the beam is collimated. One way of avoiding these problems is to use GaAlAs lasers which can be activated only on contact with tissue.

Many GaAlAs lasers have well-designed, exchangeable, sterilisable intra-oral probes. Output meters are essential, because the light from this type of laser is largely invisible. The price tag for a GaAlAs laser of around 100 mW can be between US $2,000 and $ 5,000. Price differences depend on factors such as output, ergonomics, standard of hygiene, and dose calculating electronics, to name but a few.

In recent years GaAlAs lasers of 500-1000 mW have entered the market. Prices range from $ 4,000 to $ 10,000. These lasers require proper protection for the eyes and can produce a noticeable heat sensation, especially in hairy or pigmented areas.

1.5.4 The Gallium-Arsenide laser (GaAs)

This is also a semiconductor laser, and consequently it can be quite small. It emits an infrared (invisible) beam with a wavelength of 904 nm. A laser diode emits a divergent beam (usually 10 to 20 degrees), which can be made parallel by the use of a collimating lens. The GaAs laser is always operated in a pulsed fashion, with very short pulses (100-200 ns) of high peak power (10-100 W maximum output), more or less like a flash bulb. This is often called super-pulsing.

The average output of most of the conventional GaAs treatment lasers on the market varies in direct proportion to the pulse repetition frequency. This means that at 1,000 pulses per second, for example, the average output is ten times higher than at 100 pulses per second. There are, however, some lasers that use pulse trains, in which the average output can be kept constant and independent of the set pulse frequency. This “constant power pulse” simplifies dosage calculation and shortens treatment time considerably.

Because of the GaAs laser's "flash bulb" method of working, with very intense light pulses, it reaches deeper than a laser of the same wavelength that is not superpulsed but has the same average output power. Measurements have shown that the depth of penetration can be as much as 30-50 mm, depending on the type of tissue.

In the treatment of horses, the GaAs laser has been utilised as a diagnostic tool due to the fact that the horse often feels the effect of this laser's radiation and hence reacts when a probe is held over a site of injury. chapter Chapter 7 "Veterinary use" on page 277

1.5.5 The defocused strong lasers

A more detailed description these lasers has been presented in the previous section. In therapy, they are defocused or combined with scanners so that the power density or average power is kept low enough to avoid burning. These laser types have also made it possible to investigate these wavelengths with some interesting results.

Literature:

Basford [1062] performed a double-blind, placebo-controlled, randomised clinical trial on patients with low back pain. The subjects were 63 ambulatory men and women between the ages of 18 and 70 years with symptomatic non-radiating low back pain of more than 30 days' duration and normal neurological examination results. Subjects were bloc randomized into two groups with a computer-generated schedule. All underwent irradiation for 90 seconds at eight symmetric points along the lumbosacral spine three times a week for 4 weeks by a masked therapist. The Nd:YAG laser emitted 542 mW/cm^2. Subject's perception of benefit, level of function, as assessed by the Oswestry Disability Questionnaire, and lumbar mobility were evaluated. The treated group had a time-dependent improvement in two of the three outcome measures: perception of benefit and level of function. These results were most marked at the midpoint evaluation and end of treatment but tended to lessen at the 1-month follow-up. Lumbar mobility did not differ between the groups at any time.

The aim of a study by Morrone [898] was to verify the effects of laser therapy performed with GaAlAs (780 nm, 2500 mW) on human cartilage cells *in vitro*. The cartilage sample used for the biostimulation treatment was taken from the right knee of a 19-year-old patient. After the chondrocytes were isolated and suspended for cultivation, the cultures were incubated for 10 days. The culture was divided into four groups. Groups I, II, III were subject to biostimulation with the following laser parameters: 300 J, 1 W, 100 Hz, 10 min. exposure, pulsating emission; 300 J, 1 W, 300 Hz, 10 min. exposure, pulsating emission; and 300 J, 1 W, 500 Hz, 10 min. exposure, pulsating emission, respectively. Group IV did not receive any treatment. The laser biostimulation was conducted for five consecutive days. The data showed good results in terms of cell viability and levels of Ca and Alkaline Phosphate in the groups treated with laser compared to the untreated group. The results obtained confirm previous positive *in vitro* results from the same authors, that the GaAlAs laser provides biostimulation without cell damage.

Kim [545] used 1.2 J in plastic and aesthetic surgery. The energy was delivered either by a 1,000 mW or a 60 mW 830 nm laser (1,000 mW × 1.2 sec or 60 mW x 200 sec). Both were effective, but the 60 mW laser was more effective in the initial period of wound healing, while the 1,000 mW laser was more effective in the later stage.

1.5.6 Some "exotic lasers"

Of course laser therapy has been performed with all kinds of existing lasers, such as the argon laser. Some of them may be worth mentioning:

1.5.7 The krypton laser

The krypton laser (or krypton ion laser) is a gas laser, usually emitting light at a wavelength of 647 nm (red light). It has been used in the treatment of herpes [63]. However, it is an expensive laser and is thus not often used for laser therapy.

1.5.8 The nitrogen laser

The nitrogen laser, emitting at a wavelength of 337 nm is a gas laser in the ultraviolet region of the spectrum. It has been used in a wound healing study and in the treatment of tuberculosis [715].

Chapter 2
Therapeutic instruments

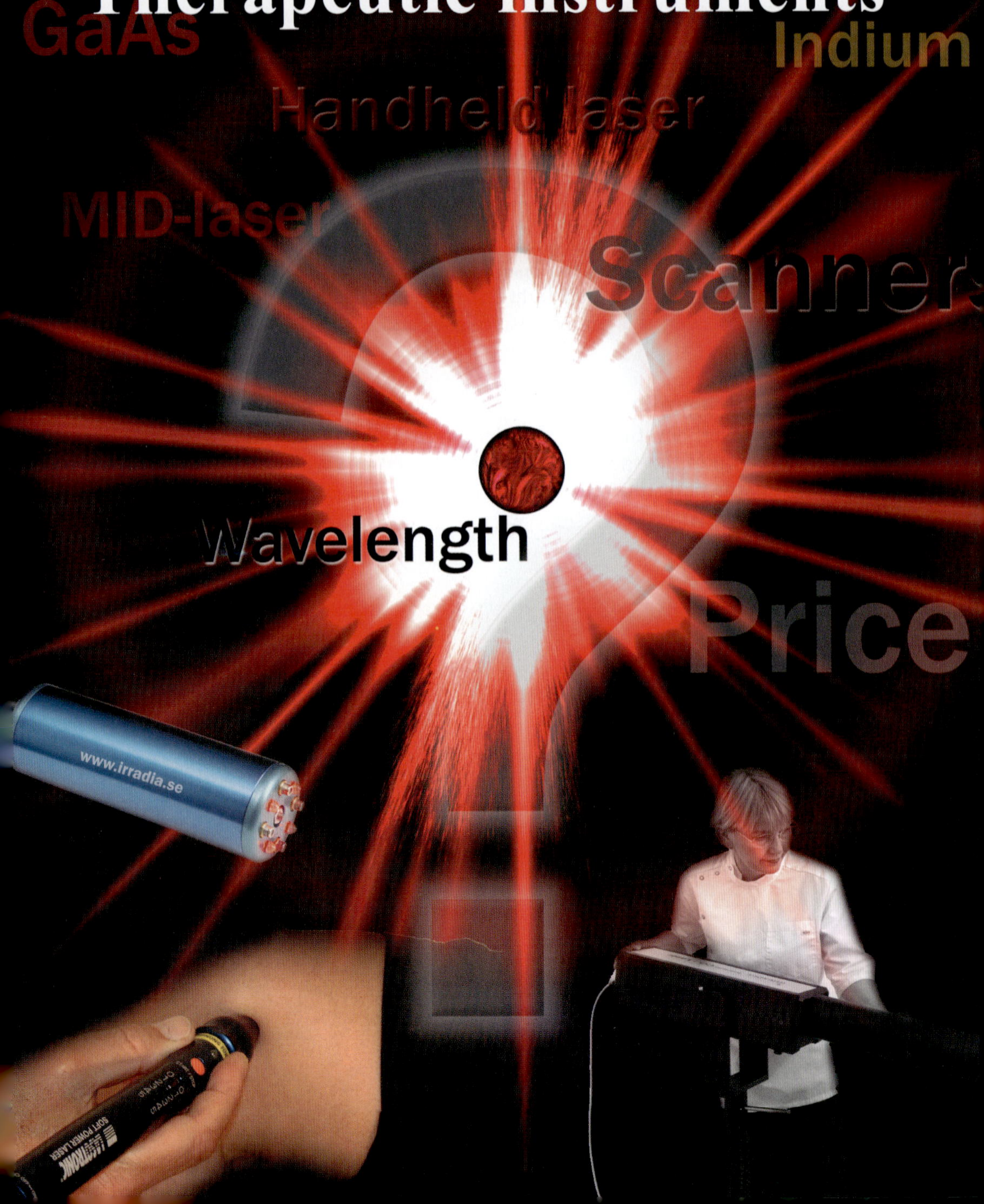

2.1 A customer's guide

In the following chapter we will only discuss laser instruments. Even though other light sources also produce biological effects, not a single article has been published showing that light emitting diodes (LED) or other incoherent sources have as good an effect as lasers when using the same parameters.

If an instrument has both LED (e.g. used as indicators or warning lights) and laser components we regard it as a laser instrument if the power from the laser or lasers clearly dominates the output power.

2.1.1 History

The first commercial therapeutic lasers appeared in the late seventies. They featured a HeNe laser with a fibre-optic cable and were often billed as "soft lasers". The purchasers consisted primarily of cosmetologists. Output powers ranged from 0.5-2 mW for many years.

GaAs lasers came onto the scene in the early 1980’s. These lasers were also quite low-powered in the beginning, 1-4 mW being typical. Pulse-train modulated GaAs lasers (“constant power pulse”) entered the market in the late 1980’s.

Low-powered GaAlAs lasers appeared in the late-80’s. 10-30 mW were typical powers. They have grown in popularity and now dominate the market. In the late 1990’s lasers of 500-1000 mW were introduced.

Carbon dioxide lasers were introduced as tools for laser therapy in the mid 1990’s.

Also in the mid 1990’s, the InGaAlP laser arrived, offering an alternative to HeNe lasers.

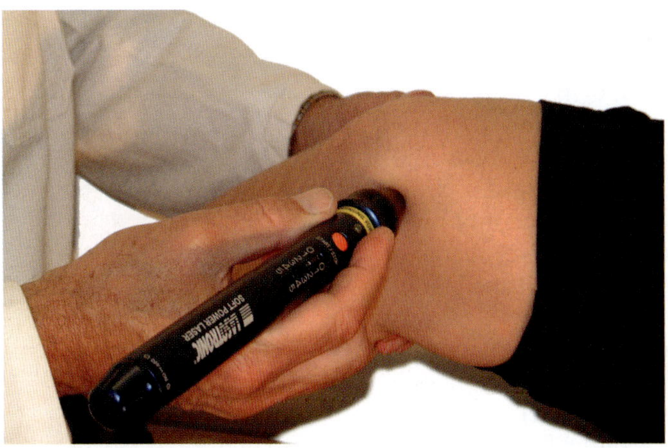

Figure 2.1 Small rechargeable 300 mW GaAlAs laser

2.1.2 What will tomorrows lasers look like

The lasers used in many clinics today are still only producing a handful of milliwatts. Equipment produced commercially in the 1970's were very low powered and generally only of HeNe type, often equipped with a fibre-optic cable conducting the light from the laser tube to a handheld probe. This cable usually reduced the light intensity by about 50%. The HeNe lasers of today can produce up to 60 mW. With an optical mono-fibre or a scanning system, most of the power from the laser tube can be utilised.

The first GaAs laser, had a typical output of 0.1 – 4 mW per laser diode. Today, there are pulse-train modulated GaAs-lasers with an average output of 100 mW, independent of the envelope frequency.

GaAlAs lasers had an output in the 1-5 mW range. Later on in the 1990's the output from these lasers rose to between 5 and 50 mW. In the new millennium, the power level has gone up to a thousand mW or more, providing new and interesting possibilities.

Many of these old lasers still are around. Taking into account losses in fibres and aging laser diodes (do test your laser!), a large number of today's laser therapists are using rather low outputs. If you don't have a power meter, you may well have a true "placebo laser"!

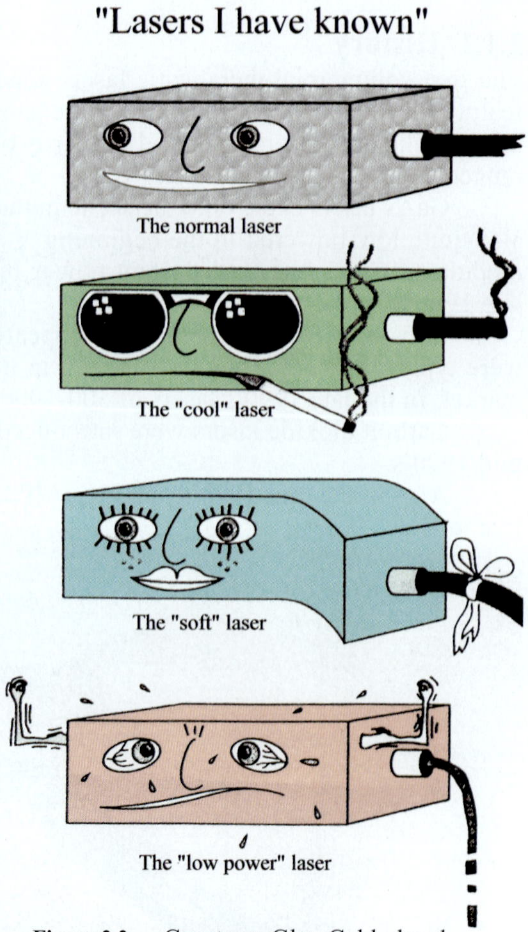

Figure 2.2 Courtesy: Glen Calderhead

The next generation of therapeutic lasers will not necessarily offer higher outputs but rather a radically different design. Holding a laser pen over an area for 10-15 minutes is not very productive work. Lasers in the form of attachable bracelets or shields have already appeared; whole-body approaches may come, laser pens for home care could be available for the general public, and so forth. Some new thinking is already mature in Russia, where adapters for irradiation via rectum and urethra are in use. We may not be able to imagine what the next generation will look like, but as soon as the market is ripe, it will be here. It is not that we do not have the technology. It is rather the small market and the small players on the market which slow down development.

Within ten years, and looking back, we will no doubt think that the lasers and techniques of the 90's were rather primitive.

2.1.3 Hand held lasers and automatic devices

A laser beam can be formed into almost any geometrical form through the use of lenses and mirrors. If the light from a laser with a narrow beam (collimated light) is to illuminate a larger surface, this can be done either by expanding the laser beam with lenses or by means of moving mirrors, scanning the beam to cover the surface area. The shape of a scanned area is usually quadratic or rectangular. In the case of expanding the beam by lenses, the illuminated area is usually circular.

In the early 80's therapeutic laser "guns" or laser scanners were in fashion. These instruments - often on big metal stands - definitely look more impressive than smaller hand held devices. An impressive laser gives a higher degree of placebo, no doubt, but the actual efficiency of those instruments was usually not related to their price and size.

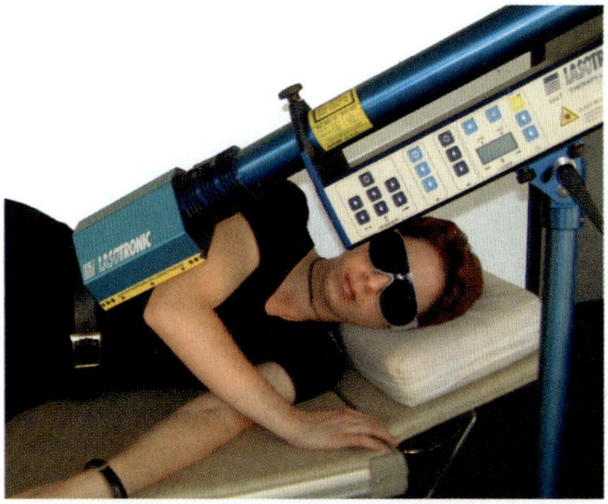

Figure 2.3 Typical scanner

The classical scanning laser was the Space Laser, using a 5-10 mW HeNe-laser mixed with light from two or more 1-5 mW GaAs-laser diodes. The value 1 mW corresponds to a 1000 Hz pulse repetition rate and 5 mW is achieved at 5000 Hz. The width and length of the area to scan could be set, as well as the scanning speed. These instruments lost a great deal of popularity when their clinical performance was not up to expectation.

The disadvantage of scanners (and laser "guns") is that they are less efficient than hand held instruments with probes that can be used for treatment with skin contact. Furthermore, they are very expensive - the price per milliwatt is especially high.

However, scanners are still useful for various conditions, such as the treatment of large wounds and other skin conditions like herpes zoster. And if used in combination with contact mode treatment, scanners have been shown to have an additional therapeutic effect. The scanners of today also have higher a output power and give a higher power density.

An advantage of a scanner is, of course, that it runs by itself so that the therapist can treat other patients in the meantime. This may, on the other hand, in turn lead to a deterioration in patient contact and information exchange between therapist and patient.

Generally, we consider the hand held devices to be more efficient than scanners in the treatment of most indications.

2.1.4 Which type of laser is best suited to which task?

There are three main types of laser on the market: HeNe (now being gradually replaced by the InGaAlP laser), GaAs, and GaAlAs. They can be installed in separate instruments or combined in the same instrument. It is not possible to give a straightforward answer to the question in the headline. There are overlapping areas of effect, and individual sensitivity. Sometimes the wavelength may not be optimal, but it may be the only possible one, due to its superior penetration of the target. The following is a brief outline of the experience of the authors and the documentation found in the literature.

2.1.4.1 HeNe laser and InGaAlP laser

The HeNe and the InGaAlP lasers are used to treat skin wounds, wounds to mucous membrane, herpes simplex, herpes zoster (shingles), gingivitis, pains in skin and mucous membrane, conjunctivitis, neuralgia, etc.

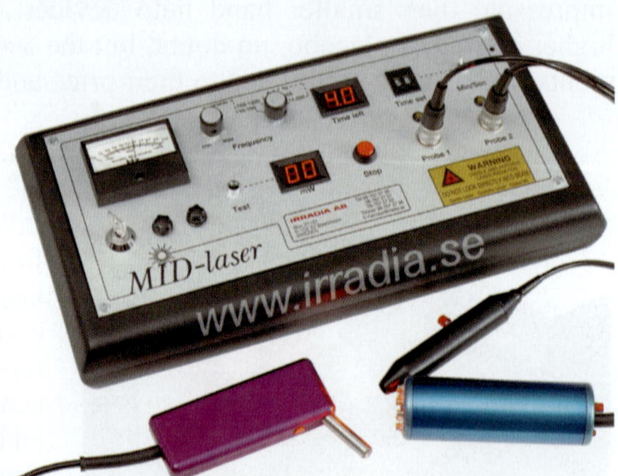

Figure 2.4 Therapeutic laser, including three different laser types

The HeNe laser has now been used for wound healing for more than 30 years and the InGaAlP laser for more than 5 years. One advantage is the documented beneficial effect on mucous membrane and skin (the types of problem it is best suited to), and another advantage is the absence of risk of injury to the eyes. Maeno [129] has treated calves with keratoconjunctivitis with excellent results, irradiating the eye through the eyelid. Schindl [350] also used HeNe lasers for experimental eye treatment. Normal HeNe output is 3-15 mW, although apparatuses with up to 60 mW are available. The optimal dosage when using a HeNe laser for wound healing is about 1.0 J/cm^2 around the edge of the wound and approximately 0.2 J/cm^2 in the open wound. The dose levels for InGaAlP lasers are higher due to the lower degree of coherence – typically twice as high.

2.1.4.2 GaAs laser

The GaAs laser is best used for the treatment of deeper situated problems and of pain and inflammations, and is less well suited to the treatment of wounds and mucous membrane. Very low dosages should be administered to mucous membrane! Most GaAs equipment is intended for extra oral use, but there are special lasers adapted for oral use. We have only found a few positive studies of GaAs lasers which demonstrate effects on wound healing. It is likely that dosage is a critical factor.

Prices are usually between US $3,000 and $5,000 for outputs between 10 and 100 mW. A GaAs laser must have an integral output meter that indicates that there is a beam and shows its power in milliwatts. This is necessary because the light is completely invisible. Protective glasses for the patient may be appropriate in view of the invisible nature of the light, especially if the beam is collimated.

In older systems, the power output is proportional to the pulse frequency. A GaAs laser that has an average output of 10 mW when pulsed at 10,000 Hz thus produces just 1 mW when pulsed at 1,000 Hz, and merely 0.1 mW at 100 Hz. If you wish to administer treatment at low frequencies with such an instrument, around, for example, 20 Hz (for the treatment of pain), the output power is, clinically speaking, unusable. However, there are GaAs lasers with "constant power pulse", meaning that the power output is held constant at all pulse frequencies. This might be of interest to a physiotherapist, for example, considering that the GaAs laser has the deepest penetration of the common therapeutic lasers. Good doses can be administered to deep-lying tissue over a short period of time. A GaAs multiprobe can also shorten treatment times for conditions involving larger areas (neck/shoulders).

The GaAs laser is, like the GaAlAs and the InGaAlP laser, a semiconductor laser. A purely practical advantage of this type of laser is that the laser diode is located in the hand-held probe. This means that there is no sensitive fibre-optic light conductor running from the laser apparatus to the probe, just an ordinary, cheap, robust electric cable. Optimum treatment dosages with GaAs lasers are lower than with GaAlAs lasers.

The GaAs laser is most effective in the treatment of pain, inflammations and functional disorders in muscles, tendons and joints (e.g. epicondylitis, tendinitis and myofascial pain, gonarthrosis, etc.), and for deep-lying disorders in general. As mentioned above, GaAs has not been shown to be as effective on wounds and other superficial problems as the HeNe laser (InGaAlP laser) and GaAlAs laser. GaAs can, nevertheless, be used successfully on wounds in combination with HeNe or InGaAlP, but the dosages should be very low in open wounds.

2.1.4.3 GaAlAs lasers

The GaAlAs lasers have become increasingly popular in the nineties. They are very easy to power electrically, and small rechargeable lasers, not much larger than an electric toothbrush, are on the market. (They can run on ordinary or rechargeable batteries.) 30-500 mW laser diodes are now relatively cheap, and a GaAlAs laser provides "a lot of milliwatts for the money". Recently, GaAlAs lasers have appeared on the market with an output of over 1,000 mW. Wavelengths normally vary between 800 and 810 nm. There are indications that the clinical effect of 780 nm differs from the very frequently used 800-830 nm.

Many GaAlAs lasers also have well-designed, exchangeable, sterilisable intra-oral probes. Output meters are essential because the light from this type of laser is largely invisible. For 800 nm wavelength the sensitivity of the human eye is only about 1 % of its sensitivity at 550 nm. In a dark surrounding, the 830 nm red light is faintly visible, however.

The GaAlAs laser normally works continuously, like the HeNe and the InGaAlP, and is used mainly on skin and mucous membranes, but can also be used on more deep-lying problems, especially the high powered lasers. Indications are difficult-to-heal wounds, rheumatoid arthritis, muscle attachments (preferably in small joints), pain and various oral conditions.

2.1.4.4 Combination probes

There are probes on the market that combine two different laser wavelengths. There are also probes that combine one or more laser diodes with LEDs of various wavelengths - known as "cluster probes". (Here we do not mean the LEDs that are used only as indicator lamps.) The authors themselves prefer equipment with only one wavelength in the probe, and there are several reasons for this. The combination of laser and LED is problematic. There is no doubt that LED light has a biological effect, though less pronounced. The incoherent light from LEDs can even counteract the effect of the laser or lasers in the probe. (See chapter 11.1.2 "Comparisons between coherent and non-coherent light" on page 335.) Also, how are we to know which of the wavelengths gives the best results under particular conditions? How do the different light sources affect each other? How is the dosage to be calculated if the probe's light sources have differing physical characteristics? Are there wavelengths that are unsuitable for some indications but will always be used because of the probe's design? How should the results of the laser + LED probes be evaluated, since they cannot be compared to "pure" laser therapy studies? In fact, a result obtained with a laser + LED probe can only be obtained with and compared to one performed with an identical probe. A comparison could be made with pharmacology, in which the preparation is refined as much as possible to isolate the desired effect.

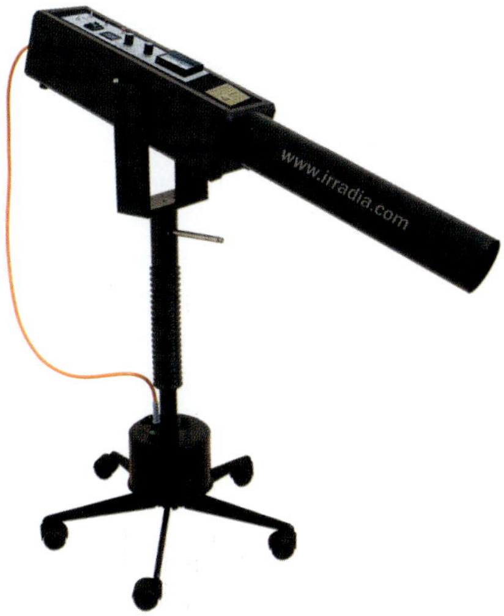

Figure 2.5 Therapeutic CO_2-laser, 10-15 W to tissue

2.1.4.5 Therapeutic CO_2-lasers

Therapeutic treatment with these lasers has become more and more popular. Instruments designed expressly for the purpose are not required. Practically any carbon dioxide laser can be used, as long as the beam can be spread out over an appropriate area and the power can be regulated to avoid burning. This can always be achieved with an additional lens of germanium or zinc selenide, if it is impossible with the standard accessories accompanying the apparatus. There are small, portable CO_2-lasers on the market today - even battery-operated units - producing up to 10-15 watts, which is more than enough power output. There is a general misconception about these lasers, implying that they can penetrate into deep areas due to their high power. In fact, the contrary applies. You will find more about this issue in chapter 11, section 1.6. The main advantage of therapeutic carbon dioxide lasers is their ability to give high doses over large areas.

2.1.5 Which laser should I buy?

There is no simple answer to this question. You have to ask yourself a number of questions: "What is the laser to be used for?", "How much am I prepared to pay?", "Must the probe be sterilisable?", "Should it be portable?", "Should it contain a microprocessor to aid in dose calculations?", "Should it be used for veterinary treatments?" and so on.

The small pen-like GaAlAs lasers are a popular choice. They are easy to handle because they have no electric cable, and can therefore be moved easily from one treatment room to another. Those with rechargeable batteries are the best choice but are more expensive than the models that run on ordinary batteries. The latter consume batteries at an alarming rate, and cannot always maintain a constant output. They are, on the other hand, very small and a little cheaper. The small rechargeable lasers are probably the most versatile for a dentist.

If you want to treat muscle, tendon, and joint problems (whether in humans or animals), a GaAs laser with a single or multiple probe is, in our opinion, an appropriate choice. Though GaAlAs still has much to offer in these areas, the GaAs penetrates deeper and has a different biological effect. A multiprobe allows shorter treatment times.

If you want to treat ulcers, skin, pain, myoses, etc., a laser with a variety of wavelengths would be a good choice, such as an InGaAlP or GaAlAs, or at least equipment to which new wavelengths can be added at a later stage.

If you are worried about the (minimal) risk of eye injury, particularly if you plan to delegate the laser work to assisting staff, you may prefer a GaAlAs laser which can be activated only on contact with tissue, or to use non collimated light.

Are you particular about dosage and not so good at mathematics? Some laser systems can calculate the dosage, or provide only the dosage you tell them to give. However, applying the "correct" dosage is not only a matter of mathematics, as will be shown later on in this book. For practical clinical purposes a "beep" indicating each Joule may be enough.

A question that is often asked is: "Should I wait until the lasers have become more sophisticated and even cheaper?" They will probably be cheaper in five years. But they will be even cheaper in ten years, and by the time you have retired, they will be cheaper still, and better...

It is clearly not an easy choice, so read this chapter carefully before making a decision - and particularly before talking to a salesperson!

2.1.6 Stronger = better?

The power output of therapeutic lasers has increased radically during the nineties. McKibbin reports that there were about 1,800 therapeutic laser units in Canada in 1990. 22% of them were HeNe lasers with an output of 1 mW or less, 35% HeNe lasers with 1-2 mW, 13% 830 nm units with an output up to 5 mW, 3% 830 nm units with an output up to 30 mW, 26% GaAs units with an output of 5 mW or less, and 1% units in the 760-780 range nm with an output up to 30 mW.

Now 2002, the situation is quite different. HeNe units are being replaced by stronger InGaAlP lasers up to 100 mW, GaAlAs units of 100-1000 mW are on the market, and GaAs units of 100 mW and more are available.

Even though it is possible to attain some effects with a 1-2 mW laser, there is no doubt that with a laser 100 times stronger, it is much easier to achieve biostimulating effects, at least if one intends to use treatment periods of the same length. Power density is also very important!

The authors used to have certain misgivings about an "inflation" with respect to the output power of therapeutic lasers. One misgiving was, and still is, the obvious risk of eye damage. The need for protective glasses has previously been exaggerated, but is now becoming more important. Another misgiving is the lack of research in the field of "high-power" therapeutic lasers. So far, insufficient data have been published on these powerful lasers. For the moment, we must rely primarily on our own clinical experience. That experience, however, is so encouraging that it cannot be ignored, even with the lack of scientific support. It would appear that "high-powered" therapeutic lasers will be able to further expand the scope of laser therapy.

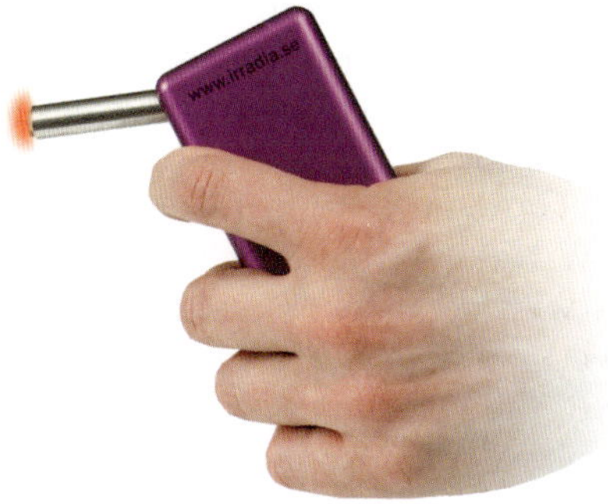

Figure 2.6 900 mW GaAlAs (810 nm) probe

The doses previously recommended for laser therapy still hold true, in a way. However, much of what we know about dosage is based upon wound healing studies. This is the field in which both stimulating and inhibiting doses have generally been observed. But a wound is superficial, and the superficial tissue will absorb most of the laser energy. So treating a condition in the inner ear through the bone behind the ear is quite a different matter. The dense bone behind the ear absorbs some 90% of the light energy. Skin and blood absorb another 5%. Thus, 100 J in contact mode means only some 5 J in the inner ear. For pain and inflammation in large joints, such as the knee, quite a few joules may be required on the surface before the actual target receives the energy needed.

Using the same amount of energy but with different energy densities will not necessarily trigger the same biological response. Kim [545] used 1.2 J in plastic and aesthetic surgery. The energy was delivered either by a 1,000 mW or a 60 mW 830 nm laser (1,000 mW × 1.2 sec or 60 mW × 200 sec). Both were effective, but the 60 mW laser was more effective in the initial period of wound healing, while the 1,000 mW laser was more effective in the late period.

Hoteya [624] previously conducted a double-blind study in the field of orthopaedics. A 150 mW GaAlAs laser was used in a group of patients suffering from chronic pain. The overall efficacy rate was 70.6%. In a later study, a 1000 mW GaAlAs laser was used. The spot size was adjusted so that the incident power density was 670 mW/cm^2, thereby avoiding any possible photo-thermal effects and any sensations of heat from the real laser as compared with the dummy laser. The overall efficacy was 75.5% with a "no change" in 24.5%. Thus, the efficacy rate was not greatly improved, but the treatment time was certainly shortened.

It is speculated that "high-powered" therapeutic lasers actually can put sufficient energy into much deeper layers of tissue, due to the high power density of the beam. Previous treatment efforts may have been somewhat less successful due to inadequate power density in deeper tissues. Increased treatment time cannot completely compensate for lower power density. For instance: 5 minutes of 30 mW = 9 J. 20 seconds × 450 mW = 9 J. The same energy is delivered, but the superior power density of the 450 mW diode will deliver energy above the response level to deep-lying areas, while the 30 mW diode will be less successful.

It is important not to over-stimulate superficial tissues with these powerful lasers. When treating wounds, the probe should be kept at a distance to reduce the power density. It should be emphasised that healthy tissues do not react adversely. Thus, the healthy tissues covering a deep target will not be damaged.

A GaAlAs 830 nm for wound healing was used by Ihara [925]. The 1000 mW laser was defocused to give a power density of 669 mW/cm^2. Five patients with persistent skin ulcers, which had proved resistant to past conservative treatment, were irradiated. The probe was held at 5 cm above the surface of the ulcer giving 2.1 - 6.3 J/cm^2 twice a week during the treatment period. The ulcers responded well to the laser therapy.

The important thing is not only the nominal output of the diode; the power density is also very important. If the spot size of a 30 mW laser is very small at the tissue, the beam may even cause a burn – especially if the skin is pigmented. The spot size of a 1,000 mW diode can be made large enough to treat even sensitive areas such as the lip without any sensation of warmth.

The examples below illustrate the fact that high power densities may be useful for pain but not necessarily for superficial cell stimulation. Again, however, it is not a matter of milliwatts, it is a matter of power density at tissue, and dosage.

Literature:

Yamada [418] reports better and faster results in treating postherpetic neuralgia with a 150 mW GaAlAs laser than with a 60 mW GaAlAs laser. The patients were treated the same number of minutes, but at different energies. The number of patients treated was small (17), and the patients in the 60 mW group also benefited from the treatment.

Shiroto [205] compared the reaction of human neutrophils *in vitro*, using 830 nm 60 mW, 830 nm 100 mW, and 904 nm 3 mW lasers. The highest stimulation was achieved with the 830 nm 60 mW laser, followed by the 904 nm 3 mW laser, while the 830 nm 100 mW laser actually retarded activity.

In a double blind study by Sattayut [924] patients with TMD for more than 6 months were treated with laser therapy. 1/3 of the patients were rendered free of symptoms (assessed at 3 months) by laser therapy alone while the other 2/3 needed additional treatment. Joint and muscular trigger points were irradiated. A GaAlAs laser, with 300 mW output and a dose of 20 J per point (100 J/cm^2) was much more effective than 60 mW and 4 J per point.

2.1.7 How much should a laser cost?

Lasers are fairly expensive instruments relative to their technical complexity, primarily because they are produced in small numbers. The most important factor is not how much the laser costs, but how good it is. An instrument costing US $3,000 without any noticeable treatment benefits (and there are such instruments, unfortunately) is in reality much more expensive than a US

$7,000 laser that effectively alleviates symptoms or cures the ailments you are treating. Many laser producers or importers have gone bankrupt or disappeared, which has left their customers in an unenviable position when their instruments break down. And remember: it is never easy to sell a second-hand laser!

2.1.8 Is a therapeutic laser really worth the money?

Are there other benefits over and above those relating to treatment? Could you, for example, successfully treat a number of conditions that are beyond your colleagues' ability, doing so without pain? Many therapists have to compete for patients and would very much like to extend their customer base. If patients can recommend their friends and acquaintances a therapist who can treat conditions that other therapists normally cannot, then that person has a much better chance of coping with the competition. However, the simple fact of using a laser does not automatically create such market advantages. Medical competence always comes first. But no matter what your degree of medical competence, a thorough knowledge of laser therapy basics is needed to achieve successful medical results with a laser. If you have both, you will be able to buy the right laser, and you will find it very profitable.

2.1.9 Do you need to update your laser?

If you already are the owner of a laser, it may be a good laser or a bad laser. To know if it is good or bad you need to find out what output power it has. And not the output power stated in the manual and not even what possibly was measured when you bought it. It is not uncommon that the output decreases by time and even that it comes close to zero. You should be able to measure the output on a regular basis with a power meter made for the actual wavelength used.

If the output is low, it can be quite money- and time saving to update your laser or even to buy a new one. How much time and money would you save in a year if you could obtain the same dose in two minutes, that you now need twenty minutes to obtain? Should you decide to buy a new laser, read the next section to get some advice.

2.2 Ten points to consider when choosing an instrument

The laser market is very complicated and full of pitfalls. How do you know which instruments are good? What is expensive? Will it be expensive in the long run to buy something cheap? It is easy to make hasty decisions when faced with a skilful salesman. Before you know it, you've signed on the dotted line.

Here are a number of questions, which you should ask both the salesman and yourself. You are well advised to read these carefully, or you may regret it later on!

1 "Laser instruments" have been sold which do not even contain a laser, instead being equipped with LEDs or even ordinary light bulbs. These instruments have been sold for between US $3,000 and $10,000. How can you acquire proof that the instrument really does contain a laser?

2 In a number of products, laser diodes have been combined with LEDs. This may be kept secret and the salesman only talks about a laser. Are all light sources in the apparatus (except guide lights and warning lights) really lasers? What output power has the laser or lasers compared to the other sources?

3 For oral work and wound healing, HeNe, InGaAlP and GaAlAs are the most common types, GaAlAs being the most versatile. Sterilisable probes are normally only available for the latter two. For injuries to joints, vertebrae, the back, and muscles - that is, for the treatment of more deep-lying problems - the GaAs laser is the best documented. Veterinary work requires a laser designed so that the light can pass through the coat and penetrate to the desired depth. It is very important that the light source is in skin contact in order to make the light penetrate into the tissue under the fur of a horse or dog. For superficial tendon and muscle attachments, the required depth can be reached with the GaAlAs laser. Many companies have only one type of laser, such as a GaAlAs, and the salesman will naturally tell you that it is the best model for everything, and that it is irrelevant which type of laser is used. However, research tells quite a different story.

4 Size, colour, shape, appearance, and price vary a great deal from manufacturer to manufacturer. Because a piece of equipment is large, it does not necessarily follow that its medical efficacy is high, or vice versa. The most important factor is the dosage that enters the tissue. Make sure the laser you buy is designed so that all the light actually enters the tissue. Ask the salesman: how is the dosage measured? Is there a power meter available? How do you know if the power of your laser has decreased?

5 Many companies that import lasers have insufficient knowledge of medicine, laser physics and technology. In fact, many such companies have gone bankrupt. If a piece of equipment is faulty, it may have to be sent to the country of manufacture for repair. How long would you be without your equipment in such a case, and what would it cost to repair? Can the importer document his expertise? Who can you speak to who has used the apparatus in question for a long period of time? Is there a well-known professional who uses this laser? What does it cost to change a laser diode or laser tube after the guarantee has expired? Can you get

written confirmation of this? Try to get a list of references that you can call and ask. How long is your guarantee - one or two years? Two years guarantee is becoming more and more common.

6 The difference between a colourful brochure and reality is often considerable. There are examples of brochures that describe an output ten times that which the equipment actually provides. How can you find out the real performance of the equipment (e.g. its output to tissue)? For pulsed lasers (usually GaAs-lasers), some manufacturers specify only the peak power of the pulse output in their technical specifications - 70 watt peak pulse output naturally seems more impressive than 35 milliwatts average output ("70 watt output" is a power that in continuous wave could cut deep in tissue). Are measurement results available from an independent agency? Is it possible to borrow an apparatus in order to measure its performance? Is there a power meter on the apparatus that can measure what is emitted and display it numerically? It is not enough simply to have a light indicator as it cannot tell you if the output power has decreased over time.

7 Some dealers might know that their products are sub-standard. Customers should beware of dealers who are overeager to get them to sign a contract. If a product is good, the dealer will have no qualms about selling it on sale-or-return basis and putting the agreement in writing. What happens if the medical effects are not as promised? Is it possible to get a written guarantee of sale-or-return?

8 In most countries, therapeutic lasers must be approved. Find out what the law says about lasers in your country.

9 Many companies organize courses and "training" events of markedly varying quality. Serious importers or manufacturers will take pains to ensure that their equipment is used properly and ensure that the customer receives some training in its use. What are the instructor's background and qualifications? Has he or she published anything? Is there a course description? What does the training material cost? Is a training course included in the cost of the equipment? Is the training material included? Is it possible to buy the training material only?

10 Development is proceeding rapidly. Suddenly, you have out-of-date laser equipment and a new and perhaps more efficient type of laser comes onto the market. What happens if your laser becomes outmoded? Do you have to buy a new laser, or can your equipment be updated with future components and probes?

1 "Laser instruments" should contain a laser as the primary light source.

2 If it has LEDs, they should only be guide lights or warning lights.

3 For oral work an exchangeable and sterilisable light conductor is best.

4 For veterinary work it must be designed to let the light pass through the coat.

5 Make sure the laser you buy has a power meter with a display.

6 Make sure that your laser instrument can be repaired after the guarantee has expired.

7 Make sure that the output as stated in the brochure is correct.

8 Is your laser approved by the authorities in your country?

9 Do you get proper training included in the price?

10 Can your equipment be updated with future components?

2.3 How do I maintain my laser?

We have seen many examples of laser instruments that have been badly treated – sometimes you wonder if the owner had his instrument hanging from a rope behind his car! This applies especially to instruments used for treating horses. Although for most people the following recommendations are obvious, we want to point them out anyway:

Avoid mechanical shock and vibrations.
Temperatures too high (> +40 ºC) or too low (< 0 ºC) may be harmful to your instrument.
Dust or smoke may collect on optical components and obstruct the path of light from source to target.
Water or high humidity may destroy electronics.
High voltage peaks in the mains can damage electronics. Be sure to disconnect your instrument in case of a thunderstorm.
Cables and mechanical switches usually break first.
Never try to repair your laser yourself. Usually this voids your guarantee.
Like most other equipment, a laser requires care and attention. If the laser has an electric cable, it should be checked regularly to prevent electrical hazards. The laser's output should also be checked on a regular basis to ensure that dose calculations are correct. A loss of power can occur when laser diodes start to age, or when light conductors age or are subjected to mechanical stress. The laser probe aperture should be washed with alcohol and soft cotton wool, for example. When the laser is used directly on skin, small

amounts of dirt and grease can enter the probe opening and gradually cause a loss of output.

If the laser beam is invisible and collimated, the laser should (for safety reasons) not be left in a state in which it is emitting light when you are not actually working with it. This can be ensured by removing the key or by separating the laser probe and battery.

If the probe is not sterilisable, it may be covered by ordinary cling film during treatment, after wich the cling film is disposed of. In any case, the aperture can be wiped with alcohol afterwards.

Chapter 3
Biostimulation

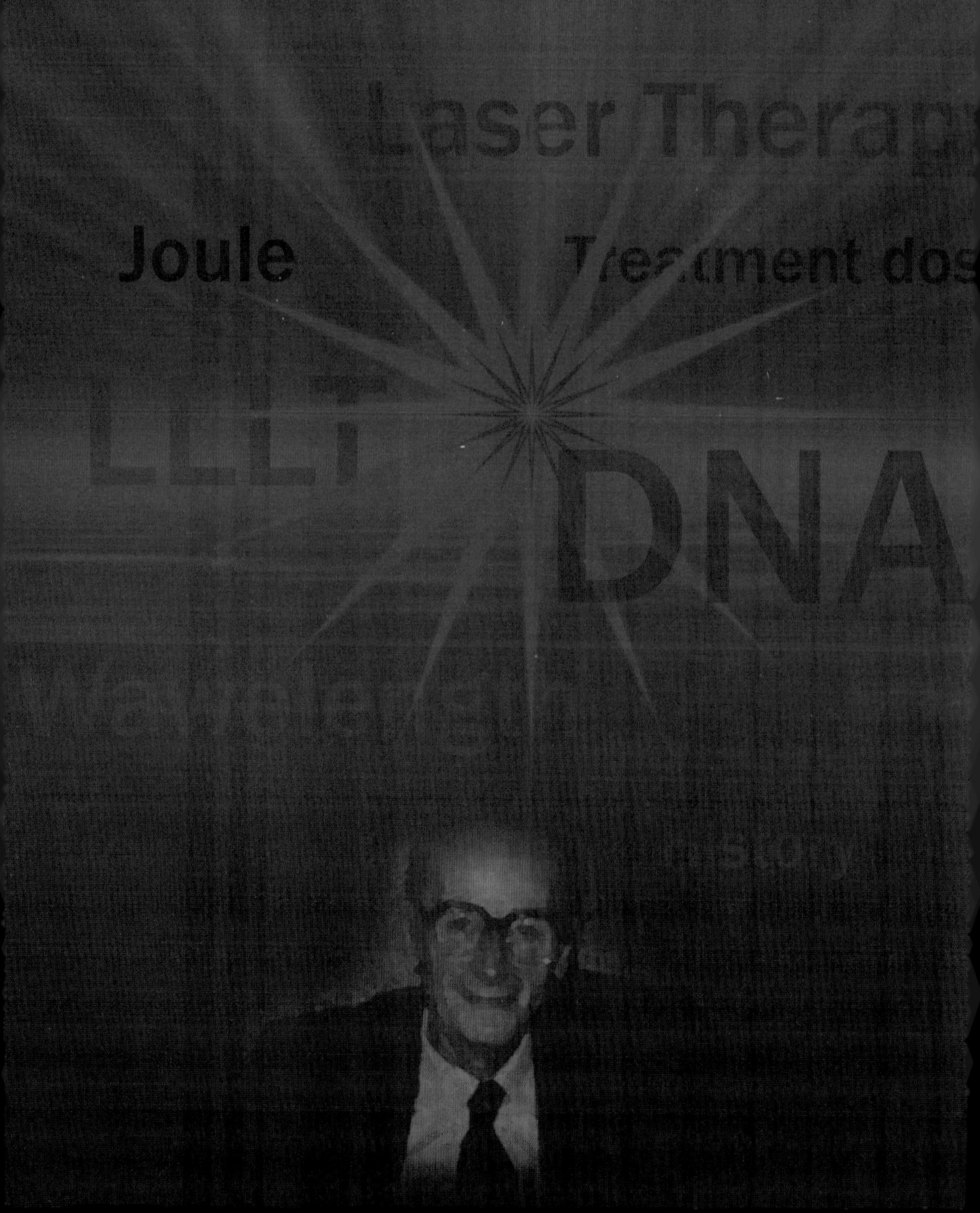

3.1 History

Initially, researchers' interest was focused on the use of lasers in surgery. Thus, rather high doses were used in early experiments.

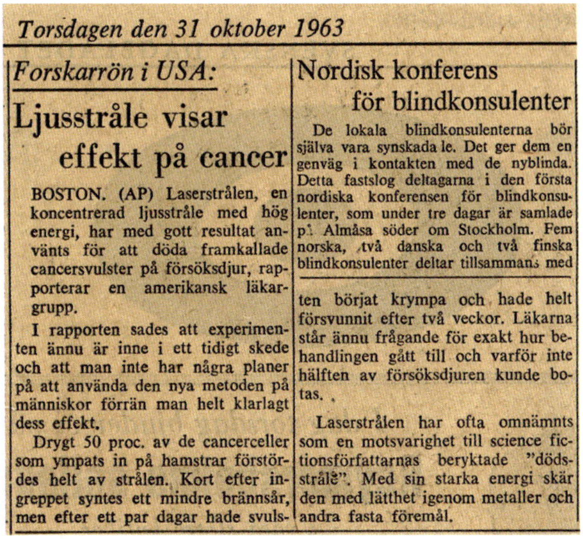

Torsdagen den 31 oktober 1963

Forskarrön i USA:

Ljusstråle visar effekt på cancer

BOSTON. (AP) Laserstrålen, en koncentrerad ljusstråle med hög energi, har med gott resultat använts för att döda framkallade cancersvulster på försöksdjur, rapporterar en amerikansk läkargrupp.

I rapporten sades att experimenten ännu är inne i ett tidigt skede och att man inte har några planer på att använda den nya metoden på människor förrän man helt klarlagt dess effekt.

Drygt 50 proc. av de cancerceller som ympats in på hamstrar förstördes helt av strålen. Kort efter ingreppet syntes ett mindre brännsår, men efter ett par dagar hade svulsten börjat krympa och hade helt försvunnit efter två veckor. Läkarna står ännu frågande för exakt hur behandlingen gått till och varför inte hälften av försöksdjuren kunde botas.

Laserstrålen har ofta omnämnts som en motsvarighet till science fictionsförfattarnas beryktade "dödsstrålë". Med sin starka energi skär den med lätthet igenom metaller och andra fasta föremål.

Nordisk konferens för blindkonsulenter

De lokala blindkonsulenterna bör själva vara synskada le. Det ger dem en genväg i kontakten med de nyblinda. Detta fastslog deltagarna i den första nordiska konferensen för blindkonsulenter, som under tre dagar är samlade på Almåsa söder om Stockholm. Fem norska, två danska och två finska blindkonsulenter deltar tillsammans med

Figure 3.1 The Swedish daily Svenska Dagbladet, October 31st, 1963

Boston (AP). An American group of physicians report that laser light, a concentrated beam of light of high energy, has successfully been used to kill cancer tumours induced in laboratory animals. In the report it is stated that the experiment still is in an initial stage and that there are no plans to use it in humans until the effect is fully documented. Some 50% of the cancerous cells that had been implanted in hamsters were completely destroyed by the laser. Shortly after therapy, a minor burn was visible but within a few days the tumour had started to shrink and was completely gone in two weeks. The researchers still do not understand exactly how the therapy worked and why the other half of the experimental animals could not be cured. The laser beam has often been referred to as an equivalent of the feared "death beam" of science fiction. With its strong energy it easily cuts metals and other solid objects.

In this article it is no doubt a biostimulation effect that is referred to. This is, according to our knowledge, the first time this effect was reported, though it was not understood. If any of our readers can find out which group in Boston did this experiment, we would be glad to know.

In 1965, Laor [589] used 700-900 J with high power densities, causing high mortality among the laboratory rats. However, doses below 20 J rarely resulted in any microscopic changes. In the same year, Derr [28] published a report on the occurrence of free radicals in irradiated biological materials. In 1967, Carney [520], using a ruby laser, demonstrated an increase in collagen synthesis in skin wounds treated with power densities of 0.4 - 2.5 J/cm^2.

In 1966, (Orvosi Heitlap 1966, 107:1012, in Hungarian, abstract in English) Mester's group at the Semmelweiss hospital in Budapest published the first scientific report of the stimulatory effects of non-thermal ruby laser light (694 nm) on the skin of rats. (See figures on next page.) These pictures were published in [733, 734]. The following year, articles were published on the effects of lasers on wounds (see figure on next page) and leukocytes in culture [10]. Mester demonstrated that cells in culture and in tissue can be stimulated by a certain dose (input energy, measured in joules per cm^2 of skin) of laser light. Too low a dose has no or an insufficient effect. Too high a dose is also less effective, or has no effect at all, while a dose that is much too large can lead to inhibiting effects. A ruby laser was used. Along with Endre Mester, Viktor Injushin in Kazakhstan was researching early about the possible biological effects of low laser energies.

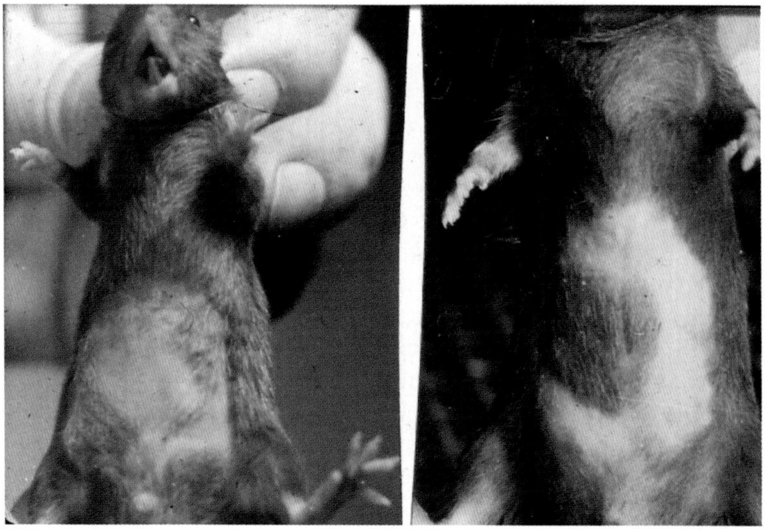

Figure 3.2 "The historic mice" I. Courtesy: Andrew Mester

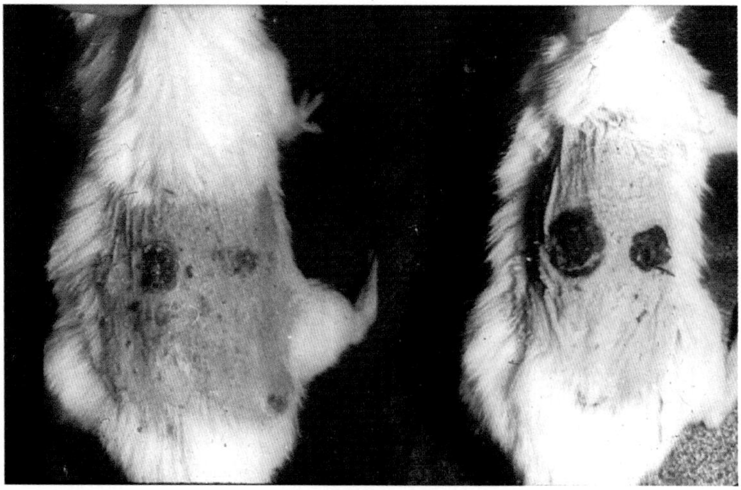

Figure 3.3 "The historic mice" II. Courtesy: Andrew Mester

3.2 A few words on mechanisms

In this chapter we will only give a brief overview of the mechanisms behind successful laser therapy. A much more detailed description is given in chapter 11.

Treatment with laser therapy is not based on heat development but on photochemical and photobiological effects in cells and tissue. What happens when this relatively weak laser light encounters our cells?

Firstly, quite a lot happens locally, where the light hits (primary response). As mentioned above, it has been observed that if laser light is administered in the right dose, certain cell functions are stimulated, and this is particularly evident if the cell in question has an impaired function. (See chapter 3.4.3 “The importance of the tissue and cell condition” on page 95.)

As will be discussed in chapter 11, it is known that chromophores, in the form of e.g. porphyrins, play an important role. It is known that small amounts of singlet oxygen build up when tissue is irradiated with laser light [28]. Rochkind's and Lubart's group in Israel has demonstrated this [29] using the NMR technique (Nuclear Magnetic Resonance). Singlet oxygen is a "free radical" which itself influences the formation of ATP (adenosine triphosphate) [30, 140], which constitutes the cells' fuel and energy store.

It is also thought that nitric oxide can play an important role [432, 469]. Additionally, it has been observed that the calcium ion balance [31] in the cell is affected. The influence of laser light on the oxidative processes has been demonstrated by Karu [180] and others. Karu [512] suggests cytochrome a/a3, a respiratory chain component, as an important photoreceptor.

This leads in turn to a number of secondary effects (secondary responses) which have been studied and measured in various contexts: increased cell metabolism and collagen synthesis in fibroblasts [8], increased action potential of nerve cells [32], stimulation of the formation of DNA and RNA in the cell nucleus [33], local effects on the immune system [34], increased new formation of capillaries by the release of growth factors [35], increased activity of leukocytes [36], transformation of fibroblasts to myofibroblasts [37], and a great number of other measured effects.

Secondly, there is a systemic effect, well illustrated through the use of CO_2-lasers as biostimulators. The wavelength of CO_2-lasers cannot penetrate the tissue for more than a fraction of a millimetre, so there is no other primary responding tissue than the outer part of the dermis. The stimulative effects found when using CO_2 are in many cases quite similar to those observed in treatment with the classic wavelengths. We can thus draw the following conclusions:

1. CO_2-lasers work through a secondary response; and
2. Deep light penetration is not a necessity per se in biostimulation, at least not for some of the biostimulative effects.

The possible reason for this is that cells in the tissue subjected to the light produce substances that then spread and circulate in blood vessels and the lymphatic system.

Literature:

In case of biostimulation with deeper penetrating laser wavelengths, the systemic effects are often due to treatment of blood cells, which in turn influence other cells, tissue and mechanisms in the system. This is illustrated by Zhuk [1141] who treated patients with chronic tuberculosis by treating the blood in a vein. The patients were divided into two groups, both getting conventional medical treatment but only one group getting laser treatment as well. The laser group showed significantly shorter recovery times. (See chapter 4.1.46 “Tuberculosis” on page 185.) Yet another illustration of the systemic effect is a report by Braverman [50]. In a study using experimental wounds, laboratory animals were treated with a HeNe or GaAs laser, or both in combination. The tensile strength of the newly healed wounds was greater in all the laser therapy groups than in the control group. There was also a group of animals on which two wounds were inflicted, only one of which was treated with laser. Even the untreated wound showed better results than in the control group. The authors of the report drew the following conclusion: "The laser irradiation can thus have released substances in the circulatory apparatus so that the tensile strength increased even in the wound on the opposite, untreated side."

The same observation has been made by Rochkind [39]. HeNe laser treatment on only the right-hand side of bilaterally inflicted skin wounds increased the healing process on both sides as compared to the control group. This also applied in the case of bilateral burn wounds.

In a crossover study, Airaksinen [302] treated patients with chronic neck and shoulder pain unilaterally with HeNe. The pressure pain threshold increased significantly on both the non-treated and the treated side, although the increase was larger on the treated side.

Inoue [405] has demonstrated that GaAlAs 780 nm laser irradiation suppressed the tuberculin reaction in sensitised guinea pigs. The suppression was seen not only on the irradiated side but also on the contralateral, non-irradiated side.

Schindl [350] induced the arthus phenomenon (an anaphylactic effect) in the corneas of 57 rabbits. The healing effect of a HeNe laser as compared to control was obvious. Consensual co-reaction could be observed in the contralateral non-irradiated eyes in the experimental group.

The above studies may explain why studies involving contralateral untreated control lesions on the same animal/patient have not always produced good or clear results. The non-irradiated “control” lesion in fact benefits from the treated lesion because of the systemic reaction just discussed.

This theory is supported by a study by Halevy [467]. Using a 780 nm 30 mW laser, 6 patients with cutaneous fissures located in the hands and feet were treated every 2-3 days. There were similar fissures on both sides of the body. On the irradiated side, 4 of the 6 fissures healed completely and in the remaining 2 there was a decrease of 40%. On the non-irradiated side, 3 healed completely and 1 healed partially.

Friedmann [513] draws the following conclusion: "Due to transmission of neural excitation and calcium waves, photobiomodulation is a systemic effect."

Villaplana [424] irradiated the anterior pituitary gland with HeNe laser through the surgically exposed lamina dura in two groups of rats (n = 30 per group). The calculated incident power at the gland was 2.75 mW. Population I Leydig cells of the central part of the rat testicles showed signs of increased but non-specific activity in the entire series of experimental animals as compared to sham-irradiated controls. Thus, laser therapy may have a systemic effect on testosterone production under these experimental conditions.

Hall [673] failed to find any systemic effect in a wound healing study in rats using GaAs. However, the parameters used did not enhance wound healing in the irradiated wound, so no local effect occured either.

Systemic effects, however, are not always found, even when there is an effect on the irradiated side. In a wound healing study on diabetic rats by Reddy [657] the following conclusions were reached: 1) the GaAs laser therapy had no apparent systemic effect on the wound on the opposite side of the treatment side; and 2) laser photostimulation decreased the healing time for full thickness skin wounds in diabetic animals, but had no effect on the biomechanical properties of the tissue once the wound was healed.

3.2.1 Photoreceptors

In order for the laser light to be absorbed, there must be receptors. Such receptors are well known in plants, but are there human light receptors other than those in the eyes and in the skin? The following is quoted from Enwemeka [1160]:

“We may have to step back in time in order to begin to understand the mechanisms involved. That low energy light particles can produce significant, and at times, life-supporting changes in various organisms, is not at all new. Our primordial ancestor, the purple bacteria, provides a vivid example. Found in abstemious habitats below that of plant life – e.g. the bottom of ponds and topsoil, depending on the species – the purple bacteria inevitably lives on a meagre amount of light. Only the reminder of light unharvested by plants penetrates to those depths. But with the carotenoids in its light-harvesting complexes absorbing light at 500 nm wavelength, and its bacteriochlorophyll absorbing at 800-850 nm, this life form is able to carry out complex life-supporting metabolic processes with relatively minimal light energy.

To date, more than three hundred photochemically reactive proteins, capable of harvesting low ligh energy, have been identified in both prokaryotic and eukaryotic organisms. Many more are being discovered yearly. In humans, the most commonly known photochemically active receptor proteins are rod and cone pigments in the eye. However, other human photoreceptors have been discovered in recent times. Examples are encephalopsins in the brain and pinopsin in the pineal gland. Given the discovery of photoreceptor proteins in the pineal gland, the hypothalamus, and other tissues of lower vertebrates, it is only a matter of time that it will become clear that other human tissues have photoreactive proteins as well". (See chapter 11.1.6 "Bright Light Phototherapy" on page 345.)

3.3 What parameters to use

For laser therapy systems, we know that the following parameters (among others) significantly affect treatment results: choice of laser wavelength, size of dose, level of power density, the laser's method of working, pulse frequency, depth of penetration, treatment methodology, treatment frequency and total number of treatments.

3.3.1 Laser parameters

There are basically two types of parameters – laser parameters and patient parameters. The laser parameters will sometimes have to be changed from patient to patient depending on the patient parameters.

3.3.1.1 Which wavelength?

It is important to use the right wavelength (i.e. laser type) for the right indications. Although it has not yet been possible to determine the "best" wavelength for each indication, the authors believe that the HeNe or InGaAlP laser (633-635 nm) is the best option for ulcers and nerve regeneration. Due to the poor penetration of light of this wavelength (up to one cm), other wavelengths must sometimes be used, although they may not be optimal.

In addition, we consider that the GaAs laser is a better choice for the treatment of deeper problems such as sports injuries and that it has a greater effect on postoperative pain and swelling than the shorter wavelength lasers. Further about this laser in chapter 11.1.5 "How deep does light penetrate into tissue?" on page 343.

GaAlAs lasers are usually the best choise for tendinitis but it can also be a good alternative for treating pain and oedema, and we have positive experience of treating chronic ulcers with this laser type. The high power density of modern GaAlAs lasers has also proved to be advantageous in physiotherapy.

It must be stressed that any wavelength, with a reasonable dose in the target area, will have a biological effect. If "the best" wavelength is not at hand, it is of course recommended to use other wavelengths. Probably, the correct dose may be just as important as the wavelength. However, that dose is sometimes not known or obtainable, e.g. due to the lack of penetration.

Karu [180] found, by measuring chemiluminescence, that the oxidative processes of blood cells were influenced by various laser wavelengths during the initial phase of acute viral respiratory illness. Of the four different wavelengths tested (660, 820, 880 and 950 nm), 660 nm was found to be the most effective. The dose range in this *in vitro* study was 0.1 - 1 J/cm^2.

Some studies have shown improved results when two wavelengths were combined. However, it could be asked whether the clinical results of these studies are sometimes just as much dependent on the combined doses as on the two different wavelengths.

3.3.1.2 Output power

Of course you should know what laser type you have as well as its wavelength. But it is just as important to know the output power of your instrument in order to calculate the right dose to administer. A significant advantage of a higher output power is that it takes less time to reach a given dose. This has a financial significance for the patient but is not a decisive factor in achieving good results. Dosage is the primary factor. Output power is, however, of great consequence in that a higher output power gives a higher power density, which very often is beneficial. Output power is also of some importance with respect to light penetration in tissue.

3.3.1.3 Average output power

When a laser works in pulsed mode, it is the laser's average output power that is significant in terms of dose calculation. (See Figure 1.7 “Different types of pulsing” on page 18.) If you do not know the average output power of your pulsed laser, you cannot calculate the dose to administer.

3.3.1.4 Power density

Power density is the same as the “intensity” of the light and is measured in watts or milliwatts per cm^2. Spreading the light over a large area gives a low intensity. As biostimulation is based on local effects, with the transport of various substances through cell membrane and tissue, power density should not be too low, even if the number of joules is high. Low power cannot entirely be compensated by increased time. Since the dose can easily become too high locally when the laser is held directly against the skin/mucous membrane, one must ensure that the treatment time is not too long when using point treatment. The power density (I) can be calculated as

$$I = \frac{A}{P} \quad [\,W/cm^2\,]$$

(See chapter 10.3 “Power density” on page 314.)

Literature:

van Breugel [228] studied the effects of HeNe laser light on human fibroblast cultures. Irradiation was administered on three consecutive days at various power densities with exposure times of between 30 seconds and 10 minutes. The laser output power varied between 0.55 and 5.98 mW. It was apparent that the most significant effects were obtained by laser output power below 2.91 mW, while 5.98 mW had no effect. The stimulative effects were strongest during irradiation periods between 30 seconds and 2 minutes. The study demonstrates that power density and exposure time are important parameters. Another conclusion is that power density is important in itself. Treating an area with 40 mW for 10 seconds is usually more beneficial than using 10 mW and 40 seconds, although the dose would be the same.

Trelles [458] found that the effects of HeNe laser light on mast cells were accomplished faster at 50 mW than at 4 mW, although all cell lines were irradiated with 2.4 J.

Further literature: [291].

3.3.1.5 Energy density

Energy density is the same as dose or fluence. The difference between power density and energy density is simply the time. As mentioned above, the power density is measured in watts per cm^2. The energy density is measured in watt-seconds per cm^2, which is the same as joules per cm^2. For calculation of energy density, see chapter 3.3.1.7 “Calculation of doses” on page 71.

Looking at a specific situation with laser light penetrating into tissue, we will have points and areas with high power density and other areas with low power density. If this distribution of light is held constant over a certain period, we will have an energy distribution that, in every point, is exactly proportional to said power distribution. If we keep the same situation going on for ten times as long, we have an energy density (i.e. dose) that is ten times higher in every point reached by the light. (See chapter 10.3 “Power density” on page 314 and chapter 10.7 “Energy density” on page 319.)

Just like the power density, the energy density is not constant - it has a two-dimensional distribution over a surface (this is also true of the area that is hit by the laser light when a treatment probe is held in skin contact) and has a three-dimensional distribution in the treated tissue volume.

3.3.1.6 Treatment dose

Treatment dose is the same as the energy density. We will in future mainly use the term dose. The dose is the most important treatment parameter. Dosage refers to the amount of energy per unit area brought to bear on tissue or cell culture. Dosage and treatment intervals can only be specified schematically. This is because the various laser wavelengths mean that different doses must be given, and treatment conditions likewise vary. People are receptive to laser treatment to varying degrees - some can "feel the laser right down to their toes", others are entirely impervious. It is appropriate to begin with a low dose for a new patient to ensure that you do not enter a biosuppressive dose range or trigger a pain response on the first treatment.

3.3.1.7 Calculation of doses

The dose is the amount of energy administered to a surface area of tissue. In the calculation we will measure area in cm². Energy can be measured in joules or calories (old measure). A joule is the same as a Ws (reads watt-second) where W stands for watt and s for second. The dose D is hence measured in joules per square centimetre (J/cm²) and is calculated as

$$D = \frac{P \times t}{A} \quad [\,J/cm^2\,]$$

where P is the laser's output power in watts, t is the treatment duration in seconds, and A is the area treated, given in cm². If the laser is pulsed, the average output power in watts should be used instead.

Choosing a variety of output powers and times, we can calculate the corresponding doses and present them in a table. The table below shows doses in J/cm², under various treatment durations, reached with three lasers with different output power. Using a 20 mW GaAs single-probe laser or a 30 mW GaAlAs single-probe laser, for example, we can calculate, using the formula in the section on dose calculation below, that when treating an area of 1 cm² for a certain duration we achieve the dose (in joules) shown in the columns in the table.

	Output power from the laser						
Time/ cm²	**10 mW**	**30 mW**	**60 mW**	**120 mW**	**240 mW**	**500 mW**	**1000 mW**
1 sec	0.01 J	0.03 J	0.06 J	0.12 J	0.24 J	0.5 J	1.0 J
3 sec	0.03 J	0.09 J	0.18 J	0.36 J	0.72 J	1.5 J	3.0 J
10 sec	0.1 J	0.3 J	0.6 J	1.2 J	2.4 J	5 J	10 J
30 sec	0.3 J	0.9 J	1.8 J	3.6 J	7.2 J	15 J	30 J
1 min	0.6 J	1.8 J	3.6 J	7.2 J	14 J	30 J	60 J
3 min	1.8 J	5.4 J	11 J	22 J	43 J	90 J	180 J
10 min	6.0 J	18 J	36 J	72 J	144 J	300 J	600 J

Dose to skin surface for different laser powers and exposure times per square centimeter area

Table 3.1: Dose to skin surface

N.B.! We have said it before; It is of the greatest importance that you know the output power of your laser! If you don't, you have no idea of the doses you give! It is not self-evident that the power of your laser is the same as when you bought it. Furthermore, the power specified in a brochure is frequently quite different from what you actually get out of your probe. The output should be measured from time to time! If you don't have a built-in power meter, you should check your laser with an external one regularly.

We often meet therapists who do not know what type of laser they are using. When asked, it is not unusual for them to respond "3B". Often they do not know what "dose" means, much less how to calculate one. Frequently, they have believed that the output power of the instrument was completely different from what it actually was.

One day we received a call from a clinic in Stockholm. They said there must be something wrong with their instrument; results were not good recently. It turned out to be a GaAs laser. The brochure stated that the average output power of the single probe (with one laser diode) was 20 mW, and the output of the multiprobe was 60 mW (with three laser diodes). Testing resulted in the following table:

Pulse frequency	Single probe	Multiprobe
10 Hz	0.002 mW	0.02 mW
100 Hz	0.02 mW	0.25 mW
1000 Hz	0.20 mW	2.1 mW
10000 Hz	1.81 mW	20 mW

Table 3.2: Output power dependent on pulse frequency

As can be seen, the output from the single probe was less than 10% of the stated nominal output at the highest pulse frequency. Neither the brochure nor the manual mentioned that the output power was dependent on the pulse frequency setting.

3.3.1.8 Dose ranges

Biostimulation has been reported in the literature with doses from as low as 0.001 J/cm^2 to 10 J/cm^2 and more. How is this possible? Can we just use any dose? Certainly not - this is where we have to start thinking! There is a great difference between irradiating naked cells in the laboratory and treating a deep lying pain condition! In fact, a "dose" is a very complicated issue. It is a matter of wavelength, power density, type of tissue, condition of the tissue, chronic or acute problem, pigmentation, treatment technique and so forth. However, there is certainly a "therapeutic dose window". Doses that are too low result in no or only a weak effect. If a dose above the highest one suitable is administered, weaker or no biological effects will result. With an even greater dose, the <u>bio-suppressive</u> range is entered (inhibiting effect result).

This is most obvious in wound healing and stimulation of hair growth. (See Figure 10.6 “Arndt-Schulz law” on page 320.)

So which are the “correct” doses? You want to know - and we seem to be beating around the bush (for good reasons). The answer is: read this book carefully, think, and do the best you can with the laser you happen to have. Doses do not have to be “perfect” to produce a good biological response. Anyway, the table below gives you a rough view of suitable doses

Indication	Laser type	Dose in J/cm^2
Open wound	HeNe InGaAlP GaAlAs GaAs CO_2	0.5-1.5 0.5-1.5 0.5-1.5 0.01-0.2 1-10
Wound periphery	HeNe InGaAlP GaAlAs GaAs CO_2	1-4 2-6 1-4 0.5-1 -
Superficial pain	HeNe InGaAlP GaAlAs GaAs CO_2	0.5-2 1-4 2-4 1-2 5-100
Deep lying pain	HeNe InGaAlP GaAlAs GaAs CO_2	- - 4-10 2-5 5-100

Table 3.3: Dose ranges for different lasers and indications

Doses for other lasers, like the Ruby laser and Nd:YAG lasers are not as well known. Mester’s group used Ruby laser and indicated 1-2 J/cm^2. Doses for acupuncture points: See chapter 3.3.3.2.1 “Acupuncture.” on page 84.

As can be seen above, it appears that lower doses are required with GaAs laser than with HeNe laser. This has been observed by e.g. Abergel [8]. In general, tissue tolerates higher "overdoses" of HeNe, InGaAlP and GaAlAs than of GaAs, which more quickly reaches an inhibiting level.

In the treatment of healthy, optimally working tissue, almost any dose can be used without noticeably macroscopic negative effects. This is e.g. the case in the use of surgical lasers cutting, evaporating and coagulating tissue, using very high power and energy densities. Right outside the destructive zone, very high levels of power density and dose occur, but this is not found to be negative.

When irradiating "naked cells", in an open wound, for example, the optimal dose is much lower than when irradiating through overlying skin. The dose and the treatment interval differ depending on whether the condition in the tissue is chronic or acute, but also on whether we primarily want to treat pain or achieve a more long-term effect. As stated before, specifying the "right" dose for a particular condition is not easy. Numerous parameters must be taken into account: wavelength and output, contact or non-contact with skin/mucous membrane, type of tissue, acute/chronic, how deep in the tissue you want to reach, the patient's general condition, the skin's pigmentation, etc. "The right dose" may sometimes be whatever the instrument is able to deliver.

Literature:

Abergel [8] investigated the effect of HeNe-laser light and GaAs-laser light on the connective tissue metabolism. In this comparison the author writes: "Similar stimulation of collagen production was also observed with GaAs-laser. With this laser a two- to threefold stimulation in two separate cell lines was achieved with energy densities that were considerably lower than those required for stimulation with HeNe-laser."

Bolton [419] irradiated human fibroblasts with a 50 mW GaAlAs laser. The proliferation of fibroblasts and the succinic dehydrogenase activity increased at doses of 2 J/cm^2, but both were inhibited at doses of 16 J/cm^2.

Igarashi [579] irradiated neonatal rats with a 830 nm laser, delivering 0.9 J twice daily from birth to day five at two points located above the hippocampus. The mean body weight of the irradiated animals on day 20 was 22% lower than that of the control animals. The density of synaptic junctions was also reduced in the irradiated animals as of day 20. (This may seem alarming, but don't worry! Suppose the weight of a newborn rat is 3 g. A newborn human weights around 3,000 g. Thus, the extrapolated dose would be 900 J. Another factor is the size of the neonathal rats; here we have millimeters when with human babies have centimeters, giving much higher power densities an local doses for the rat fetus). This study is an example of bio-inhibition.

The inhibitive effect of high doses of laser energy has also been demonstrated by Gross [779]. The effect of HeNe laser light on the cell cycle and the growth of rat kidney epithelial cells was studied. Daily doses of 11.9 - 142 J/cm^2 significantly inhibited cell growth, while less than 4.7 J/cm^2 had no effect.

Other examples of stimulation and inhibitions are [1095, 1101]. (See Table 11.3: "Examples of different dose levels in vitro" on page 349.)

3.3.1.9 Calculation of treatment time for a desired dose

The most common situation in laser therapy is that we wish to administer a certain dose **D** to a specified area **A** with our laser, having an (average-) output power **P**, and we need to calculate the treatment time **t** for the laser probe at hand. If the problem to treat is situated at a depth **d** (where d = 0 to 4 cm), the following approximate formula can be used to find the treatment time:

$$\mathbf{t} = \frac{D \times A}{P} \times (1 + d) \qquad [\text{ sec }]$$

N.B. For this formula to work, the correct units to be used are: **P** must be given in watts (not milli-watts), **D** must be given in J/cm^2, **A** must be expressed in cm^2 and **d** in cm. The treatment time will then come out in seconds. Values 1 - 4 of the parameter **d** are only applicable to the deeper penetrating laser types (GaAs laser and GaAlAs lasers). For CO_2-, HeNe- and GaAlInP-lasers, use value d=0. Usually your laser power is given in milliwatts. If you want to use the formulas in this book, you must use the power expressed in watts. To convert from milliwatts to watts, you simply divide by 1000. E.g. 40 milliwatts (40 mW) becomes 0.040 watts (0.040 W). A simple rule can be: Use 3 decimals and your power will be seen as: 0.040 W for your 40 mW probe and 0.250 W for your 250 mW probe.

3.3.1.10 "Ready reckoner"

For most people, mathematical formulas have negative associations. For the common therapist it is, however, not necessary to use a calculator for every treatment. We have made the process easy. For the treatment of larger areas, such as back, neck, shoulders, arms, knees, etc., we use "apples". If you cut an apple in two halves, the cut surface has an area of about 50 cm^2. Supposing that you know what laser type you have and its output power, you simply use the tables on the following pages. Find your laser's output power and then enter the depth of the problem: Is it deep or superficial? The table will show you the treatment time in minutes per "apple" at different depths.

Example 1: To treat an area with the size of an apple and with a problem situated 3 cm underneath said surface, using a **GaAs-laser** probe with an average output power of 50 mW at the chosen treatment frequency, you need a minimum of 3 minutes. If the area is larger than an apple – e.g. the size of 4 apples – treat 4 times 3 minutes as a minimum. Maximum treatment time: Choose twice the minimum value. Move the probe evenly over the surface.

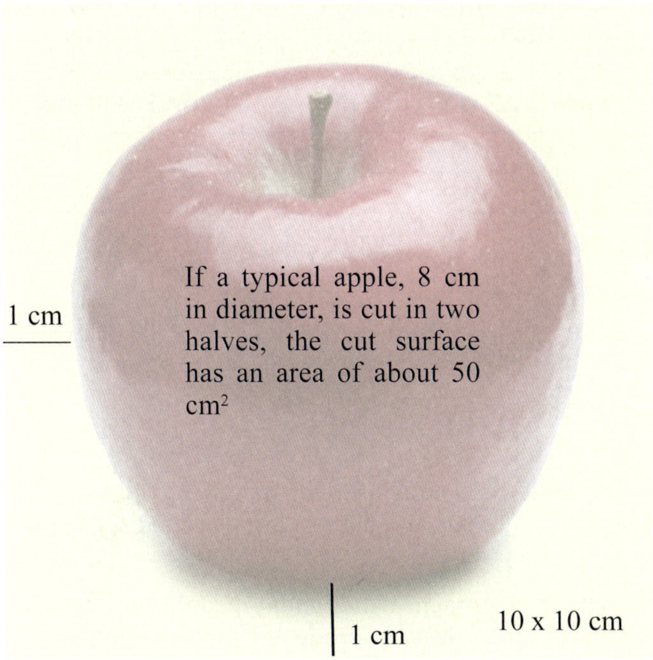
If a typical apple, 8 cm in diameter, is cut in two halves, the cut surface has an area of about 50 cm2
1 cm
1 cm
10 x 10 cm

Figure 3.4 Apple ready reckoner

Treatment time for 50 cm^2 surface area with a GaAs-laser. The output powers are average powers. Treatment should be done with skin contact

Depth	10 mW	25 mW	50 mW	100 mW	200 mW
0.5 cm	2.5 min	1 min	30 sec	15 sec	10 sec
1 cm	5 min	2 min	1 min	30 sec	15 sec
2 cm	10 min	4 min	2 min	1 min	30 sec
3 cm	15 min	6 min	3 min	1.5 min	45 sec
4 cm	20 min	8 min	4 min	2 min	1 min

Table 3.4: Treatment time with a GaAs-laser

Treatment time for 50 cm² surface area with a GaAlAs laser. If the laser is pulsed, the average output power should be used. Treatment should be done with skin contact.

Depth	10 mw	25 mw	50 mw	100 mw	250 mw	500 mw
0.5 cm	25 min	10 min	5 min	2 min	1 min	30 sec
1 cm	50 min	20 min	10 min	5 min	2 min	1 min
2 cm	*)	40 min	20 min	10 min	4 min	2 min
3 cm	*)	*)	30 min	15 min	6 min	3 min
4 cm	*)	*)	40 min	20 min	8 min	4 min

Table 3.5: Treatment time with a GaAlAs laser

*) Unrealistic depth and time

As can be seen, table 3.4, shows longer treatment time for corresponding powers and depths, reflecting the higher doses needed for the GaAlAs laser compared to the GaAs laser.

Example 2: Another approach, which many people find easier, is to ascertain the time it takes for the laser to produce 1 joule. If the laser has an output power that is 40 mW, it takes 25 seconds to produce 1 joule (calculate it by dividing 1 by your laser's power output given in watt in this example 1/0.04 = 25 sec). This means that if you radiate the area of 1 cm² for 25 seconds, you have given a dose of 1 J/cm².

3.3.1.11 Dose per point

In the treatment of trigger points and acupuncture points the dose is often said to be a number of joules per "point" and it is assumed that a point is something small. We have defined a "point" as an area that is 5 mm in diameter (= 0.2 cm²) or less. This means that if we hit the skin with the light concentrated to this small area and administer 1 joule, we have given 1 J "per point", and in this "point" (= 0.2 cm²) the dose value is 5 J/cm².
This is also explained in chapter 10.10 "Dose per point" on page 328.

3.3.1.12 Pulsed or continuous light

As mentioned previously, a laser can work continuously (most typical for InGaAlP, HeNe, and GaAlAs lasers) or pulsed (the GaAs laser).

The GaAs laser (904 or 905 nm) is always superpulsed, with two possible consequences. Firstly, the pulsing of the laser light may interfere with other pulsing phenomena in the organism, and secondly, continuous/switched and superpulsed lasers may have different active depths. A superpulsed laser always penetrates deeper than a continuous or switched laser with the same wavelength and the same average output power. The extremely intense light flashes of the GaAs laser achieve greater light intensity extending deep into the tissue.

3.3.1.13 Pulse frequency

For pulsed lasers, there is not yet much literature providing advice on which pulse frequencies are suitable for what (as regards pulsing, see chapter 1.2.10 "Continuous and pulsed lasers" on page 16 and Figure 1.7 "Different types of pulsing" on page 18.)

Although the literature in this field has not yet made clear which frequencies are particularly suited to which treatments, the many users of laser therapy have still produced a large body of empirical material. The table below shows the frequencies that, on empirical grounds, are considered particularly suitable for certain types of problem. The column to the right shows the frequencies with which many acupuncturists consider various acupuncture points should be treated. The table applies only to truly pulsed lasers.

Local treatment		**Laser acupuncture**	
Diagnosis:	Frequency range:	Point type:	Frequency:
Pain, neuralgia	0-100 Hz	Endpoints	73 Hz
General stimulation	700 Hz	Source points	146 Hz
Oedema, swellings	1,000 Hz	Sedation points	584 Hz
General stimulation	2,500 Hz	Tonification points	1,000 Hz
Inflammations	5,000 Hz	Alarm points	2,500 Hz
Infections	10,000 Hz	Beginning points	5,000 Hz

Table 3.6: Pulse frequency - laser acupuncture

When treating chronic pain, variation of pulse frequency should be considered if a GaAs laser is used. It can be beneficial to begin with a low frequency, mainly to affect the patient's pain. Later, the dose can be divided between low and high frequencies (e.g. first 20 Hz, then 20 + 5,000 Hz), with the latter dose being assumed to counter inflammation. In the final phase of treatment, 2,500 Hz can be used. This is regarded as being generally stimulating. It should be stressed here that this advice is based principally on empirical grounds and no scientific documentation exists as yet.

The frequencies discussed here have nothing in common with the different pulse frequencies recommended for laser acupuncture.

There are GaAs lasers that automatically vary the frequency during treatment, going from low to high and back. As can be seen from the above studies, it is not self-evident that this concept is beneficial.

Literature:

Mohktar [161] studied the pain-relieving effects of 16 Hz and 73 Hz frequencies, with otherwise unchanged parameters, in a double-blind study of experimental ischaemic pain. Significant effects were obtained, compared to the reference group, at 16 Hz but not at 73 Hz. The equipment used was a combined laser/LED array.

In another comparative double-blind study, also by Mohktar [162], nerve action potential was measured under irradiation at 73 Hz and 5,000 Hz, under otherwise unchanged conditions. 73 Hz gave no significant effect when compared to the placebo group, whereas 5,000 Hz did produce effects.

Kim [283] studied the effect of different GaAs pulses by irradiating 360 cultures of candida albicans with 5, 500, 1500, and 10,000 Hz. Significant differences were seen amongst the groups depending on the pulse type with which irradiation was given.

Martin [308] has shown that photobiological effects upon lower limb blood flow can be frequency-specific.

Fagnoni [509] had better results using 30 Hz rather than 70 Hz when treating patients suffering from trigeminal neuralgia.

El Sayed [529] compared the effect of GaAs at different frequencies on mast cell number and degranulation. All frequencies were effective compared to the sham irradiated groups, but only 20 Hz and 292 Hz, among the frequencies used, were significantly effective.

In a literature study on the effects of laser therapy on musculoskeletal pain Corral-Baques [1260] identified 150 papers. From these 35 reported the used frequency and only 25 all the laser parameters used. Before the 90ies the dominating wavelength was 904 but after the 90ies many 820 nm lasers were used in a pulsing mode. More than 30 frequencies were used and very few authors give a reason for using the particular frequency.

Further literature: [773, 1158]

3.3.2 Patient parameters

Of course the laser parameters depend very much on what we are going to treat. For instance, if we are going to treat an ulcer, we choose other settings than if we are going to treat knee arthroses.

3.3.2.1 Treatment area

In order to calculate dose, power density and treatment time, it is necessary to know the treatment area. In the formulas for calculation, the treatment area must be expressed in cm^2 if the outcome is to be correct.

Also, it is of importance for deciding the dose to have a knowledge of the depth below skin surface of the site to be treated.

Practical experience indicates that it may be more beneficial to treat a smaller area more intensively and then treat nearby areas later, rather than treating a larger area over a longer period of time at a single session. This may well be related to the fact that certain substances are released, which can be traced in blood and urine, that can reach disturbingly high levels when large areas are treated. It can also be a question of saturation.

3.3.2.2 Treatment intervals

Treatment intervals must be assessed for each individual case. Those expecting detailed advice on how to treat each particular case will be disappointed by what follows here. The same rules apply to laser treatment as to all other forms of medical treatment: the best results are achieved by the therapist who possesses sound medical knowledge, can listen to the patient and has a good intuition. As a general rule, however, it is better to use 3-4 treatments a week with moderate doses than using higher doses and few treatments.

Mester demonstrated that small doses with appropriate periods of time in-between are more effective than treatments that are very close. Abergel [8] has also demonstrated this on fibroblast cultures. Because laser therapy treatment has been shown to be cumulative (the dose from one treatment lasts some time, and what “remains” of the dose is added to the dose at the next treatment), it is vital that treatments are not too close together, so as to avoid a situation where the accumulated dose eventually ends up above the biostimulating range or even in the bio-inhibiting range, with consequently poorer results.

Acute problems are usually dealt with by a few treatments, which can be closely spaced. Acute herpes simplex or herpes zoster, for example, can be treated every day for a few days. Acute pain conditions can be given close treatment. Chronic complaints are usually best handled with more widely spaced treatment.

It has been shown to be beneficial to treat at closer intervals in the beginning (e.g. every other day or every third day for two weeks) and then at longer and longer intervals (e.g. once a week for a few weeks). Experience shows that it is not disadvantageous to temporarily suspend treatment after a number of introductory sessions. In some circumstances, this can actually be benefical.

Another aspect is that you always have to take the patients’ economy into account. If we haven´t noted a clear reaction after 4-5 sessions, we may suggest that further therapy is to be postponed for some weeks (or even months), to see if there will be a “late reaction”. Then we can “speed it up” with more sessions. This also convinces the patient that our primary aim is not the patients’ “money”, but the clinical results.

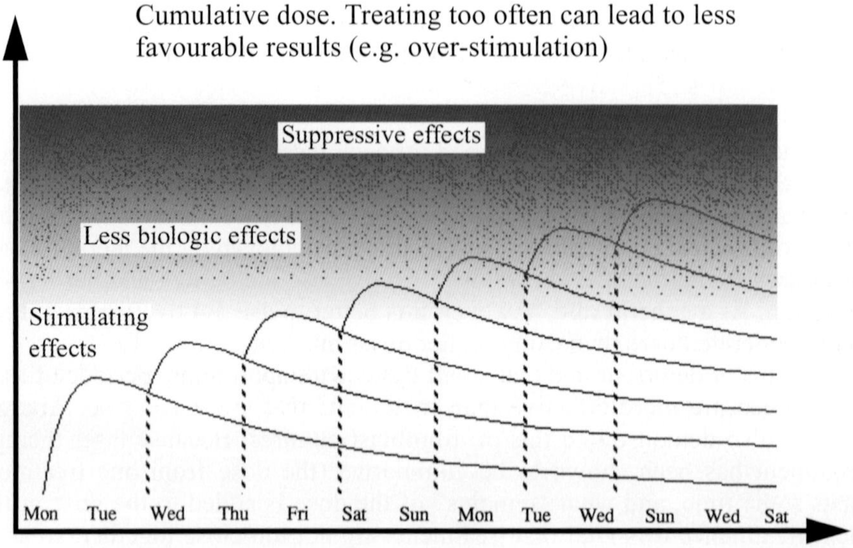

Figure 3.5 Cumulative dose

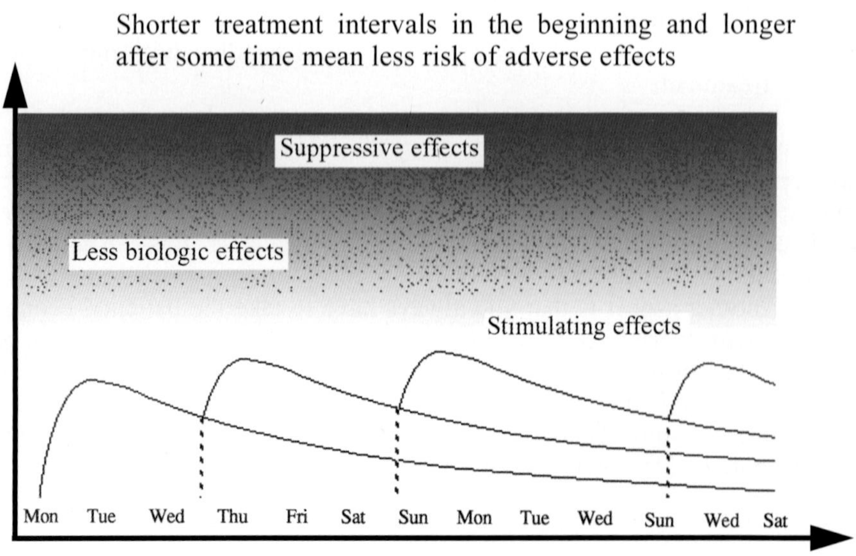

Figure 3.6 Shorter treatment intervals

3.3.2.3 Pre- or postoperative treatment?

Previously the predominant view was that there is nothing to gain by irradiating tissue preoperatively. If the tissue is healthy, laser treatment has no effect. It may be time to reconsider the conventional wisdom, however, based on the results of several studies.

All irradiation, even of healthy tissue, activates a variety of processes, leading, for example, to the production of singlet oxygen. If no trauma exists or occurs later, these products disappear quickly and the normal state returns. If trauma occurs immediately after irradiation, however, the tissues' defence systems are in a more favourable state. If the tissue is already in poor condition prior to the operation (oedema, inflammation etc.), laser energy is even more beneficial preoperatively.

Some conditions are cyclic and there are studies suggesting the possibility of treating these even in the inactive period. This has been demonstrated for herpes simplex [908] and asthma [1205].

Literature

A study by Rosner [494] entailed crushing the optical nerve of rats. The object of the study was to investigate the capacity of the HeNe laser to delay or prevent nerve degeneration. Surprisingly, the effects were equally beneficial whether radiation was applied immediately before or immediately after the nerve was crushed.

In this study the tissue was intact before inflicting a trauma. In the following studies, the tissue was in a state of imbalance: Popova [147] removed muscle tissue from rats, irradiated it with X-rays, and then replanted the tissue. Improved healing was observed in those animals given laser therapy, prior to X-ray as well as after X-ray.

A study by Pourreau-Schneider [46] showed that mucositis associated with chemotherapy in cancer patients was alleviated by HeNe laser light. Alleviation resulted both from irradiation prior to chemotherapy and irradiation following the debut of symptoms.

In an *in vitro* study by Karu [1107] it was found that the cell-glass adhesion increased in a dose-dependent manner after irradiation. The addition of different antioxidants eliminated this effect. Pre-irradiation was found to decrease (or normalise to the control level) the suppressive effects of these chemicals.

Bibikova [587] found that the process of regeneration in degenerated muscles can be markedly enhanced if the muscle is irradiated with HeNe laser prior to the injury.

Further literature: [564]

3.3.3 Treatment method parameters

There are several ways of administrating the laser light:

A. Local treatment (produces primarily local effects). This means that the laser light irradiates the affected area, e.g. a wound or an inflamed tendon.

B. Systemic or indirect irradiation (produces primarily systemic effects)

Examples of indirect irradiation are:

- irradiating acupuncture points
- irradiating trigger points
- irradiating spinal processes
- irradiating the dermatome
- irradiating the blood
- irradiating lymph nodes

In these instances we irradiate areas outside or far from the area where the patient would otherwise locate the problem.

Direct and indirect treatment can be combined. In fact, even direct irradiation is a mode of indirect irradiation. The beam will always find blood, lymph and nerves, influencing the circulating metabolites. So every local treatment is also a systemic treatment but not vice versa.

3.3.3.1 Local treatment

This means that the laser light irradiates the affected area, e.g. a wound or an inflamed tendon. The treatment technique used depends on the depth of the tissue that you want to treat.

3.3.3.1.1 Shallow problems

1 Open wounds: The probe is held 1-2 cm from the wound. The depth of penetration is insignificant, which is of course the intention. Treat the periphery of the wound in skin contact. Give the open area of the wound a lower dose than the skin periphery.

2 Tissue lying close to the skin surface: Hold the probe in light contact with the skin.

3.3.3.1.2 Deeper problems

At medium depth: Press the probe against the skin. The deeper the tissue to be treated, the higher the pressure.
At great depth: Only the GaAs and high-powered GaAlAs laser can reach to these depths, but the therapist's knowledge of anatomy is also crucial. If the patient moves his/her arm/leg to various positions, an obstructing muscle mass can be moved aside to expose openings in deep muscle attachments.

Pressing the probe firmly against the skin will also move the light closer to the target and decrease absorption through the ischemia caused by the pressure.

3.3.3.1.3 Treating inside the body

In some cases you may realize that the problem volume can not be reached through overlying skin, muscles, bone etc. A possible way to overcome this may be to use fibre optics or specialised probes to reach the place of a problem. Hence, the light can be brought into rectum, vagina, bladder, nose cavitiy etc by suitably designed probes. An optical fibre can be guided into blood vessels to treat angina etc. With an endoscope, ulcers in throat and stomac can be treated. A fibre can also be attached into a syringe needle, wich can penetrate through lacerated muscles, emitting the light at its tip. Another, very simple method that has been used for problems in rectum and vagina, is to insert a test tube of glass or transparent plastic in order to expand the tissue and then to insert a laser probe inside the test tube. The light must then be properly spread or directed so that the right target is illuminated.

3.3.3.2 Systemic treatments

Systemic treatment means that we irradiate areas outside or far from the area where the patient would otherwise locate the problem. Examples of such treatment are treatment of acupuncture points and trigger points.

3.3.3.2.1 Acupuncture.

Acupuncture with lasers is one of the most exciting areas within laser therapy. A wide range of opportunities is open to a therapist with acupuncture training. The method is sterile and painless, and therefore highly acceptable to the patient and especially to children. Practitioners with little or no knowledge can use acupuncture with some success on a narrow range of indications. If well-known and uncontroversial points are used in laser acupuncture therapy, pain, tension, nausea, and anxiety can be influenced. Both laser acupuncture and conventional needle acupuncture affect the acupuncture points, but according to experienced therapists they do not always result in identical effects. They could be said to complement each other.

Lasers only cause a negligible rise in temperature in tissue [109, 170, 189, 1221], which is why laser acupuncture should not be confused with moxa treatment. Indeed, in some cases, even a small reduction in temperature has been reported [494]. Lasers stimulate acupuncture points in a similar way to needles, although needles are more suitable for deep-lying points.

The pioneers of laser acupuncture come, unsurprisingly, from China. The oral surgeon Yo-Cheng Zhou worked with needle acupuncture between 1958 and 1965 and until 1971 experimented with acupressure on dental indications. Since 1971 he has worked with laser acupuncture, mainly as anaesthesia for extractions and minor operations. Zhou has developed an interesting technique that involves a small number of acupuncture points being subjected to high outputs. For extractions in the lower jaw, one single point is irradiated for five minutes with a HeNe laser (2-6 mW). The extraction starts immediately after, but the laser is held on the Hegu point (the thumb grip) during the whole process. Zhou also works with a CO_2-laser within the laser therapy range 0-100 mW, which he considers even more effective than the HeNe laser. His experience is that coagulation times are shorter with laser acupuncture than with normal anaesthetics and that subsequent discomfort is also reduced. Postoperative oedema and trismus are also less pronounced after laser acupuncture.

Bearing in mind that, since 1971, Zhou has performed over 10,000 tooth extractions with LAA (Laser Acupuncture Anaesthesia), the method cannot be dismissed as a placebo or something which only works on the Chinese - which was often the argument put forward before needle acupuncture was accepted in the West. LAA is not very well known amongst European authorities on acupuncture, despite the fact that Zhou, as early as 1984, published an account in English of his experience after the first 600 extractions.

The points in the upper jaw for extraction are Sibai and Quanliao, and for the lower jaw, Jiache. The Hegu grip is used during extractions from both the lower and the upper jaw. Yangbai, Yuyao, Yintang, Sibai, Quanliao, and Jiache are the main points used for minor maxillofacial operations. Zhou also uses a HeNe or carbon dioxide laser directly on the alveolus after an extraction. In the thousands of extractions performed with LAA and its subsequent local treatment, not a single case of alveolitis or postoperative bleeding has occurred. Sutures are very rarely needed.

Even though it was the Chinese who pioneered laser acupuncture, it was a Canadian - Friedrich Plog - who, quite early on, highlighted the usefulness of the HeNe laser in this context. He was already testing lasers instead of needles in 1973 [227].

Literature:

Zhao [115] studied the changes in metencephalin in rat brains after HeNe laser irradiation of the Zusanli point. During irradiation, the pain threshold rose, while levels of metencephalin and diencephalin were reduced.

Yamamoto [406] has compared the effect of needle acupuncture and laser acupuncture in a rat model, using 830 nm. A selected acupuncture point was irradiated for 90 minutes. The pain threshold was elevated and reached a maximum after 60-90 minutes. After the end of the irradiation, the pain threshold gradually returned to the previous level. The analgesic effect was antagonised by naloxene but a difference between laser and needle was found using dexamethasone.

Bradley [117] studied the effects of laser acupuncture by means of thermography. St 6 was chosen as the standard point. Four minutes of stimulation with a GaAs laser (5,000 Hz, 5 mW) and 30 minutes of needle stimulation were compared on the same subject. The facial tissue response showed up thermographically on videotape. It was observed that both needles and laser therapy caused vasodilatation in the facial region, both on the stimulated side and the opposite side. GaAs and needles produced the same results, but it took longer for GaAs stimulation to take effect. The effect was manifested immediately when using needles, and after 2-4 minutes with the laser. A comparison was also made of the effects of stimulation of a randomly chosen spot (instead of a known acupuncture point). The effects of stimulation of the acupuncture points were greater than those of the randomly chosen spots.

Kreczi [324] studied the analgesic effect of laser acupuncture in a single blind cross-over study. 21 patients suffering from radicular or pseudoradicular pain were given either laser or mock irradiation. Mean pain levels after laser treatment were significantly lower than after placebo treatment.

Smesny [445] compared the effect of needle and HeNe laser acupuncture. In a group of 112 patients with cervico-occipital headache, 50% were treated with needles and 50% with laser on identical points. Results in the two groups were equivalent (60 % in both groups).

Hoffman [494] irradiated LI 4 in 5 subjects. The typical reaction was a temperature reduction of approximately 1 °C in the region of the fingers. Irradiation of placebo points failed to induce this reaction.

King [540] used HeNe laser in auricular therapy in 80 healthy volunteers, aged 18-39 years. 41 received laser therapy and 39 sham irradiation at appropriate acupuncture points in the left ear. Experimental pain threshold at the ipsilateral wrist was determined with an electrical stimulus immediately before and after treatment. The laser group demonstrated a significant increase in pain threshold after treatment, but the control group did not.

In a double blind, randomised, placebo controlled study by Schlager [892] the effectiveness of point P6 acupuncture on postoperative vomiting in children undergoing strabismus (eye) surgery was studied. A 10 mW 670 nm laser was used and the P6 point was irradiated for 30 seconds 15 minutes before anaesthesia and 15 minutes after arriving in the recovery room. In the laser group the incidence of vomiting was 25% and in the placebo group 85%.

Further literature: [45, 111, 116, 118, 119, 175, 227, 876-891, 939]

Laser acupuncture – some thoughts by the amateur

In needle acupuncture there is always a sensory effect of the needle. This may or may not be of importance but it is a fact that the sensory input is absent in laser acupuncture. There is evidence enough to accept that laser acpuncture works, but there are even more questions involved in laser acpuncture that in needle acupuncture:

1 Is there a wavelength difference?

2 Which is the “correct” dose for an acupuncture point? Considering the difference in depth (for instance betweeen ear acupuncture points and body acupuncture points) there should be a difference. The doses used in the literature differ a lot.

3 When an acupuncture point is irradiated, there is a large “light ball” surrounding the area of the light incidence. The energy of the beam is then greatest in the center of the beam, but how crucial is it to be on the exact anatomical spot?

4 When an acupuncture point is irradiated, a certain volume of blood is also affected. Is this significant?

5 The ideal acupuncture laser should have a very small aperture to be able to pinpoint the acupuncture point and to give a high energy density. But many therapists just use the laser that happens to be at hand and they all claim that their therapy is effective.

6 In auricular acupuncture several points will be affected whenever one selected point is irradiated, even if the laser has a very small aperture. This is not the case in needle acupuncture. What is the implication of this?

7 When performing regular laser therapy, many random acupuncture points are irradiated, nolens volens. Which are the consequences?

8 Moxa (heat) is used on acupuncture points but laser acupuncture is usually not a heat phenomenon. However, some therapists use carbon dioxide lasers for acupuncture and actually burn the acupuncture point.

9 Several therapists use different pulsing systems (Nogier, Baar etc), others use continuous irradiation. Is pulsing important and, if so, what scientific documentation is there? The Nogier frequency list was made up using electro acupuncture – is it relevant to use that in the pulsing of light?

Summing up, it is obvious that a multitude of parameters are used in laser acupuncture and that there is no real concensus on these. However, since laser acupuncture seems to be an acceptable alternative to needle acupuncture, this possibility merits further research. Laser acupuncture is pain free, sterile and can safely be used on infected individuals, persons with needle phobia and on infants.

3.3.3.2.2 Trigger points

It is generally clinically advantageous to combine local treatment with trigger point treatment. The reduction in pain on palpating very often coincides with pain reduction in the inflamed area.

Further literature: [253, 302, 313, 315, 647, 670]

3.3.3.2.3 Spinal processes

Irradiation of the spinal processes corresponding to the area where the pain is located will reduce the pain. In the case of golf or tennis elbow, it may be a false golf or tennis elbow. It may be a nerve entrapment in the nerve passage leading into the spinal cord and laser treatment of C6 may reduce an oedema around the nerve and hence give pain relief.

Further literature: [540]

3.3.3.2.4 Dermatome

In cases of skin eruptions such as herpes zoster, the entire dermatome can be irradiated.

Further literature: [57]

3.3.3.2.5 Blood irradiation

An interesting treatment technique has been used in Russia for many years. The patient's blood is irradiated in order to improve the immune system and the microcirculation. The irradiation can be done through the skin via a fibre leading directly into the blood stream or via a dialysis-like machine. Wavelengths used are 633 and 890 nm.

Irradiating the blood is not a recent treatment modality [671]. In fact, as early as 1923 the US scientist Knott began to experiment with ways to irradiate the blood in order to destroy infectious organisms. In those days there were no lasers, so UV light was attempted. The works of Nobel Prize winner Ryberg Finsen spurred the idea.

This was a time when there were no antibiotics and scientists were trying every possibility in coping with infections. In initial experiments Knott irradiated the entire blood of experimentally infected dogs. He found that the irradiation cleared the blood of infection, but the dogs died in 5-7 days of profound depression and a progressive respiratory slowing and failure. This led Knott to experiment with irradiating different amounts of the blood of the dogs until he determined that the optimal approach was to irradiate 1.5-3 ml of blood for every pound of body weight (about 5% of the total blood) for about 10 seconds.

The first treatment of a human subject occurred in 1928. The patient was a woman moribund following septic abortion complicated by haemolytic streptococcus septicaemia. Treatment with UV blood irradiation rapidly returned her to normal health. Knott waited five years to make sure that the woman did not suffer from any subtle long-range effects before further treatment of a human subject was undertaken.

With the advent of antibiotics the idea of UV blood irradiation vanished. The new miracle therapy was used extensively, while the long term side effects and bacterial backlash were not yet discovered. Russian researchers [669] took a new look at the old idea in the 70s and since then the treatment has been extensively investigated in the laboratory and in the clinic.

Samoilova [482] names this "photohaemotherapy" or "photomodification" and states that it has been used for 17 years in Russia. There are reports of general effects on the immune system, including decrease of the blood viscosity, improvement of microcirculation, detoxification and oxygenation, normalisation of haemostatis, and activation of immune and proliferative processes. Some indications reported in the literature are: occlusive vascular diseases in the extremities, unstable angina, acute myocardial infarction, diabetic angiopathies, acute pneumonia, lung abscess, bronchial obstructive diseases of the lungs, drug resistant forms of schizophrenia, rheumatoid arthritis, acute calculous pyelonephritis, ischemic heart disease, circulatory encephalopathy, haemorrhagic shock, Tourette's syndrome, and OPH gestosis.

The use of lasers instead of UV light only started in the 70s (in the former Soviet Union). Laser Blood Irradiation (LBI) seemed to have effects similar to UV Blood Irradiation (UBI). Although LBI seemed to be slightly less effective than UBI, the great advantage was that LBI was easier to perform. HeNe laser could penetrate the skin, whereas UV light does not.

Several treatment methods have been used. The most common is irradiation with HeNe laser via a thin light-guide and an IV needle, which is then withdrawn. HeNe lasers of 1-10 mW are used (most frequently 1 mW) and duration of treatment varies from 30 to 60 minutes. Usually the cubital vein is used. In some cases an artery is used.

Another method is to irradiate the blood outside the body in plastic or quartz tubes. Only a small amount of the patient' s blood is irradiated. This method is mainly used for UBI.

Transcutaneous irradiation is non-invasive and has several advantages, such as better patient acceptance, ease of application and lack of cross infection risks. Some researchers claim that 1 mW intravenous HeNe irradiation equals 20-30 mW transcutaneous irradiation. Intravenous irradiation is said to cause a sensation of warmth and sleepiness. This sensation is less obvious with transcutaneous irradiation [670]. LBI also seems to improve microcirculation, thus improving the uptake of pharmaceuticals. For transcutaneous irradiation, infrared lasers are used.

An interesting aspect of blood irradiation is the effect of normal sunshine. In the Nordic countries the solar power density varies from almost 0 in winter to 100 mW/cm^2 in the summer. Some of this energy comes in the infrared and can penetrate down to the aretrioles. One hour in the sun during a clear summer day thus would give a dose from penetrating light of roughly 0.05 W $\times$ 3600 seconds = 180 J/cm^2 of the bodily areas which are at a right angle to the incoming light. That area could be rather large, suppose 50 $\times$ 60 cm = 3000 cm^2. The biological effects of the sun are obvious, but they differs a lot from that of laser therapy. However, it has been demonstrated that the effects on cells from a laser can be eradicated if the cells later are subjected to broadband light (like the sunshine). So the question is - should patients avoid gross doses of sunlight after being treated by laser?

For further reading about blood irradiation, see chapter 13.6 "The Russian experience" on page 418.

Literature

Kipshidze [472] used HeNe irradiation in 900 patients with acute myocardial infarction. All patients were treated within four hours of the anginal attack. There was a painkilling effect as well as a limitation of the ischaemic area. Antioxidant blood activity and oxygen content of blood and tissue rose. The amount of drugs used was reduced and the duration of the hospitalisation decreased by an average of 7 days.

Koukoui [481] used the same procedure for this indication, but the blood was irradiated extracorporally.

Kirichuk [483] applied transcutaneous HeNe laser light to rats that had been exposed to pathological stress. It was shown that stress-induced platelet aggregation was reduced by 34% through the irradiation.

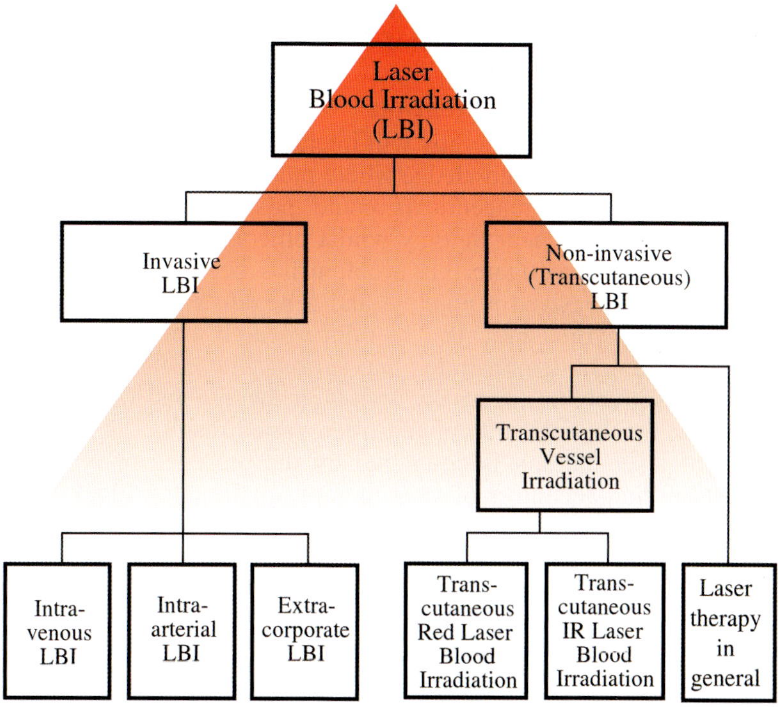

Figure 3.7 Methods of blood irradiation. Modified from Gasparyan

3.3.3.2.6 Lymph nodes

In cases of infection, the recommendation is to irradiate the local lymph nodes to boost the immune system [915]. Recent research By Almeida-Lopes [1269] also suggests that irradiation of lymph nodes in the facial area can reduce pain conditions.

3.3.4 Combination treatment

In the clinical situation, laser therapy is often used in combination with other therapies. While this is not a good research set-up, it is very often advantageous in the clinic. Laser therapy will enhance the outcome of traditional therapies.

If heat is used in combination with laser therapy, the laser treatment should come first. Heat will increase the blood flow in the tissue, thus increasing the absorption of the light in blood. The opposite then applies to cryogenic therapy.

Ultrasound is very often used in physical therapy. One study [726] has compared the effect of ultrasound, laser therapy and the two modalities in combination. The results suggest that they may counteract one another, since the outcome of the healing was better if they were used alone.

3.3.5 Interaction with medication

It is quite probable that laser therapy will interact with pharmaceuticals. This is still an untapped field of knowledge where much work remains to be done. An interaction with pharmaceuticals could possibly explain why some patients react to well to laser therapy whilst others are impervious. One of the few attempts to investigate this problem has been done by Meersman [1278]. It was hypothesised a positive and a negative interaction between laser therapy and pharmaceuticals. The pilot research work on Achilles tendinopathy management demonstrated that various chemicals commonly used will interfere positively or negatively with laser therapy and would be a logical explanation for the intermittent and often varied results. The biostimulatory action of laser therapy is countered by the presence of NSAIDs and steroids that are non-acceptors of laser therapy, as the latter block the membrane channels and antennae pigment receptors that laser therapy relies upon. The degree of reduction and total effect is variable and determined by blood levels of the chemical and individual cell receptability. Similar actions on the cell membrane and the receptor site and bonds are caused by beta blockers, calcium channel antagonists and several of the cardiac and neurological medications. These effects have till now not often been considered in research work and are significant when a meta-analysis of the literature is made and such medications is factored in. In this case many of the 'negative studies' on laser therapy are found to not have screened and excluded for the potential of pharmaceutical counter effects. In contrast, specific chemicals are found to be positive agents for laser therapy that will increase the biostimulative effect by preparing the cell receptors and membrane to be capable of a maximal effect. This facilitatory action of laser therapy acceptors is demonstrated by Plenosol, that is photoreceptive at 660 nm, whilst ubiquinon- ferrum- and copper-based local substances that can be subcutaneously infused are 810 nm and 904 nm receptive. Clinically, the total effect is that of a two-stage process that uses a combination of local injection or cutaneously absorbed substances that can be administered or applied and then irradiated with the specific wavelength. It is also demonstrated that the use of Procaine as the local anaesthetic of choice facilitates the passage of specific photo acceptor substances into the affected tissue effectively acting as a 'taxi' whilst serving its primary purpose of local anaesthetic management. The conclusion is that, where possible, medication should be excluded or included if the maximal effect of laser therapy is to be achieved. Where research is initiated to determine the effect of laser therapy, the presence of such chemicals must be considered, then noted and factored into the statistical analysis.

3.4 Other considerations

3.4.1 What about collimation?

The light from a laser diode is always divergent, usually with a fan shaped beam with an angle of divergence of around 30-90 degrees and perpendicular with an angle of divergence of 5-10 degrees when it is emitted from the semiconductor crystal. If a collimating lens is placed in front of the diode, the light's parallelity can be highly increased, more or less reaching the same parallelity as the beam of a HeNe laser. This is called collimation. The beam from a laser pointer is hence collimated this way. Parallel beams are only advantageous when treating from a distance, since the light is kept together and hits a small surface. This means that we can irradiate from a distance and still achieve a high power density on a small area. If there is no collimation, this can be compensated for by holding the probe closer to the tissue. When light, parallel or not, hits the tissue, it immediately spreads unrestrainedly [429]. Light is spread downwards into the tissue, roughly in the form of a hemisphere like a Ping-Pong ball cut in half, (see Figure 3.8 “Depth of penetration, direct contact” on page 93.) So for treatment involving tissue contact, the parallelity of the beam is of no significance. (See chapter 3.4.2.2 “Tissue compression” on page 95.)

3.4.2 Depth of penetration, greatest active depth

The depth of penetration of laser light depends, as mentioned previously, on the light's wavelength, on whether the laser is superpulsed or not, and on the output power; but also on the treatment technique used. A laser designed for the treatment of humans is rarely suitable for treating animals with fur. There are, in fact, lasers specially made for this purpose. The special design feature

3.6.4 A false picture of health

It is sometimes the case that pain disappears very quickly after a treatment session. It is then essential for the damaged tissue (e.g. an inflamed tendon) that caused the pain not to be overloaded. It is vital to inform the patient that such a false picture of health may emerge, and that the patient himself or herself is responsible for avoiding any stress to the injury. Even if the pain disappears and laser therapy shortens the healing time, the tissue must be given proper time to recover.

3.6.5 Tiredness

One "risk" associated with laser therapy is that the patient may experience extreme tiredness. This is probably due to release of metobolites, but sometimes also to the fact that the treatment eases long-standing pain. This relief allows the patient to catch up on the rest that the pain prevented him or her from getting. There are examples of trotting horses that were completely knocked out for two days after laser therapy treatment but then went back to competing as usual.

3.6.6 Pain reaction

A patient may sometimes experience pain the day after treatment. This is particularly common after the treatment of chronic complaints. It occurs because an injury is "made acute" when the process of healing starts. It is usually not a matter of an overdose. The patient should be informed of the risk of a pain reaction, that it is of a short-term nature and a positive sign. The patient may otherwise think it is some kind of "laser damage".

Except for the treatment of open wounds the risk of overdose on an individual level is actually low. Individual sensitivity should be taken into account.

3.6.7 Do high doses of laser therapy damage tissue?

Reasonable doses given in the course of laser therapy have proved to cause no macroscopic or microscopic damage to tissues. However, there has been concern about the new "high-power" laser therapy systems capable of emitting 100 – 1 000 mW and more from a point source. Could GaAlAs applied to a single small spot for 3 minutes cause macroscopic damage? If not, what about 30 minutes? And what about elevation of tissue temperature? Let us have a look at some interesting experiments.

Literature

Sasaki's [232] study was designed to evaluate concerns about possible damage to tissue following high doses of laser therapy. A 60 mW 830 nm laser was used (spot size 0.3 cm^2, power density 0.2 W/ cm^2) on rat skin and subcutaneous tissue. One group received 3 minutes on one single spot per animal (36 J/cm^2), one group 30 minutes on one single spot (360 J/cm^2), and one untreated group served as control. Macroscopic and microscopic evaluations were carried out and photographic records taken. Tissue temperature was also recorded using digitised thermography. Skin temperature in the irradiated areas rose by 1.1 °C over the first 4 minutes of irradiation and then remained constant during the remainder of the 30-minute irradiation period. Macroscopically, there were no visible signs of alteration of skin colour or texture. Histology revealed no difference in the epidermal, dermal or subdermal tissue architecture in the control specimens or in those irradiated for 3-minute or 30-minute periods.

Calderhead [245] conducted a similar experiment, evaluating possible photothermal damage to articular membranous tissue following extended exposure to a 830 nm 60 mW laser. Two groups of rats received an incident energy of 108 J on a single joint, one group through the capsule and the other group with the capsule dissected away to allow direct exposure. A third group of animals served as control. No damage was visible microscopically, and no difference was found in the histology of the control specimens or in the indirectly or directly irradiated synovial membrane specimens.

Yoshida [404] used GaAlAs at powers ranging from 300 to 700 mW, irradiating the stellate ganglion in rats. Exposure times ranged from 10 to 20 minutes. A slight oedema appeared 24 hours after the fifth irradiation at 700 mW. In other groups no pathological changes in the ganglion or in the immediately surrounding tissues were seen.

These three reports indicate that laser therapy does not cause damage to tissue, even when very high doses are given. Bear in mind, however, that these doses were given to healthy tissues and that only structural components in the tissues were studied.

Shefer [181] subjected rate skeletal muscle cells *in vitro* to HeNe laser at 180 mW/cm^2 (dose not stated). At four days post irradiation there were no histopathological changes as compared to non irradiated control cells. The same dose had previously been demonstrated to enhance satellite cell proliferation twofold [355]. It may be concluded that stimulative dose ranges do not seem to lead to any histopathological cell changes.

3.6.8 Protection against radiation injury

Podolskaya [366] has used HeNe laser on post-radiation reactions and injuries in lip skin and mucous membranes (post-radiation heilitis). The method has been more successful than previously used medical treatments. There were no complications in the laser group, while the traditionally treated group had several allergic reactions and reoperations. The pace of epithelialisation was 7 mm/week in the HeNe group, as compared to 4.1 mm/week in the control group.

Popova [147] studied the effects of HeNe laser light on the healing of muscle tissue after irradiation with 10 Gy roentgen. The muscle tissue of rats was removed, irradiated with X-rays and re-transplanted. Improved healing compared with the control group was observed whether laser light was administered before or after the transplant.

Further literature [1081]

3.7 How to measure effects of laser therapy

In many "alternative medical therapies", the effects are measured by asking the patient before and after "How do you feel?", and if, after therapy, the patient says "Much better!", the therapy is considered effective. In the case of laser therapy, several biological treatment effects can be studied by means of objective detection methods rather than subjective evaluations.

3.7.1 Thermography

One such method is thermography. With this technique, the temperature distribution on a surface is presented as a picture in which the different temperatures are shown in different colours (a "colour-coded" image). Thus, a change in blood flow can be detected second-by-second and minute-by-minute after a laser exposure.(See thermograpy pictures on page 282-283.)

Literature:

Kamikawa [319] used three different types of laser in a group of pain patients. Apart from irradiating the painful area, distant acupuncture points were used. The three lasers were: Nd:YAG of maximum 200 mW, GaAlAs 10 mW, and GaAs 10 mW. The laser beam focus was 1 mm^2. The thermographs showed a remarkable circulatory increment, extending in a wide area around the irradiated spots. Heat production in the irradiated spots disappeared soon after therapy, but the circulatory increment lasted for a while and pain was relieved. In a patient with Raynaud's disease, recordings were made at different room temperatures. At a room temperature of about 18 degrees, vascular response was easily evoked by laser therapy. At a room temperature of around 14 degrees, peripheral vasodilatation reluctantly appeared under prolonged irradiation. Fingers were used to illustrate the effect. Stimulatory effects could only be seen in the irradiated fingers. When a 150 mW Nd:YAG was used for three minutes on a spot, the temperature elevation was 3 degrees. The effect lasted for a few hours. This patient was given forty treatments, and his symptoms were reduced the following winter without further treatment.

Bradley [117] used thermography to examine the difference between the effect of needles and a GaAs laser on acupuncture points. Both needle and laser acupuncture produced an area of raised thermal emission at the site of stimulation. The effect was somewhat slower when initiated by a laser (2-4 minutes) than with needles (immediate).

Obata [185] studied the effect of 30 mW GaAlAs on a group of patients with diagnosed rheumatoid arthritis. Thermography was used on the irradiated hand to check the possible correlation between pain relief and thermographic response. A VAS scale was used to assess the degree of pain relief. Patients reacting with an immediate decrease in temperature had the best pain relief.

Further literature: [126, 232, 189, 478, 495,1208, 1246, 1249].

3.7.2 Magnetic resonance imaging

This is another objective method of quantifying the effect of laser therapy tissue repair.

Schaffer [904] explored the effect of a diode laser (780 nm) on normal skin tissue. Time-dependent contrast enhancement was determined by magnetic resonance imaging (MRI). In the examinations, six healthy volunteers were irradiated on their right planta pedis (sole of foot) with 5 J/cm^2 at a power density of 100 mW/cm^2. T1-weighted magnetic resonance imaging was used to quantify the time-dependent local accumulation of Gadolinium-DPTA, its actual content in the local current blood volume as well as its distribution to the extracellular space. Images were obtained before and after the application of laser light. When laser light was applied, the signal to noise ratio increased by an average of 0.35 (range 0.23-0.63) after irradiation according to contrast-enhanced MRT. According to the authors, it can be observed that, after biomodulation with light of low energy and low power, wound healing improves and pain is reduced. This effect might be explained by an increased blood flow in this area. Therefore, the use of this kind of laser treatment might improve the outcome of other therapeutic modalities such as tumour ionising radiation therapy and local chemotherapy.

3.7.3 High resolution digitised ultrasound B-scan

This is yet another method of objectively measuring the effect of laser therapy in wound healing, described by Dyson [923].

3.7.4 Tensile strength

Asencio-Arana [148] examined the strength and collagen concentration of high-risk anastomosis in the colons of rats after endoscopic irradiation with HeNe laser. The results showed that repeated irradiation (1.9 J/cm^2) with HeNe laser light increased the tensile strength of the anastomosis by almost 100% by the fourth day after the operation. An equivalent experiment with 6.4 J/cm^2 brought about significantly increased strength. The difference in collagen concentration, however, did not reach a significant level.

There are several positive studies on tensile strength. Braverman [50], Lyons [462], and Riendeau [68] used HeNe, while Enwemeka [463] used GaAs and Stadler [954] GaAlAs.

3.7.5 Other objective methods

Other examples of objective methods are measurements of nerve conduction velocity, nerve action potential, chemiluminescence of blood, the study of vascularisation by means of a microscope [35], and the secretion of metabolites.

3.8 "Is laser therapy effective?"

Why do we put this question here, when you allready have read more than 100 pages and are convinced? Well after all the information given in these first 100 pages, with objective test methodes and all, it is natural that you are convinced. But there are many people, still, that are not and we believe it is valuable to know this part of the "history". This can also wupport you with some arguments for discussions with "non-believers".

Many people wonder whether laser therapy really works or is simply a sophisticated form of placebo. This skepticism comes mostly from doctors, and has spread via certain media to dentists and veterinary surgeons. Many other professionals - nurses, physiotherapists, chiropractors, and masseurs, for example - have tested lasers and generally been pleasantly surprised by the results.

Unfortunately, it is not unusual that professionals in high medical positions, without knowledge or own experience of laser therapy, tell the media: "Laser therapy has no effect!" or "Laser therapy is humbug!"

3.8.1 Does laser therapy really work?

So, does laser therapy really work, or is it a sophisticated placebo? If it works, what kind of problems is it useful for? Is there any proof? Have controlled, randomised, double blind studies been published in which significant medical benefits have been proved? And if so, what mechanisms are associated with these benefits?

The following quotations are worth considering:

1. "A hard judgement has been passed on low-level lasers, which have been said to have no effect. Yet isn't it rather strange that ineffective lasers to the tune of a couple of hundred million dollars have been sold over the space of a few years? And why are there so many who can describe how the laser has helped them find a new life without pain?

It seems to be difficult, in scientific studies, to demonstrate the biological effects of the low-level laser. This raises an irreverent thought: perhaps there is something wrong with the scientific methods, or even worse, that the research scientists are not sufficiently skilled? It is unacceptable to blame placebo effects and the fact that people are dissatisfied with public health care.

In any case: a committed research scientist who sticks his neck out and says that money spent on low-level laser treatment is money wasted is taking a big risk. He cannot expect to be believed by anyone who has been successfully treated with a laser. If he is conscious of his scientific standing, he would be better advised to adopt a more humble approach".

Sten Erik Jensen, editor of Medicinsk Teknik, No 1, 1990.

2. “The work with this thesis can be described as my first exciting journey into Physiotherapy Science, and I feel like a novice seeking adventure. At the end of this journey, the turbulent story of laser therapy reminds me of a fairytale by H. C. Andersen. It is named after the main character and called “The Ugly Duckling”, which after some time turned out to be a beautiful swan. In science things are not always what they seem to be at first sight. I have learned that a touch of humbleness and an open mind are always needed in scientific work.”

Jan M. Bjordal, Master Thesis in Physiotherapy Science, Division of Physiotherapy Science, University of Bergen, Norway, 1997.

Words worth considering! There are a number of other issues to be considered, such as the animal experiments conducted where healing has been observed - are these also placebo effects? What about the researchers who have demonstrated the medical effects of low-level lasers on cell cultures, laboratory animals, and in more than 100 double-blind studies on patients: have they lied about their results, and together decided to fool the whole world? Probably not.

For those who are well acquainted with the subject and follow research developments in publications and international conferences, it is easy to answer the questions posed above:

- Laser therapy works: on chronic ulcers, neuralgia, pain, oedema,
- inflammations and on several other indications.
- There is extensive international documentation.
- A great deal is already known about the mechanisms.

3.8.2 Why the controversy?

Despite the fact that so much has been done, many people have great difficulty in accepting that laser therapy can have a positive effect on various conditions. This skepticism stems from several factors, of which the following is a selection:

- Many critics have not bothered to examine the extensive documentation but have instead relied upon the daily press or grapevines.
- Laser therapy was first described in "Eastern Europe". People within the field of medicine are more used to Americans and Western Europeans making the most important breakthroughs, and during the Cold War there was great skepticism in the West about the standard of science in “Eastern Europe”.
- Laser therapy was not approved for any indication by the Food and Drug Administration (FDA) in the USA until 2002.

- Because laser therapy does not involve risks, other than certain risks of eye injury, and does not have any side-effects or negative effects, and may therefore be used by personnel other than doctors/dentists, many persons find it difficult to believe that it can have any positive effect.
- Bogus "lasers" and laser instruments of deficient quality, which have led to little or no biological effect, have given laser therapy systems a bad reputation.
- The effects of treatment are not always evident in the short term, as they are after operations using scalpels or powerful lasers.
- It is indeed hard to accept the fact that one single therapeutic modality can have an effect on so many indications.

Furthermore,

- There are individuals who do not react well to laser therapy.
- It has taken a long time to find out how this, admittedly fairly weak, laser light, which does not provide any noticeable heat, can relieve pain and influence inflammations and infections, oedema, etc. It is only recently that we have begun to understand the mechanisms involved.

Laser therapy has been accepted in central and Eastern Europe and in Asia in an entirely different way. In Japan, where the medical authorities are known for being as strict as the FDA - if not stricter - the method has been accepted and is in widespread use. The use of laser therapy as a medical modality was approved by the Japanese government in 1987 and the application in health insurance started in 1996. Laser therapy is reimbursed in Hungary, provided that the doctor has attented a training course and received a diploma. In Norway, laser therapy is reimbursed when used in physiotherapy. A meta analysis of the laser therapy literature for tendinitis was the basis when the Norwegian government accepted the therapy in 2001.

3.8.3 Does it have to be a laser?

A good point - does it have to be a laser? Could we use a normal torchlight instead? Of course we could, but we would not achieve the same biological effects as with a laser. It is known, see chapter 11.1 “Are the biostimulative effects laser specific?” on page 334, that all light affects the living organism, but in a number of studies in which the effects of light from various sources have been compared, the laser light is shown to give the strongest effect.

Polarised wide band light (i.e. incoherent but polarised light) will indeed have a fair effect on "naked" tissues such as open wounds and mucous membranes, and, of course, on tissue *in vitro*. This has been demonstrated in early studies by Mester [23], Kana [204] and Marín [498]. However, polarisation is lost as soon as the light enters the tissue. Thus, only superficial structures will react to polarised light. If you are interested in the details and more literature, you can read more in Chapter 11.

Literature:

The effect of HeNe and monochromatic red incoherent light on the protein and glycose metabolism in hamsters was studied by Onac [447]. Both light sources had a stimulative effect but the effect of incoherent light (peak at 618 nm) was lower.

3.8.4 FDA (Food and Drug Administration)

In a panel discussion at the 2nd Congress of the World Association for Laser Therapy in 1998 in Kansas City, USA, the authors of this book pointed out that there is a clear difference between the medical authorities in the USA and Europe: In the USA everything that is not approved by the medical authority (Food and Drug Administration - FDA) is forbidden, but in Europe everything that is not forbidden is allowed. This means that laser therapy has been used by clinicians in Europe all the time - and still is.

Recently, however, the FDA has started its own investigations on laser therapy on wound healing [953, 1222]. Although the use of laser therapy in the USA is restricted, there are still many practitioners who use it. However, in order to use it they must have what it called an “IRB approval”. A local Institutional Review Board is a committee of laypersons from different professions. Such a committee can issue a permit to use an “investigational advice” like a therapeutic laser, provided the therapist produces satisfactory evidence of the efficacy and a simple design of the proposed study. Patients treated by laser therapy also have to sign a written consent to say that they accept being treated. At the begnning of 2002 three so-called 510(k) were issued by the FDA, clearing the use of laser therapy for a few indications. This may very well be followed by several others once the ice is broken.

The status of laser therapy in the United States is formulated on the web site of the FDA (March 2002):

"Biostimulation lasers, also called low level laser therapy (LLLT), cold lasers, soft lasers, or laser acupuncture devices, are being marketed with claims for pain relief and accelerated healing in other countries, where premarket approval may not be required. However, in the United States, medical lasers must have premarket approval or premarket clearance from the FDA prior to marketing for any claimed human indication, unless specifically exempted by FDA. To date, no biostimulation laser therapy devices have been approved by the FDA for humans; therefore, it is illegal to make any claims of clinical effectiveness. The Office of Compliance has issued notifications and warnings to firms suspected of illegally marketing these devices with claims of effectiveness.

Please note that FDA law and regulations contain provisions that permit limited distribution of unapproved devices for use in clinical investiga-

tions. There are numerous clinical investigations being conducted in this and other countries to determine safety and efficacy with these devices for the intended uses that are proposed.

Certain unapproved, non-significant risk Class III medical devices, including biostimulation lasers, may only be distributed in the U.S. to individual practitioners who have approval from an Institutional Review Board (IRB) for the investigational clinical use of the device, or to investigators participating in a study under an Investigational Device Exemption (IDE) approved by the Centre for Devices and Radiological Health (CDRH), as specified in the Code of Federal Regulations (CFR), 21 CFR 812. Even with IRB approval, a sponsor must comply with IDE requirements such as monitoring investigations, maintaining records, making reports, and complying with prohibitions on promotion and commercialisation of investigational devices. The investigators would have similar responsibilities, also covered in 21 CFR 812.

Although the FDA does not have jurisdiction over the practice of medicine, no biostimulation laser devices have been cleared for human treatment; therefore, no units can be introduced into commerce legally for human treatment, unless via an IDE or with IRB approval."

This text remains unchanged in spite of the recent 510(k) permits issued by the FDA. The therapies so far accepted are

1. Adjunctive use for temporary pain relief for pain associated with carpal tunnel syndrome (two permits).
2. Adjunctive use in providing temporary relief of minor chronic neck and shoulder pain of musculoskeletal origin.

Some LED manufacturers claim to have FDA clearance. This is true, but the clearance is for tissue heating (as an expensive heat lamp) and never for biostimulation.

3.8.5 "There is no documentation on that!"

A substantial body of scientific documentation is required for a new treatment method to be accepted by the medical community, which is of course positive. However, more than 30 years' clinical experience without any reports of significant side effects or injury should suffice for laser therapy not to inspire fears of unknown side effects. Over 2,500 research reports are not that many in this context, but neither are they negligible. However, do we need to know everything before we begin to use a method, if we know for sure that it is not dangerous?

Let us make a comparison with the world's most widely used medicine: acetylsalicylic acid. It has been used for generations, as its pain-relieving and antipyretic properties could be easily observed. However, the theory that acetylsalicylic acid works by alleviating pain centres in the brain has been abandoned in recent years. It is now believed that it inhibits the production of some prostaglandins. It has also been discovered recently that the substance has a positive effect on vascular illnesses. In any event, empiricism has held sway here. We do not know exactly how laser therapy works either, but whoever decides to put it to the test in a clinical environment will soon see that it works.

The reason laser therapy has received unfair treatment is historical. We can compare it with a description of NSAID (non-steroidal anti-inflammatory drugs) in a medical book. This group of medicines for the treatment of rheumatism is described as follows:

"*NSAID has a beneficial effect on inflammation and reduces morning stiffness, and alleviates swelling and pain in the joints. In spite of this, there is no proof that the substances affect the course of the illness, or that they can prevent erosion of the cartilage and joints. The clinical effects of NSAID are usually obtained within a week. If no effect is noted, it can be worthwhile to try another substance within the NSAID group, as patients show individual sensitivity to closely related substances.*"

If we substitute "laser therapy" for "NSAID" and "laser" for "substance", those who work with biostimulation will recognise the situation.

"*Laser therapy has a beneficial effect on inflammation and reduces morning stiffness, and alleviates swelling and pain in the joints. In spite of this, there is no proof that the laser therapy affects the course of the illness, or that it can prevent erosion of the cartilage and joints. The clinical effects of laser therapy are usually obtained within a week. If no effect is noted, it can be worthwhile to try another laser within the laser therapy group, as patients show individual sensitivity to different laser wavelengths.*"

Both the statements above are true and documented, but only one is generally accepted. It is interesting to quote the foreword of the Master Thesis by Bjordal [732]: "First I was surprised by the scant evidence in favour of NSAID or steroid injections in shoulder tendinitis/bursitis and lateral epicondylalgia. Next I was surprised to find that the evidence in favour of laser therapy was at the same level both in clinical effect and statistical power."

3.8.6 Confused?

Anyone who studies the literature carefully can become confused. Some wavelengths achieve the best effects on this and that, while others have poorer effects or none at all. Some doses lead to beneficial effects, but when the dose is increased, the effects wear off. If we treat a condition, some of the parameters we want to influence may be affected, but perhaps not all. If we administer treatment from a distance, we do not get the same effect as if we treat in contact or with pressure. Some frequencies produce effects on pain, others on oedema. What are we to believe? And what do we do to find the best dose, wavelength, etc.?

There is still much to learn in the field of laser therapy, and for the time being we must be satisfied with the knowledge that we have. This is often a combination of clinical experience with a degree of scientific foundation. The biological effects we produce can, in any case, be seen as an empirical mean value effect, and as long as this entails concrete and positive results we can be satisfied with this rather rigid treatment model. In the future, people are likely to think that we used laser light in a primitive fashion - but for the time being, we must content ourselves with the fact that laser therapy really works.

Is the use of laser therapy, then, only a job for trained scientists? Hardly! As usual, reality is rather more difficult than the producers of glossy brochures would have us believe, but in practice it is a lot easier than this book sometimes implies. Anyone with medical knowledge can successfully use laser therapy after an introductory course. You do not need to know everything to be a good therapist, but the more you learn the greater the success you will encounter in your day-to-day work.

3.8.7 Experience and attitudes

In the literature on the subject, a great deal of individual experience and approaches to laser therapy have been presented. One of the few attempts so far to compile the experience of a large group of professional practitioners was made by Baxter in 1990 [281]. Every physiotherapist in Northern Ireland received a written questionnaire inquiring into his or her experience with laser therapy. 397 of 533 responded, and 215 of these had experience of laser therapy. A more detailed survey was then addressed to these 215. 139 (63.1 %) responded to this survey and were asked to grade five common electronic treatment methods (interferential therapy, pulsed electromagnetic energy, short-wave diathermy, ultrasound, and laser therapy). Laser therapy was considered the best method for the treatment of pain (by a small margin) and for wound healing (by far). Laser therapy was in third place for the treatment of oedema. However, it is likely that today's laser equipment, with its considerably higher power, may give laser therapy a higher ranking for oedema, and a much greater margin of victory for the treatment of pain. The predominant indications were (in order) wound healing, soft tissue damage, pain, and arthritic conditions. All of the laser therapy users were dissatisfied with the lack of independent and clinically oriented literature in the field. Most of them had acquired their knowledge from brochures and courses run by suppliers and manufacturers. Many were also dissatisfied with the conflicting advice given by various sales representatives.

Cambier [637] carried out a similar survey of physiotherapists in Flanders in 1996. Wounds and tendinitis seemed to be the indications of choice. The results were compared with those from Baxter's study and the two studies seem to match quite well.

In the Netherlands, about 10% of dentists (approximately 600) used laser therapy in 1995. In a study by Oudoff [465], 200 Dutch dentists were asked to fill in a standard questionnaire. All of the 92 respondents used a 830 nm 30 mW laser. The dentists were positive regarding the results of laser treatment after surgery and for mucosal lesions, periodontology, and muscular disorders. They were less positive about the long-term results for toothache and hypersensitive dentine.

In Hungary, more than 30% of the dentists and family doctors were using laser therapy in 1999 [870].

3.8.8 The funding of research

It is now and then suggested that manufacturers of laser therapy equipment should prove their claims by financing research. While quite a few of the manufacturers actually have used their scarce resources to do precisely that, it is not reasonable to expect much such funding. There is no patent on laser therapy equipment, so any valuable information found in research will be available to every manufacturer on the market. Funding pharmaceutical research is quite a different matter. Pills can be patented.

Chapter 4
Medical indications

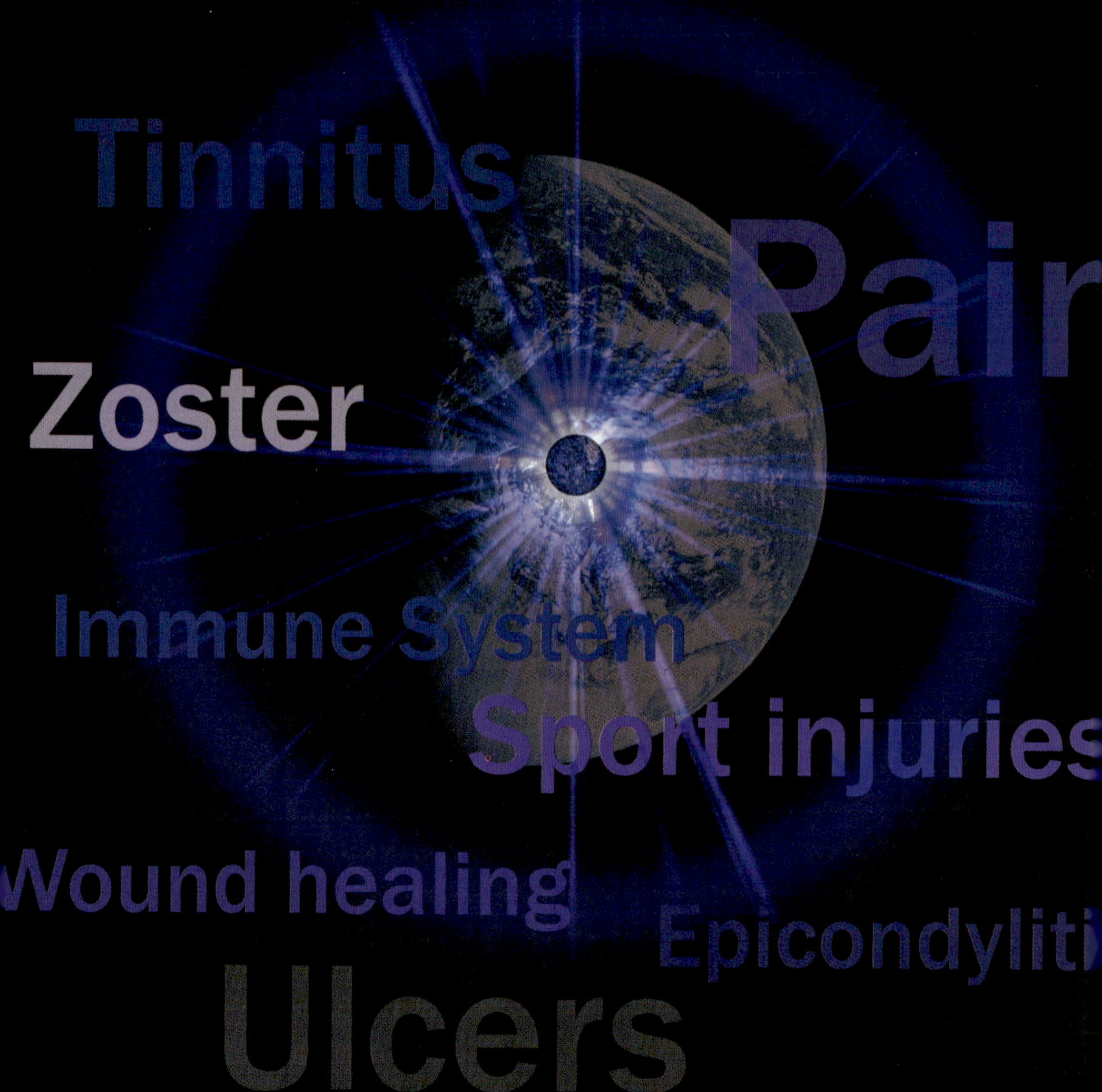

Medical and dental indications are often interrelated. In the following section, we have provided cross-references where the indication is applicable to both. Relatively little commentary is provided on the various indications. Instead we have selected some studies, letting their contents speak for themselves. We have included some indications for which the documentation is weak, in hopes of inspiring future research.

When doses in the following studies are extrapolated for clinical use, several things must be remembered. A high value for J/cm^2 does not necessarily mean that the energy used was high; the light guide may just have been thin. On the other hand, a high energy value does not necessarily mean that the energy density was high - the fibre optic “eye” may have been very large. In the research setting the "J/cm^2" unit is very important. In the clinical setting the practical but less defined “J per point” is more convenient. Extrapolating these matters from studies is laborious and sometimes not possible. Therefore we have limited the text to quoting whatever is stated in the report.

4.1 Who and what can be treated?

It is not unusual for therapists to ask: “Can I treat this with laser therapy?” As soon as we hear the question “Can I treat ...”, we can answer: “Yes”! Laser therapy is a completely safe treatment as long as it is done with lasers up to a few hundred milliwatts. But we always point out the importance of having a reliable diagnosis - a diffuse pain can be due to cancer, ilius or ...

However, the correct question is not “Can I treat that?” but “Can that be treated?” It is not true that anyone can treat anything; a combined knowledge of medicine and laser therapy is mandatory for good clinical results.

4.1.1 Allergy, acne systica gravis and eczema

Laser therapy will reduce the symptoms of local allergic reactions through its anti-inflammatory and pain relieving effect. This has been demonstrated by Sakihama [652]. The effect of HeNe laser on irritant and allergic contact dermatitis of the mouse ear and on histamine release from rat peritoneal mast cells was studied. Irradiation (12.2 J/cm^2) was performed at various intervals before and after the challenge of an irritated contact dermatitis (ICD) or allergic contact dermatitis (ACD). The laser did not influence the ICD but the allergic response was decelerated. The spontaneous histamine release was inhibited by laser irradiation, while substance P and compound 48/80-induced histamine release were not inhibited.

Literature:

Simunovic [958] used a combination of GaAlAs point irradiation and HeNe scanning to treat acne and acne scars in a two centre study on 80 patients. In the first therapy group, laser therapy was used as monotherapy and in the second it was used in combination with topical application of tetracycline. Both groups included acute as well as chronic cases. Mono therapy demonstrated relief of all local clinical symptoms. Used in combination with tetracycline, the healing process was accelerated and there was a decrease in tetracycline side effects and reduced occurrence of relapses. In all patients treated with laser therapy, scars were significantly prevented or reduced.

Ailioaie [981] and Tulebaev [555] report on positive effects on allergic rhinitis using laser therapy.

Ailioaie [1204] reports promising result in the laser treatment of children's allergic purpura. This condition, of unknown aetiology, is characterised by migratory polyarthralgia or polyarthritis, abdominal pain, vasculitis of the small vessels and in the kidney. Conventional therapy consists of NSAIDs to control subjective problems, antibiotics when indicated and corticosteroids in acute phases. The prognosis for recovery is generally good, though symptoms frequently (25-50%) return over a period of several months. In the Ailioaie study, 31 children aged 2-16 years were divided into two group (15/16) after clinical and laboratory tests. One group was given conventional therapy whereas the other was treated with a laser scanner of 670 (50 mW) and 830 (300 mW) nm in combination, 4-10 J/cm^2. Scanning was performed daily for 21 days. The clinical outcome was good in both groups but in the laser group the improvement was spectacular during the first 10 days and all final scores measured were better in the laser group. Hematuria, indicating renal involvement, was noted in 18.75% of the non-laser treated children.

Further literature: [350, 833, 1052, 1205]

4.1.2 Arteriosclerosis

Literature:

A recently documented indication is arteriosclerosis (claudicatio intermittens) of the lower limbs, described by Attia [964]. 20 patients with arteriosclerosis in the lower limbs were treated with HeNe 20 mW/GaAlAs 830 nm 250 mW, applied transcutaneously to the lumbar region by a scanner for 30 minutes, 6 days per weeks for two months. The duration of the condition varied from 1 to 8 months. Pain was relieved in 16 patients after 3 to 7 applications of treatment. At the end of the therapy, 8 patients were able to walk 1500 metres without experiencing pain in the calf muscles. Three patients discontinued therapy for reasons not related to the therapy and one patient showed no improvement.

4.1.3 Asthma

Literature:

Intravenous HeNe laser irradiation has been used to reduce symptoms in asthmatic patients [1032, 1033, 1035]. Laser acupuncture is reported to be successful for this condition. [118, 878, 879, 883].

Further literature: [340, 710, 840]

4.1.4 Arthritis

Arthritis is a very wide indication, comprising diagnoses such as rheumatic arthritis (RA), osteoarthritis (OA), morbus Bechterew and psoriatic arthritis. Laser treatment is as unlikely to cure any of these conditions as any medication, but the symptoms and quality of life of the patients can often be improved considerably. In addition to pain relief, increased range of movement and reduced swelling can be achieved to some extent. 1-2 J from the lateral side is a suitable dosage for a small joint such as a finger, with GaAs always lower in dose. For larger joints considerably higher dosage is needed. A knee, for instance, will need 15-25 J per session. Hip and shoulder arthritis require high output of the laser and a probe applied with strong pressure on suitable anatomical points to achieve a sufficient dose to the target area. Only infrared will work on deep structures while all wavelengths will work on small joints. Laser therapy affects synovia as well as cartilage. Since the cartilage in larger joints is difficult to reach with a reasonable dose, it is believed that the main effect of laser therapy comes from the influence on the synovia.

Chronic conditions may react with an increase in pain, which is why it is best to begin with a dosage on the low side. This should be explained to the patient, so that the initial occurrence of pain is not used as a reason to discontinue the treatment. The pain reaction in itself is unpleasant but is actually an indication of a positive reaction to the treatment. Prolonged treatment schedules are necessary with a total accumulated (all sessions) dose of no less than 25 J for small joints such as fingers. 3-5 sessions per week are recommended in the initial phase. Patients in the early stages are more likely to have a prolonged benefit from laser therapy [1100], whereas patients in the later stages will obtain a better quality of life but with more or less transient effects of laser therapy [1023]. However, in sharp contrast to pharmaceuticals [1059], there will be no side effects. About 90% of the prescribed NSAIDs in Canada is attributed to the treatment of arthritis [1140]. It has also been postulated that about one third of the arthritis budget has been used to handle side effects of NSAIDs. These figures support the use of a side-effect free method such as laser therapy. It would be ideal for an elderly chronic patient to have a suitable laser of his own, or one leased from the hospital. Laboratory values typically remain unchanged.

Laser therapy partly seems to influence the synovial fluid and its membranes [63, 639, 718, 751, 1018, 1022] and the articular cartilage [151, 550, 898, 1021]. The PGE2 activity is also modified [243, 1008] as well as interleukin 1-ß [188, 370].

Since the whole organism is involved, irradiating one or several joints will only give temporary relief [293, 1023]. To obtain true improvement of quality of life, all the joints involved should be treated in many consecutive sessions [397] and comparatively high energies must be used [585]. It is essential that the large and deep-lying joints be given a sufficient dosage. Such treatment is certainly time-consuming but the alternatives, on the other hand, are rather bleak. It is possible to have the patient treat himself after instructions, as suggested by Stelian [617].

Although all wavelengths will have some effects, there is a difference in the total outcome, with some wavelengths more effective than others, due to better penetration of infrared light in large joints. In a study by Giavelli [638], 406 patients with osteoarticular diseases were treated with various wavelengths. The results were as follows. In gonarthrosis patients, statistical analysis of the results showed no significant differences between CO_2 laser and GaAs laser treatments ($p = 0.975$), but there were significant differences between CO_2 laser and HeNe laser treatments ($p = 0.02$) and between GaAs laser and HeNe laser treatments ($p = 0.003$). In lumbar arthrosis patients treated with a GaAs or HeNe laser, significant differences were found between the two laser treatments, and the combined sweeping plus points techniques appeared to have a positive trend relative to the sweeping method alone, especially in sciatic suffering. In the algodystrophy syndrome in hemiplegic patients, significant differences were found between CO_2 and HeNe laser treatments ($p = 0.026$), between high and low CO_2 laser doses ($p = 0.024$), and between a low CO_2 laser dose and a high HeNe laser dose ($p = 0.006$). The differences above do not indicate that HeNe is less useful in laser therapy, only that the deep lying structures treated could not be sufficiently saturated by HeNe laser ligth.

	820, 830, 1060 nm		**904 nm**		**632 nm**	
Location	Lowest power density in mW/cm²	Dose per point in Joules	Lowest power density in mW/cm²	Dose per point in Joules	Lowest power density in mW/cm²	Dose per point in Joules
Finger/ toe	10	1– 5	3	0.5-5	10	6 – 30
Knee	10	4 – 20	3	0.5-5	10	6 – 30
Lumbar spine	100	40 – 200	15	7.5 - 37.5	Not investigated	> 30
Temporomandibular	10	1 – 5	3	0.5-5	10 – 400	6 – 30

Table 4.1: Arthritis

The table show suggested optimal range of power density in mW/cm² and dose in Joule/cm² for the most common joints for infrared GaAlAs (continuous) lasers with wavelength 820, 830 and Nd:YAG laser with wavelength 1060 nm, infrared GaAs lasers with wavelength 904 nm, and HeNe (continuous) lasers with wavelength 632 nm respectively. Modified after Bjordal [588].

Literature:

Palma has previously showed that HeNe laser light blocks the increment of Prostaglandin E1 (PGE1) and Bradykinine (B) in the Plasma Fibrinogen Level (PFL). In a new study [357], another substance related to the inflammatory process, Tromboxane (Tx), was studied. The experiment confirmed the total block of PGE1/B when HeNe was administered. However, the complex PGE1/B/Tx was only partially blocked.

The antiinflammatory effect of HeNe laser was observed by Campaña [1133]. Calcium pyrophosphate was injected into both joints of the lower limbs in rats, to mimic microcrystalline arthropaty. The untreated group showed a strong diffuse inflammatory reaction for mono and polymorphonuclears with fibro and angioblastic proliferation, with edematous lax stroma. No inflammation was observed in the laser group.

In another experiment in rats, Campaña [582] found that laser induced a similar reduction of PGE2 levels as NSAID in experimentally induced synovitis.

In an *in vitro* study by Inoue [585], GaAlAs laser treatment at low fluence inhibited mitogenic proliferation of human lymphocytes, while high-energy fluence enhanced proliferation.

Lievens [550] studied the effect of a GaAs laser on the regeneration of cartilage tissue. A 0.4 mm hole was drilled in both ears of 30 mice. One ear was irradiated daily. After one day there was no difference. After two days there was a clear activation of the perichondrium in the laser therapy group. After four days there was significant ingrowth of the perichondrium into the drill hole only in the laser group.

Further indications of an effect on the metabolism of cartilage are found in studies by Akai [466], Ruiz Calatrava [1057] and van der Veen [1058]. These studies used dosages similar to those in fibroblast studies. Researchers using higher dosages failed to demonstrate a stimulative effect [1191].

The aim of a study by Morrone [898] was to verify the effects of laser therapy performed with GaAlAs (780 nm, 2500 mW) on human cartilage cells *in vitro*. The cartilage sample used for the biostimulation treatment was taken from the right knee of a 19-year-old patient. After the chondrocytes were isolated and suspended for cultivation, the cultures were incubated for 10 days. The culture was divided into four groups. Groups I, II, III were subject to biostimulation with the following laser parameters: 300 J, 1 W, 100 Hz pulse frequency, 10 min. exposure, 300 J, 1 W, 300 Hz pulse frequency, 10 min. exposure; and 300 J, 1 W, 500 Hz pulse frequency, 10 min. exposure, respectively. Group IV did not receive any treatment. The laser biostimulation was conducted for five consecutive days. The data showed good results in terms of cell viability and levels of Ca and Alkaline Phosphate in the groups treated with laser by comparison with the untreated group. The results obtained confirm previous positive *in vitro* results from the same authors, that the GaAlAs laser provides biostimulation without cell damage. The high doses used complicate the conclusions from earlier studies.

Herman [151] used Nd:YAG *in vitro* on bovine articular cartilage. Irradiation could be shown to consistently up-regulate cartilage proteoglycan, collagen, noncollagen protein and DNA synthesis in the absence of histological or biochemical evidence of enhanced matrix catabolism. Laser-induced repair could be shown biochemically in an *in vitro* model system of enzymatically mediated cartilage matrix deposition.

Skinner [754] stimulated cultured human embryonic fibroblast cells with GaAs. Fibroblast procollagen production was monitored by the synthesis of {3H} hydroxyproline, and DNA replication was assessed by {3H} thymidine incorporation. Following laser treatment, controlled pepsin digestion measured the increase in cell biostimulation. Maximum increase of collagen production and cell biostimulation occurred after 4 episodes of laser therapy at 24-hour intervals.

The Hungarian experience of using laser therapy in rheumatoid arthritis have been summarised by Mester [894] as follows:

"Barabás [1018] irradiated the joints of rheumatoid arthritis (RA) patients. In the first open study the range of motion and circumference of the treated joints were measured, a Ritchie index was used as a semi-objective parameter, while subjective parameters as joint tenderness and pain on a visual analogous scale (VAS) were registered. Walking time was registered as a functional disability parameter. Laboratory activity parameters and the 99mTechnetium index were measured. The second part of the clinical study was double blind. Infrared (10 mW and 100 mW) lasers were used, versus dummy devices with the same appearance. The third part of the study was *in vitro* experiments. Synovial membranes of rheumatoid arthritis patients were irradiated. The DNA/RNA ratio of the RA group was compared to the control group. A significant difference was detected between the two groups. The fourth phase of the clinical studies was to detect the effects of laser irradiation in other rheumatic diseases: psoriatic arthritis, sacroileitis, osteoarthritis, entesopathy, tenosynovitis, bursitis calcarea, fibromyalgia, localised muscle spasm, periarthritis humeroscapularis etc. The different wavelengths (604, 630, 660, 670, 690, 750, 780, 790, 820, 830, 904, 1053, 1219 nm,) were compared (30 - 100 mW) with other physiotherapy modalities, such as ultrasound." The group size in the double blind study was 80 (50 laser, 30 placebo) and each finger joint received 1 J/cm^2 daily for 25 days.

In an *in vitro* study on the effect on the synovial membrane, it was found that a total dose of 25 J/cm^2 had an stimulating effect, less so with 50 and even less with 100 J/cm^2, while 250 J/cm^2 had an inhibitive effect. A continued study of 8 patients, using 100 J/cm^2 in total instead of 25 J/cm^2, confirmed this observation. The laser used was a Neodymium-Phosphate-Glass-laser, wavelength 1053 nm, energy 100 mJ per pulse.

Ortutay [518] used 1-4 J/cm^2 (830 nm) per joint with compression technique on a daily basis. Total dose per joint ranged between 25 and 40 J/cm^2. Total doses below a total of 25 J/cm^2 were ineffective, while 25-40 J/cm^2 was effective in all cases.

In another (double-blind) study by Ortutay [609] on the effect of laser therapy on psoriatic arthritis using 820 nm light, 7 of 8 patients in the treatment group had a improvement of clinical activity: increased range of movement, decreased joint stiffness and tenderness. In the placebo group, only 2 of 8 patients improved.

Palmgren [97] conducted a controlled double-blind study of the effects of GaAlAs on 35 patients with rheumatoid arthritis. Eight joints on the worst affected hand were treated with a laser 3.58 J/cm^2 or placebo laser. In the experimental group, grip strength and movement were improved, as was swelling; pain, and morning stiffness were reduced. Pain was also reduced in the placebo group, although less than in the experimental group, while other parameters were unchanged.

In the study by Rogvi-Hansen [1138] the outcome was negative, but the actual area of the articular capsule was not irradiated, although the indication studied was condromalacia patellae. This study used the treatment method used by Walker [38], irradiating the patella, the ipsilateral femoral nerve in the groin and the proximal part of the peroneal muscle. Walker used 1 mW HeNe, whereas this latter study used GaAs 17 mW.

In a clinical study comprising 224 patients, Glazewski [1079] found that "application of low-intensity laser irradiation enables us to shorten NSAIDs treatment duration, reduce dose size and obtain better therapeutic effects." Indications treated were i.a. rheumatiod arthritis, coxarthrosis, gonarthrosis and spondylosis. The lasers used were GaAs 890 nm in the range 3.6 - 7.4 mW, dose range 0.75 - 3.0 J/cm^2.

In the double blind study by Taghawinjad [335] the outcome in the verum group was not better than that of the placebo group. However, the laser used was a combined HeNe (4.4 mW) + GaAs (5 $\times$ 0.3 mW) held at a distance of 160 mm from the skin, and covering an area of 40 mm^2. The power density in this set-up is very low and the penetration insufficient.

Johannsen [605] treated 22 patients with RA in a double-blind study. The two most painful MCP joints on the most affected hand were chosen for treatment, and 2.9 J of GaAlAs light was applied to four points. Treatment was offered three times a week for a month. None of the five parameters measured showed any effect of laser therapy. The dose is on the high side.

Molina [334] compared two groups where one received ASA (acetylsalicylic acid) and the other ASA (4 g daily) plus laser therapy. During the initial double-blind phase, GaAs 6-8 J/cm^2 was applied to a total of 21 points in the hand. In an additional open phase, HeNe 6-10 J/cm^2 was administered.

The ASA/laser therapy group responded more favourably to the therapy. GaAs appeared to be more successful than HeNe.

Amano [578] applied 790 nm 0.8 J to six points for six consecutive days on the lateral side of the knee in a group of 14 RA patients due to undergo arthroplasty. During operation, small samples of the synovial membrane were removed from the lateral and the medial non-irradiated area. Histological findings in the irradiated synovial membrane showed flattening of epithelial cells, decreased villous proliferation, narrowed vascular lumen, and less infiltration of inflammatory cells by comparison with the non-irradiated synovia.

Barberis [718] treated 12 patients with chronic rheumatoid arthritis stages II and III. One knee in each patient was selected and was irradiated with HeNe, 8 J/cm^2, 11 points, 15 applications. Synovial tissue analysis showed that laser therapy reduced pre- and post-treatment levels of PGE2.

Obata [185] studied the effect of GaAlAs on a group of patients with diagnosed rheumatoid arthritis. Thermography was used on the treated hand to check the possible correlation between pain relief and thermographic response. A VAS scale was used to assess the degree of pain relief. In 10 patients, the HST (highest skin temperature) decreased immediately after irradiation. 9 of these patients experienced significant pain relief. 8 patients had an increase of HST following irradiation and 5 of these experienced non-significant pain relief.

Soriano [331] reports good results in treating a group of 938 patients with osteoarthritis, using 904 nm, 6-10 J/cm^2. Acute conditions responded better than chronic conditions. The subgroups were: NSAID + laser therapy, massage/physiotherapy + laser therapy, and laser therapy only. The results in the three subgroups were practically identical. Chronic knee and hip pain had low scores (38%), others ranged from 84% to 100%.

Stelian [617] divided 50 patients with knee OA into three groups: one received 830 nm GaAlAs, one HeNe and one placebo laser. The infrared group was double blind whereas the HeNe group had to be an open study. The patients treated their knee twice daily for ten days, a total of 22 J per day. GaAlAs and HeNe had approximately the same effect. The laser groups had significantly less pain at the end of the therapy and at checkups at 2-12 months. Their general well-being was measured with a Disability Index Questionnaire. This index was reduced by half in the laser groups but was unchanged in the placebo group.

Similar parameters but a different treatment schedule were used by Bülow [1025]. Each patient received 22.5 J per session in nine sessions over three weeks. Laser source was a GaAlAs laser of 25 mW. Although reported as negative, a closer analysis of the data submitted reveals a significant short-term effect, which is masked in the text. When these masked facts are revealed, both Stelian and Bülow present a significant but short-term effect of laser therapy for these parameters.

Haimovici [82] studied osteoarthritis in finger joints and found that both HeNe and GaAlAs improved all the parameters measured. In the same study, the effects of anti-inflammatory medication and laser were compared. The medication gave slightly better results than the laser, but the best effects of all were achieved when the two were used in combination. This underlines the fact that laser should not be seen as a single form of therapy but as a valuable means of assistance.

Obata [397] performed "Total Laser Irradiation" on 89 patients. This means that all active inflammatory joints were treated each session until pain relief was observed in all joints. The laser used was a 10 mW 780 nm unit. The erythrocyte sedimentation rate improved by more than 10 mm in 55% of the patients in the 20-session group. Lansbury's index improved by 10% in 47% of the cases. The serum immune-complex tended to decrease and the findings of synovial scintigraphy correlated well with the clinical effects.

Antipa [775] has tried to establish the efficiency of laser therapy in various inflammatory and non-inflammatory rheumatic diseases over a five-year period. 514 patients with osteoarthrosis, 326 patients with nonarticular rheumatism and 82 patients with inflammatory rheumatism were treated. Four different treatment procedures were used: 1) only GaAs; 2) both GaAs and HeNe; 3) placebo laser; and 4) classic anti-inflammatory therapy. The results were analysed using local objective improvements and the score obtained from a pain scale before and after treatment. It was concluded that laser therapy (especially HeNe with GaAs) is more efficient than placebo laser therapy and also yielded better, or at least similar, results in most of the cases than classical anti-inflammatory therapy.

Simunovic [955] reports that patients with osteoarthrosis of joints in the upper extremities had a 70% pain relief and improved function using local irradiation and irradiation of trigger points.

Lerner [826] used a HeNe laser on a group of 33 patients suffering from Mb Bechterew. Irradiation was given over the spine and joints for 20 sessions. 20 patients received laser therapy in combination with 75-100 mg of indomethacin per day, while 13 patients received laser therapy alone due to indomethacin intolerance. Therapeutic efficacy was assessed according to a number of clinico-laboratory indices. The most marked effect was observed in the combination group. The use of laser therapy alone was comparable with using indomethacin at a daily dose of 75 mg.

The double blind study by Gladkova [1078] has a rather negative outcome. However, since doses between 0.004-0.02 J/cm^2 were used, a negative outcome is to be expected.

In a double blind crossover study, Gärtner [199, 568] used GaAs and HeNe lasers to treat stage III-IV ankylosing spondylarthritis. Treatment was given for 20 to 30 minutes daily for 5 consecutive days each week for 3 weeks. Spinal ROM and laboratory tests including CRP and ESP showed no significant changes. However, pain score, morning stiffness and frequency of noctural awakening were significantly reduced. With today's more powerful lasers, the results are likely to improve.

In two meta analyses of osteoarthritis and rheumatoid arthritis Brosseau [1023, 1024, 1154] found a moderate but short term effect for rheumatoid arthritis, enough for recommending the method for clinical purposes. These two studies, however, lack a proper analysis of the dosages used, and the result of using a very low dosage in some studies confuses the true outcome of laser therapy studies. Further, the different wavelengths are "put into the same basket" although it is obvious that they have different effects.

In a meta analysis of the effect of laser therapy for osteoarthritis pain, Bjordal [588] summarises: "A literature search identified 88 randomised-controlled trials, of which 20 trials included patients with osteoarthritis and chronic joint disorders. Five trials were excluded for not irradiating the affected joint capsule. Two trials that reported significant results in favour of active laser were excluded from statistical pooling due to insufficient data presentation and lack of repeated laser irradiation. Of the remaining thirteen trials, five trials reported non-significant results. These five trials used treatment parameters outside our predefined optimal dose range, and their results were significantly poorer ($p<0.001$) than the results from eight trials giving treatment within the optimal dose range. For the 398 patients included in these eight trials, a pooled mean weighted difference of 42.9 % (range 23-62) was registered in favour of active treatment. Adverse effects were few and mild, and unblinded follow-up observations suggested that pain reduction could last for more than one month. With the reservation of possible heterogeneity in the limited patient sample, location-specific doses of laser therapy appear to be effective in reducing pain from mild osteoarthritis." This study underlines the importance of a proper dosage and subgroup analysis, an issue that has been largely overlooked by previous reviewers of laser therapy.

Further literature: [98, 99, 100, 152, 193, 210, 325, 343, 434, 453, 605, 617, 738, 1019, 1020, 1026, 1027, 1055, 1060, 1133, 1139, 1150 and 1166-1172].

4.1.5 Blood pressure

Literature:

Umeda [144] tested the effects of a GaAlAs laser on the control of blood pressure. Radiation was administered via the medulla oblongata. The results from a group of 30 patients suffering from hypertension were excellent in 20% of the cases, good in 37%, fairly good in 23%, and the treatment had no effect in 20%. In a control group of patients with normal blood pressure, no noteworthy results were achieved, except that those bordering on low blood pressure experienced a rise.

Velizhanina [698] used low level laser irradiation as monotherapy in 42 patients with early essential hypertension. Hypotensive and antioxidant effects of laser therapy plus its ability to decrease total peripheral resistance were more pronounced in patients with stage I hypertension.

Further literature: [574, 698, 971, 1166, 1215]

4.1.6 Bone regeneration

The regeneration of bone tissue is of central interest in relation to a great number of operations. Laser therapy is a valuable complement to other methods in this area. All wavelengths have been shown to influence bone regeneration, but as always the penetration of the different wavelengths must be taken into consideration. Repeated irradiation is necessary to keep the process going; a single exposure is not enough. 3-4 sessions per week for two weeks are recommended. It is speculated that the irradiation can biomodulate non-differentiated mesenchymal cells into osteoblasts and osteocytes.

Literature:

Nagasawa [106] describes two experiments on bone regeneration. In the first experiment, holes of 1 mm diameter were drilled in the femurs of 36 rats. The rats were divided into six groups of six. Before suturing, the holes in the femurs of five of the groups were irradiated with one type of laser light per group (Nd:YAG, GaAlAs, HeNe, CO_2, KrF excimer 248 nm). The sixth group was the control and was not treated with a laser. After ten days, the wound area was studied under a microscope. Some osteoclasts were visible in the untreated group, but few samples were spongy and there were few trabeculae. In the Nd:YAG group, active spongy formation could be observed, with visible trabeculae. Similar formations were observed in the GaAlAs and HeNe groups. In the group treated with a carbon dioxide laser, delayed healing was observed, while the excimer laser group showed signs of necrosis. All rats received a 100 J/cm^2 dosage, except the excimer group, in which the dosage was 2 J/cm^2.

The other experiment involved the use of BMP (bone morphogenetic protein). This is a bioactive substance, which participates in bone formation. It exists in osteoblasts and can be stored in an inactive form. Small pellets were made from calf collagen and impregnated with extracted BMP. The dry weight of the pellets was 8 mg. Pellets of this kind were implanted under the skin on the backs of rats. Six rats were treated with 100 J/cm^2 of GaAlAs laser, and six with 50 J/cm^2 of HeNe laser, after the implantation, but before the wound was sutured. A control group of six rats was not treated. After three weeks, all the pellets were removed and weighed, measured and analysed with respect to their content of Ca and P. The average dry weight of the control group's pellets was 11.6 mg, while it was 14.24 mg for the GaAlAs group, and 13.98 mg for the HeNe group. The Ca levels were 0.86 mg (control group), 1.28 mg (GaAlAs), and 1.0 mg (HeNe). The P levels were 1.04, 1.24, and 1.22 respectively. Nagasawa suggested the following explanation of the results: in addition to stimulating BMP, laser therapy also causes undifferentiated mesenchymal cells to change into osteoblasts, by means of which the osteogenetic activity increases.

Nagasawa [107] has also studied the effects of an argon laser used at an output level appropriate for laser therapy. Periapical lesions, which despite conventional endodontics had shown no sign of starting to heal two months after the start of root treatment, were treated with an argon laser (100-400 mW) directly in the root canal. In some cases, the healing process began after a single treatment.

In an *in vitro study*, Yamada [414] irradiated cultured osteoblastic cells with a HeNe laser. The cell growth rate and DNA synthesis were increased only in the growing phase of culture. During long-term culture, calcium accumulation was enhanced by laser irradiation at 1 J/cm^2, with four sessions of irradiation resulting in a 46% increase over the control. Alkaline phosphatase activity, however, was unchanged.

Ozawa [369] studied the effect of GaAlAs on bone formation *in vitro*. Osteoblast-like cells were isolated from rat calvariae of 21d rat foetuses. The cultivated cells were irradiated one time only or once a day for 21 days at various energy doses (10.8-108 J/cm^2 per day). The total area of mineralised bone nodules on day 21 was evaluated. DNA content, alkaline phosphatase activity (ALP), and the amount of extracellular collagen were also measured. Laser therapy significantly increased the number and the total area of bone nodules in a dose-dependent manner. Cell proliferation and ALP activity were higher in the early and middle culture periods, while the collagen content was higher in the middle and late periods as compared to controls. Calcium and phosphorus were both higher in the irradiation groups.

Trelles [108] studied the effects of a HeNe laser on bone fractures (of the tibia) in mice. 2.4 J was administered to one point. The fracture was treated every other day for three weeks. The healing process was studied under an electron microscope. From a histological point of view, the laser group exhibited better healing characteristics than the control group, which was not treated with a laser. The laser group also showed increased vascularisation and faster formation of bone tissue with a tighter mesh of trabeculae. The control group showed poorer vascularisation and more cartilage tissue.

David [942] failed to verify these findings using 0, 2 or 4 J every other day for 2 to 6 weeks.

Luger [536] subjected 50 Wistar rats to tibial bone fracture with internal fixation. 25 animals were treated with a HeNe laser, 35 mW transcutaneously 30 minutes daily for two weeks. The other 25 animals served as the control. After four weeks the maximal load at failure (MLF), the structural stiffness of the tibia (SST), and the extension maximal load (EML) were measured. The MLF and the SST were found to be significantly elevated, whereas the EML was reduced. Four non-unions were found in the control group, none in the irradiated group.

Lomnitski [179] studied reparative osteogenesis in 105 rabbits. The healing of drilled cavity defects in the mandibles stimulated with HeNe laser light of various powers was monitored using a histological method, and the distinctive reparative effects of the laser light were evaluated.

Yaakobi [87] made holes in the tibias of rats. HeNe laser irradiation on days 5 and 6 post-injury increased calcium accumulation twofold compared to control. Osteoblastic activity increased, too, as reflected by alkaline phosphatase activity.

Horowitz [473] performed calvarial trepanations in 18 rats. HeNe laser light was applied every day for two weeks. Through infrared spectroscopy the following parameters were found to have improved compared with the control group: 1) amount of mineralisation, 2) factor of conformation, 3) protein to lipid ratio, 4) structural stage.

Saito [569] expanded the midpalatal suture in rats. A 100 mW GaAlAs laser was used to influence bone regeneration. Irradiation during the two first postoperative days was effective, accelerating regeneration by a factor of 1.2 to 1.4 compared to the control group. Irradiation in the late period (days 4 to 6) was not effective, neither was a single irradiation.

Pyczek [832] studied the effect of low power laser light on the haematopoietic system of rats and also on the basic haematological parameters. A 5 mW HeNe and an 80 mW GaAs laser were used. Intact skin on the hind legs of rats was exposed over a section of the femur. Peripheral blood analysis was carried out before and after the experiments. These indicated that GaAs laser light induced a decrease in bone marrow mastocytes and peripheral blood basophils with an increase in the number of eosinophils. An increase in mitotic activity in the bone marrow was observed in the exposed groups of animals. No significant changes in Hb, Ht, erythrocyte or reticulocyte levels in the peripheral blood were noted, nor was there an increase in megakaryocyte emperipolesis.

The results of the rat study by Ozawa [1011] suggest that laser irradiation may play two principal roles in stimulating bone formation. One is stimulation of cellular proliferation, especially proliferation of nodule-forming cells of osteoblast lineage, and the other is stimulation of cellular differentiation, especially to committed precursors, resulting in an increase in the number of more differentiated osteoblastic cells and an increase in bone formation. The two processes can only be stimulated through laser irradiation of immature cells.

Gordjestani [1271] failed to find any stimulatory effect of bone regeneration in a rat experiment. Although this study was well designed, the dose was too high. The artificially created bony defects in the parietal bone were irradiated though the rat fur every day for 28 consecutive days with a dose of 20 J/cm^2 and a power density of 33.3 mW/cm^2. The laser used was a GaAs laser and it is generally recognised that dosage with this type of laser should be kept lower than for GaAlAs.

Akai [466] studied the influence of 810 nm laser on bone and cartilage during joint immobilisation of rats' knee models. The hind limbs of 42 young Wistar rats were operated on in order to immobilise the knee joint. They were assigned to three groups 1 week after operation; irradiance 3.9 W/cm^2, 5.8 W/cm^2, and sham treatment. After 6 sessions of treatment for another 2 weeks both hind legs were prepared for 1) indentation of the articular surface of the knee (stiffness and loss tangent), and for 2) dual energy X-ray absorptiometry (bone mineral density) of the focused regions. The indentation test revealed preservation of articular cartilage stiffness with 3.9 and 5.8 W/cm^2 therapy. Laser therapy may possibly prevent biomechanical changes by immobilisation.

In the study by Ueda [1181] osteoblastic cells isolated from fetal rat calvariae were irradiated once with a low-power GaAlAs laser (830 nm, 500 mW) in two different irradiation modes; continuous irradiation (CI), and 1 Hz pulsed irradiation (PI). The authors then investigated the effects on cellular proliferation, bone nodule formation, alkaline phosphatase (ALP) activity, and ALP gene expression. Laser irradiation in both groups significantly stimulated cellular proliferation, bone nodule formation, ALP activity, and ALP gene expression, as compared with the nonirradiation group. Notably, PI markedly stimulated these factors when compared with the CI group. Since 1 Hz pulsed laser irradiation significantly stimulates bone formation *in vitro*, it is most likely that pulse frequency is an important factor affecting biological responses in bone formation.

The aim of the work by Lizarelli [914] was to evaluate histometrically the effect of irradiation with GaAlAs, 790 nm laser in the chronology of alveolar repair of rats. Groups of five animals had their upper right incisors extracted under anaesthesia and the mucous sutured; three groups received 1.5 J/cm^2 of irradiation immediately after the extraction with laser sweeping over the operated area. After that, the animals were sacrificed at 7, 14 and 21 days after the dental extraction. The material was decalcified and processed for inclusion in paraffin. Longitudinal sections of 7 micrometers in the alveolus were made and stained with HE and the percentage of the bone tissue was assessed. The results show that laser therapy produced acceleration in osseous formation (10%) in some periods. The influence of laser irradiation on the healing process is more significant when we can apply the laser light just after the tissue trauma. Cells with a lower than normal pH, where the redox state is shifted in the reduced direction, are considered to be more sensitive to the stimulative action of light than those in which the respective parameters are optimal or near optimal. The proposed redox-regulation mechanism may be a fundamental explanation of some clinical effects of irradiation. A consequence of this is that the difference between the groups at 7 days is more significant than between the other groups.

In a clinical study by Kucerová [1042] the bone density after extraction was measured by digital X-ray. The images immediately after extraction and at 6 months were compared in laser and non-laser patients. There was no difference between these patients at 6 months. This is hardly surprising, since the remodelling of bone is more or less complete after 6 months, laser or no laser. Comparison at 2, 3 and 4 months would be more appropriate in order to determine the possible effect of laser therapy.

Pinheiro [1128] evaluated morphometrically the amount of newly formed bone after 830 nm laser irradiation of surgical wounds created in the femur of rats. 48 Wistar rats were divided into four groups with 12 animals in each group. Group A received 4.8 J/cm^2 transcutaneously, three times a week, sacrificed after 28 days. Group C received only three sessions and was sacrificed after 7 days. Group B and D served as control. There was a significant difference between group C and control but not between A and control.

Nicolau [1262] performed a similar study with 660 nm, 10 J/cm^2 on the 2nd, 4th, 6th and 8th day after surgery (DAS). The animals were sacrificed on day 5, 15 and 25. A significant difference between control and laser animals was noted with regard to resorption and formation indexes, especially during the initial phase of repair. Bone volume was significantly higher on 15 DAS and the mineral apposition rate was significantly higher in the laser group. At 25 DAS both groups had a decreased bone remodulation, although the index in the treated group was higher.

A review of the literature on laser bone stimulation has been published by Barber [1253].

Further literature: [213, 258, 413, 414, 430, 437, 438, 439, 440, 466, 484, 516, 642, 962, 1117, 1194, 1238].

4.1.7 Cancer

As explained previously, laser therapy does not cause cancer. There are, on the contrary, indications that cancer tumours in their initial stage can be positively influenced (i.e. to the patient's benefit) by laser therapy. The mechanism at work here is thought to be the general stimulation of the immune system. In the same way as bacteria and viruses, cancer cells can be stimulated *in vitro* [594] but not (in practice) *in vivo*.

Laser therapy has also been shown to ease the symptoms of cancer patients who have received drugs and/or radiation therapy giving oral side-effects (mucositis). This is an example of the use of laser therapy in oncology where the cancer itself is not treated but rather the side effects of the cancer therapy [907, 967]. Laser therapy can also, to advantage, be given as a palliative measure to cancer patients in the terminal stage.

Recent and ongoing research [986, 1081] has shown that very low doses of irradiation, ionising as well as non-ionising, can protect the cells if the low-dose irradiation is given prior to radiation therapy.

It should, again, be underlined that cancer therapy is the sole right of the specialist.

Literature:

Tamachi [44] has, in various experiments using rats, studied the uptake of 5Fluorouracil (5FU). Laboratory rats that received 6 J/cm^2 of HeNe showed a greater uptake of 5FU than those that were given 5FU only.

Konchugova [214] studied whether laser therapy, under experimental conditions, could be used to increase cyclophosphamide-developed immune suppression. The experiment suggests that laser therapy can be used to reduce the therapeutic dosage and its consequent negative side effects.

Schaffer [594] irradiated four cell cultures with 805 nm laser light with fluences between 0 and 20 J/cm^2. The cell types were (1) murine skeletal myotubes, (2) normal urothelial cells, (3) human squamous carcinoma cells of the gingival mucosa, and (4) urothelial carcinoma cells. The mitotic index of 1, 2, and 4 increased at a fluence of 4 J/cm^2, whereas a fluence of 20 J/cm^2 resulted in a slight decrease. The no. 3 cell culture showed a decrease of the mitotic index at both fluences. No differences could be observed at irradiances between 10 mW/cm^2 and 150 mW/cm^2.

78 years old patient treated for oropharyngeal carcinoma with external radiotherapy (Cobalt). Acute grade 3 dermatitis at 60 Gy (5 x 2 Gy per week). The same patient after 3 sessions of HeNe irradiation, 25 mW, 4 J/cm^2 in scanning mode.

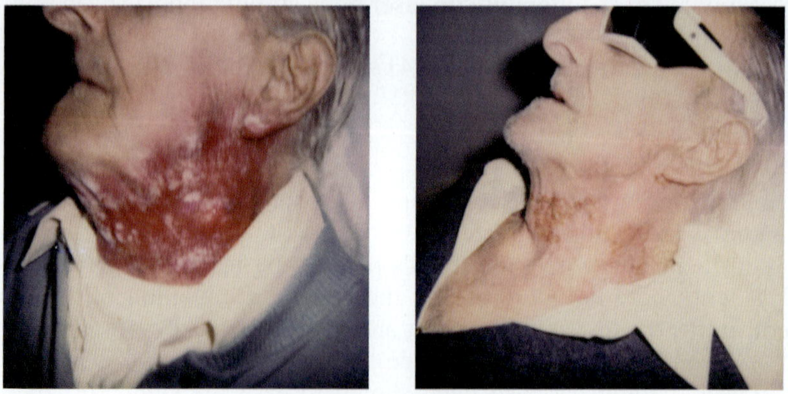

Figure 4.1 Oropharyngeal carcinoma
Courtesy: René-Jean Bensadoun

The aim of a study by Pinheiro [1211] was to assess the effect of 635 and 670-nm laser irradiation on H.Ep.2 cells *in vitro* using MTT. It was decided to evaluate the effect of increased doses of laser light on these cells. The cells were obtained from SCC of the larynx. The cultures were kept either at 5% or 10% of FBS. Twenty-four hours after transplantation, the cells were irradiated with laser light (5 mW diode lasers; 635 and 670 nm; beam cross section 1 mm at local light doses between 0.04 and 4.8 J/cm^2. For 670 nm, significant differences in the proliferation were observed between the two concentrations of FBS and between irradiated cultures and controls. Although the results were not significant, 635 nm irradiated cells also proliferated more than non-irradiated ones. This occurred under both conditions of nutrition. It was concluded, that irradiation with 670 nm laser light applied at doses between 0.04 and 4.8 J/cm^2 could significantly increase proliferation of laryngeal cancer cells.

Ulrich [489] summarises a rodent experiment: 1. Single doses of 830 nm light (1J and 100 J/cm^2) do not stimulate or inhibit growth of rhabdomyosarcomas R1H. 2. Fractionated treatment of R1H tumours with 15 or 1500 J/cm^2 for 3 weeks does not alter the growth kinetics in comparison to untreated controls. 3. Histological findings showed an increase of tumour necrosis after fractionated irradiation with 1500 J/cm^2.

In a study by Pavlova [774] the main goal was to establish the capability of laser to oppose the free radical oxidative chain reactions inherent in the effects of radiation. Adequate doses of laser were shown to produce positive effects upon the metabolism similar to those of pharmacologic radioprotectors.

Mikhailov [3] states that an 890 nm diode laser produces a tumorostatic effect at minimal power, while higher doses produce different effects.

Humzah [286] has used GaAs in cases of neoplastic ulceration with some response.

Podolskaya [366] has used HeNe lasers on post-radiation reactions and injuries in lip skin and mucous membranes (post-radiation heilitis). The method has been more successful than previously used medical treatments. There were no complications in the laser group, while the traditionally treated group had several allergic reactions and reoperations. The pace of epithelialisation was 7 mm/week in the HeNe group, as compared with 4.1 mm/week in the control group.

Pourreau-Schneider [46] used a HeNe laser to reduce the oral side-effects of fluorouracil. The drug causes painful mucositis, which in turn causes eating problems. The mucositis dictates the limit for the dosage of fluorouracil (dose limiting factor). The use of a HeNe laser was shown to reduce discomfort to a great extent, and administering laser therapy prophylactically before the treatment could also alleviate the problems.

Cowen [575] used a helium-neon laser in the prevention of oral mucositis in patients undergoing bone marrow transplant in a double-blind randomized trial. Significant reduction of the radiation-induced oral mucositis was reported using a 60 mW HeNe laser.

Barasch [611] treated 20 patients subjected to bone marrow transplantation and receiving mucositis-inducing medications. One side of the mouth received HeNe laser irradiation, the other one sham irradiation. Oral mucositis and pain scores were significantly lower for the treated side compared with the untreated side.

In the double blind study by Bensadoun [929], 30 patients were about to receive radiotherapy for head and neck neoplasms. With conventional fractionation (2 Gy/day, 5 fractions per week), mucositis becomes evident in the third week of irradiation and progresses to confluent mucositis. The severity of mucositis is a major problem in head and neck radiotherapy. In this study, patients in the laser group received HeNe laser irradiation daily

(Monday to Friday) during the seven weeks of radiotherapy, prior to each fraction. Nine points in the oropharyngeal area were irradiated, 2 J/cm^2. Except for the first week of treatment, daily grade of mucositis was higher in the non-laser group, the difference being statistically significant for weeks 4, 5, 6 and 7. In particular, the number of weeks in which patients had grade 3 mucositis was reduced. Pain and the ability to swallow were also improved in the laser group.

Migliorati [1195] used 780 nm 60 mW, 2 J/cm^2 in a group of 11 patients receiving high-dose chemotherapy and could confirm the pain relieving effect of laser therapy for this indication.

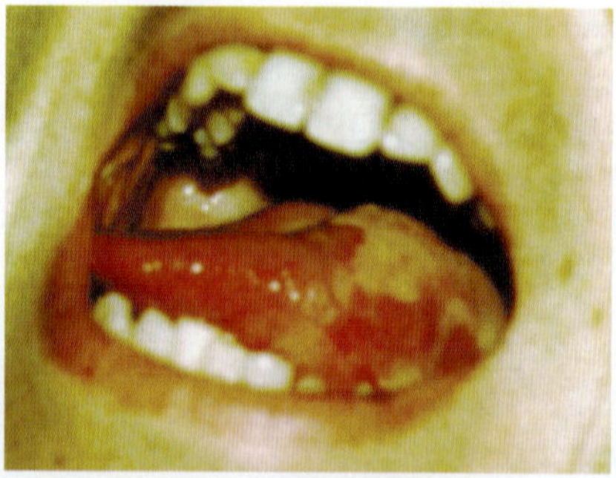

Figure 4.2 Typical mucositis
Courtesy: René-Jean Bensadoun

The study by Balakirev [1212] suggests that the application of laser therapy makes it possible to reduce the time needed for the management of radiation injury and chemotherapy complications in paediatric patients 1.5-2-fold. It was shown that exposure to laser caused mononuclear levels of donors' blood to rise, which in turn led to release, in higher concentrations, of IL-1 and FNO cytokins, major factors of immune response development.

The study by Durnov [1213] outlines the outcomes of treatment for complications associated with chemo- and radiation therapy in children with malignant neoplasms by using laser radiation. The use of this therapy may reduce the duration of the treatment of these complications by 1.5-2 times. The use of therapeutic laser radiation in the treatment of other complications that are common in paediatric oncological care is briefly described.

The study by Korolev [1214] showed that exposure of the rat adrenals 30 days after radiation (1 Gy) to infrared laser radiation arrested the development of ultrastructural disorders in the cells of the hypothalamus and the parathyroid gland and enhanced subcellular manifestations of adaptation and rehabilitation processes.

Joyce [1016] has investigated the potential ability of laser therapy to induce an adaptive response against the damaging effects of ionising radiation in Indian muntjac fibroblasts. Laser therapy at 660, but not 820 nm, at 11.5 and 23.0 J/cm^2, induced an apparent adaptive response in the form of a reduction in the frequency of radiation-induced chromosome aberrations, but not in cell survival. There was also a trend towards a reduction in the level of single-stranded and double-stranded DNA breaks induced by ionising radiation when cells were preconditioned with laser therapy. However, this did not contribute to the reduced chromosome aberration frequency. Further analysis revealed that the reduced aberration frequency was caused by a laser-induced extension of G2 delay. The adaptive response was therefore the result of cell cycle modulation by laser therapy at a wavelength where there is no known DNA damaging effect to induce the checkpoint mechanisms that are normally responsible for altering cell cycle progression.

Further literature: [1, 2, 3, 47, 371, 564, 978, 979, 980, 1072, 1073, 1076, 1176]

4.1.8 Cardiac conditions

A number of studies report on the use of HeNe laser in cardiac surgery.

Literature:

Kipshidze [717] reports that a single endoluminal irradiation with HeNe (1.8 J) prevents restenosis after balloon angioplasty in an atherosclerotic rabbit model.

Kipshidze [1124] reports that HeNe laser can influence the vascular endothelian growth factor and profileration of human endothelial cells *in vitro*. These data may have significant importance, leading to the establishment of new methods for endoluminal postangioplasty vascular repair and myocardial photoangiogenesis.

Kipshidze [344] reports further promising results in the treatment of acute myocardial infarction by guiding HeNe laser light into the heart cavity.

Itoh [723] has demonstrated that HeNe laser has a protective effect on the type of damage to the erythrocytes caused by heart-lung machines.

Lee [752] successfully used laser therapy for relief of cervicothoracic pain syndromes.

Oron [1097] found that 803 nm laser therapy reduced the formation of scar tissue following experimentally induced ischemic myocardial infarction in rats and dogs. Following the induction of the infarction, the dogs (24 in experimental group, 24 in control group) received laser irradiation epicardially with a dose of 1.08 J/cm^2. At 5-6 weeks postop. the dogs were sacrificed and infarction size was determined by TTC staining and histology. The infarct size in the laser group was reduced by 52% as compared to the control group. Catalase enzymatic activity (antioxidant marker) was higher in the laser group. The results were confirmed in a separate study of 83 rats. In this experiment, the left ventricular dilatation was also reduced by 50-60% in the laser group.

Yaakov [1197] has studied the effect of 804 nm laser on the interstitial scarring in the hearts of rats subjected to experimental heart hypertrophy. The rats were injected with isoproternol (ISO), a substance known to induce hypertrophy without marked mortality rate in the rat's heart. A careful dosage analysis was performed, resulting in a measured power of 5 mW near the heart and a power density of 4.5 mW/cm^2 on the myocardium. ISO treatment resulted in an 11% increase in hypertrophy, which was not altered by laser irradiation. However, a 57% reduction in interstitial scarring in the myocardium was evident in laser-irradiated rats as compared to non-irradiated rats.

De Scheerder [968] has used HeNe laser as an adjunct in coronary stent implantation. The preliminary results suggest that laser therapy results in a decrease of in-stent restenosis when used during primary stenting.

Infrared irradiation of the skin applied to the projections of the heart and its reflexogenic areas is also reported by other authors to be successful. There are many Russian reports on intravascular HeNe irradiation as a treatment modality for patients with heart infarction or other ischemic heart diseases. Reported effects include reduced need of nitroglycerine tablets, decreased number of angina attacks, alleviation of pain, suppression of lipid peroxidation, promotion of antioxidant protection of erythrocyte membranes, reduction of fibrinogen level, normalization of antithrombin-III, reduction of arrhythmic deaths as of two-year check-up, reduction of the activities of the hypophyseoadrenocortical and aldosteron-renin-angiotensin systems. 3-5 sessions of 30-40 minutes are frequently used.

Further literature: [408, 426, 905, 952, 991, 992, 993, 1124, 1125, 1198, 1199]

4.1.9 Carpal tunnel syndrome

Repetitive stress movements cause the Carpal Tunnel Syndrome (CTS), which is a debilitating condition causing many problems for employers and employees in industry and offices.

Laser therapy is a valuable complementary treatment modality for this group of patients. However, a correct diagnosis is necessary. For instance, carpal tunnel symptoms caused by pseudoradicular irritation from the C5-C6 region will not respond to irradiation over the carpal area. Patients could, on the other hand, be irradiated in this very area according to Wong [539, see below], if venous compression in the axilla is the cause of the symptoms, since local irradiation over the compressed area in combination with exercise will then be successful. If the carpal area has become very fibrotic, surgery is the only alternative. Under such conditions laser therapy will only give a transient pain release and reduction of oedema. Complete remission of the symptoms will only be achieved in the earlier phases of the syndrome and in combination with exercise and a change of the working conditions.

4-6 J per point over the area in question is recommended. As for many other conditions, the diversity of success in reports on laser therapy on carpal tunnel syndrome may depend on the inclusion criteria, i.e. the stage of the condition.

Laser therapy of CTS was one of the first indications to receive an FDA approval. This approval is limited to "adjunct use" for obtaining temporary relief of pain associated with CTS [1207].

Literature:

Weintraub [538], investigated whether repeated laser light exposure directed at the median nerve could reverse the symptoms and electro-physiological latencies in CTS. The study covered 30 hands displaying moderate to severe CTS. A low power, continuous GaAlAs laser was percutaneously applied at 33 second intervals to five points along the median nerve delivering 9 joules/point without discomfort or heat emission. Complete resolution of pre-treatment symptoms and abnormal physical findings was achieved in 77% of cases. Nocturnal complaints were the earliest symptom to disappear, followed by tingling, stiffness and weakness. Normalisation of distal latency was achieved in 11 CTS with a further tendency towards improvement in 23.4%. Work status was maintained with no new interventions, and after completion of the treatment trial 11 patients resumed previously impossible activities.

Wong [539] observed that CTS patients have poor posture. Upon palpation, they have pain and tenderness at the spinous processes C5-T1 and the medial angle of the scapula. In 35 such patients, treatment was focused primarily on the posterior neck area and not the wrists and hands. A 100 mW GaAlAs laser was used and directed at the tips of the aforementioned spinous processes. The laser rapidly alleviated pain and tingling in the arms, hands and fingers.

Roig [893] treated 20 patients with carpal tunnel problems with a GaAs/HeNe laser, 3.6 J/cm^2. 20 consecutive sessions, each lasting for 10 minutes, were given. At the end of treatment the outcome for pain and paraesthesia was: complete remission 7 patients, partial remission 8, no improvement 5. As for loss of muscle strength the outcome was: complete recovery 10 patients, partial recovery 5, no improvement 5.

Yu [192] treated car assembly-line workers with good results using a100 mW GaAlAs laser.

Padua [937] compared the effect of 830 nm three-diode laser therapy on primary carpal tunnel syndrome in 17 patients. Neurophysiological parameters and a patient questionnaire were used to evaluate the outcome. Immediately after therapy and at 15 days post therapy there was a positive effect, but at 2 and 12 months follow-up almost all parameters had progressively returned to the pre-treatment pattern and were similar to those of an untreated group.

Further literature: [661, 1152]

4.1.10 Cerebral palsy

Literature:

Asagai [660] reports on the use of GaAlAs (100 mW) laser treatment in a group of 1000 patients with cerebral palsy. The laser reduced muscle spasm and increased the mobility of the muscles. Although the duration of the laser therapy effect was limited to one to several hours, it can be applied in conjunction with conventional functional therapies, thereby enhancing the effects of the latter.

4.1.11 Crural and venous ulcers

Bedsores are common among bedridden patients. HeNe and GaAs lasers have been shown to be valuable in the combined treatment of crural ulcers. Treatment is time-consuming, so scanners are useful. However, point treatment should be given around the dermal periphery of the wound in combination with full-wound scanning. Power output on the open wound should be lower than on the skin.

Literature:

Rakcheev [557] carried out an animal study on 60 guinea pigs and 110 rabbits using HeNe laser on experimental trophic ulcers. As a good effect was achieved at 0.75 J/cm², a successful clinical study was performed on 56 humans.

Skoric [553] administered 1 J/cm² twice a week for seven weeks to ten patients with ulcus cruris. Complete epithelialisation was obtained in four patients, and in all other patients the ulcers became smaller (minimal 4%, maximal 52%).

Bihari [13] treated three groups of patients with crural ulcers, each group consisting of five patients. Group 1 received HeNe laser light, group 2 HeNe and GaAs in combination, and group 3 noncoherent unpolarised red light. Groups 1 and 2 showed excellent healing, with group 2 slightly better than group 1. Healing in group 3 was poor. The study was double-blind.

Lievens [352] treated ten patients aged 65-90 years, all with crural ulcers. In combination with classic treatment, they received GaAs laser light daily for 3 months. There was a statistically significant reduction in pain, wound surface, and inflammatory symptoms.

Sugrue [556] used infrared laser irradiation in a group of 12 patients with chronic venous ulcers unresponsive to conservative measures. The ulcers were treated for twelve weeks. Two ulcers healed completely and there was a 27% reduction in the other ulcers, 44% in the entire group. The most dramatic effect of laser therapy was the reduction of ulcer pain, from 7.5 to 3.5 on a VAS scale.

Soriano [559] treated 25 patients, average age 67 years, with therapy-resistant leg ulcers. GaAs laser light at 3 J/cm² was administered three days a week for a maximum of 16 weeks. The average treatment time was 10 weeks. 76% of the patients were completely healed, with the best results in the female group. There was a partial response in 8% and a poor response in 16%. Laser therapy was used in parallel with traditional treatment.

In a study extended over 6 years, Soriano [678] treated 231 patients with venous leg ulcers. The exclusion criteria were diabetes, arterial disease, vasculitis, congestive heart failure and loss of follow up at 6 months. 122 of 154 patients in the laser group and 46 of 77 patients in the control group (traditional treatment only) completed the study. Wounds were all of Size Rate 4 or larger (diameter major + diameter minor). A 40 mW GaAs laser at 10 000 Hz was used. The laser was applied with the point technique at 3 J/cm² per point around the border and onto the bed of the ulcer in non-contact. Three sessions a week were performed for 4 months, or until the ulcer was completely healed. The results were evaluated as complete healing, partial healing (more than 50%) or non-healing (less than 50%). In the laser group there was a 70% healing rate and a 14% rate of partial healing. In the control group 26% of the patients had complete healing and 22% partial healing. In the laser group, only 19% of the ulcers of great size (>16) healed completely, and if the wound was more than one year old the rate of complete healing was 40%. Wounds with an oedema failed to heal with the parameters used. In the opinion of the authors of this book the GaAs doses over open wounds used in this study are very high.

55 patients with long lasting chronic venous ulcers, suffering for more than 6 months without improvement, were treated with laser therapy by Lichtenstein [677, 1095]. 42 patients were treated with HeNe laser, 13 with 780 nm GaAlAs laser. The follow-up ranged from 6 months to 6 years. Wound closure was achieved after 7 to 40 treatments in most of the patients. Complete healing was achieved in 47 patients and moderate improvement in 4 patients. Laser therapy was used in parallel with traditional treatment.

Georgadze [558] treated 351 patients with persistent wounds and trophic ulcers in an outpatient clinic. Complete epithelialisation occurred in 236 patients.

Santoianni [560], however, found no effect of HeNe laser at 1 or 4 J/cm^2 on venous leg ulcers, as compared to a control group receiving only antiseptic local compresses.

In a study by Lundeberg and Malm [612], a 6 mW HeNe laser was used to treat leg ulcers, the stated dose being 4 J/cm^2. The area of the ulcers varied from 3 cm^2 to 32 cm^2, and to achieve the stated dose the period of therapy would thus have had had to vary from 33 minutes to 6 hours per session. The method by which the dose was calculated is therefore questionable. No indication is given of the method of treatment. If a scanning laser with an unexpanded beam was used, the power density would have been about 0.15 W/cm^2. If the beam was expanded to a diameter capable of illuminating the whole area of the ulcer at once, the power density when treating the largest ulcer would have been about 0.00019 W/cm^2, which is close to the level of moonlight when the moon is full. Unless all the parameters are accounted for, it is impossible to evaluate this study.

The same authors [613] also examined the effect of a GaAs laser on venous ulcers. The parameters stated in the report are: "The wavelength was 904 nm, average output 4 mW, peak power 10 W, pulse frequency 3800 Hz and duration 180 ns, and divergence 70 mrad. Energy density was 1.96 J/cm^2."

- First of all, the stated energy density must obviously be wrong as the treatment time was said to be 10 minutes per patient regardless of wound size. Wound size in the laser group was in the range 4-52 cm^2 (average 12 cm^2).

- Secondly, from the stated parameters, it is easy to calculate the average output power of the laser to be 6.84 mW, which in 10 minutes would give a total energy level of 4.1 J. For the smallest wound, this would mean 1 J/cm^2, and for the largest, 0.079 J/cm^2. The stated figure of 1.96 J/cm^2 cannot be correct. And since each ulcer received a different dosage (ranging, for GaAs, from the rather high to the very low), doubt is cast on the whole report. Further, according the manufacturer of the laser equipment (Irradia AB, Stockholm), a pulse frequency of 3,800 Hz is not available with any of their equipment.

The two studies above have been used in a Cochrane literature review. In all, 4 randomised studies were found, two positive and two negative. With the shortcomings of the two studies above in mind, such an evaluation has little substance. (See chapter 13.4 “The Cochrane analyses – can they be improved?” on page 412.)

Recently a single blind randomised study on stage III pressure ulcers has been presented by Lucas [943] using a 904 nm multi array with 12 diodes of 8 mW each. An energy density of 1 J/cm^2 was obtained. The same array was used for all ulcers, regardless of size. There was no statistical difference between the laser group and the control group.

In a study by Telfer [776] laser therapy was used to treat chronic leg ulcers. Seven patients with 11 leg ulcers were referred for laser therapy by plastic surgeons. They had a history of ulceration of 3 - 50 years and five of the patients had breakdown of previous skin grafts. Laser treatment was administered with 660 nm , 4-6 J/cm^2 and 880 nm, 4 - 8 J/cm^2. The patients were treated three to five times per week, 25 - 30 times per course. Three patients underwent two courses of laser therapy with a three week interval. All patients had relief of pain after 5 - 10 treatment sessions and decreased the amount of analgesics used. All ulcers in six patients were completely healed and two ulcers in a seventh patient decreased in size by 75%.

Further literature: [829, 934]

4.1.12 Depression, psychosomatic problems

Literature

From a large population of over 5000 chronic pain patients during a 70 month period, Shiroto [844] chose 1800 seriously affected patients to participate in an elective written questionnaire in addition to the usual oral pain removal assessment session. The longer-term, more chronically affected patients, because of the nature and history of their complaint, tend to exhibit less of the placebo effect than less-affected chronic, sub acute or acute pain patients. The laser used was a GaAlAs diode system, 60 mW output, 830 nm, continuous wave, and was used in the contact pressure technique. The questionnaire contained a set of questions on psychological effects following laser therapy in addition to the usual pain removal questions. The questionnaire was sent by post 4 weeks after the final treatment session. 752 patients responded. 67.7% of the respondents reported an improvement in general well-being; 60.2% reported increased physical energy; and 56.4% reported improved sleep. 47.5% and 41.5% reported increased emotional stability and improved mental vigour respectively.

The results indicate that, in addition to its effective removal of pain (76%), laser therapy has a strong systemic psychosomatic effect, which is possibly not attributable to the placebo effect, in the longer-term chronic pain patient.

The authors believe that the mechanism here may be the same as in BLT (Bright Light Treatment) of seasonal depressions; See chapter 11.1.6 "Bright Light Phototherapy" on page 345.

4.1.13 Diabetes

In some literature diabetes can be found as a contraindication for laser therapy. On the contrary, laser therapy can be used to advantage! The circulatory problems of diabetic patients are a great challenge. Schindl [145, 478, 552] has demonstrated the effectiveness of HeNe laser treatment of limbs with circulatory disorders.

Literature:

Yu [528] used an argon dye laser at a wavelength of 630 nm, 20 mW/cm^2, to treat experimental wounds in diabetic mice. Histological evaluation showed that laser therapy improved wound epithelialisation, cellular content, granulation tissue formation and collagen deposition as compared with the negative control group.

In a wound healing study on diabetic rats by Reddy [657] the following conclusions were made: 1) the GaAs laser therapy had no apparent systemic effect on the wound of the side opposite to the treated side, and 2) laser photostimulation decreased the healing time for full thickness skin wounds in diabetic animals but had no effect on the biomechanical properties of the tissue once the wound had healed.

Schindl [1136] presents a study aimed at evaluating the possible protective effect of laser therapy against high glucose-induced delay in proliferation of human endothelial cells. Human umbilical vein endothelian cells were cultured with either standard or elevated concentrations of glucose and were irradiated with a 670 nm diode laser. Irradiation was performed every other day for one week. Cell proliferation was evaluated on days 2, 4 and 7. The results demonstrated a dose-dependent protective effect of laser irradiation on high glucose-induced reduction of cell counts on day 7. These data provide further evidence for a beneficial effect of laser therapy for patients with diabetic microangiopathy.

In a double-blind placebo-controlled study, Schindl [552] gave a single dose of 30 J/cm^2 of HeNe light to 15 patients with diabetic micro-angiopathy. Following a single transcutaneous irradiation, a statistically significant rise in skin temperature was recorded through infrared thermography. In the sham irradiated group there was a small but significant drop in temperature.

In a case report by Sasaki [913] a patient with thromboangitis obliterans (Bürger's disease) was treated with a 60 mW, 830 nm laser and a defocused 20 W, Nd:YAG laser. Ulcers were remarkably improved. Agonising pain and ischemia were relieved. In the MRA findings, sudden arterial obliteration disappeared. In the thermographical findings, skin temperature increased to normal.

Grubnik [527] used HeNe laser irradiation in a group of patients with diabetic gangrene. During the amputation of the lower limb, intravenous HeNe was given. Percutaneous irradiation was applied after the operation. Laser therapy improved healing as compared to a group of similar size where no laser was applied.

Zubkova [526] reports that HeNe laser light successfully promoted healing in diabetic patients with trophic skin disorders such as ulcer, diabetic bulla, haematoma and skin chap.

Koslov [566] used laser dopplerography, TV capillaroscopy, and polarography of transcutaneous oxygen tension to study microcirculation. Patients with stage II and III arterial ischemia in the feet were studied. Laser therapy at 890 nm increased microcirculation.

In a study by Landau [658] 50 patients with chronic diabetes foot ulcers were treated with topical hyperbaric oxygen alone (15 patients) or in combination with laser therapy. 43 of the patients were cured of ulcers.

Further literature [1080, 1178, 1179, 1185, 1203, 1275]

4.1.14 Duodenal/gastric ulcer

HeNe laser treatment of duodenal ulcers using a gastroscope has been reported in at least 25 Russian studies. With the arrival of successful pharmaceutical treatment, these findings may no longer be as attractive as previously but still demonstrate the healing effect of HeNe on mucosa.

Literature:

Garkavoy [339] treated 622 patients with gastric and duodenal ulcers with a HeNe laser through a gastroscope. The treatment was administered with a power of 12 mW for 3-5 minutes a session. The healing rate of duodenal ulcers was 91% and of gastric ulcers 93% by the end of the eighth week.

Millson [708] reports that laser light in combination with different photosensitisers can kill Helicobacter pylori. Laser light or photosensitisers alone had no effect.

4.1.15 Epicondylitis

Epicondylitis is known to be a difficult-to-treat condition. Laser therapy has in the past often been used as a "last resort" and has thus been tried on the most difficult cases. But laser therapy should be one of the first treatment modalities to be used. If not sufficiently successful, others should be added in combination with continued laser therapy. All wavelengths can be used, since the condition is fairly superficial, but in our experience GaAs seems to work best. It is important to treat not only the local condition but to start treatment in the area of the shoulder joint according to the principle of "proximal priority" (see page 176).

Literature:

Some early studies were negative [230, 231], but in these cases acupuncture points and/or local points and very low doses were used. The same authors [208] later achieved promising results using local points at 3.6 J per point, but in non-contact mode. Positive findings were also reported in the early literature by Gudmundsen [242].

More recent studies using higher doses in combination with trigger points have yielded more favourable results. In a two-centre study, Simunovic [607] treated 324 patients, 50 with epicondylitis ulnaris and 274 with epicondylitis radialis. 32% of the patients were acute and 68% chronic cases. All patients had previously been treated with various methods such as TENS, supersonic vibrations, drugs and surgery. The patients were divided into three treatment groups. One received 830 nm on trigger points only, the second was treated only with the scanner, and the third group received combined treatment. The third group was the most successful. In the three groups together, complete relief of pain and restored functional ability were achieved in 82% of the acute patients and 66% in the chronic cases. One centre had more powerful lasers available. Though the same doses were used at both centres, this latter group was slightly more successful. 41 patients with bilateral problems were selected for a cross-over study. Minimal dose in unilateral cases was 20 J, which could be increased step-by-step up to 60 J.

Simunovic [1134] has also compared laser and visible incoherent polarised light in the treatment of epicondylitis, given over 12 sessions. 40% of the patients in the laser group obtained 100% pain relief. In the non-coherent group there was a maximal pain relief of 70%.

The negative outcome in the study by Krasheninnkoff [1188] might be explained by rather high a dose for this superficial condition (13.2 J/cm^2). The high drop-out rate of 25% also compromises this study. Too high a dose is also a probable reason for the negative outcome of the study by Papadopuolos [1189] – 30 J/cm^2.

Terashima [126] treated 23 patients with lateral humeral epicondylitis and 40 patients with de Quervain's disease with GaAlAs laser. In the epicondylitis group, movement pains and soreness were positively affected in 61% of cases, and in 70% of cases in the de Quervain group. Movement pains were eradicated in 13% of cases. Seen as a whole, the treatment was effective for 61% of the patients in the epicondylitis group, while 45% in the other group experienced good results.

Cieslar [627] treated 182 patients with epicondylitis humeri in a double-blind study. After 5-7 sessions, distinct pain relief was obtained, and after 10-15 sessions pain on motion and palpation had gone. Three different wavelengths were used (904, 850, and 633). The percentages of patients who had much or slight improvement was 87%. There was no significant difference between the three wavelengths used.

Konstantinovic [554] compared the effect of corticosteroid infiltration, laser therapy (GaAs 1 J/cm^2) and laser plus corticosteroid infiltration in combination. At day 7 the combined therapy demonstrated a significantly higher analgesic effect.

Nd:YAG laser was used in a study by Basford [656]. 7 sites on the most symptomatic extremity were irradiated with 13 J/cm^2 each, three times a week for four weeks. There was no significant improvement. Total delivered energy was 220 Joules, but due to a large spot size (4.9 cm^2) the dose expressed in J/cm^2 was only 0.542.

In a review of the literature on shoulder tendinitis/bursitis and lateral epicondylalgia, Bjordal [732] summarises: "The methodological quality of the four laser therapy trials for lateral epicondylalgia is slightly higher than the five best trials with steroid injections for lateral epicondylalgia. Total sample size of high quality laser therapy trials is about two-thirds of the total sample of high quality steroid injections trials on the same diagnosis. The four laser therapy trials should serve as a valid platform for making conclusions on clinical effects of laser therapy for lateral epicondylalgia. Inadequate treatment procedures or poor methodological quality were found in the three trials that reported no significant effects of laser therapy. Evidence of clinical effects from laser therapy was found at all four lateral epicondylalgia trials using acceptable methods. The results in these trials were significantly in favour of active laser therapy with confidence intervals not including zero. The trial with fewest treatments per week had the lowest success rate. Best clinical effects were seen in patients with short duration of symptoms (less than a month)."

Bjordal has also summarised data from the literature regarding the treatment of tendinitis:

- A synthesis of dose from 4 laboratory trials on inflamed collagen-producing cell cultures gives the following dose for optimal reduction of tendon tissue inflammation: Dose 3-8 J/cm^2, Intensity: 5-21 mW/cm^2.
- A synthesis from 10 laboratory trials investigating collagen proliferation gives the following optimal dose for stimulation of tendon regeneration: Dose: 0.2-4 J/cm^2. Intensity: 2-10 mW/cm^2.
- For the treatment of tendinitis an optimal suggested dosage at target location will be: Dose: 0.2-4 J/cm^2. Intensity: 2-10 mW/cm^2.
- Treatment should be applied daily for at least five days to reduce inflammation, and for at least 10 days to increase collagen production.

Further literature: [821, 1055, 1167]

4.1.16 Fibrositis/fibromyalgia

The origin of fibrositis is not known, and there is at present no effective treatment to offer this large group of mainly female patients. Laser therapy is unlikely to cure a fibrositis patient. However, laser therapy does have a very good pain relieving effect and will improve the quality of life of these patients. If the painful areas are treated, there is rapid alleviation of pain. Repeated treatment further reduces pain, and sessions can soon be held at longer intervals. 4-6 J per painful point is a suitable initial dose to test the patient's general reaction. High powered GaAlAs lasers have proved to be quite useful in treating these patients, since they provide the higher power densities that are important in pain therapy.

Literature:

Longo [636] treated 846 patients with fibromyositic rheumatism during a 15-year period. Diodes and carbon dioxide lasers were used. About 2/3 of the patients benefited from the treatment with regard to local pain, hypomobility, and phlogosis.

Thorsen [703] could not find any effect of GaAlAs laser in localised fibromyalgia in the neck and shoulder regions. The laser had a power of 30 mW and each treated point received 0.9 J and a maximum of 9 J per treatment. This is, however, a low dose and power density for this indication.

A randomised, single-blind, placebo controlled study was conducted by Gür [1226] to evaluate the efficacy of laser therapy (GaAs) in 40 female patients with fibromyalgia. The treatment was carried out daily for two weeks, weekends excepted. At the end of the therapy there was a significant difference between the two groups for parameters such as pain, muscle spasm, morning stiffness and tender points.

The purpose of another study by Gür [1281] was to examine the effectiveness of laser therapy and low-dose amitriptyline therapy and to investigate effects of these therapy modalities on clinical symptoms and quality of life (QOL) in patients with fibromyalgia. Seventy-five patients with fibromyalgia were randomly allocated to active (GaAs) laser (25 patients), placebo laser (25 patients) and amitriptyline therapy (25 patients). All groups were evaluated for the improvement in pain, number of tender points, skin fold tenderness, morning stiffness, sleep disturbance, muscular spasm, and fatigue. Depression was evaluated by a psychiatrist according to the Hamilton Depression Rate Scale and DSM IV criteria. Quality of life of the patients was assessed according to the Fibromyalgia Impact Questionnaire (FIQ). In the laser group, patients were treated at each tender point daily for 2 weeks, except weekends, at each point with approximately 2 J/cm2. The same unit was used for the placebo treatment, for which no laser beam was emitted. Patients in the amitriptyline group took 10 mg daily at bedtime throughout the 8 weeks. A significant difference was observed in clinical parameters such as pain intensity and fatigue in favour of the laser group over the other groups, and a significant difference was observed in morning stiffness. A significant difference was observed in morning stiffness, FIQ and depression in the amitriptyline group compared to the placebo group after therapy. Additionally, a significant difference was observed in depression score in the amitriptyline group in comparison to the laser group after therapy. This study suggests that both amitriptyline and laser therapies are effective on clinical symptoms and QOL in fibromyalgia and that GaAs laser therapy is a safe and effective treatment in cases with fibromyalgia. Additionally, the study suggests that the GaAs laser therapy can be used as a monotherapy or as a supplementary treatment to other therapeutic procedures.

Further literature: [333].

4.1.17 Gynaecologic indications

Literature:

Takac [143] treated women suffering from menstrual pain with a GaAs laser. He administered 20 J over each ovary and over the uterus respectively, distributing the radiation over an area of about 15 cm^2. He treated the women every day from the 12th day of the cycle up to menstruation. Of 12 patients, ten were free of pain entirely or partially and experienced greater regularity in their menstrual cycles. A closer examination of the two who did not react showed microcysts on the ovaries.

For menstrual cramps, Ohshiro [978] recommends contact irradiation over the abdominal wall plus laser acupuncture on the Shishitsu points (Zhishi in Chinese) on the bladder meridian. It is also reported that delivery pain has been relieved through GaAlAs irradiation over the mouth of the cervix. Another study by Ohshiro [1102] suggests the possibility of treating female infertility with laser therapy.

Kovács [341] has successfully used a HeNe laser clinically to treat ectopium of the portio uteri. Havlik [1039] also reports this.

Kosilov [651] treated 120 girls with neurogenic hyperreflexic bladder dysfunctions. HeNe irradiation on the projection of the bladder combined with irradiation of biologically active points was more effective than conventional treatment.

Antipa [780] studied the effects of GaAs and HeNe laser irradiation, single or in combination, compared to placebo or conventional therapy on the recovery of 118 female patients with a diagnosis of chronic pelvic inflammatory disorders. Laser therapy proved to be significantly more efficient as compared with placebo or conventional therapy. The most efficient of all kinds of irradiation was the combination of GaAs and HeNe (laserpuncture and scanning).

Fibrotic masses in the breast secondary to fat necrosis or haematoma are a complication of breast reduction mammaplasty. The treatment commonly recommended for this condition is early surgical debridement of necrotic tissue from the entire area, which causes scarring. A case report by Nussbaum [909] describes the use of laser therapy for fibrotic lumps following reduction mammaplasty. The patient was a 46-year-old woman who had breast reduction surgery 80 days prior to referral for physical therapy. At the time of referral, the largest mass was 8.0 cm in diameter. The patient reported pain and said she was distressed about the breast disfigurement. Laser irradiation was initiated at an energy density of 20 J/cm^2 and a pulse repetition rate of 5,000 pulses per second. The laser settings were adjusted during the 8-month treatment period. The final dose was 50 J/cm^2. The mass was 33% of its original size after 3 sessions over the initial 11-day period. Pain relief was immediate. The rate of resolution decreased after the initial period. The patient had some tissue thickening at the time of discharge after 6 months of treatment.

Passeniouk [963] reports that laser therapy in combination with chlorhexidine was more effective for vaginitis than daily 10 g metronidazole plus one initial dose of 150 mg fluconozole. Laser therapy as well as conventional drug therapy was carried out for 10 consecutive days. The laser group consisted of 30 patients and the drug group of 20 patients.

Laser therapy of mastitis has been successfully used for dairy cattle and Herzog [1002] reports good effects on 66 mothers, using 830 nm, 30 mW, 0.5-2 J per point. Kovalev [1003] reports positive results for this indication, using HeNe on 329 mothers. HeNe was more effective than 890 nm GaAs. Havlik [1039] also reports positive results when using GaAlAs for mastitis. On the other hand, Stoffel [1004] reports that HeNe 25 mW had no effect on bovine mastitis. However, the irradiation area of 7.5 cm in diameter produces a very low energy density. Dotsenko [1005] and Skobelkin [1272] have used defocused carbon dioxide laser successfully for human lactation mastitis.

Further literature: [142, 633, 920, 1123, 1274].

4.1.18 Headache/Migraine

This very common complaint may have a variety of different causes. Myogenically conditioned headache responds well to GaAs and GaAlAs laser treatment administered to tender points and muscle attachments, 4-6 J per point. The practitioner should also take into account peripheral tender points in the neck and shoulders. The common correlation between myogenic headache and bruxism/clenching should be observed. Ohshiro [122] recommends that all laser treatment be preceded by a system-stimulating irradiation of the vertebra that innervates the damaged area. In this case, the atlas is irradiated, directly under the base of the skull.

"Migraine" comes from the Greek "hemi crania", literally "half head". Even if not all migraines are single-sided, this is still a fairly good diagnosis. The cause of migraine is thought to relate to fast-acting dilation of cranial blood vessels. The treatment of migraine is based on irradiation of the occipital nerve paths. Further, irradiation of the carotid arteries will stimulate the vascular system of the brainstem. This should be followed by local pain point irradiation. While migraine is a typical female condition, the Horton type of headache is a typical male vascular condition which is also worth trying with laser therapy.

A clear differential diagnosis is essential when treating “headaches”.

Literature:

Wong [120, 984] treated 20 patients with migraine or symptoms resembling migraine with a GaAlAs laser. The pain disappeared after 1-5 minutes. The effect was reported to be contingent on dosage and choice of treatment point.

4.1.19 Haemorrhoids

In the treatment of first and second-degree haemorrhoids, the HeNe laser is an effective, simple and harmless clinical procedure, representing an alternative to medical therapy or surgery, according to Trelles [706]. Therapy is carried out at intervals of 5 days for a total of 6 treatment sessions. Laser therapy was effective in pain alleviation from the first session and the final result was excellent.

4.1.20 Herpes simplex

Herpes simplex (HSV1) is commonly encountered in the practice of dentistry. As students in the seventies, we learned that it disappears by itself after two weeks, but if treated it heals after fourteen days. There are now more effective treatment methods, and one of the best is laser therapy.

The results of treatment depend on the stage of the virus cycle in which treatment begins. Patients often describe how the virus has a "favourite place", and experienced patients know where and when the blisters will appear, even before anything is visible. The use of a laser produces the best results in this prodromal stage, and may even prevent the attack. It also seems that a herpes sore is reluctant to return to a place where it has been treated before.

The later in the attack we treat, the poorer the results. However, even in the later stages of an attack we can offer tangible (or perhaps even total) relief from the symptoms and an acceleration of the healing process. The dosage is determined by the patient. When obvious relief has been provided we can stop treatment. If the attack is somewhat advanced before we can begin to treat it, the treatment should be repeated one to three times - an appropriate dosage is 4-6 J per sore.

If the herpes attacks are treated every time they manifest themselves, it appears that they return at longer and longer intervals. It could be the case that laser therapy has a short-term effect on symptoms and in the long-term an effect on the onset of the virus per se. It is tempting to speculate what laser therapy can do with other virus infections.

HSV2 (genital) has been treated in two studies, but with a rather poor outcome. It may be that the few cases of genital herpes simplex improved by laser therapy were actually HSV1 patients. The poor result in HSV2 patients is surprising, considering the excellent effect of laser therapy on HSV1 and varicella zoster.

1. Picture on top shows typical labial HSV-1, three days after outbreak. GaAlAs 6 J applied with immediate reduction of discomfort. Below: The situation the following day

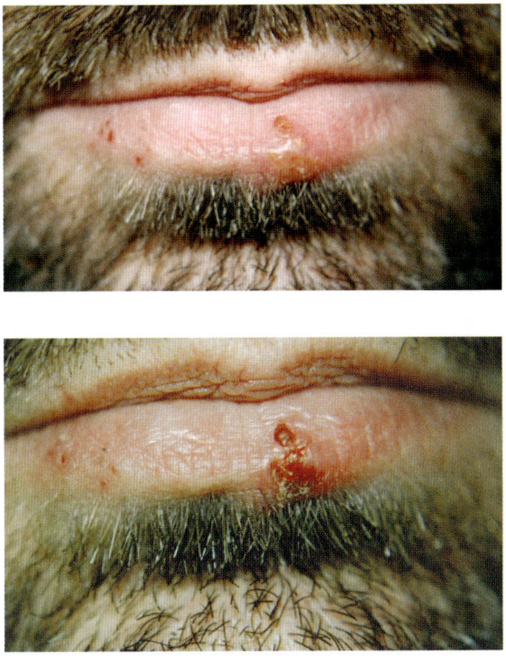

Figure 4.3 Typical labial HSV-1

Literature:

Gilioli [102] studied the effects of GaAs on herpes simplex virus *in vitro*. It was found that the viral plaque was stimulated by laser light. The stimulating effect was greater for HSV-1 than for HSV-2. The anti-viral effect in vivo presumably depends on an immune-stimulating effect.

Tardivo [358] observed the behaviour of cells infected with HSV under a GaAs laser, 30 mW. Doses of 4 and 12 J were given. A lesser cytopathic effect was noted in the irradiated cells than in the control cells, more evident at 4 J. The two cell lines were incubated for 7 days, frozen, and the released viruses inoculated in a new culture. An absence of cytopathic effect was noted in the cells infected with viruses derived from the cultures that received 12 J initially.

In an *in vitro study* by Hubacek [1036], HeNe laser had a cytopathogenous effect on HSV1 from 0.45 J/cm^2. On increasing the dose up to 6 J/cm^2, no bactericidal effect was noted.

Landthaler [239] used a krypton laser (with a wavelength of 647 nm) to treat recurrent herpes simplex in loco, zoster, and postherpetic neuralgia. Treatment consisted of 50 mW, at 90 seconds per cm^2, each area 3 cm^2. Patients with recurrent HSV had a period between outbreaks of 30 ± 19 days. After daily treatment sessions for ten days, the average period between outbreaks was 73 ± 50 days. Seven of nine patients with herpes labialis experienced significant improvement, while only one of three with herpes glutealis improved. Two of four patients with acute zoster were freed from discomfort. Five of eight with postherpetic neuralgia experienced alleviation of pain or total pain relief.

Vélez-González [360] treated 60 patients suffering from herpes simplex in the oral (HSV1) or genital (HSV2) area. Three groups in each category received (I) 200 mg Acyclovir orally plus placebo laser, (II) placebo

Acyclovir and HeNe laser light at 8 J/cm^2 or (III) Acyclovir and HeNe, in a randomised, double-blind study. Relapses on the lips and face were significantly reduced in the group treated with HeNe laser plus Acyclovir as compared with the groups treated with Acyclovir or HeNe only. The number of relapses per year before and after treatment was 5.2/2.8 for group I, 7.83/1.16 for group II, and 7.28/1.28 for group III. There was no significant difference between the latter groups. However, healing time was shorter in the combined group. The effects on the HSV2 groups were low for all three treatment modalities.

Hachenberger [60] reports the results of treating 93 patients with a HeNe laser. Pain disappeared quickly and healing occurred within three days. In no case did the herpes reappear at the same site, and relapses were less frequent.

Michels [416] summarizes eight years of experience in treating herpes simplex with HeNe laser light, 582 cases of HSV1 and 34 cases of HSV2. Healing was fast and without side-effects. 10% of the cases suffered relapses in loco, but all were patients with immune deficiency or a strong allergic background.

An important aspect of laser therapy of HSV1 has been described by Schindl [908], namely the possibility of treating patients with recurrent herpes attacks even during the symptom-free period. 50 patients with recurrent perioral herpes simplex infections (at least once a month for more than 6 months) were treated with 690 nm, 80 mW laser, energy density 48 J/cm^2, in a double blind study. Patients received daily irradiations for two weeks, 10 sessions in all. The treatment was given in a recurrence-free period and the irradiation was given at the site of the original herpes simplex infection. If both lips were involved, both upper and lower lips were treated. Patients were monitored for 52 weeks. The mean recurrence-free interval in the laser group was 37.5 weeks (range; 2-52 weeks) and in the placebo group 3 weeks (range 1-20 weeks). No side effects were noted.

In a study by Perrin [1009] it was observed that, in the ear experimental model of HSV latency, repeated exposure to infrared laser radiation of cervical ganglia following HSV inoculation appears to specifically hinder the establishment of virus latency in mice.

Further literature: [43, 61, 222, 628, 822, 1043]

4.1.21 Immune system modulation

Literature:

Takaduma [373] reports the effects of laser therapy on the immune system: "The human immune system acts as a defence mechanism against exogenous or indigenous potentially harmful bodies, such as bacteria and viruses. The major histocompatibility complex (MHC class I and class II antigens) form key elements of legitimate body components, and the organisation of MHC molecules allows T-lymphocytes to distinguish between legitimate and foreign bodies. On detection of a foreign component, T-cells activate the necessary pathways for destruction of the foreign body. Occasionally however the system breaks down and the result is a disease of an autoimmune nature. Both visible light and infrared laser therapy has been shown to act on immune system cells in a number of ways, activating the irradiated cells to a higher level of activity. Infrared laser therapy has been shown to increase both the phagocytic and chemotactic activity of human leukocytes *in vitro*, for example. This is an example of photobiological activation. Photobiological cell-specific destruction is also possible using doses of low incident laser energy on cells which have been photosensitised for the specific wavelength of the laser, such as in photodynamic therapy (PDT) for superficial cancers. Laser therapy has also been shown to act directly and selectively on the autoimmune system, restoring immunocompetence to cells. Although much more research needs to be done, there are enough experimental and clinical data to show that the laser, and laser therapy in particular, has a possibly exciting role both in immunobiological therapy for diseases of the immune system, and to activate and boost the normal reaction of the immune system components."

Kólarová [655] reports that doses of 5 to 10 J/cm^2 induced a significant increase of the phagocytic activity of leukocytes *in vitro*.

Duan [1163] has demonstrated a respiratory burst in bovine neutrophils after HeNe irradiation.

Schindl [581] describes an experiment on the immune modulating effect of a HeNe laser as follows: Escherichia coli endotoxin preimmunized rabbits were used to determine the influence of transcutaneously applied low-power laser light on differential blood count and rectal temperature. After three initial immunizations, animals were either boostered with 5 ng/kg of endotoxin or injected with pyrogen-free saline and subsequently underwent irradiation using two different wavelengths of red laser light and sham irradiation respectively. The differential blood count of laser-treated animals was characterised by significantly higher lymphocyte values and lower neutrophil values at twenty hours (boostered rabbits) and twenty-three hours (non-boostered rabbits) after irradiation. Differential blood cell counts returned to baseline levels within 23 hours in the boostered animals, whereas in the non-boostered rabbits lymphocytes showed a tendency to further increase. Recording of rectal temperature revealed a further rise after laser application, changes being of greater magnitude and longer duration in the non-boostered animals. These results seem to indicate that a single low-power laser irradiation can modulate immune responses depending on the immunological status of the organism.

In a study by Inoue [405], 830 nm laser has been shown to suppress the tuberculin reaction, one of the well-known immunological tests for the evaluation of cellular immunity *in vivo*.

Funk [565, 731] has shown that HeNe laser affects cytokine production in human peripheral blood mononuclear cells *in vitro*.

Katsuyama [662] has found a suppressive effect of diode laser irradiation on picryl contact sensitivity in a rat model. The thickness of the right ear was used as a indicator of the immune response to various doses of 830 nm laser irradiation. Laser therapy suppressed the cutaneous inflammation due to picryl contact sensitivity in an exposure-time dependent manner and this suppressive effect was restricted to within the irradiation site. Remote irradiation (proximal portion of tail) had no effect.

Yu [590] used an argon pumped dye laser at a wavelength of 630 nm to study the effect of laser therapy on the immune system. Rats with experimentally induced sepsis (cecal ligation) received laser therapy, 5 J/cm^2. At 60 days the survival rate was 79% in the laser group and 42% in the control group. *Ex vivo* lymphocyte proliferation was 180 in the laser group and 130 in the control group. Enhanced lymphocyte ATP synthesis was observed in the laser group.

Mikhailov [982] reports on the use of 890 nm laser treatment of autoimmune thyroiditis. 42 patients were given ten applications at 2.4 J/cm^2. The irradiated areas were the thymus projection zones (area of the sternum at a level of the second edge), vascular junction (left axillary area) and thyroid gland. A control group of similar size was given L-thyroxin, 100 mg/day. The clinical effect in all laser patients was a decreased feeling of squeezing in the field of the thyroid gland and a decrease of the facial oedema. The gland became softer palpatively and its size was reduced according to the utlrasound examination. The number of patients catching cold during the winter decreased. The immunoregulatory index (Th/Ts) normalised from 7.5 to 4.2%. The laser effect was still noticeable in 78% of the patients 4 months after treatment. This index was only slightly changed in the control group.

The leukocyte stimulating effects of HeNe have been described by Klebanov [1006, 1007] and Mester [23]

Further literature: [645].

4.1.22 Inner ear conditions

(See chapter 4.1.42 “Tinnitus, vertigo, Ménière´s disease” on page 178.)

4.1.23 Laryngitis

Literature

Hubacek [1036] reports positive results from treating laryngitis, using transcutaneous irradiation.

4.1.24 Lichen

Laser therapy has a good effect on the subjective symptoms of lichen conditions and it is a valuable supportive method in the conventional treatment of lichen.

Literature

[697, 724, 972]

4.1.25 Low back pain

This is certainly a difficult problem to treat, and laser therapy is by no means a panacea. It has, however, proven to be a valuable option in the hands of physiotherapists. High doses are essential. Laser therapy is a risk-free treatment modality.

Literature:

Gruszka [551] used a GaAs laser in a group of 15 patients with one or more protruded lumbar disc herniations. Previous physical therapy had improved symptoms but CAT scans had not changed. 9 J/cm^2 was given on 20 to 25 points. These points were on the lumbar spine and on points of referred radicular pain. Treatment was administered 3 to 5 times a week for 4 months. Before and after treatment, the patients' pain, gait, EMG, and CAT scan were evaluated. All patients were free from pain at the end of the treatment. Gait and neurological signs improved in all patients. EMGs improved and CAT scans showed less protrusion of the herniated discs.

Tasaki [125] treated 18 patients with low back pain with a GaAlAs laser at 30-80 mW. The sessions lasted 2-10 minutes and led to full pain relief. Pain relief took 6-8 hours to be effected among the patients who did not experience it immediately.

Basford [1062] performed a double-blind, placebo-controlled, randomized clinical trial on patients with low back pain. Sixty-three ambulatory men and women between the ages of 18 and 70 years with symptomatic non-radiating low back pain of more than 30 days' duration and normal neurological examination results. Subjects were bloc randomised into two groups with a computer-generated schedule. All underwent irradiation for 90 seconds at eight symmetric points along the lumbosacral spine three times a week for 4 weeks by a masked therapist. The Nd:YAG laser emitted 542 mW/cm^2. Subject's perception of benefit, level of function as assessed by the Oswestry Disability Questionnaire, and lumbar mobility were evaluated. The treated group had a time-dependent improvement in two of the three outcome measures: perception of benefit and level of function. These results were most marked at the midpoint evaluation and end of treatment but tended to lessen at the 1-month follow-up. Lumbar mobility did not differ between the groups at any time.

Further literature: [621, 956, 1061]

4.1.26 Microcirculation

Improving the microcirculation in tissue is one of the most important aspects of laser therapy. The self-healing capacity of the body will improve considerably if more blood is circulating in the tissue. Improved microcirculation in the region will also enhance the uptake of concomitant pharmaceutical agents.

Literature:

Schindl [145] treated three cases of Bürger's Disease, which is characterised by reduced microcirculation in the extremities. In practice, this always leads to amputation, often up to and past the knee/elbow. The illness has a very poor prognosis, and patients suffer from acute ischaemic pain. The three patients in the study refused to undergo further amputations and discharged themselves from hospital at their own risk. They remained on antibiotics during the entire treatment, but other than that, HeNe laser light was the only treatment they received. All three patients avoided further amputations, began healing and could return to work. The intense pain also disappeared. Bearing in mind these encouraging results, HeNe laser should be tested more on diabetics, in whom peripheral circulation can fall, rendering amputation necessary.

Schindl [674] treated a chronic radiation ulcer with HeNe laser, 30 J/ cm^2. A video measuring system was used to determine the number of dermal vessels in the ulcer before and after the laser treatment. After 7 irradiations the ulcer had healed completely. Light microscopy in combination with the video measuring system showed a significant increase in the number of dermal capillaries after laser treatment.

The pilot study by Al Awami [1200] was performed to evaluate the efficacy of laser therapy as a new non-drug non-invasive treatment for patients with primary and secondary Raynaud's disease. Forty patients (29 female, 11 male, mean age 51 years) with active primary (28%) and secondary (72%) Raynaud's phenomenon received 10 sessions of laser therapy distant irradiation during winter months. Assessment of subjective and objective parameters was performed at baseline one week after the last session and three months later. Variations of subjective parameters as number of daily acute episodes and severity of discomfort were assessed by a coloured visual analogue scale. A standardised cold challenge test using computed thermography of continuous temperature recordings by means of infrared telethermography was used to assess the digital blood flow. A significant improvement was noticed clinically and thermographically after 6 weeks and 3 months, respectively.

Podelinskaia [571] used a computer-aided analytical system of TV images (CASTI) to study the microcirculation in the anterior segment of the eye. Exposure to 890 nm laser therapy had a favourable impact on blood aggregation.

Saito [630] studied the effect of GaAlAs laser on the blood flow of 15 healthy male subjects. The upper side of the foot was irradiated for one minute (60 mW). Laser speckle flowmetry was performed at the start of irradiation, 30 and 60 minutes post irradiation. During the period of irradiation, blood flow was reduced significantly but increased immediately after irradiation, remaining at this level for 60 minutes. The laser specle flowmetry method itself has a potential of influencing the outcome in both groups.

Kubota [479] used the laser speckle flowgraphy to measure the microcirculation in flaps. The blood flow rate was reduced immediately following one minute of irradiation at 830 nm. 30 minutes later the flap perfusion was greater than in the control flap.

In an animal study by Kobayashi [666] the effect of GaAlAs laser on the blood flow in flaps was studied through laser speckle flowgraphy (LSF). 40 rats were divided into four groups. Two groups had random pattern flaps, two had axillary pattern flaps with the dominant vessels intact. Flaps were raised and peripheral blood flow assessed through LSF. Laser irradiation was performed in two groups, either directly on the dominant vessel or at one point on the distal part of the flap. The blood flow directly after irradiation was higher than before irradiation. At day 5 there was a clear difference between the irradiated and the non-irradiated flaps. The flaps irradiated at the dominant vessels had a slightly better outcome than those irradiated at the centre of the flap.

Studies by Bibikova [667, 587] conclude that during skeletal muscle regeneration in the toad, HeNe laser irradiation markedly promotes the process of neoformation of blood vessels and young myofibres in the injured zone.

Schaffer [904] explored the effect of a diode laser (780 nm) on normal skin tissue. Time-dependent contrast enhancement was determined by magnetic resonance imaging (MRI). In the examinations, six healthy volunteers were irradiated on their right planta pedis (sole of foot) with 5 J/cm^2 at a power density of 100 mW/cm^2. T1-weighted magnetic resonance imaging was used to quantify the time-dependent local accumulation of Gadolinium-DPTA, its actual content in the local current blood volume as well as its distribution to the extracellular space. Images were obtained before and after the application of laser light. When laser light was applied, the signal to noise ratio increased by more than 0.35 ± 0.15 (range 0.23-0.63) after irradiation according to contrast-enhanced MRT. According to the authors: "it can be observed that after biomodulation with light of low energy and low power, wound healing improves and pain is reduced. This effect might be explained by an increased blood flow in this area. Therefore, the use of this kind of laser treatment might improve the outcome of other therapeutic modalities such as tumour ionising radiation therapy and local chemotherapy".

Maegawa [1030] used a 30 mW GaAlAs laser to irradiate the rat mesenteric microcirculation *in vivo*, power density 38.2 mW/mm^2. The irradiation caused a potent dilatation in the irradiated arteriole, which led to a marked increase in the arteriolar blood flow. The irradiation also caused a power-dependent decrease in [Ca^{2+}] in the vascular smooth muscle cells.

For additional studies on microcirculation, see chapter 4.1.13 "Diabetes" on page 140.

Further literature [308, 1015, 1075, 1082]

4.1.27 Morbus Sluder

Literature:

Mb Sluder is a painful condition originating in the spheno-palatinal ganglion. Parascandalo [1071] used GaAs laser in three patients, 12 sessions, irradiating the maxillary nerve apertures. Total pain relief was obtained after five sessions, difficulties in swallowing improved after three sessions, reduction of high tear flow after several sessions. Full recovery after nine sessions.

Further literature. [1070]

4.1.28 Mucositis

(See chapter 4.1.7 “Cancer” on page 130.)

4.1.29 Muscle regeneration

Literature:

Lievens [521] summarises a study on the effects of laser therapy on muscle regeneration as follows: The effect of GaAs, 904 nm, laser irradiation on the process of skeletal muscle regeneration after simple injury to the tibialis anterior muscle of the mice is studied histologically and statistically. The right-hand side injured zones in the experimental mice were subjected to one direct by means of nuclear magnetic resonuance technique laser irradiation for 3 min every day starting on the first day post injury. The left-hand side injuries were untreated and served as a control. Morphometric analysis was performed on histological sections of injured areas at 7 and 18 days post injury. At 7 days post injury, mononucleated cells populated most of the area of injury. Thereafter, their proportion decreased gradually but more rapidly in the laser-irradiated muscles than in those on the control side. The early myotubes were evident in the control side, while they were less evident in the experimental side. The injured area was populated by myotubes in the experimental muscles, while they were less evident in the control side. At 18 days post injury, in the laser-irradiated muscles the process of muscle regeneration was almost completed. In the untreated muscles, myotubes still populated a large part of the injured zone, and there were less regenerated myofibres. It is concluded that the process of muscle regeneration is promoted when the injured area is exposed to GaAs-laser irradiation following injury to the mice tibialis anterior muscle.

In a study by Amaral [665] 15 mice received a single muscular injection of myotoxin in the tibialis anterior muscle of both legs. One group received HeNe laser irradiation with the dose of 2.6 J/cm^2, another 8.4 and the third 25 J/cm^2 on one leg, while the other was sham irradiated. The 2.6 J group showed a significant difference, with evidence of a greater concentration of mitochondria in the treated muscle, whereas the higher doses did not produce this effect. The laser treated mice showed an increase of cross-section area of the muscle fibres.

Popova [147] studied the effects of a HeNe laser on the healing of muscle tissue after irradiation with 10 Gy X-ray. The muscle tissue of rats was removed, irradiated with X-rays and re-transplanted. Improved healing compared with the control group was observed whether laser light was administered before or after the transplant.

Weiss [276] and Bibikova [277], in experiments on rats and toads respectively, observed improved muscle regeneration as a result of the use of HeNe and GaAs lasers.

Oliveira [1186] failed to find such regeneration in a rodent experiment using GaAs, 1.5 mW, 3-10 J/cm^2, daily irradiations over intact skin. Although there was no effect on the muscular regeneration, the body weight of the mice was increased in the 10 J/cm^2 group.

Buliakova [570] found that HeNe laser indeed accelerated the regenerative process in crosscut gastrocnemius muscles of adult guinea pigs. However, the regenerating muscle tissue did not connect the two muscle stumps, a narrow connective tissue scar being formed instead. The same experiment on rats was more successful, so it is likely that the regenerative ability of laser therapy depends on species peculiarities.

Schwartz [626] found a transient elevation of intracellular calcium in the myotubes immediately after irradiation, using HeNe laser light at 3-10 J/cm^2. These findings suggest the hypothesis that transient changes in calcium may accelerate the release of cytokines from the myotubes.

Shefer [1243] has demonstrated that HeNe laser can stimulate cell cycle entry and the accumulation of satellite cells around isolated single fibres, grown under serum-free conditions. It is demonstrated that laser therapy promotes the survival of muscle fibres and their adjacent cells, as well as cultured myogenic cells, inder serum-free conditions that normally lead to apoptosis.

Further literature: [356, 533, 587, 616, 702, 916]

4.1.30 Nerve conduction

Literature:

Wakabayashi [190] demonstrated that C-fibres play a part in the analgesic effect of laser therapy. A small hole was drilled in the mandibular incisor of a Wistar rat through which a probe made contact with the dental pulp. The incisor was stimulated electrically and the subsequent action potential was registered through a probe from the ipsilateral trigeminal caudal neurons. A GaAlAs laser was used to irradiate the incisor's cervical surface. The rate of firing discharges and the number of spikes evoked in the caudal neurons before and after laser treatment were compared. Laser therapy suppressed the late discharges in the response of the caudal neurons which were evoked by excitatory inputs from C-fibre afferents, but did not suppress the early discharges evoked by inputs from A-delta-fibre afferents. This indicates that GaAlAs irradiation inhibited the excitation of unmyelinated fibres of the pulp without affecting fine myelinated fibres. It is suggested that laser therapy has a suppressive effect on injured tissue by blocking the depolarisation of the afferent C-fibres.

Ohno [719] demonstrated that laser irradiation suppresses the excitation of the unmyelinated C-fibres in the afferent sensory pathway. Substance P in the rat spinal dorsal root ganglion was measured after electrical stimulation of the sciatic nerve.

The involvement of afferent unmyelinated A-delta fibres in laser therapy pain attenuation has been demonstrated by Kasai [488]. High threshold evoked responses were reduced between 9% and 19% during low-power laser irradiation in experimental animals. The data in this study suggest that low-power laser acts as a reversible direct suppressor of neuronal activity

In a study by Tsuchiya [519], a GaAlAs laser reduced the action potentials in the dorsal roots elicited from the saphenous nerve of a rat. The amplitude of slower conduction parts of action potentials (velocity <12 m/s) was suppressed. The suppression was time-dependent. After 3 minutes of irradiation, the slowest velocity group (<1.3 m/s) was totally diminished and the 1.3-12 m/s group was reduced by 12-67%. In contrast, faster components (>12 m/s) were unaffected.

Balaban [650] concludes that HeNe laser does not affect silent neurons. However, when the spontaneously active neurons, generating spikes every 7-10 minutes, were irradiated in between their spontaneous spikes, the depolarisation of membrane and generation of action potentials occurred as a function of light intensity.

4.1.31 Nerve regeneration and function

The regeneration of damaged nerves is one of the most promising indications for laser therapy. Studies on Bell´s palsy are difficult to evaluate, bearing in mind the high spontaneous remission rate. However, the rapid pain relief is a good verification of the laser effect. The swelling and the neuritis in the bony fallopian canal is believed to be influenced. This intrabony region is the major target for laser therapy in this indication. The suspected association with herpes virus also supports the use of laser therapy.

Literature:

van Breugel [353] investigated HeNe laser irradiation effects on proliferation and laminin production of rat Schwann cells *in vitro*. Schwann cell (SwC) proliferation is an essential part of Wallerian degeneration after nerve damage and thus a prerequisite for regeneration. HeNe irradiation *in vitro* showed a dose-related stimulation of SwC proliferation. Laminin production was not affected.

Mulligan [354] investigated the effect of HeNe laser irradiation on neurite elongation *in vitro*. Doses around 1.5 J/cm^2 were given to a rat neuronal clonal cell line for 5, 15, 30, 45 and 60 minutes. Neurite outgrowth was greater than control in all groups but only the 15 and 30 minute groups were statistically different from the control values.

Walker [89] and Tsai [90] achieved results which indicate that the central nervous system is photosensitive. Wu [187] conducted Walker's experiment again on a larger scale, however, and was unable to confirm the results.

Rochkind [32] has carried out extensive studies of the effects of HeNe laser light on nerve damage. In one experiment, the sciatic nerves of rats were exposed and crushed in a standardised fashion. After suturing, HeNe laser light was administered transcutaneously. The effects were monitored at intervals of one to 360 days. In the experimental group, action potential was at a high level, while in the control group (no laser treatment) it was very low. This effect was only achieved if the laser treatment was administered immediately after the injury - when it was given three and seven days afterwards, there was no difference as compared to the control group.

In another rodent study [1131] the sciatic nerves in rats were crushed in a standardised fashion and HeNe laser irradiation was performed directly after suturing. The irradiation was performed over the corresponding segment of the spinal cord and not over the crushed area. Laser therapy was performed for 30 minutes daily during 21 consecutive days. The electrophysiological activity of the injured nerves (compound muscle action potentials – CMAPs) was found to be approximatively 90% of the normal precrush value and remained so for a long time. In the control group the CMAPs dropped to about 20% at day 21 and showed the first signs of slow recovery 30 days after surgery.

In yet another experiment by the Rochkind group, Wollman [537] irradiated foetal brain cells *in vitro* using a HeNe laser. One single dose enhanced the appearance of brain cells around the treated aggregates. Two and three doses were correlated with 97% and 142% increases respectively. Rhodamine-labelled antibodies bound to receptors on cells indicated massive neurite sprouting and outgrowth of migrating brain cells in culture.

In the study by Rochkind [1236] embryonal spinal cord nerve cells dissociated from rat fetuses, cultured in biodegradable microcarriers and embedded in hyaluronic acid, were implanted in the completely transsected spinal cords in 24 adult rats. 15 rats underwent 14 days of consecutive laser irradiation (780 nm, 250 mW, 30 minutes daily). 7 rats received the same treatment but without laser. Eleven of the 15 laser treated rats showed different degrees of active leg movements and gait performance compared to 4 of the 9 rats with implantation alone. In a control group of 7 rats with no therapy after the transsection of the spinal cord, six remained completely paralysed. Intensive axonal sprouting occurred in the laser group. In the control group the transsected area contained proliferating fibroblasts and blood capillaries only.

Anders [387] found that laser irradiation with certain wavelengths alters the rate of regeneration of the rat facial nerve. The facial nerve of rats was crushed unilaterally and transcutaneously irradiated with a laser beam directed at the area of the crush injury daily for 7, 8 or 9 days. The wavelengths examined were 361, 457, 514, 633, 720 and 1064 nm. Power ranged from 8.5 to 40 mW, length of irradiation from 13 to 120 minutes. The most effective wavelength was 633 nm and 45.9 J.

In a study by Jimbo [835] the effects of GaAlAs (830 nm, 16.2 mW) laser irradiation on the distal portion of the processes of cultured murine dorsal root ganglion (DRG) neurons associated with C-fibers was studied by patch-clamp whole-cell recording of membrane potentials at the cell body. The chemical as well as laser light stimulation was limited to the processes of the neuron isolated from the cell body with a separator. The action potentials elicited by bradykinin (BK) in the cell body were reversibly suppressed by the irradiation of laser light. The laser irradiation may block the conduction of nociceptive signals in primary afferent neurons.

Walsh [977] irradiated the skin overlying the human right superficial radial nerve at three points (1.2 J per point, energy density 9.55 J/cm^2, 830 nm 50 mW). Antidromic action potentials were recorded from the nerve prior to irradiation and at 5, 10 and 15 minutes after irradiation. There were no differences between placebo laser, control and active laser groups for negative peak latency or skin temperature. Pulsing at 8, 12 Hz or 73 Hz made no difference.

The studies by Khullar [361, 900, 901, 902, 939, 1037] on the effects of laser therapy on longstanding paraesthesiae in the orofacial region found, in summary:

- A course of 20 laser therapy treatment sessions using a GaAlAs laser (=820 nm) on an area of long-standing paraesthesiae in the orofacial region induced an objectively evaluated significant improvement in fine mechanosensory perception and a decrease in the area of paraesthesiae.
- The significant improvement in mechanosensory perception was also perceived as a subjective improvement by the patients.
- A course of 20 laser therapy treatment sessions with a GaAlAs laser (=820 nm) induced no change in thermoperception in an area of paraesthesiae.
- Daily laser therapy treatment over a 28 day period with a GaAlAs laser accelerated motor nerve reinnervation as assessed by return of motor function subsequent to a standardised axonotmesis injury in the rat sciatic nerve.
- Treatment with a GaAlAs (=820 nm) laser enhanced sensory reinnervation of peripheral target tissues subsequent to an IAN axotomy injury in the rat model. The findings are demonstrated immunohisto-chemically by the presence of CGRP positive neurones

A study by Miloro [899] examined the potential benefit of perioperative and short-term postoperative laser therapy on objective and subjective neurosensory recovery after bilateral sagittal split osteotomy surgery. Six consecutive patients undergoing bilateral sagittal split osteotomy procedures were enrolled in this prospective study. A complete preoperative clinical neurosensory test, consisting of brush stroke directional discrimination, 2-point discrimination, contact detection, pin prick nociception, and thermal discrimination, was performed on each patient; and a subjective assessment of neurosensory function was made by using a visual analogue scale (VAS). The protocol for laser therapy treatment consisted of 6 J per point along the distribution of the inferior alveolar nerve at 4 sites for a total of 7 sessions delivered immediately before surgery; at 6 and 24 hours after surgery; and on postoperative days 2, 3, 4 and 7. The clinical neurosensory test and VAS were completed just before each of the treatment sessions and on days 14 and 28 by one examiner. When the results of the patients treated with laser therapy were compared with published values for neurosensory recovery after orthognathic surgery, there was a significant acceleration in the time, as well as in the magnitude, of neurosensory return. Brush stroke directional discrimination approached normal values by 14 days, whereas 2-point discrimination and contact detection showed significant improvement at 14 days and returned to near-normal values by 2 months. The results of thermal discrimination and pin prick nociception revealed few neurosensory deficits; however, those patients who were affected showed a slower recovery trend and remained neurosensory-deficient for up to 2 months. The VAS analysis revealed a rapidly progressive improvement in subjective assessment, showing a 50% deficit at 2 days and only a 15% subjective deficit at 2 months.

Yamada [1054] has compared corticosteroids, laser therapy and a combination of the two in a study comprising 7 patients in each group. The effect of laser therapy was comparable to that of corticosteroids but the combined therapy showed the best outcome. The laser was a 150 mW GaAlAs laser and the laser therapy was performed over the area of paralysis (36 J per session), the stylomastoid foramen (10.8 J) and the stellate ganglion (63.7 J). The number of sessions in the laser group ranged from 21 to 66, 5-12 weeks. In the combination group success was achieved within 14-31 sessions, 3-10 weeks.

The double-blind randomised study by Shamir [1182] evaluated the effect of laser therapy on peripheral nerve regeneration after complete transection and direct anastomosis of the rat sciatic nerve. 13 of 24 rats received postoperative laser therapy, 780 nm, applied transcutaneously, 30 min daily for 21 consecutive days, to corresponding segments of the spinal cord and to the injured sciatic nerve. Positive somatosensory evoked responses were found in 69.2 percent of the irradiated rats compared to 18.2 percent of the non-irradiated rats. Immunohistochemical staining in the laser-treated group showed an increased total number of axons and better quality of the regeneration process, due to an increased number of large-diameter axons compared to the non-irradiated control group.

Paolini [960] treated 40 patients with Bell's paralysis. One group received only prednison (corticosteroid) 60 mg/day. The other group was treated with GaAs laser on points along the nerve, followed by an array of GaAs/HeNe five days a week for three weeks, then every second day, 30 sessions in all. The outcome in the laser group was significantly better than in the pharmacological group.

Brugnera [970] treated two groups of patients with lesions to the inferior alveolar and mental nerves. 830 nm 40 mW, spot size 3 mm² was used. All paraesthesias were due to surgical interventions. The first group was identified as immediate and was treated within 2-15 days after the injury. In this group 72.7% achieved absolute recovery, 18.3% a relative improvement and 9% did not respond to treatment. In the late group, the history of injury was 30-365 days. In this group only 27.7% reached an absolute improvement.

Bernal [156] presented six years' experience of patients with facial paralysis on whom HeNe and GaAs lasers had been used. If the laser treatment was begun within two days of the occurrence of the injury, treatment with laser therapy was successful in 100% of cases and a maximum of 15 treatment sessions were required. If the patient was treated later, Meticorten (40 mg/day) was administered for seven days as a supplement. Up to 30 doses could be administered to the latter group. The degree of healing in this latter group varied, but complete rehabilitation was achieved by some of the patients.

Murakami [186] treated 52 people with idiopathic facial paralysis or Bell's paralysis. 26 were treated with stellate ganglion block (SGB), 11 received 830 nm laser therapy and 15 a combination of the two. The patients who received laser therapy or a combination of laser therapy and SGB showed a similar picture of recovery from paralysis, in contrast to the group which received SGB only. The group that received only laser therapy also showed a better initial improvement.

Patient with facial paresis following an ear operation 15 years ago. The second photo shows the situation after two laser sessions per week for one month.

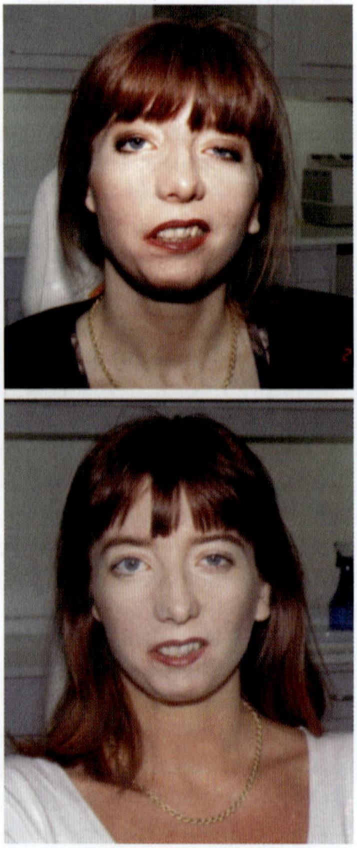

Figure 4.4 Facial paresis
Courtesy: Per Hugo Christensen

Rochkind [1038] evaluated the functional improvement of 18 patients suffering from incomplete peripheral nerve or brachial plexus injuries who received low level laser irradiation at 780 nm or placebo irradiation for 21 consecutive days. There was a significant improvement in motor function at follow up at 3 and 6 months compared to the placebo group (p=0.0001). Sensory function showed no statistical difference at 3 months but at 6 months control the improvement was significant ($p=0.035$). Electrophysiological analysis showed a significant improvement in recruitment of voluntary muscle activity ($p=0.006$) as well as a trend toward statistical significance in amplitude of compound muscle action potentials ($p=0.067$) at the end of the 21 days of therapy and at 3 and 6 months.

In a rat experiment by Byrnes [1222] the spinal cord was hemisected at vertebral level T9. 810 nm laser was applied immediately after hemisection and daily for 14 days, 1589 J/cm^2. Control rats received identical treatment, but without laser. The results indicate that laser therapy initially blocks cell invasion and activation of the injured spinal cord. Once laser therapy ceases at 14 days post-injury (the time point at which lesioned axons are reported to begin to sprout) there is a rebound increase in non-inflammatory cell invasion and activation that is visible 16 days post-injury. These alterations in the spinal cord environment may contribute to the ability of lesioned axons to regenerate following injury.

Further literature [375, 218, 493, 646, 933, 1113]

4.1.32 Oedema

A more or less pronounced oedema always appears after a surgical intervention. The anti-oedematous effect is based on a dilation of lymphatic vessels and a reduction in the permeability of blood vessels. Large doses are required if the oedema is already established - even 1-2 J/cm^2 with a GaAs laser or 10-15 J/cm^2 with a GaAlAs laser is on the low side after an operation. An established oedema may be filled with blood, and haemoglobin is one of the most powerful chromophores in the organism. Penetration is therefore shallow, particularly with a HeNe laser.

Laser energy also has a regenerative effect on lymphatic vessels, as it has on veins. As can be seen in [92] and [299] below, laser therapy can probably not be used as an oedematic prophylaxis before operation unless oedema is already present before the operation.

When treating peripheral oedemas, the proximal sites of the body should always be irradiated first. Opening the blood flow at a peripheral site could be followed by a circulatory obstruction at the proximal site, thus causing pain.

Literature:

Kiyoizumi [95] reported, in an *in vitro* experiment, that a GaAlAs laser has two different effects on oedema. The laser stimulated the synthesis of PGI_2 (prostacyclin), which has a strong vasodilating effect, and counteracted the aggregation of platelets. The accumulation of PGI_2 in the tissue reduced the oedema tendency. Laser light was also shown to counteract the occurrence of fibrin networks, which were studied with radioactive iodine. Kiyoizumi's clinical experience of skin transplants is that laser therapy reduces oedema.

Labajos [300] noted that the flow of water and electrolytes through the intestinal wall was retarded by laser therapy, 1 J/cm^2.

Lievens [92, 298] studied the effects of GaAs laser light on the vasomotricity of the lymphatic system. The everted skin of mice was observed microscopically under a cold light source. The lymph vessels were visualised by an injection of a physiological dye. The vessels did not dilate after laser treatment if the tissue had not been subjected to trauma, but did dilate as a result of laser treatment when in an oedematous condition.

In another study of regeneration of the lymphatic system, Lievens [299] used a combined GaAs/HeNe laser. A median incision along the linea alba was made on 600 white mice. The skin was turned back and pinned on a cork plate. The lymph vessels were visualised by means of an injection of Patent V Blue into an inguinal lymph node. There were 100 animals in the laser group and 500 in the control group. The results were as follows:

1. Adhesion of the wound to the underlying tissue was present in 100% of the animals in the control group after day four. The adhesion gradually disappeared after day ten. Adhesion hardly ever occurred in the laser group.
2. The regeneration of the veins was faster in the laser group.
3. In the control group, the lymphatic vessels regenerated through a network of small vessels. In the laser group, the lymph vessels regenerated into their original shape. Regeneration was much quicker in the laser group, in particular during the initial healing stage.
4. The network-regenerated vessels in the non-irradiated group were very permeable. This increased permeability could be seen in 50% of the cases even after 6 months. The vessels in the laser group showed hardly any increased permeability after the first few days.

Honmura [96] studied the effects of a GaAlAs laser on experimentally produced inflammation in rats. In all cases in the laser group, the degree of inflammation was reduced by 20-30%. Laser therapy also reduced the extent of the oedema in the acute inflammation phase. Laser therapy was effective if administered within two hours after the inflammation-causing substance was given to the rats; if it was administered later, a poorer effect on the oedema was observed. In a comparison using the inflammation-reducing substance indomethacin, laser therapy was better in one experimental model, not so good in another, but effective in both cases. Laser therapy also impeded the vessels' permeability in cases of acute inflammation and thereby reduced the acute oedema.

Røynesdal [93] studied the effects of GaAlAs in the surgical removal of impacted wisdom teeth. 6 J was administered before and after the operation. The same person operated on 25 people with bilaterally impacted wisdom teeth. The study showed that laser with these parameters had no effect on oedema, trismus or pain alleviation as compared with placebo laser.

In a study by Antipa [769] the effect of a GaAs-laser was studied on 64 patients with post-traumatic swellings, allergic vasculitis and therapy resistant varicose crural ulcers. The laser therapy was conducted in combination with classic therapy and was compared with a non-irradiated control group of 52 patients, treated only by classic therapy. Laser irradiation was directed to the skin damage by scanning. Segmental and dermatomic areas of the skin lesions were irradiated by laser acupuncture. Therapeutic protocol included an average of nine sessions. The statistical analysis shows a significant difference of the efficiency between the laser treated group and the control group, especially in the case of post-traumatic swellings, less in the case of allergic vasculitis.

Piller [928] has since 1993 treated over 700 patients with chronic secondary arm and leg lymphoedemas with GaAs scanning. Laser therapy had no effect on any parameter on normal arms and legs. In the affected arms there was a significant reduction of volume, average 233 ml. There was also a significant effect on the level of fibrotically indurated tissues in the lymphatic territories of the upper and forearm. Average reduction in legs was 199 ml, which was not statistically significant. However, as with the arms, there were significant reductions in the level of free extracellular fluids in the whole limb and reductions in the level of fibrotic induration in the lymphatic territories of lower posterior leg and upper anterior leg. These results correlated strongly with the patients' subjective indications of feelings of tension, heaviness and aching.

Prokofeva [1217] evaluated the doses of infrared laser exposure for the structures of the eye in rabbit experiments, and the potentials of such lasers in ophthalmology were assessed. Wavelength was 890 nm and doses varied from 0.0001 to 1.0 J/cm^2, corresponding to exposure duration of 0.3 seconds to 45 min. Experiments were carried out on 20 animals. The right eyes were exposed, and the left ones were control. An increase of intraocular pressure was recorded at a dose of 0.1 J/cm^2 (4.5 min) and higher. Morphological examination showed dilated, well filled and newly formed vessels in the ciliary body and iris, as well as oedema and destruction of the external layers of the retina. Exposure to a dose of 0.05 J/cm^2 and lower did not lead to destruction of any ocular structures or increase of intraocular pressure. The maximal dose causing no side effects for the organ of vision was established at 0.05 J/cm^2.

Further literature: [222, 485, 664]

4.1.33 Ophthalmic problems

Treatment of the eye with laser therapy is controversial, stemming from the early days of laser therapy and the hard-to-kill misconception that lasers in the low-milliwatt range could damage the eye. Patient and operator were recommended to use protective goggles even when treating a foot, using a laser of a couple of milliwatts.

Treating the unprotected eye is still the sole province of specialists. However, any reasonably trained person can carry out eye treatment through the eyelid. Closing the eye comes naturally when it is treated with a visible beam such as a HeNe laser. When a collimated invisible laser is used, one must make sure that the patient keeps his eyes closed. If the treatment probe is close to the eye and the beam is highly divergent, the light will not be focused in to a small point, even if the eye is open. Therefore the risk in this case is small. We therefore recommend a visible beam in this context. High-powered non-visible beams should only be used by a very qualified therapist.

Treating a stye on the eyelid for instance, is quite effective. Maeno [129] reported as early as 1989 that a HeNe laser was effective in treating keratoconjunctivitis.

Literature:

In a report by Inkova [903], 82 patients with severe post-traumatic uveitis (eye inflammation) which could not be treated by traditional anti-inflammatory therapy were exposed to laser therapy. The patients were divided into 3 groups: infrared laser exposure semiconductor pulsed laser, intravenous exposure of the blood to a He-Ne laser, and both treatments combined. The treatment efficacy was monitored by measuring lipid peroxides and superoxide dismutase in the lacrimal fluid. The treatment proved to be effective. The best results were attained by applying both methods of exposure, as shown by an earlier normalisation of the content of lipid peroxidation products and activity of superoxide dismutase.

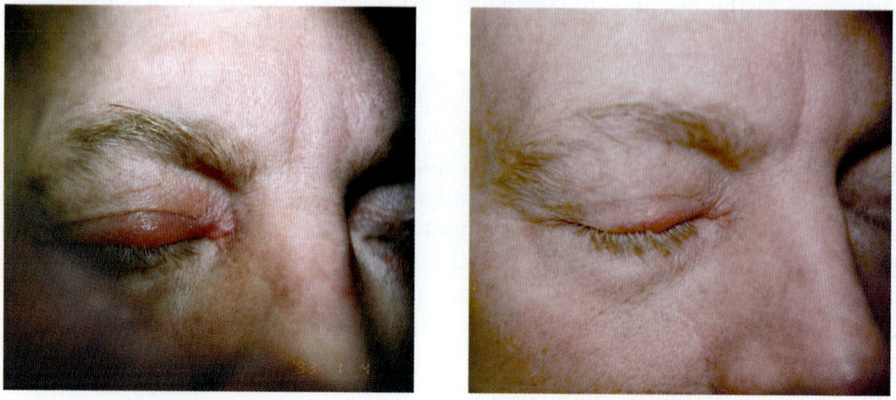

Figure 4.5 Stye day one and two, following HeNe laser therapy.

Eliseeva [654] has used intravenous irradiation in the therapy of ophthalmic problems.

A review of Russian laser therapy studies in ophthalmology is presented by Pankov [1122]. The first studies appeared as early as 1976. HeNe lasers of low output are used; some examples are 0.25 mW and 0.05 mW/cm.

Some indications treated are amotio retinae, functional amplyopia, post-traumatic iridocyclitis, endothelial-epithelial dystrophy, burn accidents, acute inflammatory and allergic diseases of the cornea, conjunctiva, iris and ciliary body. HeNe laser has also been shown to increase the lymphocirculation of the eye.

Belkin and Schwartz [599] have presented a thorough review of the literature on laser therapy in ophthalmology. The majority of the studies are from Russia. The conclusion of the review is "that many studies must be looked at with skepticism because of lack of statistical evaluation, adequate inclusion and exclusion criteria, masking procedures etc. Nevertheless, the basic science experiments described in the earlier parts of the review and the demonstrable bioeffects of low-energy irradiation measured in various body systems leave us no option but to conclude that low-energy laser irradiation does exert some effects on ocular tissues in health and disease, and that these effects exhibit definite dose-response curves. Energy concentrations less than 1 J/cm^2 are generally ineffective and those over 5 J/cm^2 can be injurious. The precise dosage, however, depends on the specific laser/tissue combination. The clinical reports surveyed here are thus not theoretically impossible, but will have to be reconfirmed".

Further literature [599, 600, 601, 602, 603, 622]

4.1.34 Pain

"Pain" could be the heading of almost any chapter in medicine. No step forward is appreciated more by the patients than the reduction of pain! The old exhortation "nil nocere" meshes well with the principles of laser therapy - lasers can prevent and reduce pain, as can be seen from much of the text above. A positive aspect of laser treatment is that pain can be alleviated as early as during the treatment session itself.

Large dosages are often required to achieve an immediate effect on acute pain. A case of alveolitis can, for example, require as much as 20 J of GaAs laser light just to alleviate the pain. Less pronounced pain, such as herpes sore, a decubital wound or a tooth neck, can require 3-4 J to achieve full relief from the symptoms. There is reason to believe that the large dosages used to alleviate severe pain also entail overdoses in the biostimulating range. The choice here is simple, however, and pain should be given priority.

Pain can be more than just suffering for the patient. It can also be an obstacle to any kind of treatment, for instance in dental surgery. A painful sore means that soft tissue anaesthetic is required to enable the dentist to manipulate the patient's lips and cheeks. Pain from the maxillary joint means that the patient cannot open his mouth sufficiently for an adequate occlusal adjustment to be performed, and it may not even be possible to take an imprint for a bite splint. Pain in the neck and back can make it difficult for a patient to lie down. In all these cases, reducing pain means that we can go straight ahead with normal therapy. Pain is often part of a vicious circle where the pain itself prevents the patient from exercise, thus aggravating the existing damage.

In the most recent meta analysis of the literature [872], there was a highly significant outcome for this kind of treatment of pain.

Literature:

Montesinos [40] studied the blood concentration of various amino acids in rats after direct laser irradiation of the pituitary gland. The mean value in the control group was 4.57 µg/ml. In the laser group treated with HeNe, the mean level after day one was 47, day three 24, and day five 53. By day seven it had dropped to 0.8 and by day 15 it had risen again to 24, then dropped once more to 22 by day 21. In the GaAs group, the level was 44 after three days and 21 after seven days. Both lasers were thus effective but worked in different ways. The peptides studied build leukoencephalins and metencephalins, which affect the apprehension of pain.

Honmura [188], however, has conducted experiments which indicate that the pain-relieving effect of laser therapy is not only opiod-related. By injecting a substance which causes pain in the paws of rats (in accordance with a well-known experimental model), it was found that the analgesic effect was just as good whether indomethacin or laser therapy was used. In one group, a single dose of GaAlAs eliminated pain for 24 hours. Naloxone is a substance that counteracts the effects of opiates. When it was used, the effect of laser therapy was reduced but not eliminated. This experiment indicates that there are other possible explanations behind laser therapy's analgesic effects.

Katsuyama [662] studied the effect of 830 nm laser in a neuropathic pain model of rat. The left side sciatic nerves of two groups of rats were ligated loosely to produce a neuropathic pain. The latency of the foot withdrawal reflex to noxious heat stimuli was measured before the ligation, immediately after laser/placebo radiation and at 14 days after ligation. The laser group received 72 J through the dermis. This group showed a significant reduction in left foot withdrawal immediately after irradiation and at 14 days, the right foot being unchanged. Placebo irradiation did not change the latency either in the ligated group or in non-ligated rats.

In an animal study by Mrowiec [432], it is suggested that nitric oxide is involved in the mechanism of low-power laser-induced analgesia. The injection of 1-NAME blocked the analgesic effect obtained by 904 nm irradiation of the skull in rats.

Wedlock [1017] sought to establish dose dependency and time course for effects of cranial laser irradiation in two rodent models of pain. These were the hot plate and tail flick tests, which are both widely used to quantify analgesic drug effects. The laser used was GaAlAs, average power output 100 mW, pulse frequency 5 kHz. Irradiation was applied to shaved heads of rats above the midbrain. In the first experiment, four groups of 10 rats received doses of 0, 6, 12, 18, and 24 J/cm^2 in random order prior to hot plate testing either immediately, 30 min, 1 h or 24 h post laser. The second study employed three groups of 10 rats receiving 0, 12, and 18 J/cm^2 in random order prior to tail flick testing at the three shorter times above. Latency to lick hind paws on the hot plate was highly significantly prolonged by laser treatment across all doses and time periods. There was a clear dose dependency for immediate observations, but at 24 h 18 J/cm^2 was the most effective dose. Laser treatment also delayed tail flick responses at both doses and all time periods, but 12 and 18 J/cm^2 doses were similar in efficacy.

Laakso [253] wanted to study the possible relationship between laser therapy and opiods. In a double-blind study, 56 patients with chronic pain conditions were treated with GaAlAs laser 820 nm 25 mW, InGaAlP laser 670 nm 10 mW, and LED 660 nm 9.5 mW. ACTH and ß-endorphin levels were significantly elevated in the laser therapy groups but not in the LED group. Responses were dependent on dose and wavelength. The cumulative effect of laser therapy was confirmed.

Shiroto [53] carried out a retrospective interview-based study of patients who had received pain-relieving treatment with GaAlAs laser light. Of the 3,635 patients treated over a period of 46 months, 82.8% regarded the treatment as effective. 76% of the 1,300 patients who received more than ten treatment applications regarded the treatment as effective. One single application could relieve pain for nine hours (16.5%) to three days (83.5%). This reference is obviously not a matter of a double-blind study or a controlled experiment, and the dropout rate is high, but the size of the group is such that the study should be taken seriously. Shiroto later [217] evaluated an extended patient group of 7,700 patients and arrived at the same results. Recently Shiroto has published the results from 8,844 patients and the results are consistent.

Zhong [303] and Choi [496] have also demonstrated the role of endogenous opiate-like peptides and serotonin in laser acupuncture anaesthesia.

Mizokami [54] studied the effects of GaAlAs laser on pain conditions at a neurosurgical clinic. The number of cases where the result of treatment was "excellent" or "good" among patients with occipital neuralgia was 81%, among patients with pains in arms/shoulders/neck 79%, and for patients with pain in the back 50%.

Irradiation of the stellate ganglion can be used as an additional treatment in pain patients. Hashimoto and Kemmutso [691, 692] have shown that even irradiation of the stellate ganglion alone can have an effect on pain. In a double-blind study, patients with postherpetic neuralgia were treated with either 150 mW GaAlAs, 60 mW GaAlAs or placebo laser. VAS pain scores and regional skin temperature were affected by laser but there was no change in the placebo group. The pain reduction was dose dependent. It is suggested that laser irradiation of the stellate ganglion is a good alternative to traditional blocks.

Phantom pain after amputations is a severe problem. Taguchi [663] reports that laser therapy has been the most effective way of releasing the phantom pain of an amputee.

In a double-blind study by Mohktar [161], experimental pain was induced in human volunteers. The pain was similar to that of an acute fracture. This type of pain is unresponsive to 900 mg of paracetamol or 600 mg of aspirin. A GaAlAs laser, however, did have a significant pain reducing effect.

Hansen [55] treated 40 patients with various chronic oro-facial pain conditions. The majority of the patients (38 female, 2 male) suffered from dysaesthesia ("burning mouth syndrome"). The patients had had their symptoms for approximately five years and were resistant to therapy. The effect was measured on a visual analogue scale (VAS) and by measuring 5-HIAA in urine. No positive effect was observed. It is interesting to note that the authors themselves state the origin of "burning mouth" as multifactor, psychosomatic or psychogenic. Thus, there would be no actual injury to the tissue, and laser, like any other modality, would have no effect. The negative 5-HIAA measurement may indeed confirm the inappropriate inclusion parameters in this study.

Eckerdal [595] used 830 nm 30 mW laser light for atypical facial pain. At the end of the trial, 76% of the patients were pain-free, and at the one-year check-up 44% were free from pain.

Bradley [436] treated 100 cases of painful oral conditions with a GaAlAs laser. A good improvement was achieved in nearly 60%.

In a double-blind study, Cieslar [626] treated a group of 522 patients suffering from various overloading syndromes of the motional system. One group was given sham irradiation, one 904 nm, another 850 nm, and yet another 633 nm laser irradiation. The diagnoses were epicondylitis humeri (1), periarthritis humeroscapularis (2), periarthritis genu (3), and aponeurosis-sitis plantaris (4). Distinct pain relief were generally obtained after 5-7 sessions. Regression of swelling and increased mobility was obtained after 10-20 irradiations. The best results were obtained in epicondylitis (87%) followed by (2), (3), and (4), the latter 61%. Indications (3) and (4) required more sessions than (1) and (2). The results obtained were significantly better by comparison with control, although the high percentage of improvement in the control group (39%) indicates that laser is a strong placebo tool. There was no significant difference between the three wavelengths.

Ceccherrelli [315] used a GaAs laser in a double-blind study on cervical myofascial pain. The patients were submitted to 12 sessions on alternate days, total dose per session 5 J. During each session, the four most painful muscular trigger points and five bilateral homometameric acupuncture points were irradiated. Pain relief was statistically significant both at the end of the treatment period and at a 3-month follow-up examination.

Toya [255] performed a two-centre double-blind study on a group of 115 patients. The groups were: extremity joint pain, cervical pain and lumbar pain. A 830 nm 60 mW laser was used in the contact mode. 82% of those in the laser group reported effective pain relief, compared to 42% in the sham treatment group.

Maricic [56] tested a GaAs laser on 53 dental patients with various pain conditions. The diagnoses included pain after extraction, neuralgia, solitary aphtha, decubitus ulcer, dentitio dificilis and hyperaemic pulp. The average number of treatment sessions was 3.4 and each session took between 3 and 10 minutes. Full relief from pain was achieved in 69.8% of the cases, an obvious improvement in 20.7%, and some improvement in 9.4%. No patient reported a total lack of pain relief.

Manne [222] studied the analgesic effects of GaAs in a blind study. 86 patients reported a pain-relieving effect in various intraoral indications.

Taguchi [189] examined the effects of GaAlAs 780 nm on a group of 124 outpatients with various pain conditions. Treatment was administered one to three times a week for an average of seven weeks. The study was conducted double-blind. A good level of pain relief was achieved in 45 out of 63 members of the experimental group, and in 8 out of 61 of the control group. Thermography was carried out 92 times on 20 different patients. An increase in the skin's microcirculation was observed after laser therapy.

Nelson [1251] studied the effect on somatosensory trigeminal evoked potentials (STEP) and latencies by intraoral laser irradiation of the maxillary nerve. After electrical input at the left infraorbital foramen on 24 experimentally blinded, pain-free subjects, HeNe laser (1.7 mW, 50 Hz, 0.1 J) was performed on 12 of these subjects and sham irradiation on the other 12, at the left maxillary third molar area. Far-field STEP latencies and amplitudes were recorded; at baseline, immediately after intervention, ten and twenty minutes after intervention. In the irradiated group an immediate average STEP amplitude decrease from baseline of 60 percent occurred, with further reduction to 65 and 72 percent at the ten and twenty minute intervals. No significant changes occurred in the sham irradiation group and no change in latencies in either group.

Further literature [443, 1045, 1055, 1261, 1276]

4.1.35 Plantar fasciitis

Plantar fasciitis can be successfully treated with laser therapy. Infrared light is needed in view of the dense skin and the depth of the target (10-12 mm). A good knowledge of the anatomy is essential, since the area of the tendon defect is less than 1 cm^2. 6-10 J over the tendon insertion, followed by 3-4 J per cm along the arch of the foot is a reasonable dosage. 3-6 sessions may be needed, depending on the initial condition of the patient.

Literature:

Basford [1028] treated 32 patients with plantar fasciitis during 12 sessions. The origin of the plantar fascia was given 1 J of 830 nm laser (30 mW) and the medial border of the fascia was swept with a total dose of 2 J. The outcome was negative, quite possibly due to the very low dosage.

Hronková [949] irradiated the place of maximum pain with a 200 mW, 870 nm laser, energy density 9 J/cm^2, ten sessions every other day. 61 patients had this therapy while 52 patients had a non-active placebo laser. In the laser group, 64% had a complete remission of pain, 26% experienced an improvement, and in 10% this therapy brought no effect. In the placebo group 18% reported a full remission of pain, 42% reported an improvement and 40% felt no effect. In a separate study, ultrasound was used for 60 patients - 1 W/cm^2 applied for 5 minutes, ten applications. 50% of the patients had a complete remission of pain, 16.6% were improved and 33.3% reported no effect. Eight of the patients who had had no effect from ultrasound were given laser therapy, not earlier than two weeks after ending the ultrasound treatment. Six of these patients evaluated their treatment as successful while the additional laser therapy had no effect in two patients.

Further literature: [626]

4.1.36 Salivary glands

Sjögren's syndrome is an RA-related condition and is characterised by low saliva and tear secretion, among other things. The treatment of Sjögren's syndrome with lasers is still in the experimental stage, although preliminary results show that the salivary glands do react quickly to local treatment. It has not yet been made clear whether laser therapy has a long-standing effect. All three wavelengths (HeNe, GaAlAs, GaAs) have been shown to stimulate the salivary glands.

Literature:

The first study of salivary stimulation was published in 1987 by Fructuoso [500]. Using GaAs laser, 6 J/cm^2, in a double-blind study, a significant improvement of the salivary production of the parotid gland was achieved. Treatment was given three times a week for three weeks, followed by one week of rest and repeated sessions, total number of sessions 25.

Nagasawa [106] treated patients with Sjögren's syndrome with a GaAlAs laser (20 mW) intraorally, five minutes per treatment. 15 to 20 treatment sessions were administered. After this treatment period, the patients' parotid gland function returned for an extended period.

Takeda [113] examined the effects of a GaAs laser on the submandibular salivary glands of rats. The rats were divided into three groups: a control group, a group treated with GaAs laser irradiation at 760 pulses per second, and a group treated with GaAs laser irradiation at 190 pulses per second. The glands were uncovered and irradiated, after which they were sutured. The effects were studied histologically one hour and 24 hours after irradiation. Increased mitosis in the duct epithelium was observed in one laser group. The greatest increase was in the granular salivary ducts, while the effects in the striated salivary ducts and in the intercalated ducts were less pronounced.

Interestingly, the 760 Hz group exhibited stimulated mitosis, while the 190 Hz group was no different from the control group. The report does not make clear whether the GaAs laser was pulse-train regulated (i.e. gave the same average power, regardless of pulse frequency), and the difference in response may thus be related to dosage.

Kats [279] treated 88 patients with sialoadenitis with HeNe laser. The treatment led to a quicker decline in inflammation and pain, high salivation, longer discomfort-free periods, and an improvement of the gland structure.

Plavnik [1109] found that HeNe laser therapy could elicit an acceleration of soluble proteins in hamster submandibular glands as a result of trophic cell stimulus.

Arao [1110] reports that the salivation in two patients with xerostomia could be stimulated with laser therapy.

4.1.37 Sinuitis

Patients suffering from maxillary sinuitis or allergic rhinitis can have difficulty breathing through the nose during dental treatment. 4-6 J is given intraorally over the bottom of the sinus at 3-4 points on the buccal and palatal side in contact mode. The sinus opening inside the nose is irradiated in non-contact mode, 2-3 J. The projections of the ethmoidal and frontal sinuses are also irradiated if they are involved. Acute sinuitis responds more quickly to treatment than chronic. During extraoral treatment, the eyes should be protected by asking the patient to close them, or by placing moistened cotton wool balls over them. Protective glasses may be obstructive. Treatment can also be through the nostrils.

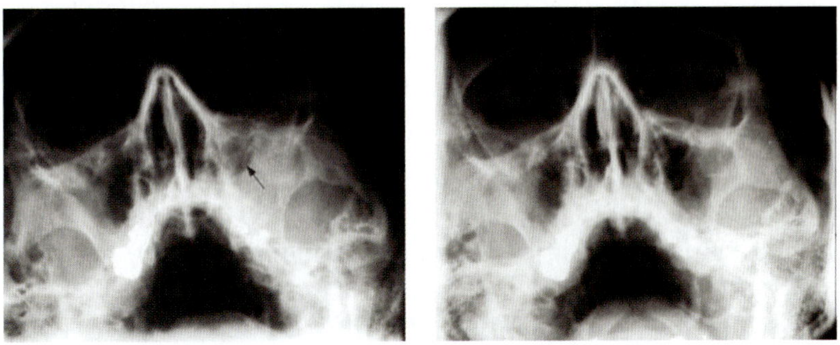

Figure 4.6 Sinuitis maxillaris before and after GaAlAs laser therapy.
Courtesy: M. Hacarova and J. Hubacek

Literature:

Moustsen [103] conducted a double-blind test using a 30 mW GaAlAs laser on a group of 60 patients. Two extraoral points on each side of the nose were irradiated, 3 J each, 3 treatments. No significant results were achieved on the sinuitis.

Roshal [104], on the other hand, treated two groups of 227 and 120 children with allergic rhinitis. HeNe laser light was administered directly on the mucosa, via fibre optics, with excellent results. The positive results of this study were confirmed by tomography and direct inspection. Although this study does not report on sinuitis, it shows the importance of reaching the inflamed mucosa with the irradiation.

Kaiser [507] used HeNe laser in a double-blind study of acute maxillary sinuitis. 30 patients participated in each group. 7 J/cm^2 was given on the skin and 4 J/cm^2 intraorally over the bottom of the sinus. The oedema of the mucosa was reduced.

Kruchinina [541] examined the effect of HeNe laser therapy in young patients with sinuitis through conjunctival biomicroscopy. Laser therapy produced a positive effect on microcirculation. The primary effects were on vessel permeability (decrease of oedema) and red blood cell aggregation. The best results were obtained in acute cases.

Further literature [340, 466, 534, 541, 542, 543, 555, 1036, 1155]

4.1.38 Spinal cord injuries

Literature:

The purpose of an experiment by Shi [839] was to elucidate the influence of the HeNe laser on the regeneration of peripheral nerves. 44 rabbits were used in the experiment. The animals were divided into 4, 8, 12, 16 weeks groups according to the observation period. Six animals were used in each irradiated group and in the control group 5 rabbits were used in each observation period. Regeneration of the axons and myelinic sheaths, the latent rate of the common peroneal nerve, the condition of the anterior tibial muscle and the toe expansion test were all observed systematically in both groups. The experimental results were: A few thin regenerated axons were seen at 4 weeks in the irradiated group, while in the control group it could be not be observed until the 8th week. A low amplitude latent rate of the common peroneal nerve was determined at the peroneal side of the anterior tibial muscle in a few animals at 4 weeks in the irradiated group, but it was not observed in the control group before 12 -16 weeks. The regeneration of the myeline sheath was evident in the irradiated group. 16 weeks postoperatively, the toe expansion test was normal in the irradiated group, while in the control group it was the same as seen at 12 weeks after operation in the irradiated group.

Rochkind [561] and his group subjected 17 dogs to laminectomy and transection of the spinal cord at TH12-L1. An autograft of the left sciatic nerve was then implanted into the injured area. Neurorrhaphy was performed on the right sciatic nerve. Seven dogs did not receive any additional treatment and served as a control. The other 10 were treated transcutaneously with 16 mW of HeNe laser light for 20 days (high doses) over the operated area. The 7 dogs in the control group became paralysed as expected. The 10 dogs that underwent the same operation but were immediately treated with a laser were able to stand after 7-9 weeks, and could walk a few steps after 9-12 weeks. The histological picture obtained from the dogs 21 days post operation showed no rejection and no prominent scar tissue at the site of contact between the spinal cord tissue and the transplanted nerve. Moreover, new axons and blood vessels originating in the spinal tissue extended into the graft. These were seen only in the laser treated group and not in the control group, in which scar tissue had developed at the site of transection.

The double-blind randomised study by Shamir [1182] evaluated the therapeutic effect of laser therapy on peripheral nerve regeneration after complete transection and direct anastomosis of the rat sciatic nerve. 13 of 24 rats received postoperative laser therapy, 780 nm, applied transcutaneously, 30 min daily for 21 consecutive days, to corresponding segments of the spinal cord and to the injured sciatic nerve. Positive somatosensory evoked responses were found in 69.2 % of the irradiated rats, as compared to 18.2 % of the non-irradiated rats. Immunohistochemical staining in the laser-treated group showed an increased total number of axons and better quality of the regeneration process, due to an increased number of large-diameter axons compared to the non-irradiated control group.

4.1.39 Sports injuries

The use of lasers in sports medicine is widespread. Top-level sportsmen and women often suffer from injuries, and it is vital for the injuries to heal quickly so that the individual can resume training. Sports injuries have the “advantage” that the subject often knows when the injury occurred and where it is. They also often have experience of how long it takes for a particular injury to heal. It is therefore easy to "calibrate" the effect of the laser. A rule of thumb is that a sports injury takes a little more than half the ordinary healing time if the healing process is stimulated with laser therapy. A common problem is that the subjective discomfort in the injured area soon disappears and the individual wants to return to training immediately. It is essential that the injured area be allowed to rest and that training be resumed gradually. Treatment should not be interrupted just because pain is gone. This is only the first sign of recovery.

Laser therapy on chronic pain conditions can increase the pain level initially. This reaction is absent when treating acute injuries. Acute injuries can actually receive higher doses than chronic cases without side effects. Common conditions such as delayed onset muscle soreness and periostitis react very favourably to laser therapy. Therapy should be started as soon as possible after training or competition. In some instances therapy before training/competition is useful. There is a strong incentive for the professional athlete to use laser therapy.

Oedema is a common element in sports injuries. If there are a number of injured places, the patient should be treated according to Ohshiro's "proximal priority principle". This means that the proximal injury is treated first, the distal last. If the distal injury is treated first, lymph accumulation increases because the proximal injury prevents drainage. The result in such a case could be increased pain.

"Power pulse" GaAs lasers with multiprobes give the shortest treatment times and have the widest range of indications. A GaAlAs laser is good for superficial and more limited injuries. However, the recent advent of high-powered GaAlAs lasers (100 mW or more) has widened the range of their indications. The handy format of medium-powered GaAlAs lasers makes them very useful for ambulatory work. (See chapter 4.1.41 “Tendinitis/bursitis” on page 176.)

Literature:

Weiss [276] and Bibikova [277] observed improved muscle regeneration as a result of the use of HeNe and GaAs lasers in experiments on rats and batrachians (a kind of frog), respectively.

Glinkowski [503] compared two groups of patients with sprained ankles. One group was treated conservatively with plaster casts for two weeks; the other received GaAs 3.6 J/cm^2 for one week. The results observed with plaster casts after two weeks were achieved within one week with laser therapy.

The studies above employed HeNe or GaAs laser. In three Danish studies by Axelsen [547], Darre [548], and Nissen [535], no effect was seen on ankle sprain, achilles tendinitis, or medial tibial stress syndrome, using 830 nm, 30-40 mW. Laser type and dose may not be suitable for these indications. The dose in [547] is very low. Winther [549] was also unsuccessful until switching to GaAs for tendinitis. De Bie failed to obtain positive results for ankle sprain as well. However, only a very small area (1 cm^2) was treated.

Simunovic [957] confirms the positive effect of laser therapy in sports injuries in a double-blind multicentre study using a combination of GaAlAs and HeNe laser.

Ohshiro [961] selected 6 Japanese sumo wrestlers and treated their symptoms. Laser therapy resulted in alleviation of their symptoms and an increased win rate.

Further literature [74, 122, 123, 281, 298, 299, 431, 709, 734, 735, 739, 1242]

4.1.40 Strain injuries

Show me a dentist, barber, secretary, masseur or a physiotherapist over 40 who doesn't have aches and pains somewhere! A better working position, more ergonomically correct equipment, and visits to gyms and swimming pools are warmly recommended, but the laser is a valuable supplement for keeping these injuries in check. Typical work-related injuries for people in the medical profession are tennis elbow and neck and low back pain. Treat tender points in the order they arose.

Literature:

Tasaki [125] treated 18 patients with low back pain with a GaAlAs laser at 30-80 mW. The sessions lasted 2-10 minutes and led to full pain relief. Pain relief took 6-8 hours to be effected among the patients who did not experience it immediately. Knowledge of suitable anatomical points for treatment is essential in order to achieve good results with this condition, which is known as being difficult to treat.

Terashima [126] treated 23 patients with lateral humeral epicondylitis and 40 patients with de Quervain's disease with a GaAlAs laser. In the epicondylitis group, movement pains and soreness were positively affected in 61% of cases, and in the de Quervain group, in 70% of cases. Movement pains were eradicated in 13% of cases. Seen as a whole, the treatment was effective for 61% of the patients in the epicondylitis group, while 45% in the other group experienced good results.

Further literature: [127, 192, 195, 199, 208].

4.1.41 Tendinitis/bursitis

Bjordal [732] has analysed the literature regarding the treatment of shoulder tendinitis/bursitis and concludes: "The methodological quality of the laser therapy-trials of shoulder tendinitis/bursitis is similar to or higher than in trials with medical interventions for shoulder tendinitis/bursitis. Total sample size of high quality laser therapy-trials is similar to or higher than total sample size of high quality NSAID-trials or steroid injection-trials on the same diagnosis. The four laser therapy-trials should serve as a valid platform for drawing conclusions on clinical effects of laser therapy." He further concludes: "There is consistent evidence of clinical effects of laser therapy in all four shoulder trials, as the results are in favour of active laser therapy with confidence intervals not including zero. The trials with fewest treatment sessions per week had the lowest success rate. Best clinical effects were seen in patients with short duration of symptoms (less than one month)."

Daily sessions for 5-6 days are needed to reduce inflammation, 8-10 to increase collagen production.

Dosage per point is adapted to the distance between skin and tendon (depth), and the number of points is adapted to the area of the inflammation. According to measurements performed by Bjordal, the various tendon locations have different characteristics that affect determination of dose. The figures below represent:

Indication	**Tendon depth to target tendon,**	**Tendon thickness**	**Area to treat**
Plantar fasciitis	10.0 - 12.0 mm	3.0 - 4.0 mm	0.1 - 0.8 cm^2
Achilles tendinitis	1.5 - 3.0 mm	4.5 - 6.0 mm	0.5 - 2.0 cm^2
Patellar tendinitis	2.5 - 4.0 mm	5.5 - 8.0 mm	1.0 - 4.0 cm^2
Epicondylitis	1.5 - 2.5 mm	2.0 - 4.0 mm	0.09 - 0.3 cm^2
Rotatorcuff	5.0 - 10.0 mm	5.5 - 8.0 mm	0.5 - 1.5 cm^2

Table 4.2: Tendinitis/Bursitis different characteristics

Literature:

In a tendon healing experiment Xu [781] used 50 white Leghorn hens. Ten were randomly assigned as a normal control group, the other 40 were used in the study. After anaesthetising, one half of the profundus tendons of the second and third toes on both sides of the feet were cut. Postoperatively, the hens moved freely in the cages. One foot was randomly chosen to belong to the treatment group, the other foot served as an unirradiated control group. The injured tendons in the treatment group were irradiated for twenty minutes daily with a HeNe laser at a constant power density of 12.74 mW/cm^2, the first exposure taking place 24 hours after the operation. The longest course of treatment was 3 weeks. The control group was not irradiated. At 3 days and at 1, 2, 3, and 5 weeks after surgery, 8 hens were sacrificed and their tendons were examined. The experimental results: (1) active, passive flexion and tendon gliding functional recovery were significantly better in the treatment group ($p < 0.01$); (2) width and thickness of the tendon at the cut site were significantly smaller in the treatment group ($p < 0.01$); (3) degrees of tendon adhesions were significantly lighter in the treatment group ($p < 0.05$). The experimental results demonstrate that HeNe laser radiation had significant effects on anti-inflammation, detumescence, progressive hematoma absorbing, inhibiting tendon extrinsic healing, reducing tendon adhesions, improving tendon intrinsic healing, i.e., stimulating epitenon and endotenon cells proliferation and migration into the gap, stimulating collagen synthesis in the tendon gap, and enhancing the late remodeling of fibrous peritendonous adhesion.

Enwemeka [124] cut and sutured the Achilles tendons of 20 rabbits. Six of these rabbits were treated locally with HeNe, seven with GaAs laser. The other seven served as a control. After 14 days, the tensile strength of the tendons was checked. The mean value in the HeNe group was 251, in the GaAs group 233, and in the control group 154.

Early mechanical loading and laser therapy have been shown to promote tendon healing. Reddy [725] combined these two parameters, using HeNe laser on rabbit achilles tendons. The findings indicate that the combination of laser therapy and early mechanical loading of tendons increases collagen production, with marginal biomechanical effects on repaired tendons.

Reddy [546] tenectomised and repaired the Achilles tendons in rabbits. The limbs were immobilised and treated with 1 J/cm^2 of HeNe light for 14 days. Control animals received sham laser treatment. The collagen content in the treated tendons was significantly higher than in the control group. Extraction of collagen from the regenerating tissues revealed that the laser-treated tendons yielded significantly higher concentrations of neutral salt soluble and insoluble collagen than control tendons.

Parizotto [653] tenectomised the achilles tendons in 32 rats and resutured the skin. After 24 hours HeNe laser was applied daily for ten days. Doses of 0.5, 5 and 50 J/cm^2 were used. HeNe laser enhanced the intra- and intermolecular hydrogen bonding in the collagen molecules. The treated tendons were more organised than controls.

Strupinska [821] treated 50 patients with achilles injuries and 50 patients with external epicondyalgia. The patients were irradiated by GaAs laser separately or together with HeNe laser. The result of the therapy was based on interviews with and examinations of patients as well as on the Laitinen pain questionnaire. The results proved an analgesic effect.

(See chapter 4.1.15 "Epicondylitis" on page 141.)

Further literature [195, 242, 736, 737, 1061]

4.1.42 Tinnitus, vertigo, Ménière´s disease

A new and promising indication for laser therapy is tinnitus. This inner ear disease is a growing problem in noisy modern society and the number of persons suffering from tinnitus is increasing. Traditional treatment for tinnitus is psychological support or various masking procedures. Acupuncture and ginko extracts have been tried with limited success. Laser therapy alone offers a new and promising treatment modality. Irradiation is given partly through the meatus, partly behind the ear, provided the problem really is located in the inner ear. Since the bone behind the ear is very compact, high power densities and prolonged treatment times are necessary to reach a sufficient dose in the inner ear when irradiating through bone.

Literature:

Witt [1084] is one of the pioneers in this field, but to the knowledge of the authors his results have not been published in any peer-review journal. Witt combines infusion of Gingko biloba (Egb 761, 17.5 mg dry extract per 5 ml ampoule) and laser. This may be a favourable combination but an evaluation of the contribution of the laser is not possible. More than 500 patients have been treated since 1989 and Witt claims that more than 60% of the patients have reached a considerable or total relief. The laser used is a combination of a HeNe laser with 12 mW output and a GaAs laser with 5 laser diodes each with 15 mW average power and output was used. Treatment technique is not stated.

Swoboda [1085] did not find any significant effect of Gingko/laser. However, the ginkgo infusion used was at a homeopathic level (D3 = 1:1000 dilution), according to Witt.

Partheniadis-Stumpf [1086] also failed to find any effect from the combined ginkgo (6 ml Tebonin) infusion and laser. However, the laser was applied at a distance of one cm above the mastoid. The non-contact mode reduces penetration considerably and the mastoid is not ideal for reaching the inner ear.

Plath [306] treated 40 tinnitus patients with 50 mg Ginkgo biloba. 20 patients received sham laser irradiation, 20 real laser. A HeNe laser with 12 mW output and a GaAs laser with 5 laser diodes each with 15 mW average power and output was used, irradiation procedure approximately the same as for Partheniadis-Stumpf. In this study, however, 50% of the patients reported a reduction of the tinnitus of more than 10 dB, as compared with 5% in the control group, in both self-assessment and audiometric findings.

A similar study has been performed by von Wedel [1087]. 155 patients were treated with Ginkgo infusion (5 ml Syxyl D3) and laser. The outcome was negative. No information about the type of laser, treatment technique or dosage is given, making evaluation impossible.

Shiomi [686] has investigated the effect of infrared laser applied directly into the meatus acousticus, 21 J, once a week for 10 weeks. The result of this non-controlled study is as follows: 26% of the patients reported improved duration, 58% reduced loudness and 55% reported a general reduction in annoyance.

The same author [687] has also examined the effect of light on the cochlea using guinea pigs. Direct laser irradiation was administered to the cochlea through the round window. The amplitude of CAP was reduced to 53-83% immediately after the onset of irradiation. The amplitude then returned to the original level. The results of this investigation suggest that laser therapy might lessen tinnitus by suppressing the abnormal excitation of the eighth nerve of the organ of Corti.

More or less the same parameters were used in a controlled study by Mirtz [1088] but in this case there was no significant effect.

Nakashima [1266] treated 68 ears in 68 patients with tinnitus. A 60 mW laser was applied for 6 minutes (21.6 J), once a week for 4 weeks in a double blind study. There was no significant difference between the two groups, which is not surprising considering the few sessions and the low energy applied. No differential diagnosis between somatosensory and other causes for tinnitus was performed.

Wilden [474, 1089] uses a different method with a considerably increased dose. A set consisting of one visible laser and three powerful

GaAlAs lasers is used, covering a large area over and around the ear in the non-contact mode. Doses between 3,000 and 5,000 J are given each session. Laser is applied as a monotherapy. More than 800 patients have been treated with this concept and positive effects are reported even for vertigo. Recent injuries in “the disco generation” are more easily treated than long-term chronic conditions. In a separate study [1090] Wilden reports improvement of the hearing capacity of these patients, as evaluated by audiometry. An advantage of the Wilden method is that several muscles with a possible somatosensory background will be affected by the large area of irradiation used.

Tauber [1091] has performed an *ex-vivo* laser penetration study. Based on these findings it was possible to calculate the energy needed to obtain a dose of 4 J/cm^2 in the cochlea itself. Irradiation via the mastoid showed values 103 to 105 times smaller (depending on wavelength) than irradiation through the tympanic membrane. 30 patients were treated five times within 2 weeks [1092]. One group was irradiated with 635 nm diode laser, the other with 830 nm diode laser. By self-assessment around 40% of the patients reported a slight to significant attenuation of the tinnitus loudness of the irradiated ear.

Prochazka [1093] has evaluated the effect of combined Egb 761 Ginkgo infusion and laser in a double blind study. 37 patients were divided into three groups. One group had Egb 761 only, one Egb761 and placebo laser, one Egb761 and real laser, 830 nm. The results in the three groups were as follows: no effect 29/26/19, less than 50% relief 44/48/29, more than 50% relief 18/26/36, no more tinnitus 9/0/26. Irradiation was performed over the mastoid and over the meatus acousticus, twice a week, 8-10 sessions, total 175 J.

Rogowski [1094] divided a group of 32 tinnitus patients into one group receiving laser therapy and one receiving a placebo procedure. Dose, wavelength and treatment technique are not stated in the available English abstract. The effect was evaluated through VAS. Within the patient group, transiently evoked otoacoustic emissions (TEOAE) were measured before, during and after therapy. No significant difference between laser and placebo was found in annoyance or loudness of the tinnitus and in changes of TEOAE amplitude. These results indicate that there is no relationship between the effect of low-power laser and changes in cochlear micromechanics.

A pilot study was performed by Gable [1224] on 3 individuals who were suffering from Chronic Otitis Externa, "Swimmers Ear" or "Tropical Ear" that had been unresponsive to conservative medical management for a minimum period of 3 months. Each patient was classed as chronic and referred by a medical practitioner for laser therapy. Each patient was irradiated over a 2 to 6 week period with a progressively increasing energy of 15 to 30 Joules via the single source of the ear canal using a 100 mW probe. Allowing for beam divergence within the confined canal, reflection and inverse square spread from the emission source to the tympanic membrane, these factors would roughly balance equating to an approximate energy density dose of 15-30 J/cm². The individual patients existing medical regime was continued unchanged. Each patient showed full condition resolution for a minimum period of 1 month post discharge. Two of the patients were swimmers, 1 competitive at state level. In both cases it enabled the individuals to return to swimming within 1-3 weeks of treatment commencement and to remain in the water during the completion of the treatment period through to full resolution and post discharge follow-up at 1 month. On a 6 month follow-up of one patient, a 9 year boy with grommets and a life history of ongoing ear infections had remained infection free for the first time for a period greater than 6 weeks. A secondary effect was a reduction of motion sickness indicating that the laser therapy has also affected the cochlear and vestibular apparatus.

A few other indications in otorhinolaryngology have been treated with low level lasers, even with intravenous irradiation. [688, 689, 690, 1095, 1096].

Further literature [874, 1174], 1227, 1228]

All the above studies assume that tinnitus and vertigo are always inner ear problems. However, these conditions frequently have a muscular origin ("somatosensory tinnitus").

The percentage of patients with a muscular origin for their tinnitus/vertigo is not known but seems to be large. A differential diagnosis is therefore very important before any therapy is applied, laser or traditional therapies. If this is not done, studies of the effect of transmeatal laser therapy become a gamble. The outcome would rather be related to the type of tinnitus dominating in the verum group than the actual effect of the therapy. An interdisciplinary co-operation between the ENT physician and a dentist is recommended.

Meniere´s disease is a condition first described by the French physician Ménière in 1861. It is a clinical entity consisting of vertigo, fluctuating hearing loss and tinnitus. Few medical conditions have been so thoroughly studied and described, yet lacking an effective therapy. Tinnitus, however, is not necessarily associated with Meniere; it is often an isolated condition. But the treatment of somatosensory Meniere and somatosensory tinnitus is very similar and in the following we make a simplification and speak only about "tinnitus".

Muscular tension is a key element in somatosensory tinnitus. The role of the laser is to create an immediate reduction of pain in the muscle with a consecutive relaxation. Thus, this intervention will make all the following therapy faster and more successful. Somatosensory tinnitus has been difficult to treat and often passes without a diagnosis. The combination of laser therapy in the traditional therapy of temporomandibular disorders (TMD) and cervical spine disorders (CSD) has been proven to be a more successful way of helping these patients, compared to traditional therapies. However, it is not to be expected that all symptoms will subdue rapidly. The skill of the dentist, the co-operation of the patient and concomitant physiotherapy are important factors. Many patients will not be completely relieved of symptoms but the majority will experience a great reduction of their problems. According to Bjorne [1263] and Estola-Partanen [1267] the treatment of somatosensory tinnitus reduces the severity of tinnitus more than the incidence. The 3-year follow up study by Bjorne [1263] showed simultaneous decreases in the intensities of vertigo, nonwhirling dizziness, tinnitus, feeling of fullness in the ear, pain in the face and jaws, pain in the neck and shoulders, and headache that were both longitudinal and highly significant. Significant reductions in the frequency of vertigo, nonwhirling dizziness, and headache were also reported by the patients as well as complete disappearance of pain located in the vertex area. A significant relief of TMD symptoms and decrease in nervousness was also achieved. It must be underlined that the success in the study [1263] reflects the outcome of the therapy before the author started to use laser therapy as an additional method. The addition of laser therapy has then further improved the progress in this category of patients. Frequently these patients can notice a change in the character of their tinnitus when the lateral pterygoid muscle is irradiated.

The suboccipital muscles should also be palpated, since these muscles and the masticatory muscles are closely functionally connected. In fact, the mandible and the upper cervical joint (C0/C1) constitute an integrated motor system.

The therapy outlined below brings new hope to a large group of "intractable" patients. It outlines the traditional therapy created by Bjorne, with the recent (2000) successful addition of laser therapy.

Somatosensory tinnitus examination and therapy acc. to Bjorne/Tunér

Anamnesis

1 Does the patient experience a feeling of fatigue in the jaws, difficulties in mouth opening, sensations of tension in the jaws/neck, hypersensitive or tender teeth, clenching of tongue/jaws, tendency for general stress, wakes up at night due to tinnitus?

2 Can the patient manipulate his/her tinnitus through movements of the jaw and neck? Usual movements evoking this phenomenon are: opening the mouth wide, protrusion and side movements of the mandible, flexion/ extension and side rotation of the upper cervical joints.

3 Can the patient manipulate his/her tinnitus by putting pressure/ stimulation in the areas of the sensory innvervation of the trigeminal nerve of the Trigeminal nerve? Usual areas evoking this phenomenon are putting pressure on tragus, over the cheek, jaw or temple, the stylomandibular ligament but also gazing with the eyes.

4 Are there other symptoms related to tension: pain in the jaws, face, neck, and headache?

Status

1 Observation of hypertrophic masticatory muscles and possible abnormal posture of the head/neck.

2 Palpation of the masticatory muscles (the lateral pterygoid muscle in particular), the TMJ, and the suboccipital muscles.

3 Range of movement of the mandible and neck.

4 Active shining bruxing facets as signs of active bruxism.

Therapy

1 Laser treatment of tender areas in the jaw and neck muscles, 5-15 J per point depending on size and location of muscle. 2-3 sessions per week acc. to the evolution of improvement, preferably with GaAlAs or GaAs laser.

2 Training in how to normalise abnormal head/neck posture, and training how to relax masticatory, neck and shoulder muscles.

3 Training of autostretching of the suboccipital muscles (the rectus capitis posterior minor and major muscles and the obliquus capitis superior muscles), the upper and middle trapezius muscles and the levator scapulae muscles. Laser therapy of tender areas in these muscles is also recommended.

4 Minute examination of occlusal function and presence of active interferences, followed by adjustment through grinding.

5 Information about the necessity of adjusting style of life.

6 Bite splint in selected cases

Most common dental occlusal backgrounds:

1 The patient is clenching/bruxing on active shining facets of the front teeth, forcing the TMJ:s to slide forwards, due to activation/tension of the lateral pterygoid muscles.

2 Cross bite (sliding areas preventing central occlusion and balanced TMJ position).

4.1.43 Tonsillitis

Literature:

In a pilot study, Petrek [524] used a HeNe laser to treat eight patients suffering from chronic tonsillitis. Three treatment sessions were given over a period of nine days. Shortly after the cessation of treatment, a significant increase of secretory immunoglobulin A in saliva was observed, followed by an increase of IgA serum levels after four weeks of follow-up. These findings correlated well with the clinical improvement in seven out of the eight patients.

Hubacek [1036] irradiated the palatal tonsils with HeNe laser, 0.6 J/cm^2 each over one week and found an increase of T lymphocytes and plasmatic cells in the tonsils after therapy.

Further literature: [700, 701, 707]

4.1.44 Trigeminal neuralgia

There are no entirely effective treatment methods for this painful condition. Laser treatment comes with no guarantee of success, but bearing in mind that the method is painless and without side effects, it should be a more attractive choice than deep blockades and strong analgesics. Patients receiving laser therapy can reduce their Carbamazapine dose. All three laser types can be used.

Both extraoral and intraoral trigger points and pain points are irradiated. 2-3 J per standard point (standard points are the various foramina, such as the infraorbital, supraorbital, mental, mandibular, palatinum major, and incisivum) is an appropriate initial dosage. Pain points can be given 3-4 J. The course of the main nerve is then irradiated extra- or intraorally. When irradiating through bone, as with the n. mandibularis inferior, the dose must be increased by a factor of 3 to compensate for loss of penetration. A pain reaction is not unusual and should be interpreted as a positive sign. Patients should be warned about its likelihood beforehand. Treat twice a week initially and then allow a longer period between treatments. Treatment should not be interrupted if and when the pain disappears, but should continue at longer and longer intervals.

Literature:

Eckerdal [452, 595] used 830 nm laser light at 30 mW in a double-blind study of the effect of laser therapy on trigeminal neuralgia. A positive effect was evident. It is necessary to find the pertinent trigger points/zones and to include the II branch of the trigeminal nerve in the treatment. Treatment was given once a week for five weeks, 2 J per trigger point. At the end of the trial, 10 of the 14 patients in the verum group were free from pain and 2 improved. At the one-year follow-up, 6 patients were still free from pain and 10 were back to the initial condition. In the placebo group, 1 patient was free from pain and 2 improved at 6 months. At the one-year follow-up, one was still free from pain and the other 13 were back to the initial state of pain. Consumption of analgesics was significantly reduced in the verum group at the end of the treatment period but was constant in the placebo group. If the patient had already received alcohol blocks, the treatment was less successful.

Further literature [191, 211, 218, 444, 452, 509, 517, 595, 635, 755, 757, 758, 762, 1057, 1070, 1111]

4.1.45 Thrombophlebitis

Literature:

In a study by Dedenko [567], a HeNe laser was used to treat thrombophlebitis. The laser produced a marked analgesic, desensitising, hypocoagulative and immunostimulating effect.

4.1.46 Tuberculosis

Literature:

Bhagwanani [715] has used nitrogen laser (337 nm) for the treatment of tuberculosis in patients resistant to traditional antibiotics. A needle is inserted into the lung and used as the carrier of the light. Ten minutes of irradiation is often enough for a clinical improvement in 90% of the patients. 60% of the patients showed improvement on their X-rays.

Agaev [716] compared the effect of HeNe laser treatment in two groups of patients with chronic destructive pulmonary tuberculosis or post-operative broncopulmonary complications. A group of 50 patients had HeNe laser treatment and a non-irradiated group of 30 patients served as control. The post surgery complication rate was 32% in the laser group and 63% in the control group.

Zhuk [1141] divided a number of patients with chronic tuberculosis into two groups. One group (group I, 174 patients) received chemotherapy and another (group II, 240 patients) chemotherapy and laser irradiation, 890 nm. Transcutaneous irradiation over the lung projection and skin irradiation of great blood vessels were used. Dose at skin varied between 0.002-0.05 J/cm^2, depending on the pulse frequency used. Within 3 months sputum smear conversation/cavity closure was observed in 60/36 % the treatment group II and 36/16% in group I. After 6 months the percentages were 85/65 % in group II and 49/29 in group I.

Further literature [710, 965, 966, 1177]

4.1.47 Urology

Literature:

In a study by Lubart [592], it was found that 780 nm laser light inhibits Ca^{2+} uptake by sperm mitochondria and enhances Ca^{2+} binding to sperm plasma membranes. The effect of light on Ca^{2+} uptake by plasma membrane vesicles in the absence of ATP was much greater than in the presence of ATP.

Sato [580] found that laser therapy increases the mobility and speed of sperm *in vitro*.

Ocaña-Quero [683] compared the effects of HeNe laser, calcium and heparin with regard to the induction of the acrosome reaction and mortality in bull sperm cells. It is concluded that the application of HeNe laser at doses from 2 to 16 J/cm^2 induced the acrosome reaction and decreased the bull sperm cell mortality percentage *in vitro* significantly better than the other capacitation agents and as compared to the control group.

Cohen [596] reports an enhanced fertilisation rate of mouse spermatozoa *in vitro* using 633 nm laser light. The results suggest that the effect of 633 nm HeNe laser irradiation is mediated through the generation of hydrogen peroxide by the spermatozoa and that this effect plays a significant role in the augmentation of the sperm cell's capacity to fertilise *in vitro*.

Lubart [1196] found that HeNe laser irradiation of human spermatozoa resulted in a significant increase in its egg penetration ability. The effect appeared only in men with low sperm penetration rates. Using the electron paramagnetic resonance technique it was established that OH radicals are produced in irradiated spermatozoa.

Kipshidze [1041] used HeNe laser on human corpus cavernosum smooth muscle cells *in vitro*. Laser induced an increase in the expression of NO and elevation of cyclic guanosine monophosphate (cGMP). This substance is important in the process of smooth muscle relaxation in the corpus cavernosum and consequently for the erection. It is suggested that laser therapy could be used in a combination with pharmaceuticals or as solo therapy for patients with coronary artery disease or hypertension.

Hasan [141] used laser therapy on male infertility. The testicles of 25 childless men were irradiated with a combination of HeNe and GaAs light. Of these 25, four were azoospermic, nine were highly oligospermic, and seven were moderately oligospermic. No result was achieved in the azoospermic group, while in the oligospermic groups the sperm count increased by between 200% and 500%. Libido also increased in 15 of the oligospermic patients. Treatment was administered twice a week, a total of ten times. As sperm creation takes two to three months, the mechanism at work here is not known. Laser therapy is, however, shown to be a supplementary method for subfertile men.

Kovalev [684] treated 55 men suffering from aspermatogenic sterility with HeNe laser. The results indicate a stimulating effect on the testicular function.

Uchida [146] treated 20 patients with chronic prostatitis or prostatodynia. GaAs laser was administered through the perineum or the rectum. In some cases, the acupuncture point Tsubo was used. Two patients were freed from their symptoms completely, and 14 experienced good to average improvement. The soreness in the prostate disappeared in most of those who received irradiation through the rectum.

Mazo [338] has also reported on transrectal treatment of prostatic problems.

The effect of different approaches to laser therapy of acute non-specific epididymitis was studied by Gomberg [681]. In a previous study by Reznikov [682], trans-scrotal HeNe irradiation had proved beneficial. Gomberg compared trans-scrotal endolymphatic and laser acupuncture for the treatment of a group of 28 patients. The endolymphatic treatment was performed via a small quartz fibre inserted into the regional lymphatic node, 0.15 J in total. The transdermal dose was maximum 2.7 J. Laserpuncture (Hegu and Zusanli) was performed using a maximum of 30 J per point. The clinical outcome as well as the polymorphonucleocyte/lymphocyte index, main population and subpopulations of lymphocytes were evaluated. Endolymphatic irradiation was found to be more efficient than trans-scrotal laser therapy. The former required 4 procedures at intervals of 24 hours, whereas trans-scrotal irradiation required 1-3 days longer. Laser acupuncture was not effective.

Induratio penis plastica is a rare affection of the penis, though occurrence is reported in 6 - 9 per cent of male population. The dual mechanism of the effect of laser treatment can be employed in implicating overproduction of fibrin (and its resorption) as well as in exerting a direct influence on inflammatory processes.

In a study by Prochazka [895], 40 patients were followed for more than a five-year period. Classic medicamentous techniques (colchicine, vitamin E) were combined with laser treatment of the following parameters: probes 200 and 300 mW, 50 J/cm^2 continuous mode + 50 J/cm^2 with beam modulated in 5 Hz frequency in one therapy bout. The therapy was applied 20 times in succession, twice a week as an introductory series of procedures, followed by a maintenance series of 3 - 5 procedures 2 - 3 times a year. In combination with ultrasound the total effect was very satisfactory.

Longo [608, 672] has treated some 100 cases of induration penis plastica with GaAs or defocused CO_2 laser. Circular and/or transversal plaque formation is a contraindication for laser therapy. In other milder forms laser therapy can improve pain, recurvatio, signs of inflammation and ecographic findings. The increase of elasticity during the erection is the first visible result of the treatment. Around 4 J per point has been used.

Johnson [770] reports the preliminary results of a non randomised trial using a 30 mW GaAlAs laser to treat patients with symptomatic Peyronie's disease. All patients in the study had the disease, consisting of a well-defined fibrous plaque causing pain and/or curvature of the penile shaft on erection that interfered with satisfactory sexual intercourse. 3 J per point was administered, beginning at the base of the penis and extending to the coronal sulcus over the dorsum of the penis at 0.5 cm intervals. An additional 3 J was delivered to each 0.5 cm of palpable plaque. The ability of the therapy to reduce the size of the fibrous plaque, the severity of the penile curvature, and the severity of pain associated with penile erection and the treatment's effect on the patient's quality of life were assessed for each patient at completion of therapy and 6 weeks later.

Strada [983] has treated nearly 300 patients with Peyronie’s disease. GaAs laser treatment in combination with ultrasound was performed once a week for five weeks. All the patients showed pain reduction at 2 months control. 60% reported reduction of recurvatio penis. A group of patients underwent phlebocavernosometry, showing disappearance of patches in 30% of the cases. Strada has also treated more than 200 patients with chronic abacterial prostatitis. A GaAs laser probe was used in an endorectal approach (every second day, 12 sessions) and a 30 mW GaAlAs laser was used in a urethral approach (every 3 days, 8 sessions). More than 65% of the patients had symptom relief even after 6 months. Spermatic fluid was analysed before and after therapy. There was an increase in total germinal cell count, improvement in motility and in morphology. Prostate ultrasound showed a mean reduction of prostate volume from 29.9 cc to 21.9 cc, probably due to resolution of oedema.

Strada also reports that urethral strictures have been treated with GaAs laser, 10 sessions. Only patients with stricture diameters larger than 3 mm were treated. Five patients improved their micturation and flowmetry.

Male genital tract chronic inflammations were treated by Gasparyan [912] using combinations of transdermal, transrectal (prostate gland) and intravenous HeNe laser irradiation. The energy of a 2 mW HeNe laser was applied via a light guide into a vein. The projections of the male genital organ and the inguinal areas were irradiated with a 890 nm 5W peak power cluster probe. For the transrectal prostate gland irradiation with a super-pulsed GaAs laser 890 nm, 15W peak power was used. 36 patients were given conventional medical therapy and another 36 were given laser therapy in combination with medical therapy. Clinical and laboratory findings were statistically better in the laser therapy group and relapse rate was lower. It is suggested that laser therapy increases the local circulation and thus also improves the effect of antibiotics.

Further literature: [142, 606, 684, 722, 920, 1202]

4.1.48 Warts

Laser therapy is widely used to treat common warts. The effect is not well documented and the results are inconsistent. The success rate in children is much higher than in adults.

Further literature: [649]

4.1.49 Whiplash-associated disorders

Literature:

Fitz-Ritson [392] compared three types of treatment for whiplash injury. The first group (17 patients) received joint manipulation and soft tissue therapy. The second group (18 patients) received the same treatment plus an exercise programme. The third group received the same treatment as group 2, plus InGaAlP laser light at 660 nm, 6 mW, and GaAlAs laser light at 880 nm, 8 mW. Extensor muscle strength was measured. The data showed a difference between group 2 and 3 (most improved) after 4 weeks, reaching statistical significance after 8 weeks.

In the experience of the authors, secondary muscular involvement can be successfully treated with laser therapy, whereas the primary problems will remain.

4.1.50 Wound healing

Non-healing skin wound before and after two days of HeNe laser therapy

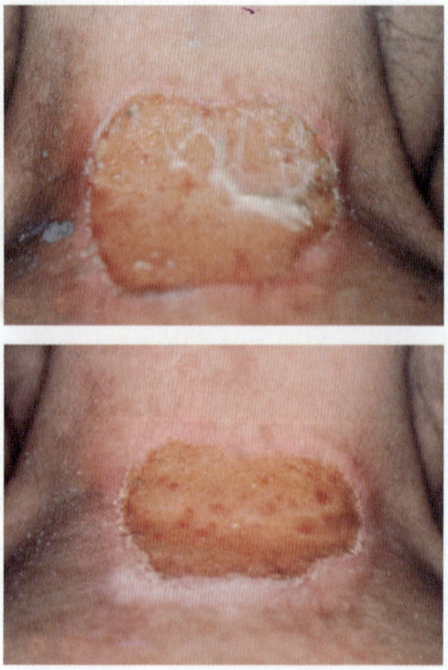

Figure 4.7 Skin wound
Courtesy: René-Jean Bensadoun

One of the most thoroughly studied areas in laser therapy is wound healing. In fact, this was one of the first indications reported, with studies by Mester and by Carney [520] as early as 1967. The first studies were made using healthy rats. This effect has been confirmed in the extensive animal studies by i.a. al-Watban [471, 475, 632]. However, the effect in a healthy individual is limited and the prime indication for laser therapy in wound healing is for individuals or tissues with a compromised state. But it is not a good idea to wait and see whether or not a wound will heal and then treat it with laser if it fails to heal. On the contrary, an evaluation of the actual state of the individual/tissue should be made in the first place and laser therapy applied if deemed favourable. We have touched upon this subject in the descriptions of various indications earlier in the book.

The technique for extraoral wounds is as follows: start by administering 3-4 J/cm^2 on points along the periphery of the wound, using the contact method. Then sweep slowly over the open wound at a distance of 1 cm, with a dosage of 0.5 J/cm^2. The open wound receives a lower dosage than the skin-covered periphery, as the laser light is not reflected, scattered and absorbed by skin in the unprotected wound and hence hits the uncovered cells directly. Treat daily for three to four days, then every other day, and evaluate the healing process. If no improvement has occurred, raise the dosage by 50%. Severe wounds with pus and exudates require higher doses. Varicose ulcers and bedsores are appropriate indications for laser therapy in combination with conventional therapies. In addition to improved wound healing, a considerable reduction in pain can be expected.

The above dosages apply to GaAlAs - for GaAs, about half the dosage should be given. HeNe has proved to be the best source for wound healing [471, 475], but the low outputs and high costs of HeNe lasers have been complicating factors. The advent of more high-powered and less expensive diode lasers in the 630-660 nm range will possibly solve this problem.

Diodes require higher doses than HeNe although the wavelength may be the same. This may be because of the superior length of coherence of the HeNe laser. Laser therapy is always a supplementary method: wounds must be cleaned and dressed as usual.

For all types of treatment where infection is present, it is beneficial to stimulate the immune system by irradiating the nearest lymph nodes [915] before treatment of the wound begins. 1-2 J per point is a common dosage. Then administer 0.5 J per point along the lymphatic vessels leading to the wound area.

It is not uncommon that a chronic wound initially appears to deteriorate, so the patient should be pre-informed about the possibility of a transient change for the worse.

If heat is used in combination with laser therapy, should the laser treatment come first? Heat will increase blood flow in the tissue, by increased absorption of light in the blood, thus reducing penetration. On the other hand, more blood will be irradiated which can lead to positive systemic effects. Penetration of the laser can be increased by using pressure technique in either case.

Laser therapy of wounds is ideal, since it promotes healing and reduces pain at the same time.

It has been argued that successful studies of rats cannot necessarily be extrapolated to apply to human skin. This is a point well taken, but studies on porcine models, dairy cattle models and humans all point in the same direction. It has also been argued that wound healing studies using healthy animals is not a suitable approach. The healing ability in healthy individuals can only be promoted slightly. whereas the best effect of laser therapy is shown in individuals with a less-than-optimal immune situation. Thus, diabetic rats have been used with greater success [922]. Since wound healing in rats is mainly dependent on contraction, a different irradiation technique should be used in laboratory studies. The entire wound should be covered by the laser beam, in contrast to the recommendations for humans, as described above. In the above study by Reddy [922] two circular wounds were created on either side of the spine. The left wound of each animal was treated with HeNe 1.0 J/ cm^2 for five days a week until the wound was closed (three weeks). Measurements of the biomechanical properties of the laser treated wounds indicated that there was an increase in maximum load (16%), stress (16%), strain (27%), energy absorption (45%) and toughness (84%) compared to control wounds of diabetic rats. Biochemical assays revealed that the amount of collagen was significantly increased in laser treated wounds. Sequential extraction of collagen from healing wounds showed that laser treated wounds had significantly greater concentrations of neutral salt soluble (15%) and insoluble collagen (16%) than control wounds, suggesting accelerated collegen production in laser treated wounds. There was an appreciable decrease in pepsin soluble collagen (19%), indicating higher resistance to proteolytic digestion.

To avoid the many interacting parameters in wound healing studies, Houghton [1098] used experimental wounds in the separated limbs of fetal mice. GaAs doses of 0.23, 1.37, 2.75 and 3.66 J/cm² improved wound healing, while 4.8 J/cm² showed no improvement as compared to control. The best outcome was noted with the two lowest doses. The 4.8 J/cm² group actually showed the best wound size change at day three, but at day 7 all the other groups were better. Collagen deposition in dermis and bone was enhanced in the 0.23, 2.75 and 3.66 J/cm² groups, but not in the 1.37 J/cm². The above well illustrates the problem of establishing a "good-for-everything" dose.

In a meta analysis of the available literature of laser therapy for wound healing [871], the laser treatment modality was found to be highly significant (d=+2.22). Further sub-analyses revealed that the efficacy for animals was +1.97 and for humans +0.54. 24 studies met the inclusion and exclusion criteria. In another meta analysis on tissue repair [872], the outcome was +1.81. The number of studies was 34.

While there are many studies, the overall methodological quality of the laser therapy literature for wound healing is low, according to a study by Lucas [1184].

Literature:

The aim of a study by Rigau [415] was to investigate the behaviour of the confluence monolayer fibroblasts culture when a central scratch of 0.4 - 1 mm and 2 irradiations are performed, by means of the study of the colony formation, haptotaxis (direction) and chemotaxis-chemokinesis (movement). An argon pumped DYE-laser, with a wavelength set at 633 nm, 2 J /cm² was used. The results indicate that all these phenomena appear sooner in the laser therapy cultures than in non-treated cultures.

In the study by Almeida-Lopes [906] human gingival fibroblasts were cultured in Petri dishes with different Fetal Bovine Serum concentrations, 5% or 10%. Four irradiations of 2 J/cm² were given at 12 hour intervals. Lasers with 670, 692, 780 and 786 nm were used. Cells in 5% FBS proliferated better than in all control groups, whereas the cells in the 10% FBS did not proliferate better than controls. The 670 and 692 visible lasers caused a higher improvement in cell proliferation that the infrared lasers. This study confirms the fact that cells in a less-than-optimal stage react better to laser therapy than cells in an optimal nutritional stage. It also confirms that visible red is the best wavelength for superficial wound healing. The fibroblasts in the 10% solution did not proliferate better when irradiated. However, the irradiation caused a polarised pattern, forming bundles in different directions, a phenomenon previously reported by Enwmeka [1161] and Tang [1162]. This may be a part of the explanation of the improved wound healing seen in laser surgery.

Webb [911] investigated the effect of a 660 nm, 17 mW laser diode at dosages of 2.4 J/cm² and 4 J/cm² on cell counts of two human fibroblast cell lines derived from hypertrophic scar tissue and normal dermal tissue explants. Estimation of fibroblasts utilised the methylene blue bioassay. Post-660 nm-irradiated hypertrophic scar fibroblasts had very significantly higher cell counts than controls.

Hubacek [1036] summarises the outcome of experimental data on HeNe wound healing: “HeNe laser emission 1.5 J/cm^2 applied five times during the course of one week improves wound healing through fibroblast stimulation in a directly irradiated wound, as well as in a remote wound. After irradiation with 1.8 J/cm^2 during a week, the production of collagen differs depending on the phase of the healing wound. Early irradiation in the first week stimulates inflammatory type III collagen. Late irradiation in the third week inhibits the inflammatory reaction and improves deposition of type I collagen.”

van der Veen [675] studied the effect of 904 nm laser on the proliferation of mice fibroblasts. At 3 mW/cm^2 average power density there was a proliferation effect on the cultivated fibroblasts as compared to control. The BrdU-labeling showed an increased DNA activity. There was also a perfect match between the increased number of fibroblasts and the DNA activity.

Yu [586] studied the effect of 660 nm laser therapy on the production of basic fibroblast growth factor (bFGF). Fibroblasts irradiated with 2.16 J/cm^2 demonstrated increased cell proliferation and enhanced production of bFGF. At 3.24 J/cm^2, no proliferation or production of bFGF could be detected.

Yu [584] found that HeNe laser irradiation of keratinocytes *in vitro* stimulated interleukin-1 alpha and interleukin-8 production and their respective mRNA expression. Both these cytokines play a profound role in the enhancement of keratinocyte proliferation.

Webb [615] wanted to test the claim that laser therapy could prevent or improve previously created hypertrophic scar tissue. A 17 mW 660 nm laser diode was used at dosages of 2.4 or 4 J/cm^2. Two cell lines derived from hypertrophic scar tissue (HST) and normal dermal tissue explants (NDT) were irradiated and a cell count was taken. The irradiated hypertrophic cells exhibited significantly higher cell counts than control on days 1-4 for HST and days 1-3 for NDT.

Hrnjak [676] irradiated human embryonic fibroblasts with 0.5, 1, 1.5 or 2 J/cm^2. A single HeNe laser irradiation exhibited a significant stimulation effect on the fibroblast proliferation.

In a rabbit study by Nicolopoulos [721] a subtotal meniscectomy of the medial meniscus was performed in 24 animals. In group A the operation was performed with a surgical blade and in group B and C with CO_2 laser. The animals in group C received GaAlAs laser, 48 J/cm^2 every day until sacrifice. It was concluded that: 1) less damage was produced by CO_2 laser than by surgical blade; 2) the healing potential of rabbit meniscus following laser resection was accelerated with the use of laser therapy post-operatively.

Krypton laser light (670 nm) is rarely used for biostimulation. However, al-Watban [632] reports the results of wound healing experiments in rats. The optimal wound healing effect of 30% was found at 20 J/cm², zero stimulation was found at 100 J/cm², and a maximum 14% deceleration was found at 260 J/cm². The more widely used lasers showed better results than Krypton laser in the range of 9-20%.

al-Watban [471], [475] used several wavelengths (442, 514, 632, 670, 780, and 830 nm) in a study of wound healing in rats. It was found that 633 nm had the best effect, but all wavelengths had a positive effect. The doses should be decreased with increasing wavelength. Depending on wavelength, healing was accelerated from 15% to 29% in time and from 32% to 50% in size reduction. Since wound healing in rodents is mainly through contraction, it is necessary to irradiate the entire wound with the beam, unlike in humans, where irradiation of the periphery is more important.

In a study by Bisht [897] linear skin wounds were produced on either side of the dorsal midline in rats and immediately sutured. Wounds on the left side were irradiated daily with helium neon laser at 4 J/cm² for 5 min, while those on the right side were not exposed and served as controls. The mean time required for complete closure in the control group was 7 days while irradiated test wounds took only 5 days to heal. The mean breaking strength, as measured by the ability of the wound to resist rupture against force, was found to be significantly increased in the test group. Early epithelisation, increased fibroblastic reaction, leukocytic infiltration and neovascularisation were seen in the laser-irradiated wounds.

In an experiment on 218 white rats, Efendiev [833] established an effect on the site of a future incision with the infrared laser irradiation in continuous mode. Output power ranging between 1 to 150 mW (dosage between 0.06 and 9.3 J/cm²) induced pronounced stimulation of the processes of collagen formation and significant increase in strength of scars. When the power density was increased, the reparative processes in the wounds were slowed and disturbed.

Morrone [921] reports that 780 nm laser therapy showed better qualitative and quantitative healing in traumatised muscles as compared with controls in a rabbit experiment.

Gomez-Villamandos [425] induced duplicate pharyngeal mucosal ulcers in 12 horses. Using a fibroendoscope, one of the two injured sides was treated daily with a HeNe laser at 8 J/cm². On day 7, histological samples were taken from two horses. Irradiated lesions cicatrised after 10.5 days and non-irradiated lesions after 18. A histological study showed coagulation, necrosis and oedema at the control site. However, in the samples from the irradiated lesions, no inflammatory oedema, numerous active fibroblasts, connective tissue or intensive epithelial regeneration were observed.

Guo [619] reports on the outcome of HeNe laser treatment of 53 cases in pediatric surgery. The results in children were better than in adults.

In a double-blind study, Palmgren [351] investigated the effect of laser therapy on infected abdominal wounds after surgery. A GaAlAs laser, 820 nm, 15 mW output, was used to treat 9 patients, while 9 patients were given sham irradiation. The dose was 1.6 J/cm^2. Healing time to half wound size was significantly shorter in the laser group (6.8 days versus 14 days in the placebo group). The wound healing per day was 2.45 cm^2 in the laser group and 1.67 cm^2 in the placebo group.

In a study by Schaffer [907] three women with painful mastitis from irradiation after breast cancer with ionising radiation and a male with a radiation ulcer were treated with GaAlAs laser 780 nm, 5 J/cm^2. The healing of the ulcers was controlled using MRI measurement before and after treatment. In all patients a complete clinical remission was noted following laser therapy. The results were confirmed by a decrease in inflammatory changes as depicted in MRI imaging.

The same indication is reported by Schindl [967]. Three patients with radiation ulcers following breast cancer therapy were treated with HeNe laser, 30 J/cm^2, three times weekly. At 36 months control no patient showed recurrence of the radiation ulcers or any neoplasm.

Almeida-Lopes [969] divided 150 patients who had undergone maxillofacial surgical CO_2 laser treatment into three groups: one control without laser therapy, one with 688 nm laser therapy and one with 830 nm laser therapy. The laser therapy groups were irradiated immediately after surgery, at day 7 and 14 with a fluence of 2 J/cm^2. The results showed that the laser therapy groups healed quicker than the non-irradiated group. There was no statistical difference between the 688 and the 803 group.

The regeneration of the liver after partial hepatectomy, followed by laser therapy, is reported by Castro e Silva [598]. 70% of the liver in Wistar rats was removed by scalpel. Before suturing, a dye laser of 590 nm, 50 mW/cm^2, was used for five minutes in the experimental group. The animals in the experimental as well as in the control groups were sacrificed at 24, 48 and 72 hours after the procedure. At 24 hours there was a dramatic increase in ATP production per mg of mitochondrial protein in the laser group. At 48 and 72 hours there was no difference. The quantification of the liver regeneration was estimated by counting the nuclei stained in the PCNA immunohistochemical assay. The increase in the labeling index for the laser treated group was remarkable after 24 hours but the difference was small at 48 and 72 hours. This study illustrates the regenerative effect of laser therapy and also the need for repeated irradiation to keep the process going.

The effects of laser therapy on burns are described in [1029, 1048, 1049, 1050]. In a study by Schlager [1067] the effect of 635 and 690 nm on experimental burn wounds in rats was studied. There was no effect using the parameters of the study. This study has been criticised by al-Watban [1068] for lack of information about the procedures and parameters.

A cumbersome task in wound healing therapy is the changing of dressings. If a dressing could be transilluminated by laser light without losing too much of the light energy, the therapy would be much facilitated. Lilge [1066] has addressed this problem.

Marino [951] treated 34 geriatric patients suffering from bed sores with HeNe scanning, 7.3 mW, 0.024 – 0.054 J/cm². Photographic and planimetric evaluation was performed every 15 days. Daily sessions were performed until at least 80% of the initial area was reduced. The number of sessions needed was related to the general clinical condition of the patient and higher doses were more successful.

A systematic review of the literature by Lucas [1046] was limited to infrared studies. Only four randomised clinical trials were found and only one [13] showed any effect. A meta analysis was performed for three of the studies and no significant effects could be found for decibitus ulcers, venous leg ulcers or other chronic wounds. The dosage calculation inaccuracy for the study [613] was not observed. In two of the three studies, the light sources are not lasers. One study [1063] is a non-coherent light study. Another study [1064] was excluded because of a different definition of the outcome, making a comparison difficult. It should, however, not have been included in the first place, since it is not a laser study but a study of the effect of combined laser and LED.

High powered lasers can easily be defocused and used within the regular therapeutic doses. In a study by Kubota [1116] a 1000 mW, 830 nm, laser was used to treat skin ulcers. The power density was 669 mW/cm² and the dose 6.3 J/cm².

Although laser therapy of wound healing is best used for non-healing wounds, the study by Medrado [1270] suggests that the quality of the wound healing process in perfectly healthy tissue is still influenced by laser therapy. Cutaneous wounds were performed on the back of 72 Wistar rats. 24 rats received one single irradiation of 4 J/cm², another 24 received 8 J/cm² and 24 served as control. The wavelength was 670 nm, 9 mW, and continuous mode. The lesions were analysed after 24, 48, 72 hours and 5, 7 and 14 days. After 14 days all wounds had healed in a similar morphological fashion. However, histology and immuno-histochemistry in the three groups were different. Both laser groups revealed improved healing parameters compared to the control group, and all parameters were best in the 4 J/cm² group. During the first days signs of acute inflammation were less intense and subsided earlier in the laser treated animals. The degree of oedema, vascular congestion and the exudation of neutrophilic polymorphoneuclar leukocytes were particularly affected. After 72 hours the laser groups showed prominent granulation tissue. The vascular proliferation was most apparent when immuno-histochemically sections marked for smooth muscle actin were examined. Fibroblast proliferation and collagen deposition accompanied vascular proliferation. Collagen fibres appeared more regularly organised (in densely packed parallel bands) in the laser groups. This study seems to verify the common opinion that wounds in healthy tissue will heal in normal time, laser or no laser. However, the symptoms of oedema and pain will be reduced and the quality of the scar area will improve. Apart from the reduction of post-accident symptoms, the scar tissue will improve, which may have implications in aesthetic surgery. It is also worth observing that one single irradiation immediately after accident/surgery has a positive effect.

Further literature [704, 828, 935, 975, 976, 1149, 1164, 1165, 1246, 1248, 1273]

4.1.51 Zoster

Zoster (shingles) is a much-feared condition, not only for the acute pain that it causes but because it can also lead to longer periods of pain after objective healing. This "postherpetic neuralgia" (PHN) is most common in older patients. The Norwegian and Danish word for zoster is "fire of hell", which is rather apt. Laser has an effect both on the acute zoster outbreak and on the post-herpetic pain. Shingles affects not only the midriff but, for example, the trigeminal nerve. This can make it impossible to close the eye, or cause difficulty of motor control, sores in the throat and oral cavity, and pulpitis sensation. In general, laser therapy relieves the symptoms, and a series of treatments reduces the patient's suffering considerably. There is reason to believe that treatment in the acute phase reduces the risk of PHN. One of the suggested effects of laser therapy on zoster is that it restores the intraneural blood flow, preventing the death of larger nerve fibres and thus arresting the development of PHN [692].

Literature:

Moore [57] treated 20 patients suffering from PHN for whom conventional treatment had failed and who had experienced pain and discomfort for at least six months. Ten patients were treated with a GaAlAs laser. Another ten received placebo laser treatment followed by GaAlAs laser light (a "cross-over study"). The experiment could thereby be conducted in a double-blind fashion while still administering equivalent treatment to all patients. The placebo group experienced little improvement after the first four treatment sessions, but after four "real" laser applications they came very close to the results of the laser group. Pain intensity and spreading were measured. With 10 as a starting value for pain intensity, the average result was 2 and 3.3 respectively in the two groups. Pain distribution was initially set to 100, and the end result was 31 and 41. 15% of those treated experienced either little or no effect. When the experiment ended, the initial laser group had better scores than the second. This confirms the ongoing positive effect of laser therapy even after the end of a treatment period.

In a retrospective report covering 300 patients over 9 years, Moore [404] summarises: cephalic zoster patients experienced less pain reduction (61%) than thoracic patients (78%), with an equivalent difference in pain recurrence of 22% and 33% respectively. In a cost-efficiency calculation, laser therapy was some 28% less expensive. The use of laser therapy in the acute phase greatly reduces the incidence of postherpetic neuralgia.

In another study by Moore [476], comprising 20 PHN patients with malignant disease, all patients obtained at least 50% pain reduction after 8-

10 treatment sessions. This category of patient often does not tolerate the usual medication for PHN due to the high incidence of side effects. Power density was 3W/cm^2.

McKibbin [58] treated 39 PHN patients with a GaAs laser. Patients estimated pain on a VAS scale of 1 to 10, the average value for the whole group being 8.5. At the end of the treatment period, the average value was 3.3 and one year after treatment it was 2.8 (44% were entirely free from symptoms).

Hong [59] reports on the outcome of the treatment of 20 PHN patients who had not responded to conventional therapy. 60% of the cases were deemed to be successful after a year. The laser used was a GaAlAs.

Hachenberger [60] irradiated 41 cases of postherpetic neuralgia, 93 herpes simplex patients and three herpes progenitalis patients. He observed that these related complaints all responded well to HeNe laser treatment. None of the 93 herpes simplex patients experienced a recurrence in the same place during the observation period of three years.

Iijima [183] treated 18 outpatients suffering from postherpetic neuralgia with a HeNe laser. Up to 50 doses were administered! Judged on a scale of one to four, the number of effective cases was 94.4%. VAS dropped from 6.2 to 3.6, and the total pain intensity from 100 to 44.6%. The results agreed with those of a previous study comprising 36 patients [184].

Otsuka [421] also reports positive results of HeNe (with GaAlAs as an adjunct in difficult cases) during the acute phase of zoster.

Epidural or stellate ganglion blocks have been used to ease postherpetic pain. Otsuka [423, 523] has also used laser therapy near the stellate ganglion and found effects similar to those of traditional injections. Thermograms illustrated a facial temperature increase. Irradiation near the carotid artery had a similar effect. The same author also reports a stimulative effect from stellate ganglion irradiation in patients with Raynaud's disease.

Hashimoto and Kemmutso [691, 692] have also shown that even irradiation of the stellate ganglion alone can have an effect on pain. In a double-blind study, patients with postherpetic neuralgia were treated with either 150 mW GaAlAs, 60 mW GaAlAs or placebo laser. Laser affected VAS pain scores and regional skin temperature, but there was no change in the placebo group. The pain reduction was dose dependent. It is suggested that laser irradiation of the stellate ganglion is a good alternative to traditional blocks.

In a double-blind study on the effect of GaAlAs laser on postherpetic neuralgia, Sato [398] found that the regional body temperature in the laser group increased from 31.9 °C to 32.6 °C, while it did not change in the placebo group.

Further literature [418, 421, 1051].

4.2 Anecdotal indications

Many indications have been tested clinically but still lack any scientific support. Some of these are minor indications such as insect stings and restless legs, but some are important, such as osteoporosis, vitiligo and strawberry haemangiomas.

At a meeting held at the University of Oslo in February 1999, Wintsch [844] reported on the treatment of allergic rhinitis with laser therapy. In the discussion afterwards, he was criticised and his report was regarded to be "anecdotal" as it was neither blinded nor controlled. Calderhead then pointed out that a single case report may be of low value, but when there are many case reports showing similar results, there may be something of interest behind them. Many important discoveries have started with case reports or even anecdotal reports. (Literature on rhinitis: [555, 781])

In every profession, unconfirmed reports and tales of pure fiction circulate. Let us look at some of the more dubious examples that now and again pop up in the therapeutic laser field.

4.2.1 Obesity

Obesity has been alleged to be affected by laser therapy. When treating a person with GaAs on an area of the abdomen, therapists have been able to observe a slight "depression" in the fat layer where the probe is held - the laser has in some way affected the tissue. However, the patient has not lost any weight, and furthermore, where would all the fat have gone if no weight was lost?

However, what we usually regard as "fat" is not just fat. The "fat" in a thigh contains only about 30% fat – the rest is fat cells, water and glycogen. In some cases it can be regarded, more or less, as an oedema. As laser treatment of oedema can be very effective, local treatment of "fat" can seem to be effective.

4.2.2 Wrinkles

Wrinkles are the laser therapy critic's favourite subject. We have not been able to find the source of the assertion that therapeutic lasers can remove wrinkles. The assertion is probably as incorrect as the critic's explanation of the alleged effect: "The laser can possibly cause a local inflammatory reaction in the skin which leads to local oedema, which in turn temporarily flattens out the wrinkles". Laser therapy does not cause any local inflammatory reaction in the skin. But the critics have obviously seen a temporary smoothing of wrinkles, as they are theorising about the underlying cause.

However, as mentioned previously, see chapter 3.5.1 "Laser therapy with carbon dioxide lasers" on page 98, it has been demonstrated that superficial burning ("laser peeling") with a CO_2-laser beam or an Er:YAG laser is effective in skin resurfacing for the treatment of wrinkles. Chernoff [294, 295] performed over 50 exfoliations to smooth out perioral, lip, and periorbital wrinkles and scars. The thermal damage depth was between 75 and 150 μm. The result is astonishing (far better than what can be achieved with chemical peeling and mechanical dermabrasion). There is no question that biostimulation is a decisive factor in the process.

This is even more strongly underlined in the recent reports about so called "non-ablative skin rejuvenation". Here, laser powers and fluencies have been used at levels that do not cause pain, and often not even a heat sensation. Examples of such lasers are: 590 nm pulsed dye-laser [1145], 1064 nm Nd:YAG-laser [1146], 1320 nm Nd:YAG-laser [1147] and 1540 nm Nd:glass laser [1146]. This is obviously a question of biostimulation effects. (See chapter 1.4.1.1 "Carbon dioxide lasers in surgery" on page 29.)

4.2.3 Cellulites

Laser therapy has a stimulating effect on various pathological skin conditions. Whether or not cellulites is a pathological condition is open to discussion. No documented reports on the effects of laser therapy for this indication have been published. See also paragraph above.

4.2.4 Hair loss

In one of Endre Mester's first experiments on rats [733], it was found that, on the shaved parts of the body, the coat grew back faster in areas that had been treated with a ruby laser. This led to a certain amount of interest in the possibilities of stimulating hair growth in humans. It is generally thought that the stimulation of hair growth with laser therapy is a fiction, but this is only partly correct.

There are basically two types of "hair laser". The first looks like a hood hairdryer, and contains a HeNe laser tube with a maximum output of 6 mW. The laser light is distributed via hundreds of small fibre-optic conductors over the whole of the inside of the hood. Nowadays, a number of GaAlInP laser diodes are generally used, with a somewhat longer wavelength (670 nm). One problem is that there is a loss of energy in any area with hair, even if the hair is thin. These "hood hairdryer lasers" seem to work in many cases, but no convincing documentation has been put forward.

"Hair laser" number two is a normal HeNe or GaAlInP laser probe. Since the probe is held in direct contact with the scalp, the dosage level reached locally is much higher than in the "laser hairdryer". Nevertheless, this still requires many treatment sessions and there is no guarantee of a successful result.

Literature: [332, 631]

4.2.5 Problems with orgasm

The Swedish evening paper Aftonbladet, February 9th, 1986.
In 1986 it was reported that the French sexologist, Dr Jacques Waynberg, was using infrared laser to treat anorgastic women. These women have diffi-

culties in reaching an orgasm and the irradiation of the clitoris region was said to stimulate the local blood flow. 10-16 sessions were said to improve the condition.

This is probably an example of biostimulative laser effect. The article does not specify laser type and doses, but it is most likely a defocused CO_2-laser since the article states that "the clitoris is heated by the laser, but there is no pain". Treatment time is usually four minutes. Dr Waynberg suggests that the effect is due to the increased blood circulation.

Chapter 5
Dental laser therapy

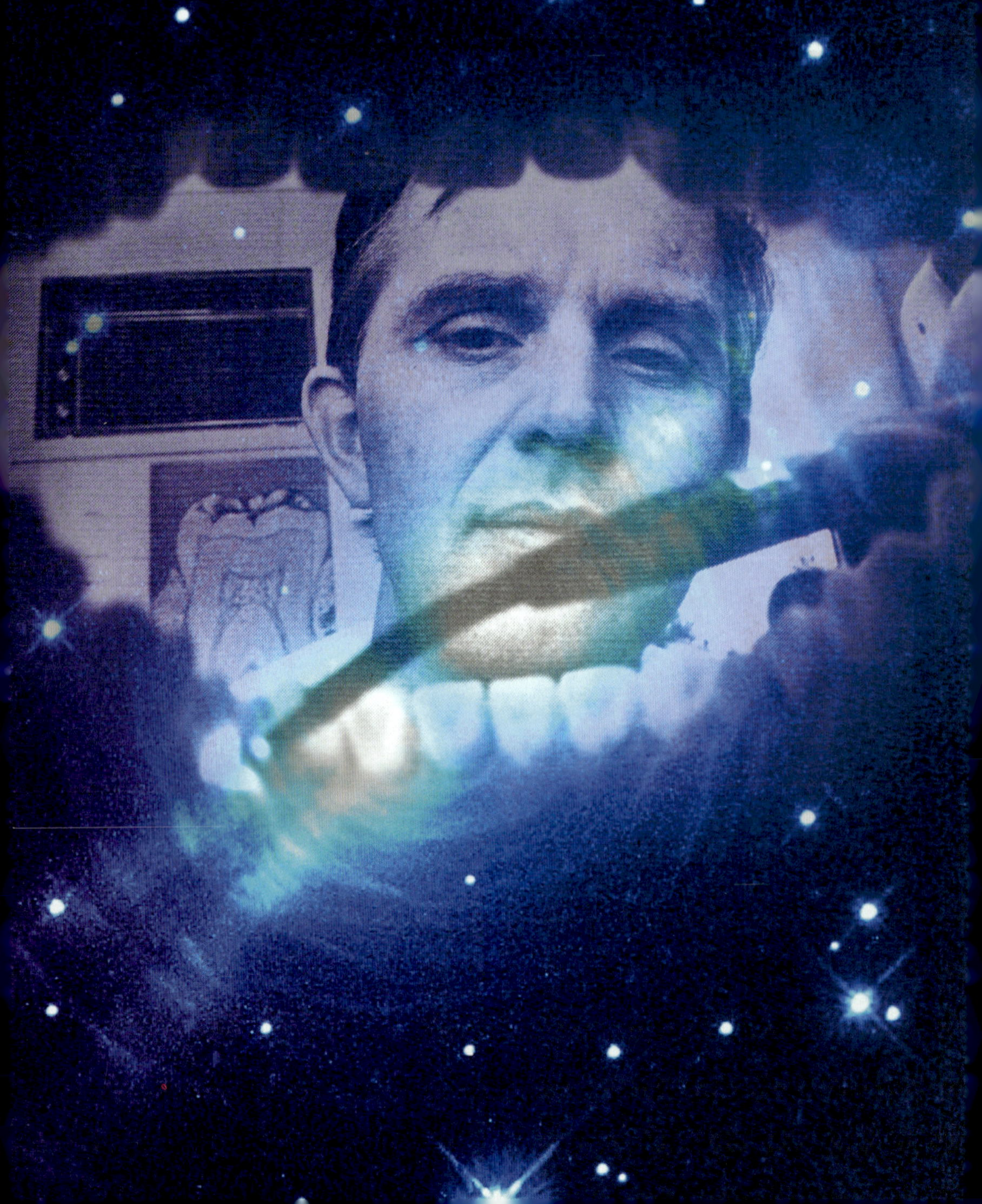

The therapeutic laser is just one of many modern tools which we can use in our everyday work. It is also a fairly new tool which relatively few dentists have acquired yet. But in the not too distant future we may come to see it as a natural part of our equipment, no more unusual than the curing light or the ultrasonic scaler.

The effect mechanisms behind laser therapy are more complex and difficult to understand than those behind the curing light or the ultrasonic apparatus, however. Much more research needs to be conducted before we can fully understand all the important aspects of laser therapy. However, the method has been in use for over 30 years without any reports of patients being harmed, so why make patients wait? Also, more than 90% of the available literature on dental applications of laser therapy reports positive effects.

5.1 What is “a god dentist”

A "good dentist", in the patient's eyes, is one who does not inflict pain either during or after treatment. Even if we cannot always fulfil these desires, we should at least be able to make use of all available means of reducing the number of occasions on which our treatment causes pain. Laser therapy is an excellent way of reducing or eradicating pain.

A "good dentist" is also, of course, one who protects or restores the health of the patient's teeth and soft tissue. This part of the book shows how laser therapy can help the dentist to do this, sometimes as a part of treatment, sometimes as the only available method. Indeed, the owner of a suitable laser will be able to treat indications such as paraesthesias and trigeminal neuralgia, indications previously referred to specialists and not very successfully treated by them.

Many colleagues have asked for more exact information regarding dosage, treatment schedules, suitable wavelengths, etc., for their laser treatments. This can often be provided in individual cases, but in general it is better to avoid oversimplified advice. Other publications have done so in an instructive and practical fashion, but only in describing the use of a laser of a certain output and wavelength. In this book, we have chosen to describe all of the four different types of laser routinely used in laser therapy, which makes it more difficult to give general dosage advice. Furthermore, there will probably be fairly large inter-individual differences when it comes to dosage requirements. On the following pages, a number of dosage examples will be given, but it should be born in mind that they are approximate mean values for a certain type of laser.

A dentist should be able to answer patients' questions about lasers, even if he himself does not use one. Many patients have heard about lasers but probably think they are only used in surgery. Some are likely to know that it is possible to drill in hard tissue with a laser, or to vaporise and cut soft tissue.

Do not imagine, after reading the above, that laser therapy is so complicated that you will be unable to achieve a reasonable understanding of it and its concepts. In practice, everyone can quickly achieve good results for several indications, and the growing body of experience of laser therapy will bring even better results.

5.2 On which patients can laser therapy be used?

Laser therapy can be used, with few exceptions, on all patients, but we should remember that this form of treatment is no different from other forms of medical treatment. Not all patients react in the same way to laser therapy, and one patient may not always react the same way, depending on the condition of the tissue and immune system.

Let us look at anaesthetic injections by way of comparison. Some patients are thought to need double quantities of anaesthetic, while others need very little. In some cases, the effects disappear very quickly, in others they remain for an unusual length of time. Even a patient who normally finds it easy to be fully anaesthetised may suffer when the dentist treats his deep pulpitis - it may be that nothing helps.

In general terms, we can expect up to 80% of patients to respond positively to laser therapy. If a patient does not respond to treatment, bear in mind that the degree of success of the treatment is contingent on a number of parameters. A poor result can be due to too small a dosage, too great a dosage, incorrect diagnosis, too few treatment sessions, unsuitable pulse frequency or power density, etc. Remember: the more experienced the practitioner, the more success he or she will have with laser therapy.

Experience shows that practitioners use laser therapy not only on patients, but on themselves, on relatives and on friends, and maybe even treat complaints outside their own domain. The next step could be that practitioners may even begin treating their patients for non-odontological problems, in which case they will appear to their patients as unusually skilled professionals, even if, by definition, they are working outside their normal sphere of business. Experience also shows that many practitioners have too much respect for the new tool in the beginning. Remember that it is only light! Bearing the few contraindications in mind, a great new field is now opening up.

5.3 Dental indications

A caveat is in order here. This chapter may seem like rather heavy reading, as it contains numerous short summaries of articles that discuss studies of different laser therapy fields. We prefer this structure, despite its drawbacks, as the aim of this book is not just to inform the dental profession about the uses of laser therapy but to show that there is a great deal more scientific documentation on the subject than most people realise.

The following is a body of information (in alphabetical order by subject) about a number of areas of use for laser therapy. The text is intended as a source of inspiration for the laser user, not a set of detailed treatment instructions.

The suggested dosages should be seen as average doses, and clinical judgement should always be the basis for dosage calculation. It should also be noted that most complaints require repeated treatment. This is often impossible from a practical point of view. The patient may not be motivated enough to visit every other or every third day, or the dentist may think it difficult to charge for such drawn-out treatment if assisting personnel are unable to administer it. In practice, then, laser treatment often takes place in connection with the patient's ordinary appointments, in which case treatment is hardly ever optimised.

5.3.1 Alveolitis

Laser therapy directly after extraction helps to prevent alveolitis. If alveolitis is already established, 4-5 J before the alveolus is debrided and plugged with medication is recommended. Irradiate the alveolus and the surrounding area directly. If the alveolitis is very painful, do not hesitate to use 15-20 J.

Literature:

A study by Hedner [43] has shown that 47% of patients with "dry socket" manifested a reaction of herpes simplex type 1 after the extraction of the third molar in the lower jaw. This raises an interesting hypothesis: does the alveolitis-preventive effect of laser therapy depend in part on the antiviral effect of the laser?

Further literature: [106, 111, 116, 218, 544]. (See chapter 4.1.20 “Herpes simplex” on page 147.)

5.3.2 Anaesthetics

Some patients are difficult to anaesthetise. By administering 2-3 J over the apex, circulation is increased and the anaesthetic is more quickly absorbed. This also means, of course, that duration is reduced. The duration of the numbness in the lip after anaesthesia can therefore be reduced by laser therapy. This can be advantageous in pediatrics.

Teeth with a large volume of pulp can be successfully anaesthetised with a defocused surgical laser such as the argon, Nd:YAG och Er:YAG. Lasers with an output within the biostimulative power density range cannot give this full anaesthetic dosage but can still be used to raise the pain threshold. When treating caries in young teeth, the following method can be tested. The enamel should be drilled as usual - this does not usually present any problems as far as pain is concerned. The laser should then be applied into the cavity and 8-10 J administered. The pulp will not be anaesthetised but the pain threshold will be raised. The method can be used on co-operative patients.

An injection per se rarely causes complications, and the perforation of the mucous membrane is hardly noticed if thin 30 gauge hypodermic needles are used. 2-3 J over the injection area can further reduce the patient's awareness of the injection.

Unfortunately, we now and again hit a vessel with the needle, and in addition to the usual treatment with pressure and cooling, 6-8 J can reduce the oedema and the subsequent pain. Treatment is administered both extraorally and intraorally.

Intraligamental anaesthesia can lead to postoperative pain if the injection is given too rapidly. 3-4 J under the papilla reduces or eliminates the pain. Prophylactic treatment before the anaesthesia wears off is recommended.

Literature:

Vélez-Gonzáles [105, 504] injected a salicylic solution subcutaneously in rats and compared absorption between irradiated and non-irradiated animals. Using HeNe laser with doses ranging from 1.9-4.9 J/cm^2, absorption was found to increase in a dose-dependent fashion.

Tamachi [44] administered HeNe to rats that had been given experimental cancer. The uptake of the cytotoxin 5 FU in the cancer cells was higher in the group treated with a HeNe laser than in the group that received only 5 FU.

Omura [1047] discusses the problem of insufficient drug uptake in some patients. The situation can, in the author's experience, be improved by using several treatment modalities, such as acupuncture, electrical stimulation and laser therapy.

Yang Li [1135] has observed that animals in wound healing studies frequently have reacted with a negative response if anaesthetics such as ketamine and ether have been used. It is speculated that there is some reagent competing against laser for the same receptor in the fibroblast.

5.3.3 Aphthae (canker sores)

Aphthae are not as easy to treat as herpes simplex. The symptoms of most patients can, however, be alleviated by laser treatment, and the healing period can be reduced. Carbon dioxide, Er:YAG and Nd:YAG lasers can also alleviate symptoms if a defocused beam is used. The dosage is determined by the patient's response to pain relief. When the patient feels a distinct reduction in pain, you are on the way to the "right" dosage. Several treatment sessions are often necessary to prevent any discomfort to the patient until the aphthae have disappeared. 4-6 J is a good "starting point".

Aphthae treated with Er:YAG laser, before and immediately after irradiation.

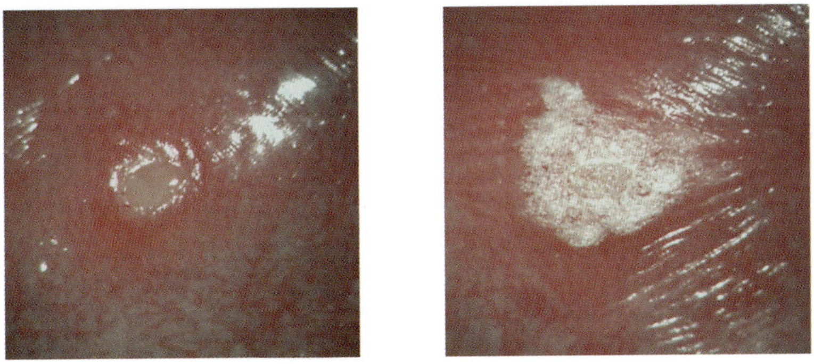

Figure 5.1 Aphthous
Courtesy: Continuum Lasers

Literature:

Guang Hua Wang [64] demonstrated a pain-alleviating effect when a HeNe laser was used on aphthous ulcers. A 1% and a 10% KCl solution were applied to the aphthous ulcer, after which the SRT (Shortest Response Time) was measured. The procedure was repeated three times, after which the SRT was 100%, i.e. an immediate response. The trial group (25 people) was irradiated with a HeNe laser immediately after the third application of KCl solution. The SRT increased markedly in the trial group but not in the control group. The application was repeated every five minutes for 45 minutes. The laser output was 25 mW, and the treatment time was ten seconds.

Manne [222] treated 12 cases of aphthae with a GaAs laser. In 11 cases the aphthae disappeared three days after a single treatment session, and in the last case five days after two sessions.

Fagnoni [486] treated 32 aphthae cases with a HeNe laser, 300 mJ/cm^2. Approximately 22% of the lesions healed within one day, 41% in two daysand 31% in three days.

Takashi [238] reports the positive effect on aphthae using a HeNe laser.

Colvard [525] successfully used a therapeutic CO_2 laser to treat aphthous sores.

Further literature: [56, 531, 623, 635, 1036].

5.3.4 Bleeding

A laser is useful in the treatment of postoperative bleeding. Although the mechanism behind this is unclear, the literature shows that laser therapy brings about an initial vasoconstriction, but that it is followed by a vasodilatation [44, 121, 152, 479, 630]. Logically speaking, this should lead to increased bleeding, but clinical experience shows the opposite, which is why other mechanisms must be involved. HeNe laser radiation is absorbed better in haemoglobin than GaAlAs and GaAs and thus seems most suitable. The low power of most HeNe lasers is an obstacle, however. 1-2 J is administered in each alveolus directly after the extraction. GaAlAs has been shown to counteract the appearance of fibrin networks [96], which could be one reason why HeNe laser has a better effect on this indication.

Literature:

Fine [305] studied the effect of an IR laser on the bleeding of heparinised mice. The bleeding stopped after five minutes. The animals in the control group bled to death.

Trelles [262] reports that vasodilatation of both arterioles and venules is one of the biological effects characterising the action of laser therapy on tissue. Vasodilatation does not occur immediately but a few minutes after irradiation and then continues even if the affected tissue is cooled.

Kubota [479] used the laser speckle method to measure the microcirculation in flaps. The blood flow rate was reduced immediately following one-minute irradiation with 830 nm. 30 minutes later the flap perfusion was greater than in the control flap.

Juri [505] summarises a rodent study as follows: It is concluded that HeNe laser radiation blocks the usual increment of plasma fibrinogen level after tissue injury, probably by interfering with the interaction of PGE_1 + Bradykinin.

Brill [1083] suggests that HeNe laser irradiation inhibits platelet activation and aggregation through the involvement of intracellular secondary messengers – cGMP and/or NO.

Iakovleva [834] studied the effect of HeNe laser exposure, power 1 mW, at the tip of the light-guide, on the blood anticoagulative system in narcotised mongrel dogs during the postresuscitation period after 4-min clinical death from massive blood loss. The anticoagulative system of the blood plasma was depleted during the reanimation period (the activities of plasmin and fibrinogen-heparin complexes and the level of heparin dropped). Intravascular laser exposure of the blood (for 30 min. during blood loss after drop of the mean arterial pressure to 40 mm Hg and at the beginning of the second hour of the postreanimation period) boosted the activities of plasmin and fibrinogen-heparin complexes but failed to increase the level of heparin in the postreanimation period.

Further literature: [106].

5.3.5 Caries

Every operation on the hard tissue of teeth involves trauma for the dental pulp. It is subjected to thermal variations, vibrations and then chemical influence from insulating and filling materials. The normally very short-term symptoms a patient experiences after an operation involving the hard tissue can be eliminated by administering 1-2 J per root after the operation. 1-2 J can also be given over the gum papilla to eliminate postoperative irritation from wedging. This kind of prophylactic operation may seem trivial to the dentist - perhaps we ourselves should sit a little more often in the dentist's chair in order to feel more motivated to treat this "insignificant" discomfort that we cause.

Hyperaemia after composite fillings and the cementation of ceramic inserts is an all too common problem. In most cases, the problem is of a transitory nature, but who wants a hyperaemic tooth for several weeks? The majority of these problems can be avoided if the tooth is given 2-3 J per root immediately after filling/cementation. A number of telephone calls are also avoided. More serious hyperaemia should be treated repeatedly, but this is clearly preferable to root treatment on a tooth that was problem-free before we started to treat it!

Several studies have shown that CO_2 and various YAG lasers have the ability to decrease the solubility of enamel. Hsu [838] has shown that even rather low intensities of CO_2 laser (85-170 J/cm^2) can induce this effect and that it is dramatically increased in the presence of fluoride. The interesting question is - how low intensities are necessary? Early Russian studies indicate that HeNe laser in combination with a fluoride varnish will decrease the decay. Recent studies in the USA and South Africa seem to confirm these findings.

An innovative concept of killing cariotic bacterias is to combine various dyes, such as TBO, with laser light in the laser therapy range [778, 930].

Literature:

Kazmina [410] investigated the caries preventive action of a HeNe laser. 350 children and 50 adults were divided into three groups. All groups were treated conventionally to restore oral health. Normal preventive measures were taken. The first group received no further treatment and the second group received additional treatment with a fluoride lacquer, three sessions, repeated twice a year. The third group had the same treatment as group two but had additional treatment with a HeNe laser twice a year. The laser employed had a power output of 17 mW (from a tube) and a bundle diameter of 5 mm and was thus able to irradiate the entire tooth. Each tooth was irradiated for one minute per session. At the four-year control the CFE index was used (Caries-Filling-Extraction). The index for the untreated group one was 1.0, indicating one new carious lesion per patient. The fluoride lacquer group had an index of 0.29 and the lacquer/laser therapy group had an index of 0.02.

Kunin [625] used a HeNe or GaAs laser in combination with fluoride lacquers. Percentual reduction in enamel solution rate was studied in four groups. Group 1 received fluoride varnish only, group 2 semiconductor laser treatment only, group 3 HeNe and varnish, group 4 semiconductor laser and varnish. The reductions were 12.7, 19.5, 27.2 and 23.8 respectively.

Low levels of laser light also seems to have a positive effect on the bonding mechanisms between dental substances and composite bonding materials materials, according to Kunin [1103].

Okamoto [841] has demonstrated that cariogenic bacterias are sensitive to HeNe laser light, but only in the presence of various dyes, mainly phenylmethane dyes. There was a dose dependent suppressive effect on the bacteria and it is suggested that HeNe laser may be suitable for clinical applications in preventive dentistry.

In an *in vitro* study, Hicks [837] evaluated the effect of combining low level argon laser treatment and acidulated phosphate fluoride treatment on caries initiation and progression in human root surfaces. The combination of low level laser and fluoride treatment increased the caries resistance of root surfaces when compared with no treatment and with laser irradiation treatment alone.

The enhancement of the fluoride effect when using laser therapy has also been noted by Liu [1104].

van Rensburg [836] used a GaAlAs laser with an energy of 5.45 J (30 mW for 180 seconds) and an energy density of 27.54 J/cm^2 to irradiate two fluoride containing orthodontic bonding materials. SEM evaluation showed that the laser irradiation had no superficial physical ultrastructural effects on either of the two materials. However, the fluoride release of one material could be enhanced for up to seven months by a sole application of laser. Fluoride release from the other material was also increased but was not statistically significant

Iwase [77] studied plaque build-up in 20 hamsters fed on a sucrose-rich diet. One molar in each of the animals was given HeNe laser treatment for two minutes, five times a week, for five weeks. Prior to this, plaque had been allowed to build up freely for four weeks. After a total of eight weeks, the amount of plaque around the treated tooth was measured and compared with the amount of plaque on the contralateral tooth. In 19 of the 20 cases, there was a smaller amount of plaque on the treated tooth, and in the last case a greater amount.

Further literature: [842]

5.3.6 Dentitio dificilis

Conventional treatment is supplemented with local laser therapy over the operculum, buccal and lingual bony wall and any tender points in the musculature. Complementary use of laser therapy leads to a much faster reduction of discomfort than conventional treatment on its own. Laser therapy is also effective in alleviating pain during the eruption of deciduous teeth. The submandibular lymph nodes should be included in the treatment [915]. Herpes virus is suspected to be involved in the symptoms during eruption of deciduous teeth, which would further explain the good effect of laser therapy.

Literature:

Manne [222] treated 12 cases of juvenile pericoronitis with GaAs. In eleven cases, there were quick positive reactions, while one case was unsuccessful despite two applications within the space of 24 hours, and extraction was necessary.

5.3.7 Endodontics

A pain reaction can arise after over-instrumentation in root canals when treating both vital and non-vital pulp. This pain is short in duration but still causes the patient discomfort. 2-3 J over the apex eases the symptoms in most cases. This treatment can be administered prophylactically to some advantage when it is known that over-instrumentation has occurred.

In other respects, laser therapy can be recommended for pulp capping and pulp amputation of milk teeth. Laser therapy appears to stimulate the odontoblast calcium and collagen production, leading to secondary dentine formation.

Literature:

Paschoud [109] exposed pulp horns and studied the effects of HeNe laser light in direct pulp capping with three different pulp capping preparations, all based on calcium hydroxide. Pulp capping preparations only were used in three control groups. When capping with Pulpdent and Contrasil, a dentine bridge was developed over a shorter period by those treated with a HeNe laser than by the control group. No positive results were achieved in combination with Dycal.

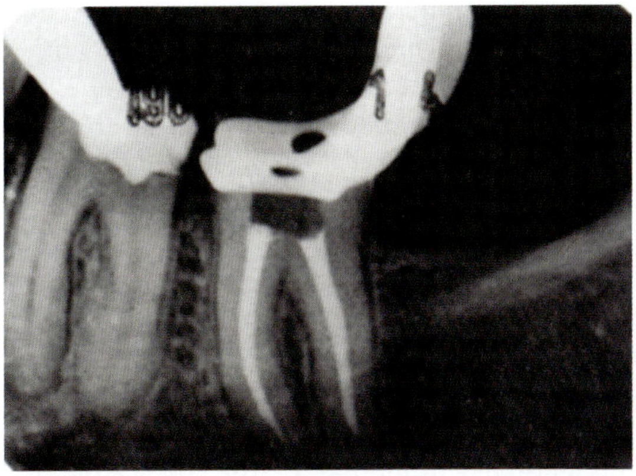

Figure 5.2 Endodontics

The conclusions drawn were that calcium hydroxide preparations can create a dentine bridge during pulp capping, and that HeNe laser light further stimulates new formation of dentine. The properties of the preparation itself are central to the result. The intrapulpal temperature was also taken during this experiment. After two minutes it had increased by 0.5 °C, after which it increased no further.

Dcabrowska [714] performed 30 pulp cappings or amputations in combination with calcium hydroxide and laser therapy. 36 teeth were treated with calcium hydroxide only. The laser treated group had a more favourable outcome.

Kurumada [577], on the other hand, used GaAs laser light without calcium hydroxide on vital pulpotomies. Laser irradiation induced enhancement of calcification in the wound surface and stimulated formation of calcified tissue.

Nagasawa [107] has observed that Nd:YAG and argon laser irradiation within LLL doses strongly stimulates the formation of secondary dentine.

Thwee [1118] performed pulpotomy in Wistar rats and exposed the open pulp to HeNe laser irradiation. After irradiation, the pulp was coated with a calcium hydroxide coating. A large amount of dentine-like calcified barrier was formed in the laser irradiated group.

Ohbayashi [1107] isolated human dental pulp cells and irradiated the cells with two doses of GaAlAs laser. In the laser groups there was an increased collagen production, increase in the calcified nodules and enhancement of osteocalcin and alkaline phosphate activity.

Liu [1114] confirms the pain-relieving effect of laser after post-endodontic filling pain.

The results of the study by Utsunomiya [1010] suggest that laser irradiation accelerates wound healing of the pulp and the expression of the lectins and collagens. Furthermore, D-glucose-, D-mannose-, N-acetyl-D-galactosamine-, and N-acetyl-neuraminic acid-binding sugars and type I, III, and V collagens play an important role in the healing of pulp.

The effect of bone repair in periapical lesions has been studied by Sousa [1238]. 15 patients with a total of 18 periapical lesions were divided into two groups. One group received endodontic treatment and/or periapical surgery. The patients in the other group were submitted to the same procedure and in addition the lesions were irradiated by GaAs laser, 11 mW average power, 9 J/cm². This therapy was performed during 10 sessions with an interval of 72 hours. Bone regeneration was evaluated through X-ray examination. The results showed a significant difference between the laser and the control group in favour of the laser group.

5.3.8 Extraction

After extraction, the alveolus is irradiated along with the lingual and buccal bony wall. Faster coagulation, less postoperative discomfort and quicker healing can be expected. A normal consequence of using elevators during extraction is that neighbouring teeth become sensitive, which makes chewing difficult. 2-4 J over the apex usually reduces this discomfort, and the treatment can be administered prophylactically immediately after the extraction.

For reduction of oedema, relatively high doses of GaAs or GaAlAs light are needed on a large area around the wound. The laser decreases the permeability of the lymphatic vessels and induces dilatation of these vessels.

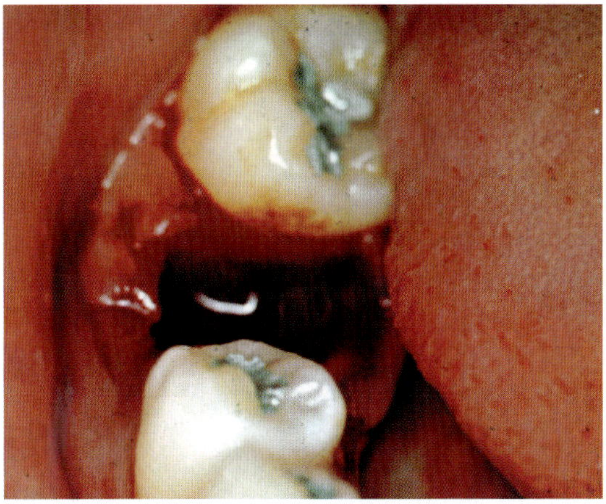

Figure 5.3 Extraction

It has not yet been possible to determine the "best" wavelength, although a HeNe laser seems to be the best option for coagulation, which is vital for continued healing. GaAlAs and GaAs lasers have more effect on postoperative pain and swelling than HeNe.

When removing impacted wisdom teeth, or after operations involving stress on the maxillary joint, 2-3 J over the joint directly after the operation is recommended. HeNe can be used here, even if the dosage is more quickly reached with GaAs/GaAlAs. For postoperative oedema and pain, doses of 15-25 J are needed locally and extraorally. The dose must be correlated with the amount of trauma.

Literature:

Filho [399] extracted the upper left incisor of 24 rats. 12 of the extraction wounds were given HeNe laser with 3 J/cm^2. Clinically, the rats exposed to the laser beam showed a better healing rate than the unlased rats from the control group.

Takeda [110] studied the effects of a GaAs laser on tooth extraction. 24 rats were used in the experiment, in which irradiation was administered immediately after extraction. The wound was then studied under a microscope on days 0, 2, 4 and 7. Five minutes after the extraction there was no histological difference as compared with the control group. On day 2, fibroblasts had begun to proliferate from the remaining periodontal membrane in the clot. This proliferation was more pronounced in the laser group than in the control group. The ossification process was more advanced in the laser group on day 4, and on day 7 the laser group's trabeculae were thicker and greater in number.

Fernando [216] compared the effects of 830 nm laser light during the simultaneous extraction of two similarly impacted lower wisdom teeth. Postoperative pain and swelling were studied. 4 J was applied directly into the empty socket. In a double-blind study, no difference was observed between the treated and untreated sides.

Verplanken [128] treated 44 patients with GaAs laser immediately after tooth extraction, with a control group of 27 patients. The distance between the bucco-lingual and mesio-distal wound walls, the colour of the coagulum, and postoperative pain and swelling were measured. The author summarised the results as follows: "We could observe a significant stimulation of the healing process as a result of laser therapy."

Wahl [693] was not able to find any effect of a 6 mW HeNe laser on the postoperative outcome after removal of the third molar.

Tay [1137] studied the effect of laser therapy following third molar surgery. 55 patients with bilateral and similarly impacted third molars were selected for surgery under general anaesthesia by one surgeon at one sitting. A 30 mW GaAlAs laser was used. The patients were divided into laser and placebo laser groups. The laser group received 10 J at four sessions during the first 24 hours postoperatively, a total of 40 J. The contralateral side served as control. There was a significant reduction of pain in the laser group, with the greatest reduction found after the initial dose of 10 J.

C-reactive protein plasma concentration can be monitored to evaluate the degree of inflammation in tissue. CRP plasma concentration is usually low, increases quickly at the onset of acute inflammatory processes and quickly falls when effective control of the process occurs. Freitas [1268] used this method to monitor the possible anti-inflammatory effect of 830 nm laser after the removal of impacted third molars. 12 patients were irradiated with 4.8 J per session 24 and 48 hours after surgery. A control group (n=12) was treated with sham laser. CRP values were more symmetric and better distributed for the irradiated group 48 hours after surgery but there was no statistical difference between the groups.

Further literature: [1132, 1193]

5.3.9 Gingivitis

Laser therapy can be used as supplementary treatment for gingivitis. In combination with conventional treatment, laser therapy quickens healing and reduces postoperative pain. The need for complete debridement and good oral hygiene must be emphasised. Preoperative laser therapy reduces pain associated with scaling.

Literature:

Chomette [70] studied the histology of biopsies of human gingiva taken five minutes, 15 minutes, one hour and 24 hours after HeNe laser irradiation. As early as an hour after irradiation, the fibroblasts' enzymatic activity had increased. An increase of the number of fibroblasts and cell organelles was also reported, along with increased collagen production. No similar change was observed in the control biopsies.

Chomette [71] also studied the healing process in 14 patients from whom gingiva biopsies had been taken. In patients with no gingivitis before the biopsy, (laser group) cicatrisation took place within 14 days, and in the control group (no gingivitis, no laser treatment) within 21 days. Even in the presence of gingivitis, the laser groups exhibited quicker and better cicatrisation.

Loevschall [75] examined the effects of GaAlAs laser on human oral fibroblasts. This study showed increased incorporation of thymidine in the fibroblasts, which suggests that laser therapy can stimulate DNA synthesis.

Kim [948] conducted an *in vitro* study of the GaAlAs laser's stimulating effect on gingival fibroblasts from human subjects. The cell cultures were treated daily for four days, and the treatment period in the three groups was 30, 60 and 90 seconds. The number of cells in the experimental group rose with increased exposure to laser irradiation, although the rise was not statistically significant in comparison with the control group. It was also found, when comparing the protein content of the different cultures, that a very significant increase had taken place in the experimental group treated with 90 seconds GaAlAs irradiation. In terms of DNA content, the only significant difference was in the group that had received 60 seconds GaAlAs irradiation.

Rydén [42] studied the effect of a GaAs laser on experimental gingivitis in 10 healthy human volunteers. After three weeks plaque accumulation, one side was given a total dose of 1 J, divided between day 21 and day 24. The degree of gingivitis was examined by identifying the vessels in the area, using photography, on day 0, day 21, day 28 and day 42. No statistical difference was found between the laser group and the control group with respect to the number of vessels. The laser treated and the sham irradiated teeth were only about 1 cm apart.

Schindl [674] treated a chronic radiation ulcer with HeNe laser, 30 J/cm^2. A video measuring system was used to determine the number of dermal vessels in the ulcer before and after the laser treatment. After 7 irradiations, the ulcer had healed completely. Light microscopy in combination with the video measuring system showed a significant increase in the number of capillaries after laser treatment.

Kusakari [121] reports that laser therapy increased blood flow during the first stages of human gingivitis without any morphological changes of the blood vessels.

A study conducted by Yarita [182] found no change of morphology in the initial stages of gingivitis in humans. In a group that had received laser treatment, however, increased blood flow was observed.

Kozlov [368] has studied the microcirculation in patients with periodontal disease of various degrees, using biomicroscopic techniques and laser Doppler flowmetry. The intensified tissue blood flow observed after HeNe laser irradiation was caused by intensification of blood microcirculation and the activation of neovascularisation. Tissue blood flow stimulation was caused by precapillary dilatation and opening of "reserved" capillaries. Doses between 10 and 30 J/cm^2 had adverse effects. The best effect was observed in patients with moderate periodontal disease. The key to the four studies above is the condition of the tissue. Experimental gingivitis in healthy subjects reacts differently to laser therapy than a true disease would.

Kubota [479] measured the microcirculation in skin flaps using the laser speckle method. One minute after irradiation the perfusion was less, and 30 minutes later it was greater than in the control flap.

In a histopathological study, Abramovici [640] studied the effect of a HeNe laser on the healing process of open gingival wounds in cats. The irradiation initiated a massive inflammatory cell exudate together with an anti-oedematic effect after the second postoperative day. A substantial acceleration of the healing process was noted on the sixth day. The biostimulatory effect seemed to act photodynamically at both the intracellular and extracellular levels, thus promoting the proliferatory capacity of fibroblasts and the capillary bud formation necessary for a rapid differentiation of connective tissue.

Lee [136] examined the gingivitis of 13 dental students. GaAlAs laser light was administered to one side of the jaw on days 1, 3, 5 and 7. A histological evaluation was carried out on day 4. The sulcus bleeding index decreased on the experimental side, but the pocket depth and plaque index were unchanged. On the side treated with laser, a reduction in motiles and spirochetes was observed, along with an increase in non-motiles. From a histological point of view, the inflammatory infiltration decreased in density and extent after laser therapy.

In the study by Sakurai [1008] laser irradiation inhibited PGE2 by LPS in hGF cells through a reduction of COX-2 mRNA level. The findings suggest that laser therapy may be of therapeutic benefit against the aggravation of gingivitis and periodontitis through bacterial infection

Amorim [1225] selected seven patients who were to undergo gingivectomy on both sides of the jaw. In these patients laser therapy (685 nm, 50 mW, 4 J/cm^2) was applied on one side only, the other side serving as control. The healing process was monitored clinically and biometrically, using photographs for a period of 35 days. The analysis was performed by three specialists in periodontology. Biometrical evaluation showed improvement of the healing for the period of 21 and 28 days in the laser group. Clinical evaluation showed better reparation mainly after the third day.

Further literature: [72, 76, 77, 164, 165, 166, 641].

5.3.10 Herpes zoster

(See chapter 4.1.51 “Zoster” on page 196.)

5.3.11 Hypersensitive dentine

Painful necks of teeth often respond well to laser treatment. Recent desensitising agents have greatly reduced the problem of hypersensitive dentine. While these products effectively reduce minor sensitivities, laser therapy is superior for cases with more profound pulpitis. The seriousness of the hypersensitivity decides the dosage and number of sessions needed. The tooth neck should be treated until the patient feels a distinct improvement (check with the air syringe). With GaAlAs/GaAs lasers and its greater penetration, it is possible to irradiate directly over the apex, through mucous membrane and bone. With HeNe laser it is only possible to use the tooth neck, except for the upper incisors. A combination irradiation over the coronary pulp, tooth neck and apex is recommended. A hypersensitive tooth that does not respond to 4-6 J per root in 2-3 sessions is a candidate for endodontics.

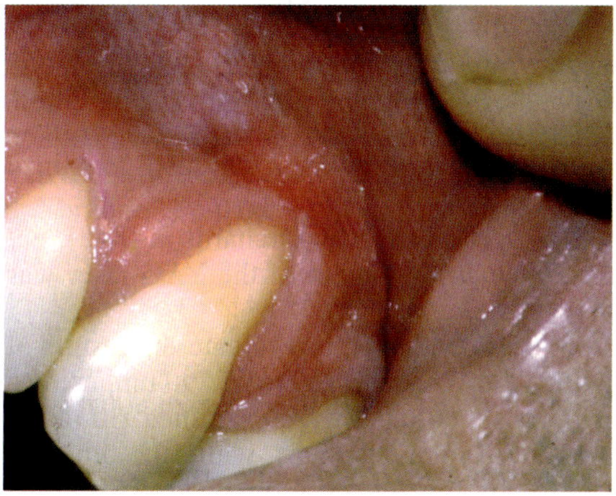

Figure 5.4 Hypersensitve dentine

With the advent of porcelain inlays/onlays and large composite fillings, the number of postoperative complaints has increased considerably. The patients are disappointed and some of them have to undergo endodontics. Such postoperative sensations can be eliminated or reduced by using laser therapy before cementing and filling. If post-operative problems appear, the laser could solve many of them in one or a few sessions. This is indeed much more profitable than free endodontics.

There are a great number of studies in this field. For a literature review, the article by Kimura [1055] is recommended. These studies also confirm the safety of the therapy.

Literature:

Kaihøj [65] treated 84 sensitive tooth necks with a GaAlAs laser. In 17 cases, there was no result, 12 showed some effect, 34 experienced good results, and 21 perfect results. Treatment was administered on days 1, 21, and 90, with a check-up three to six months after the last treatment. No supplementary treatment was undertaken.

Wakabayashi [66] used a GaAlAs laser (30 mW, 780 nm) to treat sensitive root surfaces. Laser treatment was effective in 61 out of 66 cases. In the control group treated with a placebo laser, the treatment was effective in 17 out of 64 cases. The most painful teeth were less responsive to treatment, and pain was more recurrent here.

Gomi [80] studied the pain-relieving effect of three types of laser in 130 cases of hypersensitive dentine (I) and 120 cases of pain during cementation of inlays (II). In experiment (I), HeNe laser treatment was effective in 71% of the cases in which it was administered once, in 79% of the cases in

The effects of 680 and 830 nm lasers on osseointegration was studied by Blay [1220]. 30 adult rats were divided into three groups; two laser groups and one control. The rats in the two laser groups had pure titanium Frialit-2 implants implanted into each proximal metaphysis of their respective tibias, inserted with a 40 Ncm torque. The initial stability was monitored by means of a resonance frequency analyser. Ten irradiations were performed, 48 hours apart, 4 J/cm^2 on two points, starting immediately after surgery. Resonance frequency analysis indicated a significant difference between frequency values at 3 and 6 weeks, as compared to control. At 6 weeks the removal torque in the laser groups was much higher than in the control group.

Further literature: [91, 121, 213, 583, 931, 1218, 1219]

5.3.13 Jaw fractures

Fractures of the facial skeleton are treated locally over the fracture itself every other day for one to two weeks.

Literature:

Kats [112] studied the effects of a HeNe laser (30-480 mJ/cm^2) on fractures of the jaw. In the trial group of 19 patients, quicker healing and a moderation of the inflammatory process were observed as compared with the control group of 27 patients.

Glinkowski [420] used GaAlAs, 830 nm and GaAs, 904 nm lasers in a study of standardised tibial fractures in mice. Bone radiographs were studied using a laser densitometer. Both wavelengths accelerated healing, but 904 nm was more successful.

Further literature: [108, 944], (See chapter 4.1.6 "Bone regeneration" on page 126.)

5.3.14 Leukoplakia

This condition does not always produce subjective symptoms. If the patient does have leukoplakia symptoms, they can be alleviated with laser therapy. Whether laser therapy can actually cure the condition has not been reported, but a stimulation of the immune system in the area affected is worth trying.

Literature: [209]

5.3.15 Lingua geographica (glossitis)

This condition is sometimes free of symptoms, sometimes associated with varying types of subjective discomfort. 3-4 J laser therapy over 5-6 points relieves the symptoms. Its effect on long-term healing is not clear, but there is no effective treatment of any other kind that can heal this condition.

Literature:

Mezawa [114] studied the effects of GaAlAs laser light on nociceptors in cat tongues. A decrease in nociceptor activity could be demonstrated after one minute's irradiation. No further change was noted in the 5-10 minute interval, and the authors drew the conclusion that a plateau was reached after five minutes.

Hubacek [1036] reports successful treatment of glossodynia using GaAlAs laser, 4-6 J/cm², 4-10 sessions.

5.3.16 Lip wounds

Angular cheilitis caused by a low vertical dimension can be successfully treated with laser therapy but will reappear if the fundamental cause is not dealt with. Wounds on lips usually heal quickly with laser therapy in cases of trauma and mechanical/chemical irritation. Lip fissures are well worth treating. A typical symptom is that they begin to bleed after having been very dry - this is the beginning of the healing process. HeNe or small doses of GaAlAs laser are recommended.

Literature: [1201]

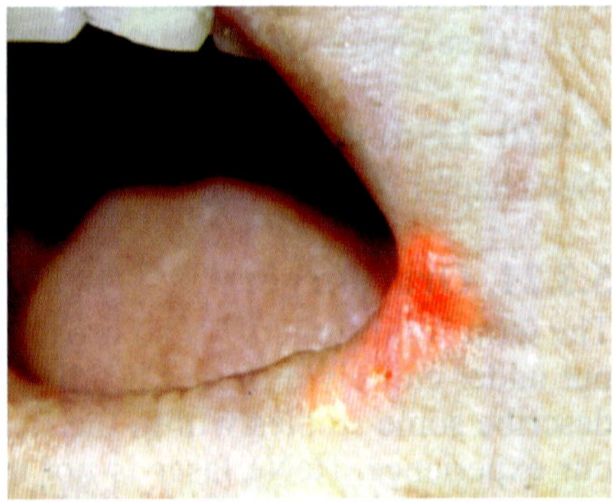

Figure 5.5 Angular chielitis

5.3.17 Mucositis

(See chapter 4.1.7 "Cancer" on page 130.)

5.3.18 Nausea

A common complication in dentistry is nausea. Some patients are very sensitive to operations behind the premolars and taking impressions may be very difficult. In these cases, the laser can be applied to the sulcus mento-labialis in the contact mode. 1-2 J will reduce nausea in a great number of cases. If not successful, the acupuncture point P6 on the wrist can be used. The effect will arise a couple of minutes post irradiation.

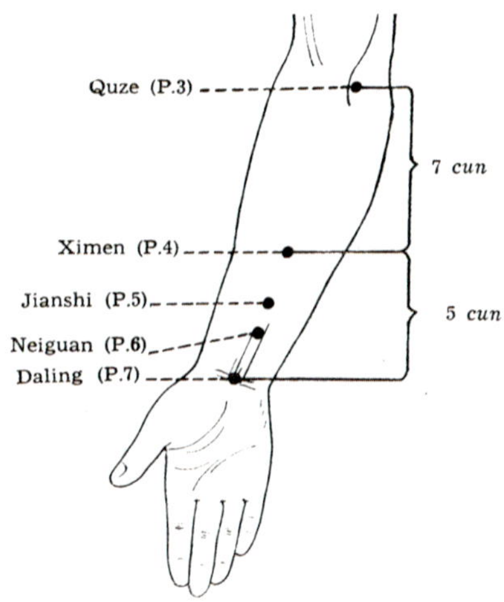

Figure 5.6 Location of the P6 point

5.3.19 Nerve injury

Damaged nerves heal slowly. Feared complications in odontology are damage to n. alveolaris inferior and n. lin-way as part two. Mast cell degranulation in the control specimens was average 49%, in the laser specimens 87% and in the combined TBO/laser specimens 88%. With these parameters the TBO did not have any additional effect.

Further literature: [708, 778, 827, 841, 842, 930, 1115]

5.4.2 Composite curing

A common wish among dentists is to be able to cure dental composite material quicker and more thoroughly. Experiments in curing have been conducted with argon lasers (488 nm), nitrogen lasers and HeCd lasers (443 nm). There are commercial systems based on argon lasers, but the high price is a disincentive to general use. The argon laser is capable of curing a layer of 2 mm within 10 seconds, compared to the recommended 40 seconds with traditional blue curing light. Laser curing will improve the physical properties of the resins. It can, however, increase shrinkage and brittleness [455]. With the advent of plasma arch and LED-based curing lights, laser curing seems to have lost its appeal.

5.4.3 Tooth bleaching

Argon (488 nm), GaAlAs, Nd:YAG and CO_2 lasers are used in combination with in-office tooth bleaching. The laser will cause teeth to bleach faster, but will not bleach teeth better than at-home bleaching or bleaching without laser [843]. The laser excites the hydrogen peroxide molecule in the bleaching gel. The short wavelength and the higher photon energy of the argon laser makes it a first choice. Halogen lamps, plasma-arch lamps and other heat lamps emit short wavelengths as well as longer invisible infrared thermal wavelengths and are more likely to create unfavourable pulpal responses.

5.4.4 Dental casts

Dental casts take up a great deal of storage space, particularly for the orthodontist. It is now possible to make holograms of these gypsum models, thus leaving more space on the orthodontist 's shelves. Measurements can also be taken from holograms in the same way as from gypsum models. Furthermore, one hologram can be superimposed over another and the differences between them studied.

5.4.5 Caries detection

Laser fluorescence can be used to detect occlusal caries. A diode of 655 nm has been successfully used to diagnose hidden occlusal caries.

5.5 Case reports

Case reports are of limited scientific value and are often referred to condescendingly as "anecdotal accounts". Of course, case reports should not be seen as anything other than treatment effects observed in particular cases, and perhaps by only a few therapists. They can, however, serve as useful guides for the clinician and as examples of what can be attempted. They are the kind of stories you might relate to a colleague during a coffee break between lectures but would not consider mentioning in the lecture itself. They are, in any event, the cases you sometimes remember most clearly, and they are useful from a practical point of view. Below is a more readable rounding-off of this chapter - some case reports from the author's experience.

1 A.B. A 20-year-old woman with pain in the maxillary joint and teeth which ground acutely. She could not open her mouth more than 17 mm with deviation. GaAs laser light was administered bilaterally (8 J) over the joint area and the immediately surrounding tissue, after which the patient could open her mouth 22 mm with greatly reduced pain and deviation. An imprint for a bite splint could be taken without any problems.

2. C. A 54-year-old man suffering from painful candida-infected leukoplakia bilaterally under the tongue. HeNe laser light had a good, but only temporary, pain relieving effect. After surgical removal of the leukoplakia, HeNe was administered on the side where the postoperative pain was greatest. This side healed more quickly. The patient later experienced pain in the area on occasion, but this could be eradicated after one or more laser treatments.

3 F.Å. A 56-year-old woman with few teeth remaining in the lower jaw, full upper jaw prosthesis, and partial prosthesis in the lower jaw. She was encouraged by a doctor to seek the help of a dentist for her long-standing headaches. The prostheses were highly abraded, and new prostheses with a larger vertical dimension and better occlusal stability were made. The patient returned five days after the new prostheses were fitted for the treatment of a small decubital wound. The headaches remained. By way of an experiment, a GaAs multi-probe (19 Hz) was placed against the right temple. The patient immediately said that it "felt good". After three minutes' irradiation (11 J), mainly on the most painful side, the patient said that most of the pain was gone. Out of scientific curiosity, the frequency was increased to 5,000 Hz, at which the patient experienced a sensation of pressure. At 6 Hz, the patient did not feel anything in particular. The changes in frequency were made without the patient's knowledge, but she could tell immediately when it "felt good" and when it "tightened". At a new appointment the next day, the headache had disappeared completely. 8 J was administered, and the patient was still able to notice differences in pulse frequency. At a check-up after three months, the patient was still untroubled by headaches.

4 B.S. A 43-year-old woman with "fibromyalgia" as a preliminary diagnosis. The patient was in need of dental care, but lying in a dentist's chair even for as little as ten minutes increased her pain considerably. She could be treated

in a sitting position, but this would make the planned treatment, involving porcelain inlays, more difficult. GaAs irradiation along the spine and on the trigger points of the back once a week and immediately before treatment made a 45-minute treatment session possible, and the patient experienced a much improved pain situation for one to three days after each laser treatment.

5 L.J. A 34-year-old man who needed emergency treatment for a fractured upper incisor. His usual dentist did not have the time to treat him. On the same day, the patient had injured his left hand and the tips of three fingers had been cut off. He arrived via the hospital's casualty department with bandaged fingers and in great pain, and would not take analgesics on principle. During the dental treatment, the patient held a GaAs multiprobe against the palm of his left hand and soon noticed a pleasant sensation. After four minutes (14 J) the pain had disappeared, leaving the patient both pleased and surprised.

6 T.D. A 23-year-old male football player. The patient noticed the laser therapy equipment in the dentist's surgery and wondered whether it might help his periostitis. He could play football for only 30 minutes or so without the pain in his legs becoming unbearable. Scanning laser treatment with HeNe once a week and immediately before a match increased the pain-free period by 100%.

7 M.D. A 49-year-old woman. At the age of 28, she had developed pains in the soles of her feet, which gradually spread to the palms of her hands. After a few years, the pain had spread throughout her skin. No certain diagnosis had been offered, despite many doctors' appointments. The patient had not taken the recommended pain-relief medication in order to avoid side effects. It was sometimes impossible for her to walk because of the pain. The problem came to the attention of the dentist when he touched the patient's cheek, at which she felt pain. 6 J of GaAs was administered over one side of the face. The patient experienced an obvious reduction in pain, and a new "itching" sensation in the cheek. When the patient came to the next appointment, she no longer had any pain in the side of her face treated with laser. The whole face was now treated, along with the palms of the hands and the soles of the feet, with a GaAs multiprobe. A total of 14 J was administered. At the next appointment, the patient reported a large, general reduction in pain. The arms and legs were also treated (20 J). At the following appointment, only mild pain in the part of the soles of the feet where the pain began remained. After six laser therapy applications, the patient no longer experienced pain and a few months later said she was enjoying her "best year in ages". After 7 years, there has been no recurrence.

8 J.S. A man in his 50s with shoulder pain since several years. Steroid injections had had a good but not long lasting, effect. Sleep was impaired, and he could not have his cameras hanging over his shoulder the way he was used to. After three treatments, he was able to sleep on the affected side, after six he was completely pain free. Full Range of Movement. A tennis elbow was cured in three sessions en passant.

9 A.M. This female patient had been suffering from pain in her neck and shoulders for about ten years. Due to the difficulties in moving her neck, GaAlAs laser treatment was administered prior to dental treatment, 10 J per point. This had a satisfactory effect. The patient said that the centre of her stiffness was in the right trapezius. As this part was treated the pain and stiffness were considerably reduced. At the following dental appointment the patient pointed out that her tinnitus on the right side had almost gone. This condition was not previously known by the therapist. Since there was some, although lighter, tinnitus on the left side as well, both sides of the body were treated, this time including the masticatory muscles. At the next appointment the tinnitus was almost gone in both ears, and the patient remarked: “my vertigo is much reduced!” This condition was also unknown to the therapist. Five follow up sessions were performed. The patient was almost free of problems at four months’ checkup. After five months the problems started to reappear since the patient had continued the kind of work that initially caused the problems.

The few examples above are cases in which laser treatment has helped when it has been difficult to find other forms of treatment which work, bearing in mind the circumstances. The latter cases, which do not really come under the "dental laser treatment" heading, do nevertheless give some indication of the various conditions in which a dentist can have the opportunity to use the laser.

Chapter 6
Dental research

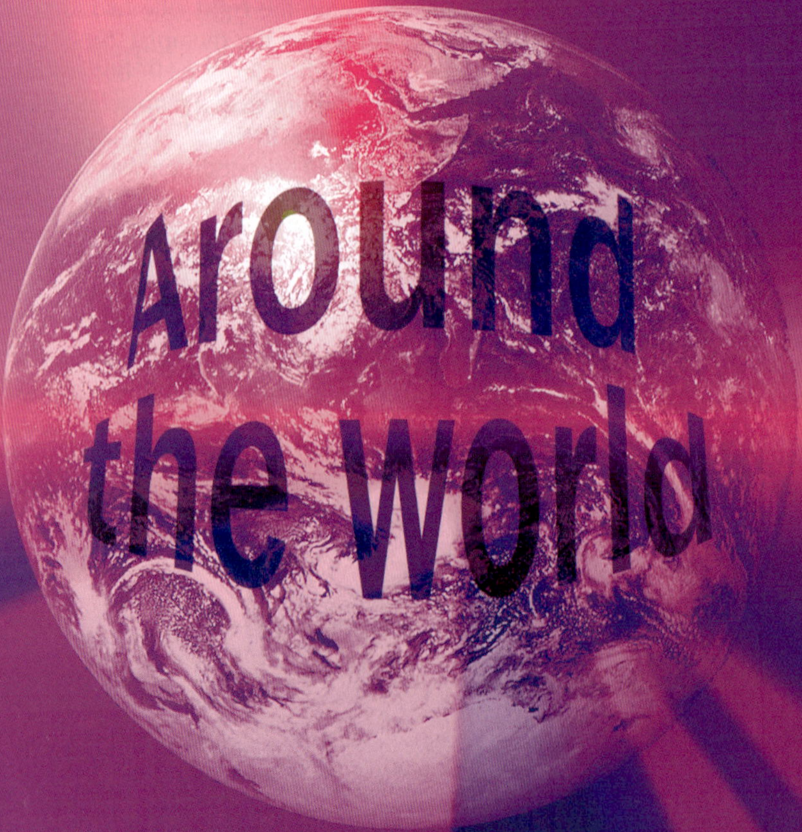

A large number of dental faculties and institutions have shown an interest in low level laser therapy. We will here give a brief account of what has been published. This embraces reports from 98 dental institutions in 38countries. Those reports that are independent of any faculty, or where the connection is not clear, are shown in italics. 336 of the 353 studies (94 %) show positive effects of laser therapy. Some of the reports described here as positive did not actually find effects amongst all the parameters studied. We regard them as positive in this context in that they have found positive effects of laser therapy in one or more of the parameters studied.

Studies have been classified as "dental" if the indication studied is dental or if the researcher is a dentist.

The dental literature on laser therapy comprises only some 15% of the total laser therapy literature. Many of the trials are uncontrolled and some are only available as abstracts or proceedings reports. Several lack an acceptable account of important parameters. It is interesting, though, that more than 90% of those who have tried laser therapy in dentistry register positive responses.

Argentina

Córdoba University, Faculty of Dentistry, Córdoba

Juri H et al. Effects of Nd:YAG laser irradiation on PGE2 level in experimental arthritis. Proc X Internat Congr Soc Lasers in Surgery and Medicine, Bangkok 1993, p. 314. Nd:YAG laser treatment was given to rats with experimental arthritis. 8 J in three sessions reduced the synthesis of PGE2 in arthritis.

Plavnik L, Crosa M, Malberti A. Effect of low power laser radiation on guinea pig submandibular glands: a structural and biomechanical study. J Dent Res. 2000; 79 (5): 1010.

Australia

University of Queensland, Dental School

Skinner S M et al. A preliminary study of the effects of laser radiation on collagen metabolism in cell culture. Aust Dent J. 1996; 41 (3): 188-192. Increased fibroblast procollagen production *in vitro* using GaAs doses between 0.099 and 0.522 J/cm^2.

Walsh L J. The use of lasers in implantology: an overview. J Oral Implantol. 1992; 18: 335-340.

Walsh L J. The current status of low level laser therapy in dentistry. Part 1. Soft tissue applications. Austr Dent J. 1997; 42 (4): 247-254.

Sandford M A, Walsh L J. Thermal effects during desensitisation of teeth with gallium-aluminum-arsenide lasers. Periodontol 1994; 15 (1): 25-30.

Gerschman J A et al. Low Level Laser by dentine hypersensitivity. Australian Dent J. 1994; 39: 6. Tactile and thermal hypersensitivity significantly reduced through 830 nm treatment in a double-blind test.

Royal Perth Hospital, Plastic Surgery and Maxillofacial Unit, Perth.

McNamara D C, Rosenberg I, Jackson P A et al. Efficacy of arthroscopic surgery and midlaser treatment for chronic temporomandibular joint articular disc derangement following motor vehicle accident. Austr Den J. 1996; 41 (6): 377-387. GaAs laser was a positive adjunct to conventional TMD therapies.

Austria

Universitätsklinik für Kiefer- und Gesichtschirurgie, Vienna

Schenk P, Porteder H, Zetner K. Elektronenmikroskopische Untersuchungen von oralen Schleimhautepithelien nach Bestrahlung mit dem Helium-Neon-Laser. Dtsch Z Kiefer Gesichts Chir 1985; 9: 278-283. HeNe on gingiva from dogs showed the following when examined microscopically: an increased number of vesicles and vacuoles, mitochondrial enlargement and dilatation of the endoplasmic reticulum. An increased dosage led to ultrastructural changes in various organelles.
Porteder H et al. Einsatz des Helium-Neon-Lasers zur Förderung der Wundheilung. Österr Z Stomatol 1983; 80: 333-339. A clinical report on the use of a HeNe laser in intraindividual comparisons of various oral surgical operations.
Porteder H et al. Postoperative HeNe laser irradiation in the face and neck region. Proc. 7th Congr Internat Soc Laser Surg Med, Munich 1987, abstr 223. Positive wound healing effect of HeNe laser irradiation following face and neck carcinoma surgery.

Belgium

University of Ghent, Department of Orthodontics.

Gordjestani M, Dermaut L, Thierens H. Infrared laser and bone metabolism: a pilot study. Int J Oral Maxillofac Surg. 1994; 23: 54-56. Bone regeneration in rats unsuccessful at GaAs 20 J/cm^2 for 28 consecutive days.
Verplanken M. Stimulation du processus de guérison des plaies d'extraction par thérapie au laser mou. Rev Bel Méd Dent 1987; 42F (5): 134. A GaAs laser was used in connection with tooth extractions. The healing process was studied with respect to swelling, coloration, and wound closure. All the parameters studied were favourable in the laser group.

Brazil

UNESP, Faculdade de Odontologia, São José dos Campos, S.P.

Filho W, Nogueira T et al. Effects of irradiation with a HeNe laser on the healing of the hard tissue. Surgical and Medical Lasers. 1989; 2-3 (2): 71 (abstract). The left upper incisor in 12 rats was extracted and 3 J/cm^2 was given to the wound area using a HeNe laser. Clinically, the rats exposed to the laser beam showed a better healing rate than the unlased rats from the control group.
Nogueira T et al. An experimental investigation of low power laser effects on wound healing. Surgical and Medical Lasers. 1990; 3 (3): 129 (abstract). Rat skin wounds did not react favourably to e.d. 6 J/cm^2 HeNe laser light. However, favourable indications were found when using e.d. 90 J/cm^2.

Bauru School of Dentistry. University of São Paulo

Conti P C. Low level laser therapy in the treatment of temporo-mandibular disorders (TMD): a double-blind pilot study. Cranio. 1997; 15 (2): 144-149. GaAlAs laser Three times 4 J did not significantly improve TMD symptoms.

University of São Paulo, Dentistry School

de Paula Eduardo C et al. Benefits of low-power lasers on oral soft tissue. Proc SPIE. 1996; Vol 2672: 27-33. (Lasers in Dentistry II). 790 nm laser has successfully been used in the treatment of Herpes Simplex 1 and aphtous ulcers. For some lesions Nd:YAG laser has been added.

Sobral M, Carvalho R, Garone Neto N. Prevalencia de hipersensibilidade dentinaria cervical. Revista Odontológica da Universidade de Sao Paulo. 1995; 9 (3): 177-181.

Sant'Anna G R, Duarte D A, Brugnera Jr A et al. Dye-assisted laser therapy as a disinfecting approach to caries dentine. *In vivo* microbiology study. Proc. 3rd Congr World Assn for Laser therapy, Athens, Greece, May 2000, p. 62.

Groth E B. Treatment of dentine hypersensitivity with low power of Ga-Al-As. J Dent Res. 1995; 74 (3): 794, abstr. 163. 25 teeth with dentine hypersensitivity were treated twice with 7 J at each session and checked after 2-4 weeks. A significant reduction was achieved compared to control teeth.

Migliorati C, Massumoto C, de Paula Eduardo F et al. Low-energy laser therapy in oral mucositis. J Oral Laser Applications. 2001; 1 (2): 97.101.

Sousa G R, Ribeiro M S, Groth E B. Bone repair of the periapical lesions treated or not with low intensity laser (904 nm). Laser Surg Med. Abstract Issue 2002. abstract 303.

Sawazaki I, Ribeiro M S, Mizuno L T et al. A comparative study of the effects of low laser radiation on mast cells in inflammatory fibrous hyperplasia coloured or not coloured by the toluidine blue. Laser Surg Med. Abstract issue 2002, abstract 301.

Silveira L B, Ribeiro M S, Garrocho A A et al. In vivo study on mast cells behaviour following low-intensity visible and near infrared laser radiation. Laser Surg Med. Abstract issue 2002, abstract 304.

Silva Junior A N, Pinheiro A, Oliveira M G et al. Computerized morphometric assessment of the effect of low-level laser therapy on bone repair: an experimental animal study. J Clin Laser Med Surg. 2002; 20 (2): 83-87.

Brugnera Junior A, Garrini A E, Pinheiro A et al. Laser therapy in the treatment of dental hypersensitivity – a histologic study and clinical application. Laser Therapy. 2000; 12: 16-21.

Nicolau R A, Jorgetti V. Rigau J et al. Effect of low power laser Ga-Al-As (660 nm) in the bone tissue remodelation in mice. Proc. 4th Congress of the World Association for Laser Therapy, Tokyo, Japan, June 27-30. 2002; page 127.

University of São Carlos, Sao Carlos, Sao Paulo

Lizarelli R, Lamano-Carvalho T, Brentegani L. Histometrical evaluation of the healing of the dental alveolus in rats after irradiation with a low-powered GaAlAs laser. In Lasers in Dentistry V, John D. B. Featherstone, Peter Rechmann, D.D.S., Daniel Fried, Editors, Proc SPIE. 1999; Vol 3593: 49-56.

led to the same vascular changes when compared thermographically. The study was conducted on patients with temporomandibular joint disorders (TMD).

Bradley P F, Reynolds P A. Low reactive level laser therapy in Oral and Maxillofacial Surgery. Review of 100 cases. Laser Therapy. 1994; 6: 67. GaAlAs laser treatment was effective in 60% of the cases.

Bradley P F, Rebilini Z. Low intensity laser therapy (LILT) for temporomandibular joint pain: a clinical electromyographic and thermographic study. Laser Therapy. 1996; 1: 47. Study comprising 75 cases. In osteoarthritic cases, 830 nm laser therapy was almost comparable to an intraarticular injection of cortisone. In cases with a duration of less than 8 weeks of symptoms, laser therapy could be used alone, in other cases in combination with other treatment modalities.

Bradley P, Groth E, Gursoy B et al. The maxillofacial region: recent research and clinical practice in low intensity level laser therapy (LILT). In: Lasers in Medicine and Dentistry. Ed. Zimunovic Z.; 2000; p 385-401.

Sattayut S. A study of the effect of low intensity laser therapy on painful temporomandibular disorders. 1999. University of London PhD thesis.

Sattayut S, Bradley P F. Low intensity laser therapy (LILT) for TMD myofascial pain: results from a pilot study. Proc. 6th Int Congr Lasers in Dentistry. Ed. J Frame. University of Utah Press.

Rajab A A. A study on the effect of low intensity laser therapy on the osseointegration of hydroxy apatite implants. 1999. University of London PhD thesis.

Institute of Dental Surgery, Department of Microbiology, London

Burns T et al. Killing of cariogenic bacteria by light from a gallium aluminium arsenide diode laser. J Dent 1994; 22 (5): 273-278. Exposure to GaAlAs in the presence of suitable dye may be able to kill bacteria in carious lesions prior to restoration.

University of London, Department of Microbiology.

(The following are only a few examples of the extensive research done by these authors in this borderline between PDT and laser therapy):

Wilson M, Burns T, Pratten J, Pearson GJ. Bacteria in supragingival plaque samples can be killed by low-power laser light in the presence of a photosensitizer. J Appl Bacteriol 1995. 78 (5): 569-74.

Wilson M, Pratten A. Lethal photosensitisation of Staphylococcus aureus *in vitro*: effect of growth phase, serum, and pre-irradiation time. Lasers Med Surg. 1995; 16 (3): 272-276.

University of Glasgow, Division of Neuroscience

Orchardson R, Witters C J. Effect of HeNe and pulsed Nd:YAG laser irradiation on intradental nerve responses to mechanical stimulation of dentine. Lasers in Surg Med. 2000; 26 (3): 241-249. Nd:YAG between 0.6-1.5 W could either enhance or suppress intradental nerve responses. The HeNe light guide alone had no effect, understandably.

Indonesia

Fakultas Kedokteran Gigi Universitas Airlangga, Laboratorium periodontia.

Rubianto M. The effect of low level laser therapy on the healing of periodontal tissues following curettage. Majalah Kedokteran Gigi (Dental journal). 1997; 30 (1).

Israel

Nissan J, Binderman I. Effect of soft laser on bone healing of surgical defect in rat mandible. J Dent Res 1993; 72 (4): 776, Abstract 53.

Italy

Ospedale A. Cardarelli. Div di Odontostomatologia e Traumatiolgia Maxillo-Facciale, Naples

Parascandolo S et al. Azione della Laser-Terapia nella nevralgia essenziale del trigemino. Int Congress on Laser in Med and Surg, Bologna June 1985. Monduzzi Editore S.p.A., Bologna, Italy. Preliminary positive results of the treatment of trigeminal neuralgia.

Cassese M et al. Laser-terapia nelle sindromi algico-disfunzionali delle articolazioni temporo-mandibolari. Int Congress on Laser in Med and Surg, Bologna June 1985, p. 337. Monduzzi Editore S.p.A., Bologna, Italy. A report on the successful laser treatment of TMJ disorders with a GaAs laser.

Parascandalo S et al. Azione della Laser-terapia nella sindrome di Sluder: considerazioni clinico-etiopatogenetiche. Int Congress on Laser in Med and Surg, Bologna June 1985, p. 325. Mb Sluder is a painful condition originating in the spheno-palatinal ganglion. GaAs laser was used in three patients, 12 sessions, irradiating the maxillary nerve apertures. Total pain releif was obtained after five sessions, difficulties in swallowing improved after three sessions, reduction of high tear flow after several sessions. Full recovery after nine sessions.

Grulliero A et al. Dolore post-operatorio in chirurgia orale. Int Congress on Laser in Med and Surg, Bologna June 1985, p 329. Conventional methods more successful than GaAs laser therapy for postoperative pain, except for pain after surgical removal of leukoplakia, where laser therapy was more successful. No effect on alveolitis.

Ruffolo P et al. Impiego della Laser-terapia nelle leucoplachie del cavo orale. Int Congress on Laser in Med and Surg, Bologna June 1985, p 279. Positive effect of GaAs laser therapy on leukoplakia.

Parlato M et al. Analgesic laser therapy in dentistry. Arch Stomatol (Napoli). 1989; 30 (6): 1183-1187. Report on clinical analgesic effect.

Caruso F et al. Laser in periodontology: theoretical-experimental approach. 3. Experimental study of the effects of HeNe (633 nm) and infrared diode (904 nm) lasers on the gingival mucosa of rats. Arch Stomatol (Napoli). 1990; 31 (2): 277-289. Increase in epithelial keratin and a variation of the disposition and of the number of prekeratin grains in the treated site. No alterations in the nuclei.

Università di Torino. Instituto Policattedra di Clinica Odontostomato-logica

Fagnoni V et al. Studio sulla guarigione di ferite chirurgiche eseguite sulla mucosa orale di coniglio trattata con soft-Laser. Int Congress on Laser in Med and Surg, Bologna June 1985, p 269. Better results on mucosa using HeNe than GaAs laser.

Fagnoni V et al. Laser therapy in dentistry and stomatology. Observations on 200 cases treated, Medical Laser Report 1984; 1: 36-40.

Fagnoni V et al. Considerazioni clinico terapeutiche sull'íeffetto della luce laser di bassa potenza nel Herpes Simplex Labiale. Laser Abstracts. 1984; 1: 28-33. 54 cases of lip herpes simplex treated with HeNe or GaAs laser, 3-6 J/cm^2. Subjective symptoms disappear after first treatment and the anatomic lesion in 5 days.

Fagnoni V et al. Use of HeNe soft-laser in 32 cases of mouth aphtha. Laser Abstracts (Rivista Europea di Laser Terapia Medica e Chirurgia). 2 (2): 25-29. HeNe laser 300 mJ per lesion, recovery within 1-3 days in all cases but two.

Fagnoni V et al. Il laser di bassa potenza come coadiuvante nella terapia della sindrome algico-dizfunzionale dell'íarticolazione temporo-mandibulare. Laser Abstracts. 1985; 3: 16-26. Successful cases of TMJ treatment with HeNe/GaAs laser on local and acupuncture points.

Fagnoni V et al. Trattamento delle nevralgie trigeminali con laser di bassa potenza. Laser Abstracts. 1985; 2: 23-36. Laser therapy for trigeminal neuralgia using 1 mW GaAlAs, pulsed 30 Hz. Frequencies above 70 Hz less effective.

Fagnoni V et al. Verifica sperimentale delle variazioni degli oppioidi endogeni plasmatici in pazienti affetti da nevralgie trigeminali e trattati con laser di bassa potenza. Laser Abstracts. 1985:3 (2): 35-42. Plasmatic ß-endorphin was reduced in patients suffering from trigeminal neuralgia following 904 nm laser irradiation.

Fagnoni V et al. Studio sulla guarigione di ferite chirurgiche della mucosa di coniglio precedentemente irradiate con laser I.R. a dosaggi diversi. Laser Abstracts. 1985; 3: 32-37. Rabbit oral mucosa wounds were irradiated with 4 J/cm^2, 904 nm laser, using either 5 mW for 1 minute or 0.5 mW for 10 minutes. Both groups had poor healing compared to control.

Fagnoni V et al. Verifica sperimentale sulle variazioni termiche nella cavità pulpare di denti humani estratti, durante irraggiamento con laser di bassa potenza. Laser Abstracts, 1985; 3 : 27-31. Effect of 880 and 904 nm laser treatment on the pulpal temperature of human extracted teeth. 420/720 J at these wavelengths did not elevate the temperature. Increased dosage of a maximum of 2160 J resulted in a threshold increase of 7.5 under these *in vitro* conditions.

Fagnoni V et al. Su di un caso di emangioma della mucosa orale trattato mediante irraggiamento con laser di bassa potenza. Minerva Stomatologica. 1983; 32 (5): 701-703. Treatment of a case of haemangioma with laser therapy.

Fagnoni V, Fontolan D. Importanza della laser-terapia di bassa potenza per la riduzione dei tempi di guarigione dopo interventi di chirurgia parodontale. Laser Abstracts. 3 (2): 25-33. Faster wound healing after periodontic surgery.

Fagnoni V et al. Study of behaviour of dental enamel in acid solution after treatment with fluorine combined with low power laser. Laser Abstracts. 2 (1): 30-34. Teeth were prepared and exposed to 20% lactic acid. Microscopic comparisons were made between 1) areas exposed to acid only, 2) prefluorized areas exposed to acid, and 3) prefluorized areas exposed to 67.2 J/cm^2 GaAs laser light prior to acid exposure. The laser-treated areas were surprisingly unaffected by the acid.

University of Modena, Department of Dentistry and Oral Surgery, Modena

Palano D et al. A clinico-statistical investigation of laser effect in the treatment of pain and dysfunction of temporo-mandibular joint (TMJ). Minerva Stomatol. Pain relief through HeNe and GaAs treatment.

Debernardi G et al. Ricerche istologiche sull'íazione tessutale della luce laser sulla mucosa orale dei ratti. Laser Abstracts. 1984/85; 1: 9-18. HeNe laser 1 mW was used on the intact mucosa of rats, irradiating on six consecutive days with 0.3 and 0.9 J/cm^2 respectively. No histologic changes compared to control.

Debernardi G et al. Ricerche istologiche sull'íazione della luce laser sulla mucosa orale di coniglio. Laser Abstracts. 1984/85; 1: 19-26. 904 nm laser irradiation of healthy mucosa of rabbits. With 5 treatments and a total dose of 60 J/cm^2 the microscope revealed necrotic areas with copious inflammation.

Università degli Studi di Firenze, Instituto di Odonto-gnato-stomatologia, Florence.

Bernardini U D, Longo L. Terapia laser nella nevralgia del trigemino. Proc. Atti dell'í VIII Congresso Nazionale A.I.S.D., Verona. 1985: 80-81. Positive results in treating tri-geminal neuralgia with GaAs laser. Symptoms may increase after a few treatments but subside by the sixth session.

Università degli studi di Bologna, Instituti policattedra di clinica odontostomatologica, Bologna.

Pelliccioni G A et al. Effetti biologici del LASER su colture cellulari. Laser Abstracts. 1986; 4: 26-33. No effect on fibroblast cultures using GaAs laser 300 Hz, 0.3 mW or 6000 Hz, 6 mW.

Re F, Viterbo S. Indicazioni sull'íuso della soft-laser terapia in odontostomatologia. Minerva Stomatol. 1985; 34: 563-572. Positive experience regarding dental pain states using HeNe laser acupuncture.

Bertelli E, Ceccariglia A. Laser therapy: clinical aspects of analgesic effect in dentistry. G Anaest Stomatol. 1990; 19 (3): 21-24.

Toscani A, Bombelli G. Laser therapy in post-extraction alveolitis. Dent Cadmos. 1987; 55 (9): 73-74.

Cardioli G P et al. Use of 904 nm laser in dentistry; first clinical experience. G Stomatol Ortognatodonzia. 1985; 3: 87-89.

Benedicenti A. La valutazione dell' incremento di ATP endocelulares in linfociti sottoposti a biostimulazione con luce laser 904 nm infrared. Parodontologia e Stomatologia (Nouva) 1983; 22 (1): 9-36.

Japan

Niigata University, School of Dentistry

Kusakari H, Orikasa N, Tani H. Effects of low power laser on wound healing of gingiva and bone. Laser Bologna '92, p. 49. Monduzzi Editore S.p.A., Bologna, Italy. *In vitro* and *in vivo* studies showed some improvement in collagen production, bone regeneration and synthesis of protein and DNA.

Kusakari H. The use of lasers to dental implants. Proceedings of X Congress of Lasers in Surg and Med, Bangkok 1993,.p. 332. Positive results of laser therapy in implant operations on dogs.

Orikasa N et al. Effects of GaAlAs laser in bone histomorphometry. Lasers in Dentistry, Proceedings of the Intern Congr of Lasers in Dentistry, Tokyo August 1988. p 105. Excerpta Medica, Elsevier Sci. Publ. B.V., Amsterdam. The effects of various wavelengths and dosages on new bone formation.

Yarita T et al. Effect of low power laser on gingival microcirculation. Proceedings of X Congr Int Soc Laser Surg Med, Bangkok 1993, p. 235. In the first stage of gingivitis, blood flow increased if GaAlAs laser was used. No morphological changes were reported.

Iwate Medical University, School of Dentistry, Department of Oral Pathology, Morioka

Takeda Y. Irradiation effect of low-energy laser on alveolar bone after tooth extraction. Experimental study in rats. J Oral Maxillofac Surg 1988; 17: 388. A histological study confirmed that laser therapy increases the formation of new bone and the proliferation of fibroblasts.

Takeda Y. Irradiation effect of low-energy laser on rat sub-mandibular salivary gland. J Oral Pathol 1988; 17: 91. Increased mitosis in the salivary ducts after treatment with GaAs laser. The changes were most significant in the granular salivary ducts, less in the striated, and least in the intercalated ducts. Qualitative epithelium differences existed between the control and experimental groups.

Ebihara A, Takeda A, Araki K et al. Clinical evaluation of GaAlAs-semiconductor laser in the treatment of hypersensitive dentin. Jap J Conservative Dent. 1988; 31: 1782-1787.

Keio University, Department of Dentistry and Oral Surgery, Tokyo

Asanami S et al. The activatory effect of low incident energy HeNe laser radiation on hydroxy apatite implants in rabbit mandibular bone. Laser Therapy 1993; 1(5): 29. Better osseointegration in the hydroxy apatite implants after the use of HeNe laser once a day for four days following the operation.

Ikeuchi S et al. Effects of low power HeNe laser on the healing of full-thickness skin defects. Lasers in Dentistry, Proceedings of the Inter Congress of lasers in Dentistry, Tokyo 1988; p 85. Elsevier Publishers, Amsterdam. Bilateral wounds were inflicted on rats. One wound was treated with a HeNe laser. Raised hydroxyprolin content and DNA and more mature tissue were found in the treated wound.

Mutomura K et al. Effects of various laser irradiation on callus formation after osteotomy. J Japan Soc for Laser Medicine. 1984; 4: 195-197. Bone promoting effect of laser therapy demonstrated.
Mutomura K et al. Effect of photoirradiation on bone tissue. J Japan Soc for Laser Medicine. 1985; 5: 603-605. Increased periosteum activity and osseous formation.
Mutomura K et al. Effect of argon-dye laser on fracture healing. J Japan Soc Laser Medicine. 1986; 6: 171-174. Promotion of fracture healing in the initial phase and accelerating osteogenesis using laser therapy .
Kono K. *In vivo* study of low power laser irradiation on new bone formation of rat calvaria defect - influences of an irradiation term and an irradiation time. J Jap Stomatol Soc. 1992; 3: 35. Laser therapy promotes bone repair.

Nihon University, School of Dentistry, Department of Endodontics, Tokyo

Mezawa S et al. The possible analgesic effect of soft-laser irradiation on heat nociceptors in the cat tongue. Arch Oral Biol 1988; 33(9): 693. 60% reduction in the lingual nerve's activity after GaAlAs laser irradiation.
Hatano Y. Lasers in the diagnosis of the TMJ problems. In: Lasers in Dentistry, Eds, Yamamoto Y et al. 1989; p. 169-172. Elsevier Science Publishing B.V.
Ochiai S et al. *In vitro* studies of the effects of laser irradiation on streptococcus mutans, In: Lasers in dentistry. Eds. Yamamoto Y et al. 1989; p. 247-252. Elsevier Science Publishing B.V. Nd:YAG irradiation of s. mutans colonies at 1529 J cm^2 strongly reduced bacterial growth. HeNe laser at 28.7 J and GaAlAs laser at 573 J did not change growth as compared to control. Production of lactic acid was not changed in the HeNe or GaAlAs groups.
Shimizu N et al. Prospect of relieving pain due to tooth movement during orthodontic treatment utilizing a GaAlAs diode laser. Proc. SPIE. 1995; Vol 1984: 275-280. GaAlAs laser treatment reduced the production of prostaglandin E2 and interleukin-1ß in human periodontal ligament cells *in vitro* when subjected to stretching forces.
Shimizu N, Yamaguchi M, Goseki T et al. Inhibition of prostaglandin E2 and interleukin 1-ß production by low-power laser irradiation in stretched human periodontal ligament cells. J Dent Res.1995; 74(7): 1382-1388
Saito S, Shimizu N. Stimulatory effects of low-power laser irradiation on bone regeneration in midpalatal suture during expansion in the rat. Am J Ortod Dentofac Orthop. 1997; 111(5): 525-532. One-time or late irradiation (days 4-6) had no effect. However, irradiation during days 0-2 was most effective.
Ozawa Y et al. Stimulatory effects of low-power laser irradiation on bone formation *in vitro*. Proc SPIE. 1995; Vol 1984: 281-288. GaAlAs laser treatment increased bony formation, DNA content, alkaline phosphatase activity, extracellular collagen formation, calcium and phosphorous content when osteoblast-like cells from rat foetuses were irradiated *in vitro*.
Ozawa Y, Shimizu N, Kariya G et al. Low-energy laser irradiation stimulates bone nodule formation at early stages of cell culture in rat calvarial cells. Bone. 1998; 22 (4): 347-54. The results suggest that laser irradiation may play two principal roles in stimulating bone formation. One is stimulation of cellular proliferation, especially proliferation of nodule-forming cells of osteoblast lineage, and the other is stimula-

tion of cellular differentiation, especially to committed precursors, resulting in an increase in the number of more differentiated osteoblastic cells and an increase in bone formation. Both bone-formation-stimulating roles may be exhibited by laser irradiation to immature cells only.

Kawamura M et al. Effect of Nd:YAG and diode laser irradiation on periodontal wound healing. Innov. Techn. Biol. Med. 1990; 11(1): 113. Diode and Nd:YAG lasers at high doses may inhibit epithelial downgrowth after periodontal operations.

Ohbayashi E, Matsushima K, Hosoya S et al. Stimulatory effect of laser irradiation on calcificed nodule formation in human dental pulp fibroblast. J Endodontics. 1999; 25 (1): 30-33. GaAlAs laser stimulated the formation of calcified nodules in pulp fibroblasts and further stimulated the activity of collagen, alkaline phosphate and osteocalcin.

Senda N, Ito K, Sugano N et al. Inhibitory effect of yellow He-Ne laser irradiation mediated by crystal violet solution on early plaque formation in human mouth. Lasers Med Sci. 2000; 15 (3): 174-180.

Nishikata J, Hirano Y, Ito K et al. The bactericidal effects of the He-Ne laser on streptococcus mutans. J Jpn Soc Periodontol. 1992; 34: 410-415.

Ito A et al. Studies of Nd:YAG low power laser irradiation on stellate ganglion. In: Lasers in dentistry. Ed. H Yamamoto. 1989; p. 271. Elsevier Science Publishers B.V.

Showa University, School of Dentistry, Department of Endodontics, Tokyo

Wakabayashi H, Hamba M, Matsumoto K et al. Effect of irradiation by semiconductor laser on responses evoked in trigeminal caudal neurons by tooth pulp stimulation. Lasers in Surgery and Medicine. 1993; 13: 605-610. GaAlAs laser affects afferent C fibres.

Wakabayashi H et al. Treatment of dentine hypersensitivity by GaAlAs soft laser irradiation. J Den Res 1988; 67: 182. GaAlAs reduces dentine pain.

Wakabayashi H, Tachibana H, Matsumoto K. A clinical study on the hypersensitive dentin by 40 mW GaAlAs semiconductor laser. J Showa Univer Den Soc. 1992; 12: 10-16.

Wakabayashi H, Hamba M, Matsumoto K et al. Electrophysiological study of irradiation of semiconductor laser and the activity of the trigeminal subnucleus caudal neurons. J Jap Soc Laser Dentistry. 1992; 3: 65-74.

Tachibana H, Wakabayashi H, Matsumoto K. A clinical study on the hypersensitive dentine by 20 and 40 mW GaAlAs semiconductor laser. J Showa Univers Dent Soc. 1992; 12: 343-347.

Matsumoto K, Funai H, Wakabayashi H. Study on the treatment of hypersensitive dentine by GaAlAs laser diode. Jap J Conserv Dent. 1985; 28 (2): 766-771

Matsumoto K, Tominari H, Wakabayashi H. Study on the treatment of hypersensitive dentine by laser. Place of laser irradiation. Jap J Conserv Dent .1985; 28 (2): 1366-1371.

Matsumoto K et al. Study on treatment of hypersensitive dentine by HeNe laser. Showa Shigakkai Zasshi. 1988; 8 (2):180-184. Also in: Jap J Conserv Dent. 1986; 29: 312-317.

Matsumoto K, Wakjabayashi H, Funato A. Histopathological findings of dental pulp irradiated by GaAlAs laser diode. Jap J Conserv Dent. 1985; 28 (2):1361-1365.
Matsumoto K, Nakamura Y, Wakabayashi H. A clinical study on the hypersensitive dentine by 60 mW GaAlAs semiconductor laser. J Showa Univ Dent Soc. 1990; 10: 446-449.
Kinoshita F et al. Clinical evaluation of low-energy, semi-conductor laser therapy in oral surgery - a double-blind study. Josai Shika Daigaku Kiyo. 1986; 15 (3): 735-742
Kimura Y, Wilder-Smith P, Yonaga K, Matsumoto K. Treatment of dentine hypersensitivity by laser: a review. J Clin Periodontol. 2000; 27: 715-721.
Watanabe H, Nakamura Y, Wakabayashi H et al. Study on laser transmission through tooth structures by 40 mW Ga-Al-As semiconductor laser. J Jap Endodont Ass. 1991; 12: 40-44.
Watanabe H. A study of HeNe laser transmission through enamel and dentine. J Jap Soc Laser Dent. 1993; 4: 53-62.

Tokyo Dental College, Department of Orthodontics.

Harazaki M, Isshiki Y. Soft laser irradiation effects on pain reduction in orthodontic treatment. Bull Tokyo Dent Coll. 1997; 38 (4):291-5. Pain after the insertion of orthodontic apparatus came after eight hours in the experimental group and after 3.5 hours in the control group. The pain was also milder in the laser therapy group

Hashimoto K. Clinical application of various lasers in oral surgery. In: Lasers in dentistry. Eds. Yamamoto Y et al. 1989; p. 63-70. Elsevier Science Publishing B.V., Amsterdam. The effect of GaAlAs laser on symptoms from nerves, inflammatory diseases and muscular problems investigated in a double-blind study. 25 out of 38 patients in the laser therapy group scored excellent-good-fair (4+11+10), 5 (0+2+3) out of 28 in the control group.

Thwee T, Kato J , Hashimoto M et al. Pulp reaction after pulpotomy with He-Ne laser irradiation. In: Abstract handbook. Vol 4. Internat Soc Laser in Dentistry. 1994. Denics Pacific Ltd, Hong Kong. HeNe laser in combination with calcium hydroxide created a dentine-like calcified layer after pulpotomy in Wistar rats.

Hiroo Metropolitan General Hospital, Tokyo

Nagasawa A. Laser therapy activation of bone production in alveolar bone disease. In: Low reactive-level laser therapy. Practical application. T. Oshiro. 1991; p. 87-93. John Wiley & Sons, Chichester. Also: Medical and Surgical Lasers. 1989; 2-3 (2): 65 (abstract).
Nagasawa A et al: Fundamental studies in reactive histological changes in pulp tissue of lased teeth. J Jap Soc Laser Med Surg.
Nagasawa A et al: Clinical Applications of laser therapy in Dental and Oral Surgery in the Urawa Clinic. Laser Therapy. 1991; 3(3): 119-.
Nagasawa A et al. Bone regeneration effect of low level lasers including argon laser. Laser Therapy. 1991; 3: 59-62.

Ohu University, Graduate School of Dentistry, Ohu

Kurumada F. A study on the application of Ga-As semiconductor laser to endodontics. The effects of laser irradiation on the activation of inflammatory cells and the vital pulpotomy. Ohu Daigaku Shigakushi. 1990; 17 (3): 233-244. (in Japanese)

D-mannose-, N-acetyl-D-galactosamine-, and N-acetyl-neuraminic acid-binding sugars and type I, III, and V collagens play an important role in the healing of pulp wounds.

<u>Chen M et al.</u> *Application of a pain alleviating effect of low power laser irradiation to patients in orthodontic treatment. J Jpn Soc Laser Med. 1933; 14: 5-11 (in Japanese).*

<u>Yoshida T et al.</u> *Pain reduction effect of soft laser in orthodontic therapy. Proc. Annual Meeting Jpn Orthodont Soc. 1992: 69.*

<u>Motomura K et al.</u> *Effects of various laser irradiation on callus formation after osteotomy. J Jpn Soc Laser Med. 1984; 4: 195-196.*

<u>Yamada K.</u> *Biological effects of low power laser irradiation on clonal osteoblastic cells (MC3T3-E1). J Jpn Orthop Assn. 1991; 65: 787-799.*

<u>Tominaga R.</u> *Effects of HeNe laser irradiation on fibroblasts derived from scar tissue of rat palatal mucosa. Kokubyo Gakkai Zasshi - The J of the Stomatol. Soc of Jpn. 1986; 57: 580 (in Japanese).*

<u>Kinoshita F et al.</u> *Clinical evaluation of low-energy, semi-conductor laser therapy in oral surgery - a double-blind study. Josai Shika Daigaku Kiyo. 1986; 15 (3): 735-742 (in Japanese).*

<u>Miyajima K, Yoshida K, Iwate T et al.</u> *Effects of HeNe laser irradiation on gingival fibroblasts. Aichi-Gakuin Dent Sci 1994;7:1-5.*

<u>Kanamura N, Saitoh H, Uematsu N et al.</u> *Pain-relieving effects of soft laser (He-Ne) irradiation on various oral lesions. Jpn J Conserv Dent. 1986; 29: 1548-1555.*

<u>Sudoh A, Ogino H, Yamasaki A, Yamaguchi T.</u> *Effect of low power laser irradiation on experimental tooth movement. J Dent Res 1995; 74 (Special Issue): 457, abstract 453. Orthodontic tooth movement in cats was observed, exerting a force of 100 g and irradiating with GaAlAs laser once a day. The laser irradiation accelerated the tooth movement. Osteoclastic activity was higher on both sides of the tooth as compared to controls.*

<u>Yamaguchi M et al.</u> *Clinical study on the treatment of hypersensitive dentine by GaAlAs laser diode using the double blind test Aichi Gakuin Daigaku Shigakkai Shi - Aichi-Gakuin Journal of Dental Science 1990; 28 (2): 703-707. (In Japanese). 30 mW 790 nm laser light was used to treat dentinal hypersensitivity. After one day, these results were 36.9% and 13.9%, and after 5 days, 43.3% and 19.4%, in active and placebo group, respectively. A overall evaluation indicated these results to be 60.0% and 22.2% respectively.*

<u>Kawakami T et al.</u> *The effectiveness of GaA1As semiconductor laser treatment to pain decrease after irradiation. Higashi Nippon Shigaku Zasshi. 1989; 8 (1) :57-62 (in Japanese). A 790 mW, 830 nm laser was used on a variety of pain situations. 3J was usually applied. Pain was classed I-III with III as the highest grade of pain. The results were as follows: 1. In the hypersensitivity of dentine, the treatment was not effective with 2 cases of grade III, but with all cases of grade I and II (35 cases) the pain decreased just after irradiation. 2. It was effective in all cases of pain, like pain after root canal filling and pain after extraction of teeth. 3. It was effective in all cases with gingivitis, stomatitis and gingival ulcers after infiltration anaesthesia.*

Ishikawa T. Clinical evaluation of GaAlAs semiconductor laser diode (Uni-Laser) irradiation in treatment of solitary aphta, erosion and hypersensitive dentine. Shikwa Gakuho. 1987; 87 (2): 295-303.

Iida M, Ando Y, Watanabe H , Ishikawa I. Effect of GaAlAs-semiconductor laser irradiation on dentine hypersensitivity of exposed root surface and influence to micro-flora in dento-gingival region. J Jap Soc Laser Dent. 1993; 4: 3-7.

Arao M et al. The clinical study of low power laser treatment for temporomandibular arthrosis. Proc. 4th Int Congr Lasers in Dentistry. Ed. Hong-Sai L. 1995, p. 245-250. Munduzzi Editore, Italy.

Hamachi T, Iwamoto Y, Hirofuji T et al. Clinical evaluation of GaAlAs-semiconductor laser in the treatment of cervical hypersensitive dentine. Jap J Clin Periodontol. 1997; 24: 808-813.

Setoguchi T, Mastunaga M, Chinjyo N et al. The effects of soft laser application and strontium chloride application on dentine hypersensitivity induced by periodontal treatment. Jap J Conserv Dent. 1990; 33: 620-627.

Korea

Seoul National University, College of Dentistry, Department of Oral Diagnostics

Kim K-S et al. An experimental study on the effects of low power laser (GaAs) on the wound healing in rat tongue and skin. J Korean Acad Oral Med. 1985; 10 (1): 91. Epithelium and fibroblast regeneration increased but the wound surface was not reduced compared to control.

Kim K-S et al. Study on the effect of low power laser irradiation in treating of gingival inflammation. J Korean Acad Oral Med 1987; 12 (1): 5.

Kim K-S; Kim, Saeng Kon. An experimental study of the effects of low power density laser on the human gingival fibroblast. J Korean Acad Oral Med 1987; 12 (1): 17. GaAlAs laser on human fibroblasts led to a significant rise in their number and in DNA content, although the two effects were the result of different dosage levels.

Kim K-S et al. Comparative study of the clinical effects of bite splint, laser acupuncture and laser therapy for temporomandibular disorders. J Dental College, Seoul Nat Univ. 1988; 1 (12). GaAlAs laser had a better effect on temporomandibular disorders than treatment with bite splint or laser acupuncture.

Kim K-S et al. Effects of low level laser irradiation with 904 nm pulsed diode laser on the extraction wound. J of Korean Academy of Oral Medicine. 23: 301-307 (1998).

Lee Cang Woo, Kim K-S. Study on the effect of low density power laser radiation in treating gingival inflammation. Clinical, microbiological, histological study. J Korean Acad Oral Med 1989; 12 (1): 5-6. GaAlAs laser treatment led to reduced bleeding from the pockets but the pocket depth did not change. Spirochetes were reduced, as was the histological inflammation.

Kim K-S et al. Effects of low incident energy levels of infrared laser irradiation on the proliferation of streptococcus mutans. Laser Therapy. 1992; 4: 81-85.

Kim K-S, Yoon S-H, Kim J S, Lee J H. Effect of Ga-As diode laser irradiation on tooth pulp responses. J Dent Res 71 (IADR Abstracts) 1992; 657, abstract 1133.

Kim K-S et al. Effects of low incident energy levels of infrared laser irradiation on the proliferation of candida albicans, Part I: a long term study on pulse types. Laser Therapy. 1994; 6: 161-166.

Kim K-S et al. Effects of low incident energy levels of infrared laser irradiation on the proliferation of candida albicans. Part II: A short term study during cell growth. Laser Therapy. 1995; 7: 61-66. Laser therapy had no bioactivating or inhibiting effect on healthy fungi, regardless of pulse type.

Kim K-S et al. Effects of low incident energy levels of infrared laser irradiation on the proliferation of Candida albicans. Part III: A study on the interirradiation interval. Laser Therapy. 1995; 7: 151-156.

Kim K-S et al. Effects of low level laser irradiation (LLLI) with 904 nm pulsed diode laser on osteoblasts: a controlled trial with the rat osteoblast model. Laser Therapy. 1996; 8: 223-232.

Lee P-Y, Kim K-S. Effects of low reactive level laser irradiation (LLLI) on the wound infected by staphylococcus aureus. J Korean Acad Oral Med 1996; 21 (1): 14.

Kim K-S et al. Effects of low-level laser irradiation on the rat osteoblast function. J Korean Acad Oral Med. 1996; 21 (1): 2.

Kim K-S et al. Effects of low level laser irradiation (LLLI) with 904 nm pulsed diode laser on staphylococcus aureus. Laser Therapy. 1997; 9: 121-130.

Lee K-H, Kim K-S. Effects of low level laser irradiation on the ALP activity and calcified nodule formation of rat osteoblastic cell. J of Korean Academy of Oral Medicine. 1996; 21: 279-292 .

Wonkwang University, School of Dentistry, Department of Oral Diagnostics and Oral Medicine

Kwon Soon-Oh et al. A study on the effects of low-power laser irradiation on the sciatic nerve regeneration in rats. J Korean Acad Oral Med 1991; 2 (16): 31. Laser treatment of damaged sciatic nerves was effective but the differences between the various dosage levels were unclear.

Dankook University, Department of Dentistry, Choongnam

Kim, Dong-Woon. The healing effects of low power density laser to the experimental periodontitis. Histopathological study. Thesis for M.S. 1993. GaAs laser reduced epithelium downgrowth in the pocket after a flap operation. The inflammation was reduced and periodontal ligament regeneration was stimulated. Dose not indicated.

Lee P Y et al. Effects of low incident energy levels of infrared laser irradiation on healing of infected open skin wounds in rats. Laser Therapy 1993; 5: 59. Bilateral wounds were inflicted on rats and all wounds were infected with S. aureus. The group treated with laser showed less swelling and better wound contraction.

Pusan National University, College of Dentistry, Department of Oral Medicine

Kim S-Y, Park J-S. The effect of low level laser therapy at the trigger points in masseter and other muscles. J Korean Acad. Oral Med. 1996; 21 (1): 3.

Chonbuk National University, School of Dentistry, Department of Oral Medicine

Shin K-B et al. Report of cases on the therapeutic effects of low-level laser in dental field. J Dental Science, Chonbuk Nat Univ 1990; 8 (1): 339-346. In case of cervical abraded and/or root-exposed dentine hypersensitivity the applied low-level laser manifested some thermal pain-relieving effect. In cases of traumatic muscular trismus the applied low-level laser manifested a prominent muscular tension-releasing effect.

Shin K-B et al. An experimental study on growth pattern and ultrastructure of human gingival fibroblasts treated by low level laser. J Korean Acad Oral Med 1992; 17 (2): 129-149.

Shin K-B et al. An experimental study on the effect of low level laser and some cytokines on gene expression of human gingival fibroblasts. J Korean Acad Oral Med 1994; 19 (2): 57-71.

Shin K-B et al. Effects of low level laser on proliferation and gene expression of fibroblasts and immune cells. J Korean Acad Oral Med 1995; 20 (1): 53-65.

Cho K-A, Park J-S, Ko M-Y. The effect of low level laser therapy on pressure threshold in patients with temporomandibular disorders. A double blind study. J Korean Acad Oral Med. 1999; 24 (3): 281-300.

Kuwait

Ministry of Public Health, Dental Centre, Department of Crown and Bridge

Wafa F et al. A clinical study of laser therapy in fixed prosthodontic pain control after tooth preparation to receive a crown. Laser Therapy 1990; 2: 83. 60 patients who received crown therapy also received laser therapy and the postoperative analgesic effects were evaluated.

The Netherlands

University of Amsterdam, Academic Centre for Dentistry, Department of Masticatory Function

Hansson T L. Infrared laser in the treatment of cranomandibular disorders, arthrogenous pain. J Prosthet Dent. 1989; 61: 614. A pilot study found that GaAs laser treatment can reduce pain as well as the treatment period if combined with conventional bite splint therapy.

Bezuur N, Habets L, Hansson T. The effect of therapeutic laser treatment in patients with cranomandibular disorders. J Cranomandib Disord. 1988; 2: 83. 27 patients with long-term maxillary joint problems were treated with GaAs laser. 80% of the patients with arthrosis experienced total pain relief. In this group, the maximum jaw-opening ability increased gradually during the year when the study took place. Laser treatment was administered on five consecutive days and given directly over the maxillary joint. Even the group with myogenic problems experienced a reduction in pain and an increase of the maximum jaw-opening ability, despite the fact that the muscles were not treated. The effect on this group was, however, milder and is thought to be related to the partial arthrosis diagnosis of these patients.

University of Nijmegen, Department of Orthodontics and Oral Pathology

in de Braekt M M H et al. Effect of low level laser therapy of wound healing after palatal surgery in beagle dogs. Lasers in Surg Med 1991; 11: 462. Von Langenbeck's palatinal repair method was simulated on beagles. GaAlAs laser 830 nm improved neither the tissue's contracting ability during healing nor the general quality of the healing.

in de Braekt M M H et al. The effect of low-level laser treatment on maxillary arch dimensions after palatal surgery on beagle dogs. J Dent Res. 1991; 70: 1467-1470.

Norway

University of Oslo, Faculty of Dentistry, Department of Oral Surgery and Oral Medicine

Røynesdal A K et al. The effect of soft-laser application on postoperative pain and swelling. A double-blind cross-over study. Int J Oral Maxillofac Surg. 1993; 22: 242-245. 6 J GaAlAs laser light administered before and after the removal of totally impacted lower third molars. No effect on pain reduction, swelling or jaw-opening ability could be observed using this laser.

Midamba E D, Haanaes H R. Effects of low level laser therapy (laser therapy) on inferior alveolar, mental and lingual nerves after traumatic injury in 15 patients. A pilot study. Laser Therapy 1993; 5: 89-94. GaAlAs laser reduced paraesthesia by 78% in the alveolaris inferior and lingual nerve in a group of 15 people suffering from long-term paraesthesia.

Midamba E D, Haanaes H R. Low reactive-level 830 nm GaAlAs diode laser therapy (laser therapy) successfully accelerates regeneration of peripheral nerves in humans. Laser Therapy 1993; 5: 125-129. An expanded study on a group of 40 patients with paraesthesia as above. The average improvement was 71%.

Khullar S M et al. Preliminary study of low-level laser for treatment of long-standing sensory aberrations in the inferior alveolar nerve. J Oral Maxillofacial Surg. 1996; 54: 2-7. A significant improvement in mechanoreceptor sensory response after GaAlAs treatment was observed in patients with post-surgical damage to the inferior alveolar nerve. In this double-blind study the post treatment degree of thermal sensitivity, however, was comparable in the laser and the placebo groups.

Khullar S M et al. Effect of low-level laser treatment on neurosensory deficits subsequent to sagittal split ramus osteotomy. Oral Surg Oral Med Oral Path. 1996; 82 (2): 132-138. Double-blind study. 20 treatments with GaAlAs 4 × 6 J improved lip and chin mechanoreceptor neurosensory deficit. No improvement in thermoreception was observed.

Khullar S M et al. The effects of low level laser treatment on recovery of nerve conduction and motor function after compression injury in the rat sciatic nerve. Europ J Oral Sci. 1995; 103: 299-305. 20 rats received crush injuries of the sciatic nerve. 10 animals were treated with GaAlAs 6 J daily for 28 days. At 21 days post injury the laser group had a significantly better Sciatic Functional Index than the non-treated group. However, no differences were found histologically or between evoked cAP parameters. Consequently, the effects of laser therapy recovery must have occurred more peripherally to the point measured.

Khullar S M et al. Low level laser (LLL) treatment enhances sensory reinnervation of peripheral target tissues subsequent to inferior alveolar nerve (IAN) axotomy in rats. In: Reinnervation after nerve injury: the effects of low level laser treatment. Dissertation at Oslo University, Norway, 1997. The dental pulp is innervated by unmyelinated C fibres and myelinated A-fibres, both of which are known to contain calcitonin gene related peptide (CGRP). Axotomy of the IAN was performed in rats and one group received laser. A statistically significant greater number of CGRP immunoreactive nerve profiles were seen in the laser group at the area of evaluation.

Khullar S M et al. Upregulation of growth associated protein (GAP) 43 expression and neural co-expression with neuropeptide Y (NPY) following inferior alveolar nerve (IAN) axotomy in the rat. J Periph Nerv Syst. 1998, 3 (2): 79-90. Single sided axotomy was performed in rats. Ten days post injury a pronounced upregulation of GAP 43 immunoreactivity could be demonstrated in neurons located in the mandibular region of the trigeminal ganglion, as compared to the control side, and this was still evident on day 21.

Khullar S M et al. Enhanced sensory reinnervation of dental target tissues in rats following low level laser (LLL) irradiation. Lasers Med Sci. 1999; 14 (3): 177-184.

Poland

Medical Academy of Bialystok, Department of Conservative Dentistry

Dcabrowska E et al. Intravital treatment of the pulp with simultaneous laser biostimulation. Rocz Akad Med Bialymst. 1997; 42 (1): 168-176. 30 pulp cappings and amputations were performed in combination with calcium hydroxide and laser therapy and were compared to 36 procedures without laser. The laser treated group had a more favourable outcome.

Medical University of Lodz, Institute of Dentistry, Lodz.

Grzesiak-Janas G, Grazyna A A. Low-power-laser therapy in Costen's syndrome. Proc SPIE. 1996; Vol 2781: 126-128. (Lasers in Medicine) Low power laser therapy in "Costen's syndrome" is reported to have a significant influence on the regression of pain symptoms.

Grzesiak-Janas G, Janas A. Conservative closure of antro-oral communication stimulated with laser light. Journal of Clinical Laser Medicine and Surgery. 2001; 19 (4): 181-184.

Machnikowski I et al. Application of therapeutic laser in treatment of the selected chronic illnesses of the oral cavity. Protet Stomatol. 1989; 39 (3): 147-150. Fast regression of the pathological changes during treatment of chronic recurrent aphthae and herpes simplex as well as diminution of suffering in most cases of trigeminal neuralgia.

Portugal

Peres F, Felino A, Carvalho J F. Analgetic effect of 904 nm laser radiation (IR) in oral surgery. Rev Port Estomatol Cir Maxilofac. 1985; 26: 205-217

Romania

University of Medicine and Pharmacy, School of Dentistry, Department of Oral Rehabilitation.

Colojoara C, Mavrantoni A, Miron M. Clinical and bacteriological study on the effect of Nd:YAG laser in gingivitis therapy. In: A window of the laser medicine world. Proc SPIE. 1999, Vol 4166: 233-244.

Disciplina de Propedeutica Stomatologica, Universitatea "Ovidius" Constanta.

Bechir A. Comparative study and results obtained in reducing painful sensitivity in vital pillars with combined therapies. http://www.infomedica.ro/anul%202000/10_2000/rez10_2000_7.htm

Russia

Moscow Institute of Medicine and Stomatology

Kats A et al. Use of laser in non-specific inflammatory processes of the temporomandibular joint. Stomatologiia (Mosk); 1983; 5 (62): 42-45. HeNe laser used in a group of 61 patients. Energy density used was 0.4-0.8 mW/cm^2, treatment time 4-10 minutes. Reduction in pain, head noise and numbness reported.

Kats A et al. Comparative estimation of the patient's treatment with sharp purulent diseases of adjacent jaw tissues with laser irradiation. J Stomatology. 1985: 4: 38.

Kats A et al. Remote results of the complex treatment of chronic sialadenitis with the use of helium-neon lasers. Vestnik Khirurgii 1985; 135: 39. 88 patients with chronic sialadenitis were treated with HeNe laser. Pain and inflammation disappeared. Saliva secretion increased, the length of time between periods of discomfort increased, and the gland structure recovered.

Kats A. Low energy laser radiation in the combined treatment of salivary gland inflammation. Stomatologiia. 1993; 72 (4): 32-36. 95% of the patients treated with laser therapy showed positive results.

Kats A et al. Changes in the blood flow in the course of laser therapy for an uncomplicated fracture of the mandible. Stomatologiia (Mosk). 2: 41.

Kats A et al. Laser therapy in fracture of the mandible. Vestnik Khirurgii. 1986; 136 (6): 93-96. HeNe laser light promoted jaw fracture healing.

Kats A et al. Small-scale laser unit and its use in dental surgery. Med Tekh. 1984; 4: 50-54. Report on the clinical effect of laser therapy in 3000 patients.

Kats A et al. The effect of functional tests and of low-energy helium-neon laser on the local blood circulation in the area of the partoid glands. Stomatologiia. 1994; 73 (2): 42-44. The use of laser exposure as a functional test in the examination of the salivary glands is substantiated. The study was carried out in a group of 97 patients with chronic nonspecific sialadenitis.

Ivanov A et al. Effect of Helium-Neon laser radiation on the course of temporomandibular joint arthritis and arthrosis. Clinical improvement in 89% of the 109 patients treated. Stomatologiia. 1985. 64; 81-83. Positive results on clinical symptoms.
Lukashevich I G. HeNe laser in facial pain. Stomatologiia (Mosk.). 1985; 64 (1): 29-31.
Lomnitski I, Bibiashevski E V. Substantiation of the optimal exposure to monochromatic red light for stimulating osteogenesis. Stomatologiia (Mosk). 1982; 60 (2): 14-16.
Lomnitski I. The mechanism of stimulation of reparative osteogenesis with laser radiation. Stomatologiia (Mosk). 1983; 5: 18-20. Animal study.
Lomnitski I. Clinical X-ray characteristics of the healing of mandibular fractures following the use of HeNe laser radiation. Stomatologiia (Mosk). 1985; 3: 38-40.
Urazalin ZhB et al. Laser therapy in the combined treatment of mandibular fractures. Stomatologiia. 1983; 62 (1): 3435.
Supiev T K. Action of laser radiation on the course of an inflammatory process in the maxillofacial area. Stomatologiia (Mosk). 1984; 5: 17-19.

Voronezh State Medical Academy, Voronezh

Kalivradzhiyan E et al. Usage of low-intensity laser radiation for the treatment of the inflammatory processes of the oral cavity mucosa after applying removable plate dentures. Proc SPIE. 1995; Vol 1984: 225-230. Laser therapy utilised in the early treatment of pressure zones under removable dentures.
Sokolova I et al. Low-intense laser radiation in complex treatment of inflammatory diseases of parodontium. Proc SPIE. 1995; Vol 1984: 234-237. 60 patients treated for periodontal disease; 30 with laser (890 nm) and conventional methods, 30 with only conventional methods. Laser therapy reduced healing time.
Podolskaya E et al. Radiation damage of lips and its treatment by low-intensity laser irradiation. Proc SPIE. 1995; Vol 1984: 245-246. Laser therapy gave favourable effects in the treatment of adverse postirradiation reactions in lips and mucous membranes in cancer patients.
Kazmina S et al. Laser prophylaxis and treatment of primary caries. Proc SPIE. 1995; Vol 1984; 231-233. Improved caries prevention with fluoride lacquer and HeNe laser as compared with fluoride lacquer alone at four-year follow-up.
Kunin A A. Use of helium-neon laser in treating periodontal diseases. Stomatologiia (Mosk). 1983; 62 (1): 26-27.
Kunin A A et al. Changes in microbic associations qualitative contents in caries and its complications with the use of low intensive laser radiation. Proc SPIE. 1995; Vol 2630: 104-117. Microflora in pulpitis and periodontitis was reduced after HeNe laser irradiation.
Kunin A A. et al. Fluorine lacquer coating and HeNe laser exposure to prevent deciduous teeth caries. J Stomatology. Moscow. 1991: 71-72.
Kunin A A et al. Laser methods of caries prophylaxis. Proc SPIE. 1995; Vol 2630: 94-103. HeNe and 890 nm laser in combination with standard prophylactic measures enhanced anti-carious effect in a group of 350 children.

Kunin A A et al. Biological effects caused by low-power laser light in the treatment of the dentition, periodontium and mucosa of oral cavity, and lip diseases. In: Progress in Biomedical Optics, Proc. of Effects of low-power light on biological systems. Proc SPIE. 1997; Vol 3198: 37-46.

Kunin A A, Bykov E I, Podolskaya E E et al. Clinical and morphological indications for laser treatment of patients with precancerous diseases of the oral cavity. Proc SPIE. 1996; Vol 2929: 185-197.

Kunin A A, Minakov E V, Sutchenko A V et al. Diagnosis and indications for low-intensity laser therapy of the pathology of the oral cavity mucosa of patients with hematologic and gastroenteric disease. Proc SPIE. 1996; Vol 2929: 165-176.

Kunin A A, Erina S V, Pankova S N. Comparative estimation of the effectiveness of laser and other methods of stomatological disease treatment. Proc SPIE. 1996; Vol 2929: 146-155.

Kunin A A, Erina S V, Sokolova I A et al. Indications for laser therapy in diverse models of periodontitis. Proc SPIE. 1996; Vol 2929: 156-164.

Kunin S, Pankova Y, Oleinik T et al. The influence of low level lasers together with modern filling materials and bonding systems on mineral metabolism of hard tissues. Proc. European Conf Biomed Optics, Munich, Germany, June 2001, p. 18.

Kolesnik A G et al. Prophylaxis and treatment of initial caries with the use of lowintensive lasers. News of Lasers in Surgery and Medicine. Moscow. 1989.

Kolesnik A G et al. Experiments in anticaries activity of lowintensive laser light. News of Laser Medicine and Surgery, part 2. Moscow. 1990.

Korzhova V V et al. Specifities of treatment of early stages of caries of pregnant women with the use of laser phoresis. J Stomatology. 1993; 3: 10-20.

State Research Centre for Laser Medicine, Moscow.

Kozlov V et al. Lasers in diagnostics and treatment of microcirculation disorders under parodontitis. Proc SPIE 1995; Vol 1984: 253-264. Microcirculation in patients with periodontal disease of various degrees was studied using biomicroscopic techniques and laser Doppler flowmetry. The intensified tissue blood flow seen after HeNe laser irradiation was caused by intensification of blood microcirculation and the activation of neovascularization. Tissue blood flow stimulation was caused by precapillary dilation and opening of "reserved" capillaries. Doses between 10 and 30 J/cm^2 had adverse effects.

Mikhailova R I et al. The laser therapy and laser acupuncture of patients with chronic recurrent aphthous stomatitis. Stomatologiia (Mosk. 1992; 3-6: 27-28.

Sluzhajev J F. Mechanisms of biological effects of the laser on the strong dental tissues. News of Laser Medicine and Surgery. Mosk. 1990.

Sluzhajev J F et al. HeNe laser effect on dental enamel solubility in health and caries. J Stomatology. 1990; 5: 6-9.

Pilikin A S. Effect of helium-neon laser radiation on the microcirculation of the oral mucosa. Stomatologiia (Mosk). 1984; 63 (4): 12-13.

Prokhonchukov A A et al. The laser therapy of diseases of the periodontium and oral mucosa. Stomatologiia (Mosk). 1996; 75 (3): 55-62.

Prokhonchukov A A et al. 30 years of experience in using lasers in dentistry. Stomatologiia (Mosk). 1995; 74: 68-73.
Shargorodskii A G. The comparative efficacy of different physiotherapy combinations in treating mandibular fractures. Stomatologiia (Mosk). 1994; 73 (1): 24-26.
Zazulevskaia L I et al. Physiochemical research on the bone tissue of the alveolar process in experimental periodontitis. Stomatologiia (Mosk). 1991; 70 (1): 9-12.
Melnichenko E M et al. The clinico-experimental validation of the use of low-intensity laser radiation for the treatment of exacerbated recurrent herpetic stomatitis in children. Stomatologiia. 1992; (2): 76-78.
Mukashev T K et al. The use of helium-neon laser radiation in the combined treatment and prevention of dental caries in children. Stomatologiia 1991; (2): 67-69. The possibility of improving the efficacy of the known anticarious agents with HeNe laser exposure was investigated in 455 caries-susceptible children. The results suggest that a combination of treatment and prophylactic measures with HeNe laser exposure led to a reduction of the carious process intensity, essentially improved the efficacy of the known anticarious agents and promoted the elimination of focal demineralization.
Bazhanov N N et al. The efficacy of using a helium-neon laser, ascorbic acid and methylene blue in the combined treatment of patients with maxillofacial phlegmons. Stomatologiia. 1990; (5): 35-7. A combination of 5% ascorbic acid, 1% methylene blue aqueous solution and HeNe laser was used to treat 188 patients with maxillofacial phlegmons. The treatment accelerated injured tissue regeneration, permitting early secondary suturing and shortening the invalidity periods.
Korytny D L: Use of Helium-Neon laser in therapeutic stomatology. Stomatologiia (Mosk). 1978; 57 (5): 5-21.
Oasevich I A, Shargorodskii A G. (Low-intensity infrared laser radiation in the diagnosis and combined treatment of acute nonspecific lymphadenitis of the face and neck in children) Infrakrasnoe nizkointensivnoe lazernoe izluchenie v diagnostike i kompleksnom lechenii ostrogo nespetsificheskogo limfadenita litsa i shei u detei. Stomatologiia (Mosk). 1999; 78 (2): 28-30.
Pavlova T N. The use of blood, irradiated with a helium-neon laser, in the combined treatment of patients with phlegmons. Stomatologiia. 1993; 72 (1): 16-18.
Chistov V B. The effect of low-intensity radiation from a helium-neon laser on the alkaline phosphatase activity in an uncomplicated mandibular fracture and in traumatic osteomyelitis. Stomatologiia 1989; 68 (6): 13-5 The osteal alkaline phosphatase (AP) activity was examined in 167 Wistar rats with uncomplicated regeneration and traumatic osteomyelitis of the mandible exposed to low-intensity HeNe laser. Laser exposure stimulated the bone AP activity in the animals with traumatic osteomyelitis and uncomplicated regeneration.
Pavlova T N. The use of blood, irradiated with helium-neon laser, in the combined treatment of patients with phlegmons. Stomatologiia. 1993; 72.
Mozgovaia L A et al. The socioeconomic efficiency of using low-intensity laser radiation in pediatric dental practice. Stomatologiia. 1996: 27-28.
Lutsyk L et al. Use of a helium-neon laser in the combined treatment of oral mucosa diseases in children. Stomatologiia (Mosk). 1981; 60: 6-15.

Christov V B. The effect of low-intensity radiation from a helium-neon laser on the alcaline phosphatase activity in an uncomplicated mandibular fracture and in traumatic osteomyelitis. Stomatologiia (Mosk). 1989; 68 (6): 13-15.
Britova A A et al. The effect of laser reflex therapy on lysosomal enzymes of saliva in patients with parodontitis. Zdravookhraneniye Kazakhstana. 1990; 4: 53-55.

Singapore

National University of Singapore, Faculty of Dentistry

Lim, Hong-Meng; Lew, Kenneth; Tay, David. A clinical investigation of the efficacy of low level laser therapy in reducing orthodontic postadjustment pain. Am J Orthod Dentofac Orthop. 1995; 108: 614-22. 830 nm 30 mW laser therapy reduced pain in a VAS scale estimation but the reduction was not statistically significant.
Tay E J, Lee L I, Yee S, Loh H S. Laser-induced reduction of post-operative pain following third molar surgery. Lasers in Surgery and Medicine. 2001; Suppl 13: 17. 10 J applied during four sessions within the first 24 hours post-operatively, total dose of 40 J, was effective in reducing postoperative pain.

South Africa

University of Pretoria, Faculty of Dentistry, Centre for Stomatological Research.

van Rensburg S D, Wiltshire W A. The effect of soft laser irradiation on fluoride release of two fluoride-containing orthodontic bonding materials. J Dent Assoc S Afr. 1994; 49 (3): 127-31. A GaAlAs laser with an energy of 5.45 J (30 mW for 180 seconds) and an energy density of 27.54 J/cm^2 was used to irradiate two fluoride containing orthodontic bonding materials. SEM evaluation showed that the laser irradiation had no superficial physical ultrastructural effects on either of the two materials. However, the fluoride release of one of the materials could be enhanced for up to seven months by a singe laser treatment. Fluoride release from the other material was also increased but was not statistically significant

Spain

Faculty of Odontology, Department of Oral Medicine and Maxillo-facial Surgery, Madrid

Carrillo S et al. A randomised double-blind clinical trial on the effectiveness of helium-neon laser in the prevention of pain, swelling and trismus after removal of impacted third molars. Int. Dent J 1990; 40: 31. Trismus was reduced more by HeNe laser light than by ibuprofen if the treatment was administered in conjunction with the extirpation of impacted wisdom teeth. There was no effect on pain and swelling.

Hospital Provincial de Madrid

Lopez V J. The laser in the treatment of TMJ dysfunction. Revista Actualidades de Estomatologia Clínica. 1986 (July): 35-39. 168 patients with arthralgia were treated with a combination of bite splints and HeNe laser light. Ten treatments were administered directly over the joint over a three-week period. 90% of the patients were freed from pain as a result. 53 patients were free from pain after a single treatment.

Universidad de Oviedo, Escuela de Estomatología

Rodriguez N, Felechosa A S et al. Effectos de la radiación laser sobre el periodonto. Aproximación en un modelo animal. II. Effectos de las altas dosis de irradiación. Invest. Clin. Laser 2a Epoca 1989; 1 (1-2): 15. The effects of laser therapy on the periodontal tissue of mice were studied. Epithelium changes were most pronounced after ten days.

Universidad Nacional, Faculdad de Odontología, Córdoba.

Ibañez J C, Medico R O. Laser therapy in temporomandibular dysfunction. Rev Fac Odontol Univ Nac (Córdoba). 1989; 17 (1-2): 21-30.

Universitat Rovira i Virgili, Facultad de Medicina i Ciencia de la Salut, Reus.

Rigau J. Acción de la luz láser a baja intensidad en la modulación de la función celular. 1996; PhD thesis. [Action of low intensity laser light on the cellular function].

Kaiser C et al. Estudio en doble ciego randomizado sobre la eficacia del HeNe en el tratamiento de la sinuitis maxilar aguda: en pacientes con exacerbación de una infección sinusal crónica. (Double blind randomized study on the effect of HeNe in the treatment of acute maxillary sinuitis in patients with exacerbation of a chronic maxillary sinuitis). Bolet'in CDL. 1986; 9: 15.

Kaiser C et al. Helium-neon (He-Ne) laser irradiation versus placebo in the treatment of acute maxillary sinuitis. Avances en Odontoestomatología. 1987; 3 (2): 73-76

Sweden

Karolinska Institutet, Department of Periodontology, Stockholm

Rydén H, Persson L et al. Effect of low level energy laser irradiation on gingival inflammation. Swed Dent J 1994; 18: 35-41. GaAs laser, 0.5 + 0.5 J, had no effect on the formation of new vessels in experimental human gingivitis in healthy volunteers.

Hall G et al. Effect of low level energy laser irradiation on wound healing. An experimental study in rats. Swed Dent J 1994; 18: 29. Bilateral wounds in rats, one of which was treated with GaAs laser. No effect on wound healing using Mester's dosage recommendations for HeNe laser.

Anneroth G et al. The effect of low-energy infrared laser radiation on wound healing in rats. Br J Oral Maxillofac Surg 1988; 26:12-. Wounds in rats were treated with GaAs laser. No effect.

Switzerland

Université de Genève, Geneva.

Paschoud Y, Holz J. Effet du soft-laser sur la néoformation d'un pont dentinaire après coiffage pulpaire direct de dents humaines à l'hydroxyde de calcium. Rev mens. suisse odonto-stomatol 1998; 98: 345. HeNe laser light together with a calcium hydroxide preparation led to an improved dentine bridge in cases of pulp capping. Only two of the three preparations used brought about this effect in the laser group.

La Carita Hospital, Locarno

Simunovic Z. Application of HeNe laser therapy in major and minor surgery. Lasers in Surgery and Medicine 1987; 7: 125. A report on experience.

Simunovic Z. Curing stomatological and maxillo-facial diseases with MID laser therapy. 1984. QLT; 1. Report of clinical experience of GaAs lasers for periodontology, mucositis and trigeminal neuralgia.

Simunovic Z, Simunovic K. Status after multiple teeth extractions treatment with low level laser therapy: A randomised clinical study with control group. Lasers in Surgery and Medicine. 2001; Suppl 13: 11.

Taiwan

Pharmaceutical Industry Technology and Development Center, Taipei Hsien.

Hsu J et al. Combined effects of laser irradiation/solution fluoride ion on enamel demineralization. J Clin Laser Med Surg. 1998; 16 (2): 93-105. A comparison between CO_2 lased and unlased portions of enamel showed increased acid-resistance with increasing laser energy density and, at the highest energy density of 170.0 J/cm^2, there was little or no lesion development in the fluoride-free dissolution medium. The demineralisation of enamel was reduced dramatically in the presence of 0.2 ppm fluoride for both lased and unlased enamel; only modest lesion development was observed for unlased enamel and, at an energy density as low as 85.0 J/cm^2, the surface of the enamel was found to be completely protected.

Thailand

Khon Kean University, Bangkok

Sattayut S, Hughes F, Bradley P. 820 nm gallium aluminium arsenide laser modulation of prostaglandin E_2 production in interleukin 1 stimulated myoblasts. Laser Therapy. 1999; 11 (2). 820 nm GAAlAs laser, when applied at higher energy levels (19 J/cm^2 versus 4 J/cm^2), can reduce the level of prostaglandin E_2 (PGE_2) synthesis stimulated by interleukin 1 (IL-1) in an experimental model of differentiated muscle cells. Authors suggest that this mechanism underlies some of the analgesic effects attributed to low intensity lasers in cases of musculoskeletal pain.

Turkey

Istanbul School of Dentistry, Istanbul

Kokino M, Alatli M et al. An investigation of the stimulating effect of Laser on callus in the treatment of fractures. Int Congress on Laser in Med and Surg, Bologna 1985, p 387. GaAs laser had a stimulating effect on callus formation.

Kokino M, Alatli M. Effect of Laser irradiation on tendon healing. Int Congress on Laser in Med and Surg, Bologna 1998, p 405. GaAs laser has a marked effect on tendon healing.

Gazi University, Faculty of Dentistry, Ankara

Delilbasi E et al. The quantitative investigation of infrared laser effect on the level of copper and zinc in various tissues. Clin Phys Physiol Meas. 1988; 9 (4): 375-377.

Zinc level increased in muscles but decreased in submandibular glands, copper decreased in both. In irradiated skin both levels increased.

Marmara University, Department of Oral and Maxillofacial Surgery

Gürsoy B et al. Penetration studies of low intensity laser therapy (laser therapy) wavelengths. Laser therapy, 1996; 8 (1): 18-22. Comparison between 660 and 830 nm laser penetration in tissue, using CCD camera, radiometer and isotropic detectors. A 200 mW 830 probe reached a depth of 3.5 cm with a lateral spread of 5.5 cm.

United Arab Emirates

Clinic for Laser & Physiotherapy, Dubai

Makk A, Pollera M. Multicenter study related to laser treatment of T.M.J. A retrospective analysis of 10 years' experience. Abstracts LASERMED, Munich 1995: p. 104. HeNe and GaAlAs laser of 2 mW each successfully used in patients with TMD problems.

USA

Baylor College of Medicine, Texas Children's Hospital, Department of Pathology.

Hicks M J et al. Root caries *in vitro* after low fluence argon laser and fluoride treatment. Compend Contin Educ Dent. 1997; 18 (6): 543-8. This *in vitro* study evaluates the influence of combining low fluence argon laser treatment and acidulated phosphate fluoride treatment on caries initiation and progression in human root surfaces. The combination of low energy laser treatment and fluoride treatment increased the caries resistance of root surfaces when compared with no treatment and with laser irradiation treatment alone.

University of Illinois, School of Dentistry, Department of Material Science

Braverman B, Bapna M S et al. Effect of HeNe and infrared laser irradiation on wound healing in rabbits. Lasers in Surgery and Medicine 1989; 9: 50. HeNe and GaAs laser improved the tensile strength of wounds.

University of California, School of Dentistry, San Francisco

Pogrel A et al. Effect of low-energy Gallium-Aluminium-Arsenide laser irradiation on cultured fibroblasts and keratinocytes. Lasers in Surgery and Medicine. 1997; 20: 426-432. 830 nm 5-100 mW laser at doses of 0.12-4.24 J/cm^2 did not show any effect on cell proliferation, adhesion or migration.

Center for Dental AIDS Research, Waukegan, Ill.

Neiburger E J. The effect of low-power laser on intraoral wound healing. N Y State Dent J. 1995; 61 (3): 40-43. 670 nm laser treatment was as effective as 633 nm in significantly speeding the rate of healing in rats. A controlled clinical case of HeNe treatment of human aphthous stomatitis lesion is reported.

Neiburger E J. Rapid healing of gingival incisions by the helium-neon diode laser. J Massach Dental Soc. 1999; 48 (1): 8-13. It is unclear if it is a HeNe laser or an GaAlInP laser, but it had god effect.

Chapter 7
Veterinary use

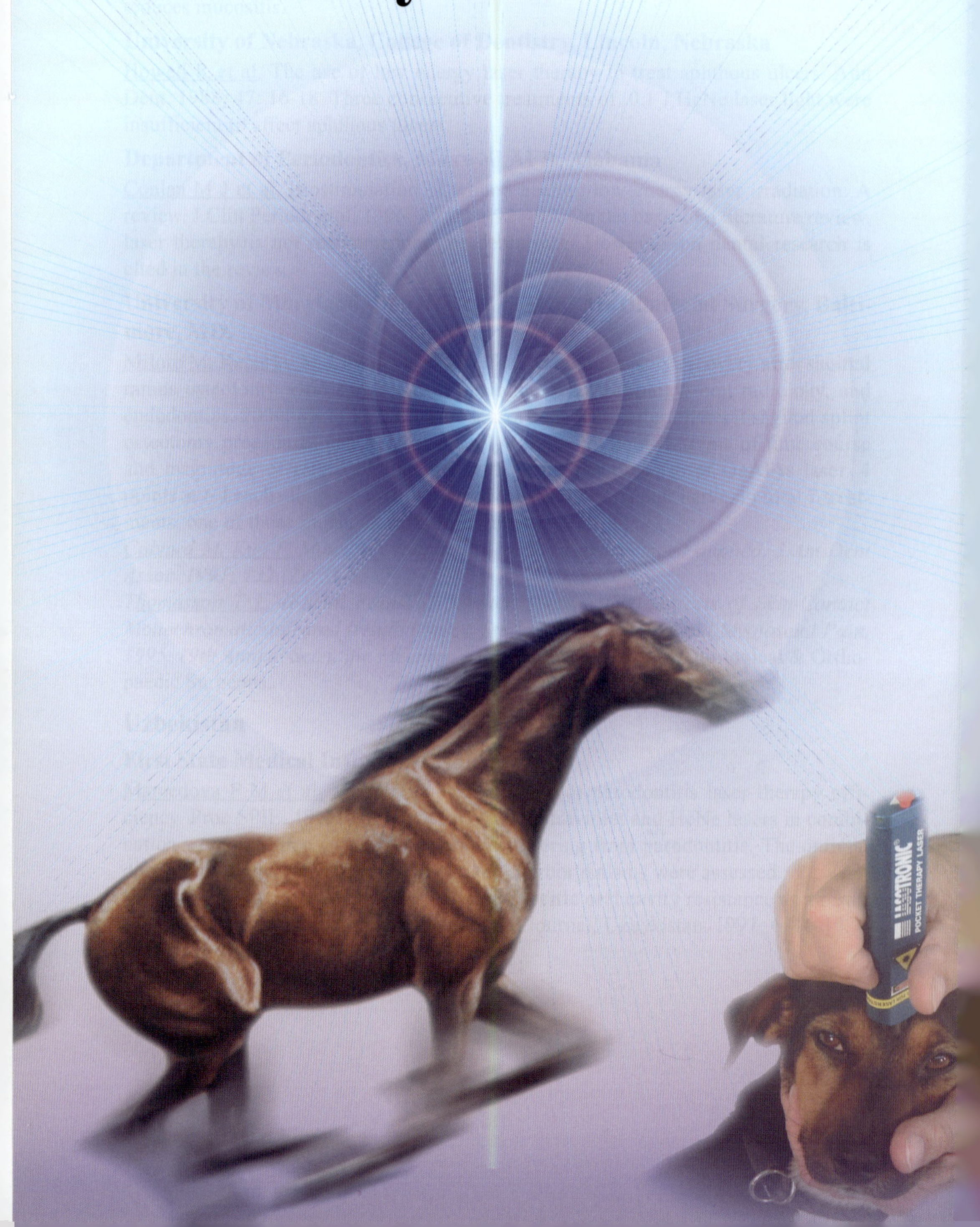

Veterinary medicine is another field in which the laser enthusiast can find further uses for his or her laser. All the common laser types are effective, and GaAs is particularly good for deep-lying tissue.

The scientific documentation in the field of veterinary medicine is extensive, with over one thousand published studies on animals. In most cases, effects have been observed. Most of these studies have involved animals for whom a veterinarian would not ordinarily be called in the event of problems - rats, mice, rabbits, guinea pigs, etc. However, at the present time much documentation is also available on dogs and horses.

Fortune hunters and unscrupulous sales representatives managed to give the laser treatment of trotting horses a bad reputation during the 1980s. In the veterinary field, as in so many others, the reaction was to throw the baby out with the bath water. It is not the laser that is at fault, but often the deficient knowledge of the user and the poor quality of the equipment. A sound knowledge of equine medicine is necessary to achieve good results, in the same way as in human medicine.

Horses are more sensitive to laser light than humans. High local power density - and especially super pulsed lasers - brings about a reaction (including sometimes a pain reaction) when the light enters the vicinity of an injury or problem area. This is particularly true of GaAs lasers and at high pulse or pulse-train frequencies. If the horse reacts strongly, it is suitable to start with a low pulse frequency before going to the higher levels. This reaction in horses can also be used to locate a problem. In trotting and sport in general, the practitioners of laser therapy with the right training and the right equipment are enthusiastic about the results. The economic incentives are obvious. Dogs, cats and other household pets can also be treated with lasers with good results.

In recent years (1996-1999), Lindholm [562] has treated more than 500 horses with a defocused CO_2-laser. The results have been 80% positive in treatment of vertebral joint problems, but the treatment is significantly less effective for tendinitis. The clinical outcome of defocused CO_2-laser therapy for acute traumatic arthritis reveals at least an equal therapeutic effect compared with conventional therapy.

A common problem, and one that is even more pronounced in the treatment of race-horses because of the amounts of money involved, is, as we have discussed elsewhere, that laser treatment can radically alleviate pain after just one or two applications. In a couple of cases, when people without medical expertise have observed that the horse's limp has disappeared and

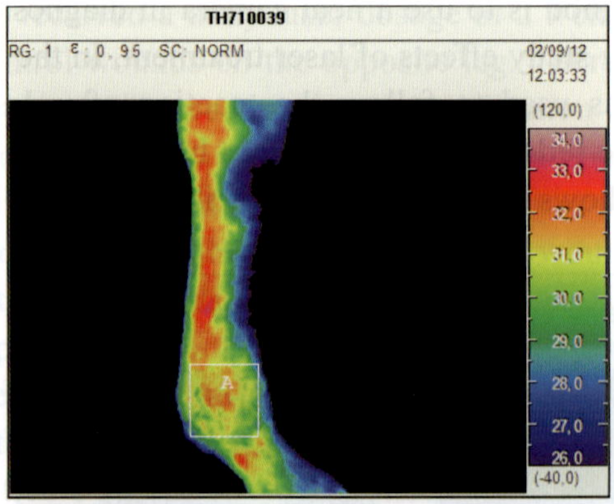

It is amazing how quickly the inflamed tissue reacts. The fur is not cut or shaved off, hence the temperature difference is even higher on the skin under the fur.

Laser parameters: The average output power of the laser probe is measured to 62 mW (four GaAs-laser diodes, each with 13 watt peak power, 150 ns pulse duration, pulsetrain modulated with basic frequency 16 kHz, 50% duty cycle and envelop frequency 2500 Hz). The instrument was made by Irradia AB Sweden, www.irradia.se

Treatment parameters: Treatment was done over the whole inflamed area. That area was about 5 × 40 cm (200 cm^2). Treatment time was 4 minutes. This gives a treatment dose of about 0.075 J/cm^2, which is rather normal for the GaAs-laser type.

The heat photography is done by Lindströms Digital Infrared Thermal Imaging, (L DI T I), Haninge, Sweden (www.lditi.com).

For more information see "Thermography" on page 105.

Chapter 8
Contraindications

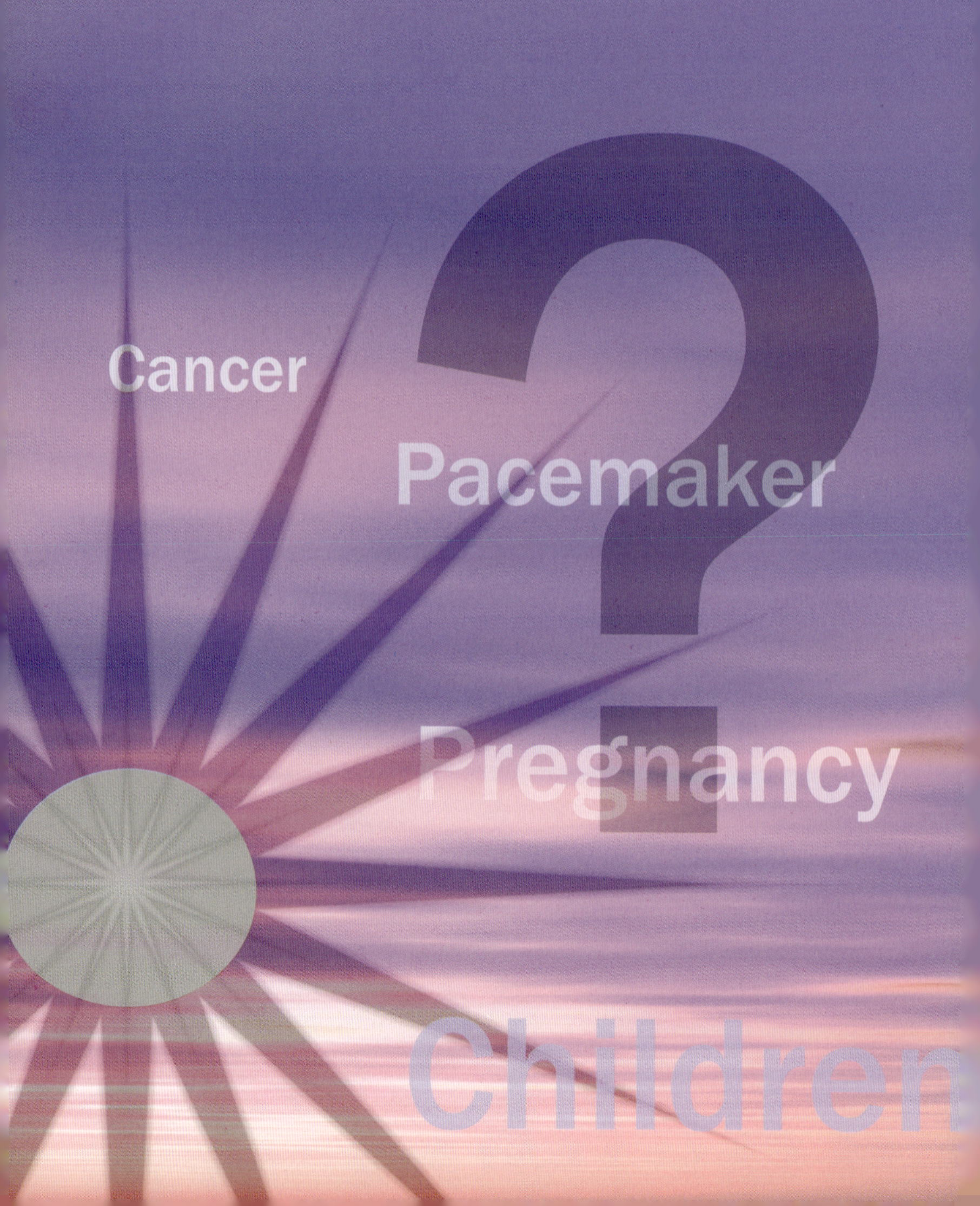

Older literature on lasers often repeats certain alleged contraindications related to laser treatment. We have analysed some of these.

8.1 Pacemaker

As pacemakers are electronic and cased in metal they cannot be influenced by light, and this is therefore a misconception. Try influencing your CD player with a laser!

8.2 Pregnancy

Pregnancy is another alleged contraindication. In this case, normal medical judgement with respect to the effect on the foetus should prevail. Large doses over the abdomen should perhaps be avoided, but the foetus will certainly not be any the worse off for its mother being rid of a sensitive tooth neck or a herpes sore. Avila [194] has demonstrated cell damage in chicken embryos after irradiation with a HeNe laser through an opening in the egg. We should bear in mind that the small chicken embryo received 5 mW of laser light for five minutes from a short distance through more or less transparent tissue. To give a human embryo the same dose per kilo of body weight via the mother's skin, weeks of treatment would be needed! The problem with both pacemakers and pregnancy is that they have long been presented as contraindications. If a complication unrelated to the use of a laser arises during or shortly after laser treatment, it is easy to blame the laser and the therapist is left with the burden of proof. It pays, therefore, to be prudent.

8.3 Epilepsy

Epilepsy is another alleged contraindication. Because pulsed visible light, particularly at pulse frequencies in the 5-10 Hz range, can cause epileptic attacks, one should obviously be careful with instruments that use flashing visible light. It is rare, however, for low-level lasers to have pulsing visible light. Nothing is said in the literature on the subject of invisible pulsing light affecting epileptics, but some anecdotal accounts would suggest that it is best to be careful with GaAs when treating such patients. Simunovic [444] reports on GaAs treatment of an epileptic person who could only tolerate frequencies below 800 Hz.

8.4 Thyroid gland

The thyroid gland is a sensitive gland and it may be wise to avoid administering large doses of laser light over it. Studies on rats [159] indicate that the subject can suffer from disorders if treated with large doses. Hernandéz [285] has shown that GaAs induces a decrease in the mRNA of thyroglobulin, changes in the cytoskeleton of thyroidal cells, and a reduction in thyroidal

Chapter 9
Laser therapy on the Internet

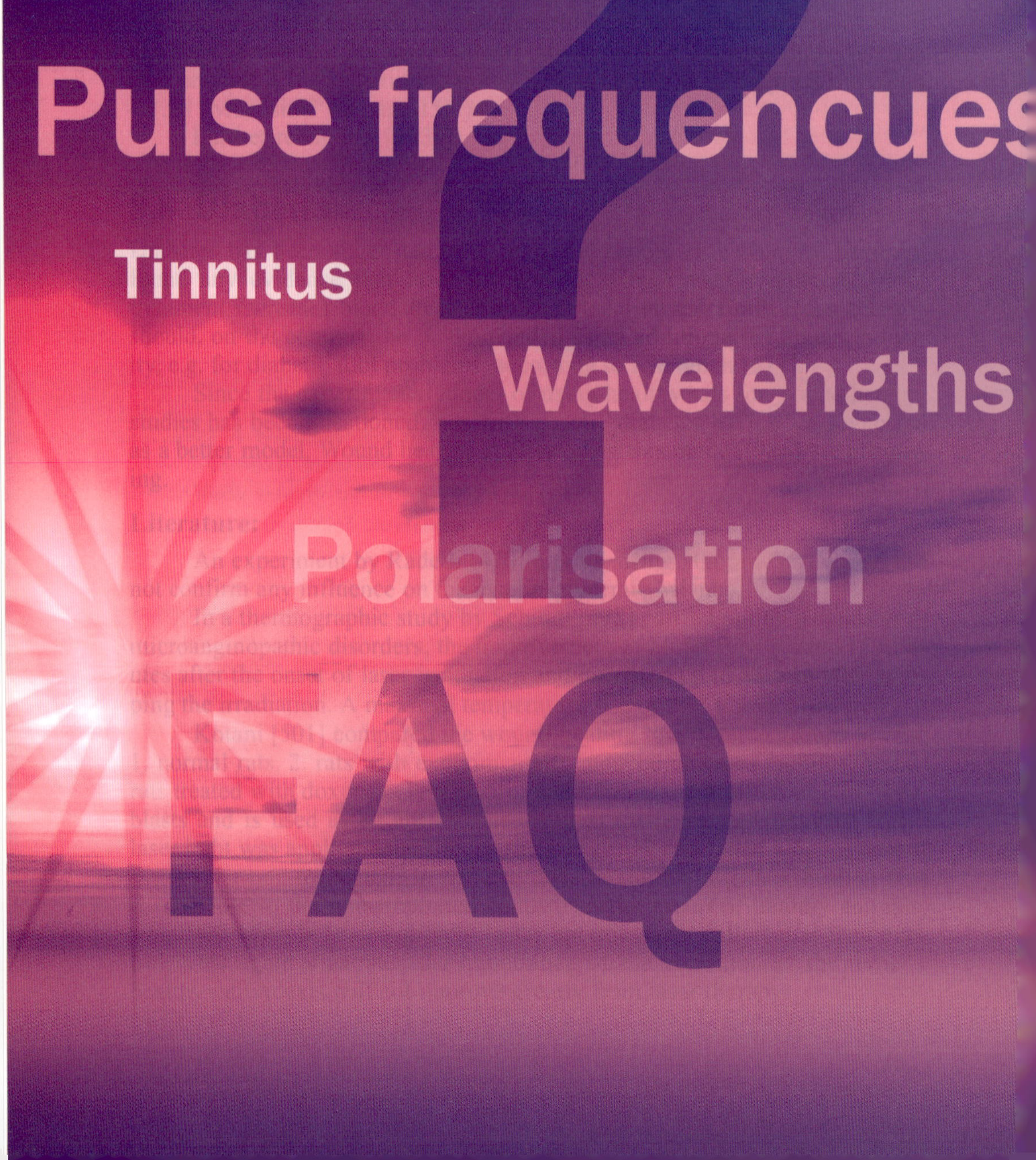

9.1 Laser therapy on the Internet

LaserWorld, the home of the Swedish Laser Medical Society offers abstracts of the literature, questions and answers about laser therapy, guest editorials, links to congresses, associations, manufacturers, publishers and much more. The URL is www.laser.nu or www.laserworld.org.
International Medical Laser Information Center, IMLIC is a joint effort of the majority of the medical laser associations of the world. The URL is http://homepage1.nifty.com/jmlic

9.2 Internet discussion groups

The Internet is a rich source of information about laser therapy. Joining one of the discussion groups can be of great help. The members of these groups are therapists, doctors, dentists, manufacturers, physiotherapists, researchers, administrators etc. and everyone has a chance of extending his own knowledge. The following offers some examples of discussions held during 2002 and where the authors of this book were active.

9.2.1 Tinnitus

Can anyone comment on results of laser therapy for tinnitus? Who makes a unit for tinnitus? And does anyone in the US use one?

WS

I use a scanner (480/20 mW GaAlAs/HeNe) for tinnitus, vertigo and hearing loss in conjunction with chiropractic, allergy testing and nutritional support. As always: Sometimes the results are phenomenal, sometimes they are poor.

Dr. Z

Dear David, We have done a double-blind placebo controlled trial with 830nm 150mw GaAlAs diode laser on unselected tinnitus patients in a Private ENT practice. There was no statistical significant difference between the treated or untreated groups. There were, however, a few remarkable results - as most people will find if they utilise LLLT for tinnitus. One theory holds that cases with active Meniere's disease are more likely to benefit - this would fit in nicely with the anti-inflammatory effects of laser therapy. I am not aware at this stage of a study looking at this specific subset of patients. I am therefore not using it as routine therapy for the general tinnitus patient.

Neels

9.2.2 Wavelength

With regards to the red light (630 nm - 680 nm), I have a couple of observations. No matter the power or the frequency used those wavelengths seem to be much less irritating, I can use a 200 mW, 660 nm probe with less problem than a 10 mW, 904 nm. With an active inflammation, wound, trauma, or

cost? What about like-for-like treatment times? What about not like-for-like but rather the best LED parameters vs the best laser parameters?
Ars longa, vita brevis, as they used to say.
James

Regarding LED, I can add that there is yet another good study on LED: Neuman I, Finklestein Y, Lubart R: Low energy phototherapy in allergic rhinitis and nasal polyposis. Laser Therapy. 1996. 1: 37 (abstract). It has later been published in full.

These three studies clearly show the benefit of LEDs, if within the therapeutic window with dosage and wavelength. But they are all on superficial structures. For deeper structures the laser is probably needed. However, we know that irradiation reaching only the skin (like defocused CO_2 laser therapy) can have an effect on deeper structures. So there must be messenger metabolites involved. This means that LEDs might influence deep structures even though the actual light does not, in sufficient quantities. Lasers, on the other hand, can reach superficial and deep targets at the same time.

Future research will show what would happen if we apply paragraph 3 below (What about not like-for-like but rather the best LED parameters vs. the best laser parameters?). That would really be interesting.

I don't mind discussing LEDs on this list. This topic needs discussion since they are widely in use and still lacking good scientific support. So did lasers 10 years ago. So the main thing is that the discussion is based on facts, not on loud marketing.

Many years ago I visited The Voice of Free China in Taipei and talked to "The Dragon Man", a producer on the international service. He needed listeners' letters to keep his bosses happy, so when the letters were few, he intentionally said something stupid on the air. And the letters poured in. This discussion list really came to life.
Jan

It does not matter if it is a laser or and LED unit. Once it enters the skin it is scattered and is no longer a coherent collimated beam. The big advantage of the LED's is that the angle of the beam is already between 20-40 degrees so it covers a much larger area. With an LED cluster you can cover a much larger area in a shorter time and a LED unit has the ability to use several wavelengths in a single probe, which the laser cannot duplicate. Of course you could buy several lasers with different wavelengths but then you are still limited to the number of wavelengths available. I know the manufacturers would much rather sell the lasers because they make a lot more money and the cost to manufacture is not much more than the LED units.
LED instrument producer.

The Producer's contributions are NOT valuable, misleading and in violation of the marketing claims the company is allowed to make, given their intended use allowed them by the FDA. I suggest they be removed from the list.

JS

There are similar affects of a LED and a LLT. But your conclusion is flawed. We do not know "scientifically" how either work. We know Light is a particle, we know Light is a wave. Therefore you conclude that 1: particle = wave, and 2: more is better. I am interested in not only HOW it works but WHY.

Ed

Well, for the information of more serious persons on this list, here are a few comments:

- In all (about 20) studies comparing lasers and LED, laser has come out on top. LED often effective, but less, but sometimes not at all and sometimes negative effect.
- The argument that cluster LED probes can have many wavelengths is devious. Every pill (wavelength) must have a meaning and interactions must be considered. Same thing goes with wavelengths.
- I doubt that laser manufacturers earn more money than LED manufacturers, but certainly LED's are cheaper. But what matters is not price but efficiency.
- Laser clusters are available as well but are only advantageous when treating large areas. Therapy must often be pinpointed. Laser therapy is not a hit-and-run story.
- I am not against the use of LED, it is a useful therapy if used in selected indications. But I am against those trying to fool people into believing that lasers and LED's are the same and using the laser scientific studies as references, trying to imply that what goes with lasers goes with LED's. Much more could be written about this, but why speak to the deaf?

Jan

Thank you Jan. I was also bothered by that post from the Producer company. That piece of equipment is an LED device and no power or wavelength parameters were given making it less than useful!

The main problem with laser therapy for tinnitus is the diagnosis. Since many cases of tinnitus are related to muscular tensions, irradiation directed into the cochlea only will not be helpful in these particular cases. The temporomandibular joint will benefit somewhat, but it is necessary to irradiate all muscles involved, quite often in the neck and in the lateral pterygoid. These cases generally require TMD therapy, sometimes physical therapy and often relaxation programmes. Without a differential diagnosis the outcome of laser therapy will be guesswork.

which has not received FDA permission to market, is the risk something adverse will occur or the claimed benefit will not occur.

What the user cannot do is to publicly adverse the specific device for any claims. Again this becomes the issue of advertising unapproved devices for unapproved uses. What you tell an individual patient is between you and them, what you say publicly either in print or by Internet can become a FDA issue.

Richard

Does this mean that a physician cannot mention their thoughts/ results on what it can to for their patients?

David

Any claim other than as a heat source would be considered advertising of unapproved uses. It appears that a number of companies are doing this. This is a difficult issue for the Agency since we can only take an action, usually a Warning Letter telling company to cease such advertising when we have a specific complaint or we ourselves become aware of this. Continually monitoring such advertising is difficult and manpower intense and we do not usually have staff sufficient to do this.

Richard

The way I understand it NO MEDICAL DEVICE can be legally marketed in the USA for use on humans without either a PMA or a 510(k) unless it is a preamendment device (one marketed in the U.S. before May 28, 1976) since preamendments products were exempted (grandfathered). I should qualify that by saying class III and most class II devices. Which includes LLLT / LED therapy devices.

James

Since no laser therapy devices have to be approved for marketing in the US no claims can be made since these device would be considered unapproved devices and therefore cannot be legally marketed. The only way a laser therapy device can be marketed in the US is as an investigational device being used in an Institutional Review Board (IRB) approved clinical study.

Richard

Ah, but where do we stand on the sale and use of LED devices. Diomedics make an LED device, which they claim has FDA approval (under the old 510(k) for Infra-red heating lamps) and I'll bet you they are interpreting the term LLLT as Low Level Light Therapy. So how do their claims stand in view of the above? They are openly selling it and making all kinds of claims.

Melyni

This clearance was not granted for a Low Level Laser Therapy device, the clearance was based on the fact the device created heat at a level and duration that would make the device equivalent to heat lamps, which have this indication. There are no Low Level Laser Therapy devices approved/cleared for marketing that use non-thermal biostimulation mechanisms for their claimed benefit. The decision to find the Light Force Therapy device equivalent was based on comparison to Infrared Lamps which would mean evidence was provided that the system generate heat to result in a specific increase in skin temperature. This clearance was not based on any claim of photostimulation.

Richard

The first company to receive a 510(k) from the Federal Drug Administration (FDA) was Majes-Tec Innovations in the USA and its Erchonia laser. The company is to be congratulated for this approval, which has taken many years and dollars to obtain. The Laser Therapy community in general is also to be congratulated, the approval being a first small step on the road to an opening of the huge US market for laser therapy. Such an opening is important not only because it will allow laser companies to make money (and improve their products) but because it might spur new research and improve the scientific documentation. There are a number of concerns to be discussed regarding this 510(k) and the consequences of the very same.

A) The machine. As far as can be gathered from brochures, the Erchonia laser is a 635 nm diode laser with a maximum output of 10 mW. The retail price is above US$ 10.000. Through an optical lens the energy over the fibre eye opening is 1 mW (/cm^2 ?). The approval is for "adjunctive use in providing temporary relief of minor chronic neck and shoulder pain of musculoskeletal origin".

B) The history of laser therapy. Mester in Hungary in the late 60ies, using ruby and HeNe lasers on non-healing wounds, performed the first human studies. Powers were 5-25 mW (no more was available in those days) and the doses 0.5-1.5 J/cm^2. When these observations finally reached the West, something odd happened. Although more powerful laser devices were now available, "soft lasers" of 0.1-2.5 mW were produced and sold. One of the most well known lasers was the Dynatronic 1120, having 0.9 mW from HeNe tube and less than 0.3 from fibre. Some researchers (Walker et al, Snyder-Mackler et al) published positive and very interesting reports on the use of such lasers. Few, if any, control studies could confirm these results. And the sad thing is that most of the research done in the 80ies was then down in the same dosage marshland, using dosages around 0.001-0.01 J/cm^2. No wonder the outcome was negative in most instances! The original doses applied by Mester's group seem to have been completely forgotten or ignored. Now it seems we are back where we started, using red light of extremely low intensity. So it is interesting to have a look at the laser that the FDA has approved.

level laser and other photonic therapies. To this end, I respectfully offer the following information, comments and questions. The following paragraphs come from the Erchonia "Operation and Maintenance Manual":

The Erchonia PL3000 laser device is a single diode, 635 nanometer, variable hertz device. The variable hertz feature offers the end user the option of selecting a "constant" or "pulse" wave.
The Erchonia laser emits a 635 nanometer wavelength with a tolerance of +/- 5 nanometer. The internal battery initiates a specially created and patented electric diode that emits a 1-milliWatt red laser beam.

Laser devices are typically constructed to emit a "spot" of light. The Erchonia laser utilizes internal mechanics that collects the light emitted from the electric diode and processes it through a proprietary patented lens, then redirects the beam with a line refractor. This process produces a line 3 mm wide with a length of approx. 104 mm at 4" away, and approx. 152 mm at 6" away. These measurements result in 0.0002 joules per minute / cm^2 (4 minutes) and 0.0001 joules per minute / cm^2 (6 minutes).

Professional Use Instructions

The Erchonia laser device is to be administered externally for the treatment of minor neck and shoulder pain, using the following protocol:
1. One minute of pulsed laser applied to the sagittal suture (top of the head). NOTE: probe is to be held 4" to 6" inches away from the target area for this and all remaining steps of the protocol.
2. Two minutes of pulsed laser applied to the left cervical, shoulder and torso area. Apply laser starting in the cerebral region, at the top of the ear, lasering left cervical anterior and posterior muscles, working the laser down into the left shoulder and torso anterior and posterior muscles.
3. Repeat step 2 to right cervical shoulder and torso area.
4. One minute of pulsed laser applied to right shoulder during passive external rotation of the shoulder. Laser the anterior muscles of the right shoulder (pectoralis group) with the patient's arm bent at the elbow.
5. One minute of pulsed laser applied to the right shoulder during passive adduction of patients right arm and shoulder. Laser the posterior muscles of the right shoulder.
6. One minute of pulsed laser applied to the right cervical muscle and trapezius muscle during passive left lateral flexion of the cervical spine. Starting in the neutral position of the head, the doctor applies laser to the right cervical muscles and right trapezius muscles.
7. One minute of pulsed laser to the right sternocleidomastoid and scalene muscles during passive range of motion. The doctor lasers the right sternocleidomastoid and scalenus muscles.
8. Repeat step 4 to the left shoulder.
9. Repeat step 5 to the left shoulder.
10. Repeat step 6 to the left cervical spine.
11. Repeat step 7 to the right cervical spine.

The Erchonia PL2000 was used in a multi-site, double blind clinical study, where the effectiveness of the use of the device was measured in a group of 43 subjects who received the treatment against a group of 43 subjects who received a placebo (fake treatment). Analysis of the primary outcome measure from the study using a one-tailed z-test found that the difference in the proportion of individual successes for subjects in the test group who had received the actual laser treatment and the proportion of individual successes for subjects in the placebo group who received the "fake" treatment was statistically significant.

NOTE: I could not find information on definition of treatment success, statistical results, or treatment parameters.

The FDA also addressed your questions on dosage levels during the Erchonia application evaluation. Dr. Tracey Bourke from the US FDA asked TUCO for a clarification of their fluence values. The question:

"Please clarify the fluence values given. Values of 0.0002 joules and 0.0001 joules as described under the PL3000 section do not make sense as presented. Also take into account that different distances result in different fluence if the same treatment time is used."

TUCO's answer:

"In order to clarify the fluence values given on page 2 of the Operator's Manual, it is necessary to know that these values, as they exist, were added to address a previous concern of the FDA relating "spot" dimension and joule value. These calculated results represent a sampling of the line in a squared centimeter, based on distance from the body, in order to inform the FDA of the joule value of a "spot." If the intent of the questions is to determine the total joules per treatment then the answer would be 0.6 joules per minute over the total area of the beam."

I share the same concern when you state in item C of your message that "...but since the FDA was satisfied, we can safely believe that everything is OK when it comes to the design and scientific quality. Yet, there are problems."

Let's remember that the FDA CDRH must follow certain rules and procedures in the evaluation of 510(k) applications. Just because an application obtained a 510(k) notification does not necessarily mean that the device is OK from the clinical perspective. A 510(k) notification for pre market approval means that the applicant has met the FDA requirements of safety and effectiveness to obtain the right to distribute a medical device in the US. It does not say that a 510(k) device is "approved" for medical or therapeutic use. It is a fine line that we need to be aware of as we spread the word about LLLT in a fair and constructive manner. So, item D in your message is right on the heart of the issue: "Good or just a bit effective."

It is illustrative to see the results of the MicroLight 830 study as submitted to the FDA. In a document prepared by MicroLight dated January 20, 2002:

"In 1998 the MicroLight Corporation embarked on a double blind study for the use of low level lasers in the treatment of Carpal Tunnel Syndrome. The study protocol targeted approximately 135 patients diagnosed with carpal tunnel syndrome with moderate to severe symptoms, with a mean Symptom Severity score of at least 2.0, with a score of at least 30 on a 100 point VAS pain scale, who have failed conservative therapy for at least one month and who have not had previous carpal tunnel release surgery. One half of the subjects received treatment with the active laser and one half received treatment with a placebo laser.

Patients were treated three times a week for five weeks. Follow up times were 1, 6, and 12 weeks after the last treatment, at which time information was recorded on each patient. Treatment was considered successful if a patient showed a 30% or more reduction in VAS pain score at the 12 week follow-up point. By this definition, the MicroLight laser successfully treated 55.8% of the patients in the active group, compared to 40.0% success for patients in the placebo group. No adverse effects from the MicroLight 830 treatment were noted."

It would have been useful to know the significance level of the t-test, or the sample standard deviations. So, was the MicroLight result good or just a bit effective? We know that it had to be effective enough in its narrow definition to get the 510(k) notification. Does the FDA 510(k) notification mean that the MicroLight 830 is an effective medical device?

I am currently conducting randomized clinical trials with IR low level laser devices for 2 clients. It is possible to extend the studies at no cost to compare other devices including the Erchonia and/or MicroLight. Any suggestions?

In summary, I strongly believe that we, as practitioners and researchers, must address the question of appropriate dosage that you raised in your message in item 4.

Nelson.

9.2.9 Miscellaneous

In the book by Tunér and Hode, I have seen the name HeLa cells. What are they?

Eva

Hi Eva, I made some research and found out that HeLa cells stands for **Hen**rietta **La**cks. She died, 31 year of age 1951. Before she died, a sample of cervical cancer cells was taken from her cervix. The sample of the HeLa cell culture survived and multiplied so well in culture, that they were soon being shipped to research labs around the world for study. Although Henrietta Lack is dead, her cells live on in research labs around the world! In fact, some biologists believe that HeLa cells are no longer human at all and consider them to simply be unique and should rather be celled microorganisms!

Lars

I recently heard that the placebo effect now can be measured. Then I don't mean statistically from tests with active and placebo group, but physically in the brain. But how about positive and negative placebo, can that be verified too?

Alex

Interesting question. I made some research and found that this was shown in an experiment performed in the institution of neurology at the Karolinska Institute in Stockholm during 2001. In that experiment, all the test persons were subjected to painful heat. Some of the test persons was given pain relive in the form of opioides before they were subject to the painful heat and other test persons did only receive placebo pills and at further occasions they got no medicine at all.

The patients' brain activity pattern was investigated by means of positron emission-tomography (PET). Comparison between the patients brain activities showed that the anterior cortex of cingulum was active in connection with pain relief. Surprisingly it was also active for the persons who thought that they got pain relief, but not for the persons who neither got, nor thought that they got a pain-relieving drug. The investigators, Predrag Petrovic and Martin Ingvar, also found that the activity in the anterior cortex of cingulum was coupled to activities in deeper areas of the brain, especially in pons. I don't know if there is a difference between negative and positive placebo.

Lars

Chapter 10
The difficult dose and intensity

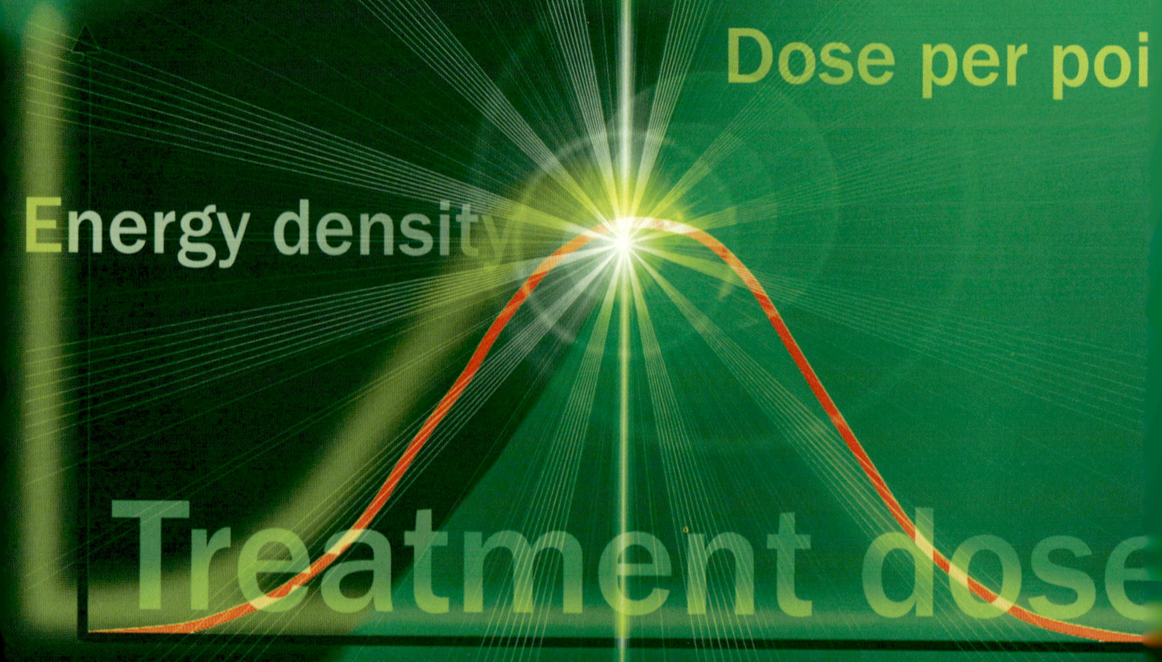

We have previously pointed out that this book is not intended to be a tutorial in physics. However, we want to clarify some definitions in order to better understand the problems of dose and power density.

10.1 Basics about energy

For many people, the word energy means something else than it does for a physicist. A healer may say that he transfers "energy" to the patient. But that "energy" cannot be measured in the scientific sense. In this book, we will stick strictly to the form of energy that can be measured in joules (J). One of our most fundamental laws, valid in the entire universe, is the so called "principle of energy". This law says:

Energy can never be created and never be destroyed.

Energy can occur in many forms. It was traditionally synonymous with "work". Climbing up a hill takes a lot of work/energy. If my body weights 75 kg and I transport it from one level and up to a level 10 meters higher, I have performed an amount of work and increased my **potential energy** by

75 kg × 10 m × 9.81 m/s² = **73,600 joules** = potential energy

Where 9.81 m/s² is the earths gravity constant
In this case I convert **chemical energy** in my body into potential energy. If I fall down from this height, I will convert that potential energy into kinetic energy.
If I travel with the speed of 10 m/s (36 km/hour) and my weight is 75 kg, then I have a **kinetic energy** of

0.5 × 75 kg × (10 m/s)² = **37,500 joules** = kinetic energy

If I heat water with my electric heater and use 220 volts and 5 amperes for 100 seconds, then I have consumed **electrical energy** from the electric mains supply.

220 volt × 5 amp × 100 sec = 110,000 Ws = **110,000 joules** = electric energy

In this heater, this amount of energy is converted into the same amount of **thermal energy** which we can feel in the form of heat in the water.

A **laser** (or other radiation source) emits **radiation energy** in the form of a flow of photons, each with a well-defined energy. If its output power is 250 mW (= 0.25 W) and it is kept radiating for 2 minutes (= 120 sec), its emitted energy will be

0.2 W × 120 sec = 24 Ws = **24 joules** = radiation energy

Another example of energy conversion is when potential energy of the water in a water dam is first converted into the kinetic energy of moving water in a waterfall, which in turn is converted into electrical energy by means of a turbine connected to an electric generator. Even matter itself is a form of energy - **material energy** - following the famous equation

$$E = mc^2$$

formulated by Albert Einstein. In a nuclear reactor, matter is converted to thermal energy.

10.2 Output power

When you work with a laser, there are two fundamental things you need to know:

- Your laser type and its wavelength
- Its output power (for pulsed lasers - average and peak power)

If you don't know the output power of your laser, then you have no idea about the doses you administer - maybe you are just giving "homeopathic" doses or maybe you are giving too large doses.

Power is measured in watts, which is the same as joules per second, which is an energy flow. A strong laser has a high output power and a weak laser has a low output power. Power is in some way synonymous with "strength". However, power is not the same as intensity (see power density in next paragraph).

We have pointed out earlier that it is important to find out the real output of your instrument, which often is not what your brochure or manual claims. Output can decrease by ageing or by dirt in the aperture. The laser diode may even be broken (especially if it is infrared and invisible). The best precaution is to have a power meter, either built into the instrument or as a separate device.

10.3 Power density

Power density is briefly described in chapter 1.2.13 “Power density” on page 17 and in chapter 3.3.1.4 “Power density” on page 69. It is more or less the same as the "intensity" of the light and is measured in watts per cm^2 or milliwatts per cm^2 (in some literature watts per m^2). Intuitively we understand that if we spread out the light over a large area we will get a lower light intensity than if we concentrate it to a smaller surface. The power density (I) can be calculated as

$$I = \frac{A}{P} \qquad [\ W/cm^2\ ]$$

From this equation we can see that with constant output power from the laser (P), the power density (I) is inversely proportional to the surface (A) that it illuminates. In a practical situation, the power density is not constant over the illuminated surface - it has a two-dimensional distribution over the surface (even when a treatment probe is held in contact with the skin) and has a three-dimensional distribution inside the treated tissue.

In the picture below, we illustrate how the power density varies with the distance from the source in a divergent beam of a diode laser.

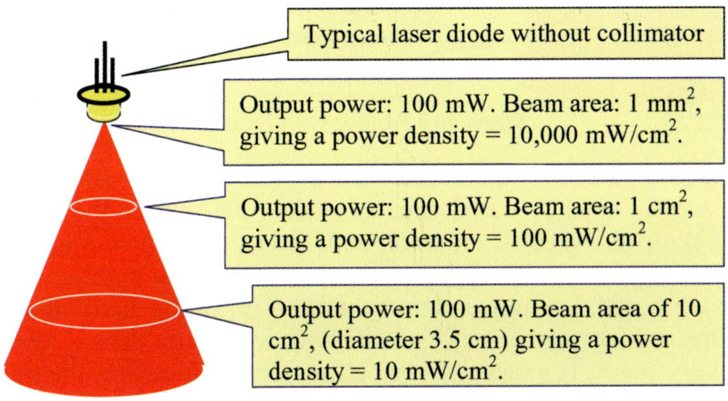

Figure 10.1 Typical diode collimator

Before leaving this subject, we illustrate the situation when a beam is focused - at the focal point we have an extremely high power density.

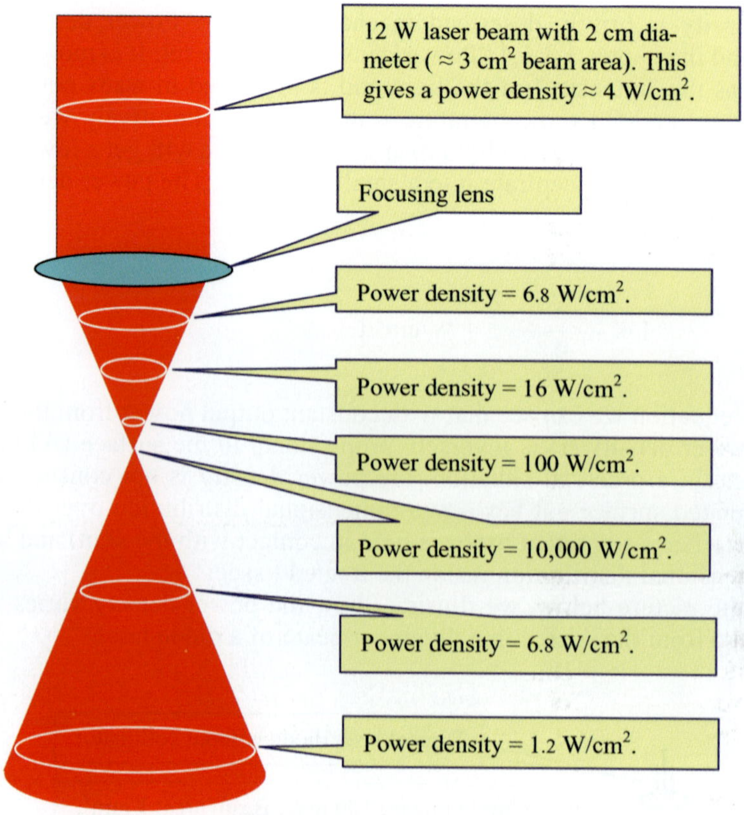

Figure 10.2 Laser with focusing lens

We have already mentioned that there are probes with focused light. When a surgical laser is used to cut tissue, this takes place near the focus point. Again: Looking at a specific situation with laser light penetrating into tissue, we will get scattering of the light, points and areas with high power density and other areas with low power density will occur. If this distribution of light is held constant for one second, we will have an energy density distribution that, in every point, is exactly the same number of joules as the number of watts in power distribution. If we keep the same situation going for ten seconds, we have an energy density (i.e. dose) that is ten times higher in every point reached by the light.

Like the power density, the energy density is not constant - it has a two-dimensional distribution over a surface (this is also true for the area hit by the laser light when a treatment probe is held in skin contact) and has a three-dimensional distribution in the treated tissue volume. (See chapter 3.4 "Other considerations" on page 92.)

10.4 The laser beam

The opening or glass surface through which the light comes out is called the "aperture". The beam from a laser tube or a laser probe does not usually have the same intensity in all parts of the aperture.

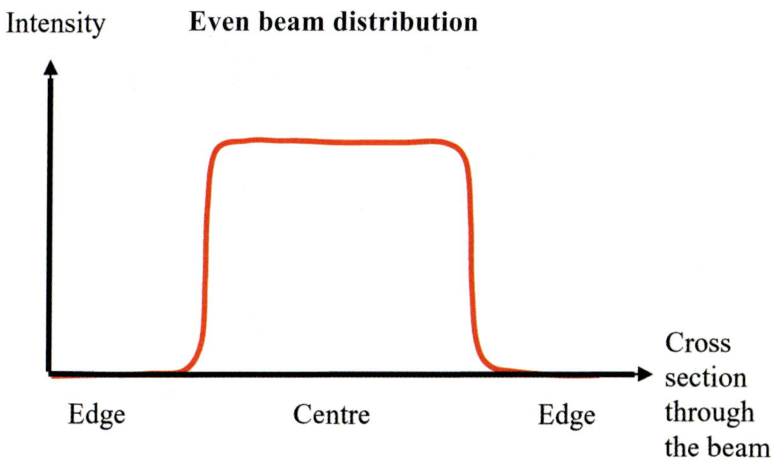

Figure 10.3 Even beam distribution

Usually it is stronger in the middle than at the edges. This often takes the shape of a so called Gaussian distribution (see the figure below).

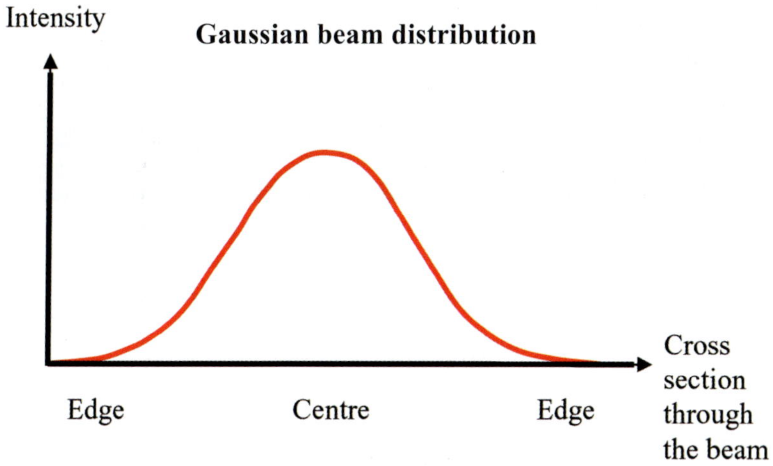

Figure 10.4 Gaussian beam distribution

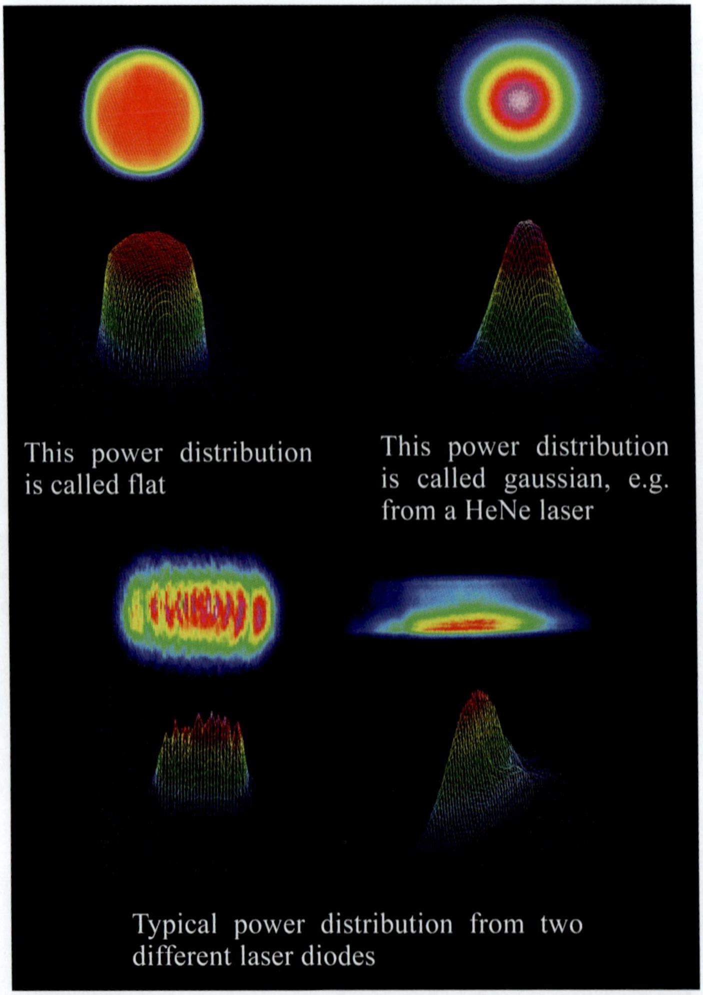

In this figure we show two ways to demonstrate the power distribution in a laser aperture. Top figures in colour coded two dimensional picture and below each figure, the corresponding three dimensional picture.

Figure 10.5 Measured power distribution in typical probe apertures
Courtesy James Caroll

The intensity distribution within the aperture is mainly of interest in scientific work, such as *in vitro* treatment, because in the treatment of tissue the light is strongly scattered. (See Figure 3.8 "Depth of penetration, direct contact" on page 93.) If, however, the beam is spread out over a larger surface (one or several square centimetres), then the intensity distribution is of importance.

10.5 The laser probe

In a practical situation, we have to look at our particular kind of laser probe (handpiece). There are many ways to design a probe:

a. In a gas laser (HeNe, Argon) a fibre is often used. It usually has a small diameter and ends at the top of the probe.
b. For diode lasers, the laser diode is usually situated inside the probe itself. In some probes the laser diode is unprotected and mounted at the very end of the probe in such a way that the glass surface of the diode is in contact with the skin during treatment. When irradiating from a distance, the light is divergent, which is advantageous from the point of view of eye hazards. But when the laser diode glass surface is in direct contact with the skin, we have a very small "light-spot" (typically in the order of one mm^2) which gives a very high power density. Further, the probe can be pressed against the skin, leading to tissue compression, which in turn causes the blood to move away from the beam. This will on the one hand increase the penetration depth and on the other lead to less effective treatment of blood cells than if the probe is not compressing the tissue.
c. In other probes the laser diode is mounted at some distance from the probe-end and there will be a distance (air) between the glass aperture of the laser diode and the skin. Depending on the distance and the angle of divergence of the laser light, the "light-spot" may be small or big with correspondingly high or low power density.
d. In some probes, the light from the laser diode is collimated by means of a collimator (lens system), resulting in a parallel and usually narrow beam. This gives us a choice of two options. In the first case, the glass surface of the collimator is at the extreme probe-end, making contact possible between skin and glass surface (compare point b). Here the cross section of the beam is usually larger than in case b. A typical cross section of such a collimated beam is in the order of 2 x 5 mm = 10 mm^2 = 0.1 cm^2. Remember that a collimated beam can be dangerous to the eyes, especially if it is invisible.
e. In the second case, the glass surface of the aperture can be situated at some distance from the probe-end with no possibility of skin contact. Instead of pressing against the skin with a glass surface, we often get a ring-shaped contact area. A consequence of this can be that some blood is trapped inside the ring, preventing penetration into the tissue. In this case the collimated beam can be dangerous to the eyes of patient and therapist, especially if it is invisible and carelessly aimed.
f. Another option is focusing the light from the laser diode through a lens. This focus can be placed inside the probe at the very end of the probe (possibly equipped with a glass surface) or slightly outside the end of the probe. Between the lens and the focal point the beam is convergent and after the focal point the beam is divergent, which is favourable from the point of view of risk to the eyes. The advantage of a focused beam is also that at or in the neighbourhood of the focal point the power density is high - at the focal

point itself it can be extremely high (See Figure 10.2 “Laser with focusing lens” on page 315.)

g. A laser probe can have more than one source, in which case it is usually called a multiprobe. Multiprobes can have the laser diodes unprotectedly mounted at the end, (See Figure 7.1 “Laser probe for veterinary use.” on page 281.), or mounted inside in a multiprobe. In a multiprobe, the laser diodes are usually spaced over an area.

h. Combination probes where different types of lasers are mixed (e.g. visible and non- visible wavelengths, pulsed with non-pulsed etc). In this case it has not been shown that simultaneous treatment with two or more laser types is advantageous.

i. Combination probes where one or several laser diodes are mixed with LEDs (here we don't mean LEDs which work solely as indicator lights). These require more research before we can safely accept them as useful. (See 11.1.2 “Comparisons between coherent and non-coherent light” on page 335.

10.6 Pulsed lasers

These have been discussed in, chapter 1.2.10 “Continuous and pulsed lasers” on page 16. A matter previously not commented on is the fact that if the laser is pulsed the power density is a function of time and can be divided into two figures: The peak power density (which in itself is not constant over the illuminated surface) and the average power density (with the same spatial distribution).

Specifically looking at the GaAs-laser, the peak power density is extremely high. Assume, for example, that the peak power of a GaAs-laser diode is 10 watts and that the diode is held in skin contact. Then, typically, the light is concentrated over a very small surface, e.g. 1 mm^2. This means that the power density in this small area is in the order of 10 W/mm^2 = 1000 W/cm^2. However, the average power density is of course much lower.

10.7 Energy density

Energy density is also named "dose" or "fluence". The difference between power density and energy density is simply the time. As mentioned above, the power density is measured in watts per cm^2. The energy density is measured in watt-seconds per cm^2, which is the same as joules per cm^2. For calculation of energy density. (See chapter 3.3.1.7 “Calculation of doses” on page 71.)

Looking at a specific situation with laser light penetrating into tissue, we will have points and areas with high power density and other areas with low power density. If this distribution of light is held constant over a certain time, we will have an energy distribution that, at every point, is exactly proportional to the power distribution. If we keep the same situation going for ten times as long, we have an energy density (i.e. dose) that is ten times higher at every point reached by the light.

10.8 Treatment dose

Again, the treatment dose (or the fluence) is the same as the energy density. We will mainly use the term dose. The dose is the most important treatment parameter. Dosage refers to the amount of energy per unit area applied to tissue surface or cell culture surface.

Biostimulatory effects of laser are governed by the arndt-Schulz law of biology, i.e. weak stimuli excite physiological activity, strong stimuli retard it. Many therapists have the feeling that the more energy the better the result. But as can be seen from the diagram below, what was originally a stimulating laser dose may become an inhibitory dose if you continue the irradiation beyond the optimal value. The optimal dose for biostimulation, based on current clinical experience, is 0.5 - 1 J/cm^2 in an open wound and 2 - 4 J/cm^2 when treating through overlaying skin. Dosage should also be adjusted according to individual response.

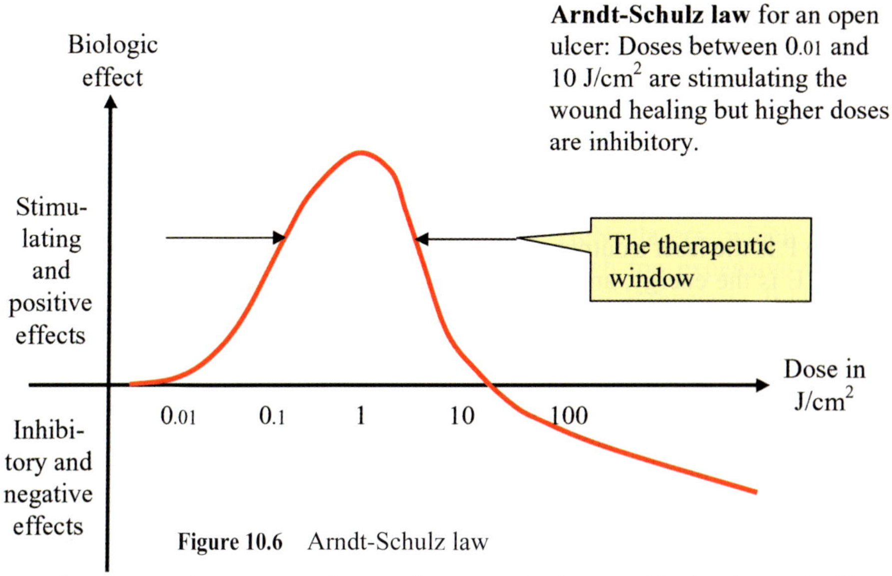

Figure 10.6 Arndt-Schulz law

Dosage and treatment intervals can only be specified schematically. This is because the various laser wavelengths and different treatment conditions mean that different doses must be given. People are receptive to laser treatment to varying degrees - some can "feel the laser right down to their toes", others are entirely impervious. It is appropriate to begin with a low dose for a new patient to ensure that you do not enter a biosuppressive dose range on the first treatment.

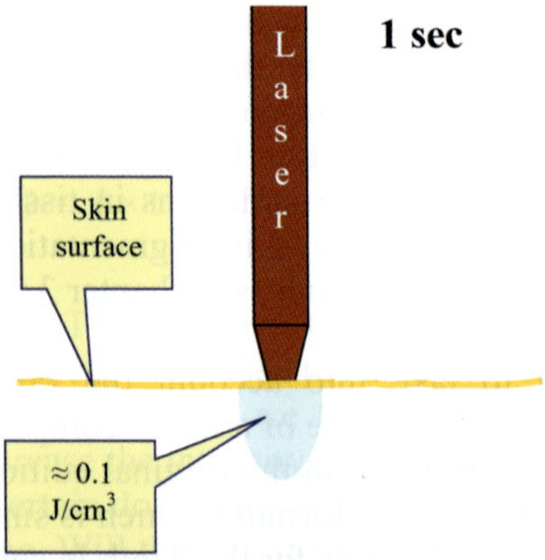

When you hold the laser probe against the skin for **one second** and the laser probe has an output power of 100 mW, 0,1 joule enters into the tissue. The distribution of that energy is usually egg shaped as can be seen in the figure to the left. In the light blue area a bio-stimulative dose within the therapeutic window will occur.

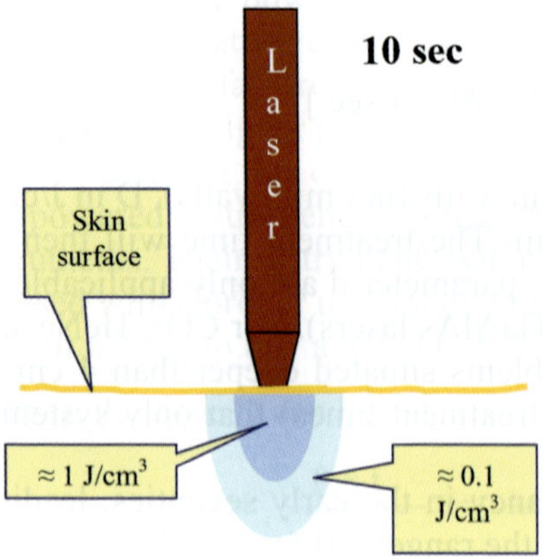

If we keep this set-up unchanged and keep the probe in the same position, with the same output power, for **ten seconds** instead of one second, we have put ten times more energy into the tissue and we will get a larger volume of tissue receiving doses within the therapeutic window. Also note that the dose decays exponentially from the area right beneath the probe and out against the outer regions.

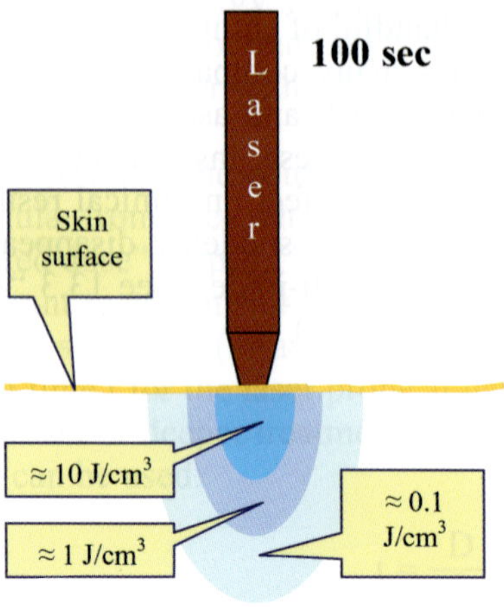

In order to illustrate this further, let us assume that we keep this set-up unchanged and increase the time, holding the probe still and in skin contact for **one hundred** seconds instead of ten seconds. Now we have administered ten times more energy into the tissue, i.e. one hundred times more energy of laser light than in the case shown in the top figure. We will then get an even larger volume of tissue receiving doses within the therapeutic window.

Figure 10.7 Laser on skin

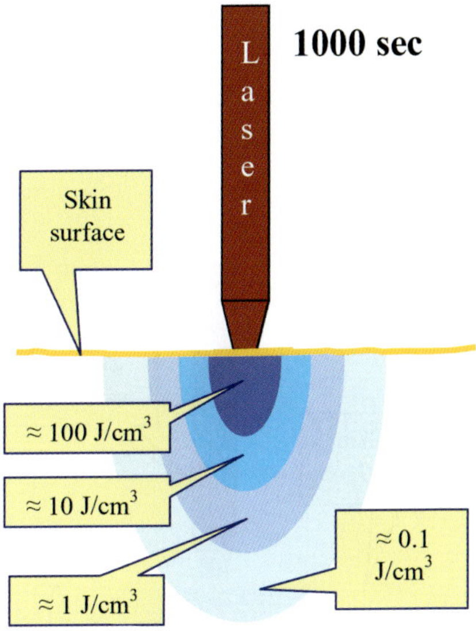

When we previously talked about dose, we always used the unit J/cm^2. But the observant reader has already noticed that in the figures shown here, the dose is expressed in joules per volume, e.g. J/mm^3 or J/cm^3. In reality this is a more correct way of expressing the energy density in a volume and in most cases we do treat volumes. Only in the treatment of cell cultures can the volume be regarded as so small that joules per surface unit may be acceptable. Even when we treat a superficial ulcer we also, in reality, treat a volume rather than a surface.

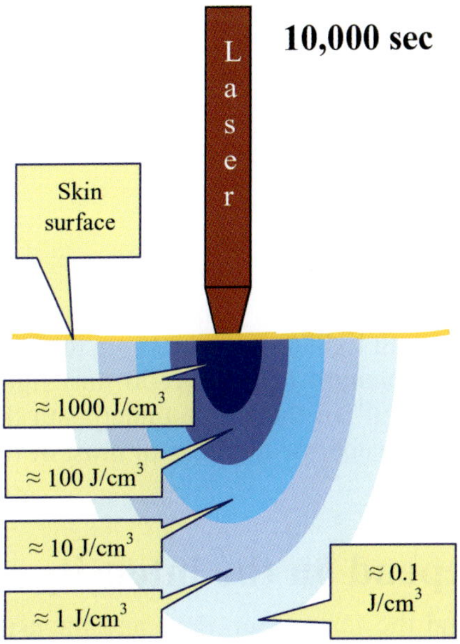

In the figures to the left, the different colours represent different dose levels. The darker the colour the higher the dose (of course there are no such sharp edges in reality - it is a smooth and gradual change). In the volume in the figure to the left, the darkest blue area is shown as receiving about 1000 J/cm^3, but this does not mean that the shown volume is 1 cm^3, nor does it mean that it is the same dose everywhere in the volume; it is an average value.

In the bottom figure the difference in dose between the darkest and the lightest blue volume is in the order of 10,000 times. This may mean that no stimulatory effect, or even an inhibiting effect, may occur in the volumes receiving the highest doses.

Figure 10.8 Lasers on skin

However, this is not necessarily a problem as long as the tissue in those volumes is healthy - the laser light is not harmful to healthy tissue even at very high doses.

In an attempt to illustrate how the dose is distributed in treated tissue, we have shown a typical situation for two lasers with different wavelengths, one being less absorbed in tissue than the other. .

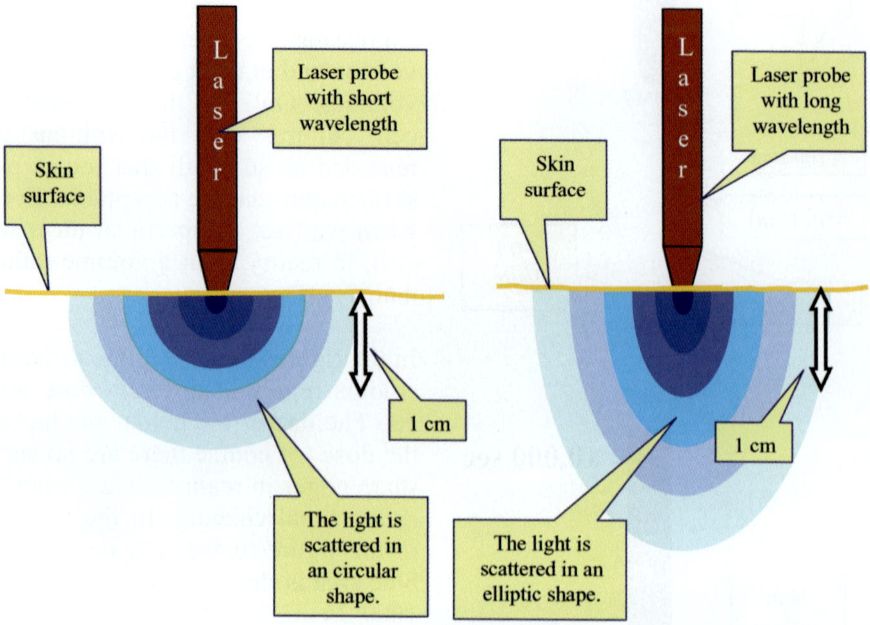

Figure 10.9 Lasers on skin, short - long wavelength

Two examples of treatment: Short wavelength light (wavelengths up to about 700 nm) is scattered more than long wavelength (700 to 1100 nm) light, resulting in different shapes of the "light ball" in the tissue underneath the skin surface. This is also the reason for the deeper penetration of most of the infrared lasers.

10.9 The dose does not depend on the intensity

What is not obvious is that with one and the same laser, dose and intensity are independent, even without changing the output power. To simplify the situation, we assume that the light from the laser diode is divergent and that the light cone is circular, (See Figure 10.1 "Typical diode collimator" on page 314.), and not elliptical and that, within the circle, it gives an even distribution of light all over the area hit by the beam. At different distances from the laser diode, the power density varies considerably. Just outside the glass covering of the laser diode (or end of a fibre) the power density is very high; it then decreases rapidly with the distance (inversely proportional to the square of the distance from the source).

If we want to treat a circular leg ulcer with a diameter of 3 cm (area 10 cm^2) we can choose the following alternatives:

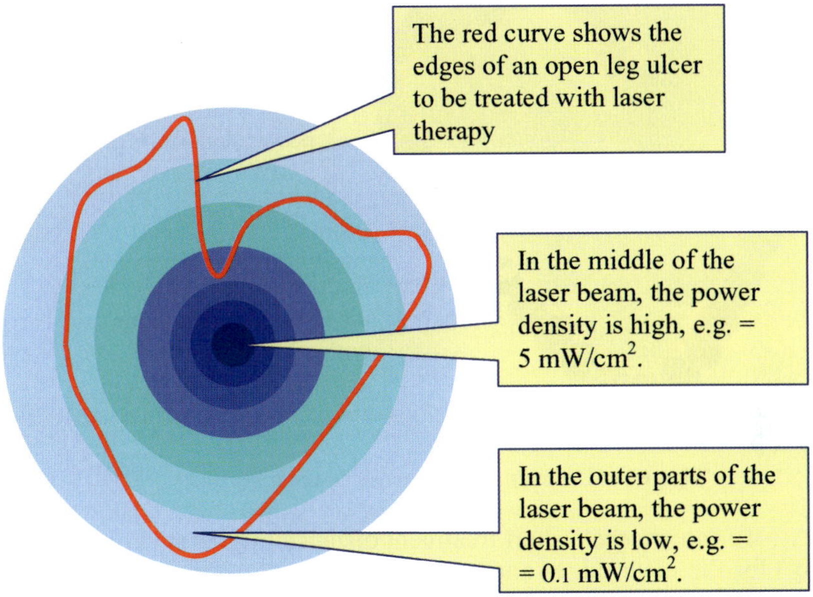

Figure 10.10 Treatment of an open leg ulcer

1. We can use a treatment distance such that the beam covers the entire ulcer (as in figure 10.9), or …

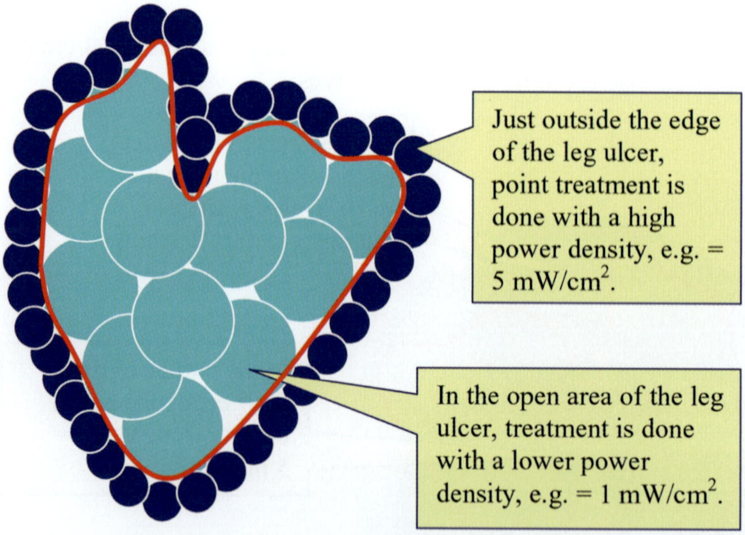

Figure 10.11 Treatment outside of an open leg ulcer

2. … we can choose a short treatment distance (higher power and energy density) for the ulcer edges and a longer distance for the open parts of the ulcer (as in figure 10.10).

When treating an open wound, almost all the energy delivered reaches the intended target. The wound is naked and easily inspected, and the laser light goes directly into the relevant tissue without first passing through covering layers of skin, which, through absorption, diffusion, and reflection, remove a large percentage of the light. If the laser light is collimated (parallel light that does not spread en route from the source to the target), it makes no difference if it is delivered from a distance, since air does not absorb the light. If the laser light is not collimated, however, it should be delivered close to the surface to achieve proper power density and to avoid unnecessary complications in calculating the light intensity in the tissue.

Ready-reckoner.

For most people, mathematical formulas give negative associations. For the common therapist, it is, however, not necessary to use a calculator for every treatment. We have made the process easy. For the treatment of large areas, such as back, neck, shoulders, arms, knees, etc., we use "apples". If you cut an apple in two halves, the cut surface has an area of about 50 cm^2. Supposing that you know the laser type you have and its output power, you simply look up your laser in the table below and enter the depth of the problem: Is it deep or superficial? The table will show you the treatment time in minutes per "apple" at different depths. (See Figure 3.4 “Apple ready reckoner” on page 76.)

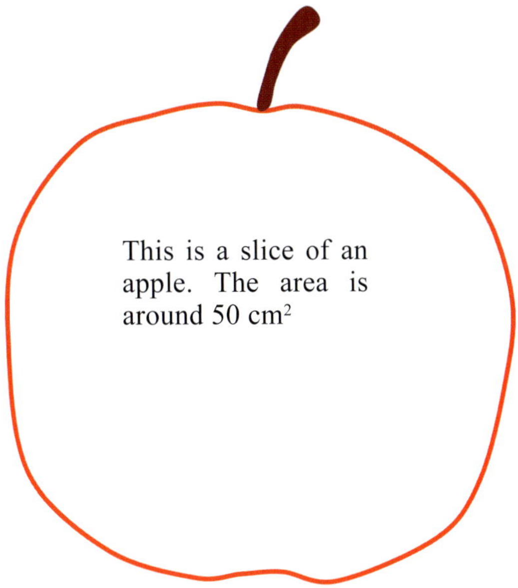
This is a slice of an apple. The area is around 50 cm²

Figure 10.12 Apple

Example 1: For an area the size of an apple using a GaAs-laser probe with an average output power of 60 mW at the chosen treatment frequency (N.B. in many GaAs-lasers, the output power is frequency dependent) and a deep problem, you should treat for a minimum of 3 minutes. Is the area larger than an apple - e.g. the size of 4 apples - treat for 4 × 3 minutes as a minimum. Maximum treatment time: Choose twice the minimum value.

10.10 Dose per point

In the treatment of trigger points and acupuncture points the dose is often said to be a number of joules per "point", the assumption being that a point is something small. We have defined a "point" as an area that is 5 mm in diameter (= 0.2 cm^2) or less. This means that if we hit the skin with the light concentrated to this small area and administer 1 joule, we have given 1 J "per point", and if this "point" is 0.2 cm^2, the dose value is 5 J/cm^2 .

Diagrammatically this may appear as below:

If this is one square centimetre (1 cm^2) and 1 joule of energy is applied equally over its total area, then the energy density is 1 J/cm^2 in every point over the total area.

$100 \text{ mW} \times 10 \text{ sec}/1 \text{ cm}^2 = 1 \text{ J/cm}^2$

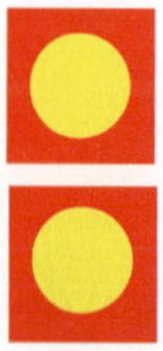

If the red spot shown in the figure is the area of light from a laser probe applied in contact with the skin, held still during the exposure time and having an area of 0.1 cm^2. Then the energy density is 10 J/cm^2 in every point over the spot area if 1 joule of energy is applied.

$100 \text{ mW} \times 10 \text{ sec}/0.1 \text{ cm}^2 = 10 \text{ J/cm}^2$

However, the average over the whole 1 cm^2, is 1 J/cm^2.

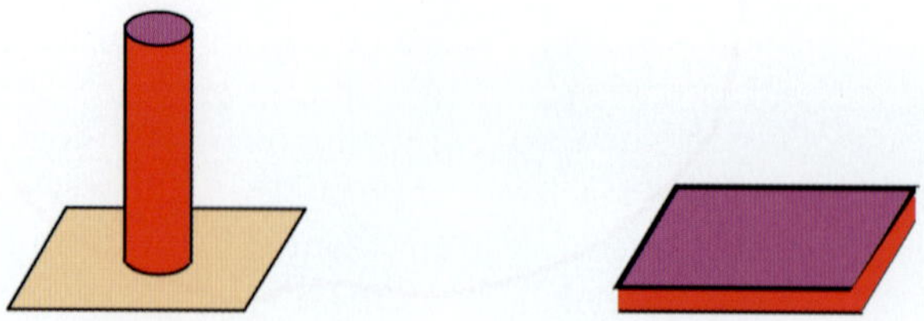
Unevenly distributed light = unevenly distributed dose
Evenly distributed light = evenly distributed dose

Figure 10.13 Distributed light

Point treatment is used in the treatment of trigger points and in laser acupuncture. (See chapter 3.3.3 “Treatment method parameters” on page 83.) A suitable dose for a trigger or acupuncture point is one to four joules.

10.11 More about treatment technique

When treating a certain area, different techniques may be used. Some therapists use the "spot" technique, meaning that they hold the probe still, move it slightly, hold it still, etc. Others use a scanning technique, sliding the probe over the skin. Different figures can be used and it does not really matter what technique you use as long as you have a good idea about the doses you give. Whether one treats clockwise or anti-clockwise is of no relevance

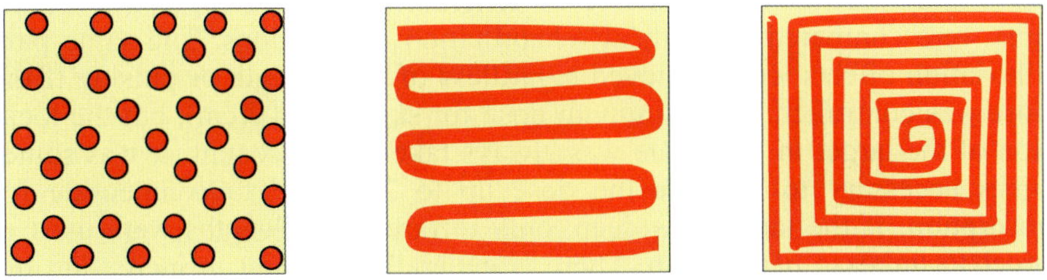

Figure 10.14 Treatment technique

The question at hand is not how many joules are delivered during a treatment session - that information may in fact be entirely irrelevant. The question is how many joules actually reach the diseased tissue. The two figures may be widely divergent.

When treating a known anatomical point located just beneath the skin, there are large dose differences depending on whether the light is delivered from a distance with a narrow collimated beam, from a distance with a divergent beam (spread out over a larger area), in contact with the skin, or in contact with added pressure. The difference between remote, contact and pressure treatment is great. The amount of energy (number of photons) reaching the inflamed tissue may vary a lot. Saying that "3 joules per point" were delivered may be meaningless for purposes of comparison. One therapist may end up delivering a dose (and/or power density) 100 times greater than that delivered by a colleague, although the same "dose" was given! Or, even if the dose is the same, taken as an average over a certain area, the power density can differ very much, giving different treatment results.

If the diseased tissue is deeper still, a new problem arises: where in the tissue is the treatment target?

Another important factor which comes into play is the skill of the therapist. If the diagnosis is correct, it is easier to know which tissue to irradiate. If the therapist has a good knowledge of anatomy, he or she will also know how to reach the tissue with the lowest possible energy loss. It may be necessary to place the patient in a particular position so that intervening muscles move out of the way and reveal the target. In such situations, the dose delivered by a qualified therapist may exceed that delivered by an unqualified colleague by a thousand-fold. Comparing the number of "joules delivered" in such a case is meaningless. It may very well be the case that therapist number one has found the right point and applied pressure to ensure minimum power loss. Therapist number two has irradiated from a distance, through an intervening layer of muscles, covering the target area by chance and luck. If therapist number two thinks that lasers are ineffective, we can understand why.

Technique and expertise mean a lot. This is shown clearly in a study by Ortutay [518]. The outputs of 13 different laser wavelengths (604-1219 nm) were compared in medical rehabilitation applications. The same pain alleviation effects were achieved regardless of wavelength or pulsing if the dose was controlled. The minimum dose for skin was 4 J/cm^2, but the location of the target in the tissue was always taken into account. It was sometimes necessary to increase the dose up to 20 J/cm^2 to compensate for absorption. If the target was deep, only infrared wavelengths were used in order to increase penetration. There is generally no point in increasing the dose if the wavelength has a low penetration factor; the penetration of the particular wavelength must be taken into account. However, as mentioned before, pain treatment needs higher doses than e.g. wound healing.

This study clearly shows that a "joule" is very much a relative concept. The dose recommendations in this book make the assumption that the joule is delivered in a more or less optimal manner. This means, in most cases of local treatment, that it is delivered as close to its anatomical target as possible.

Chapter 11
The Mechanisms

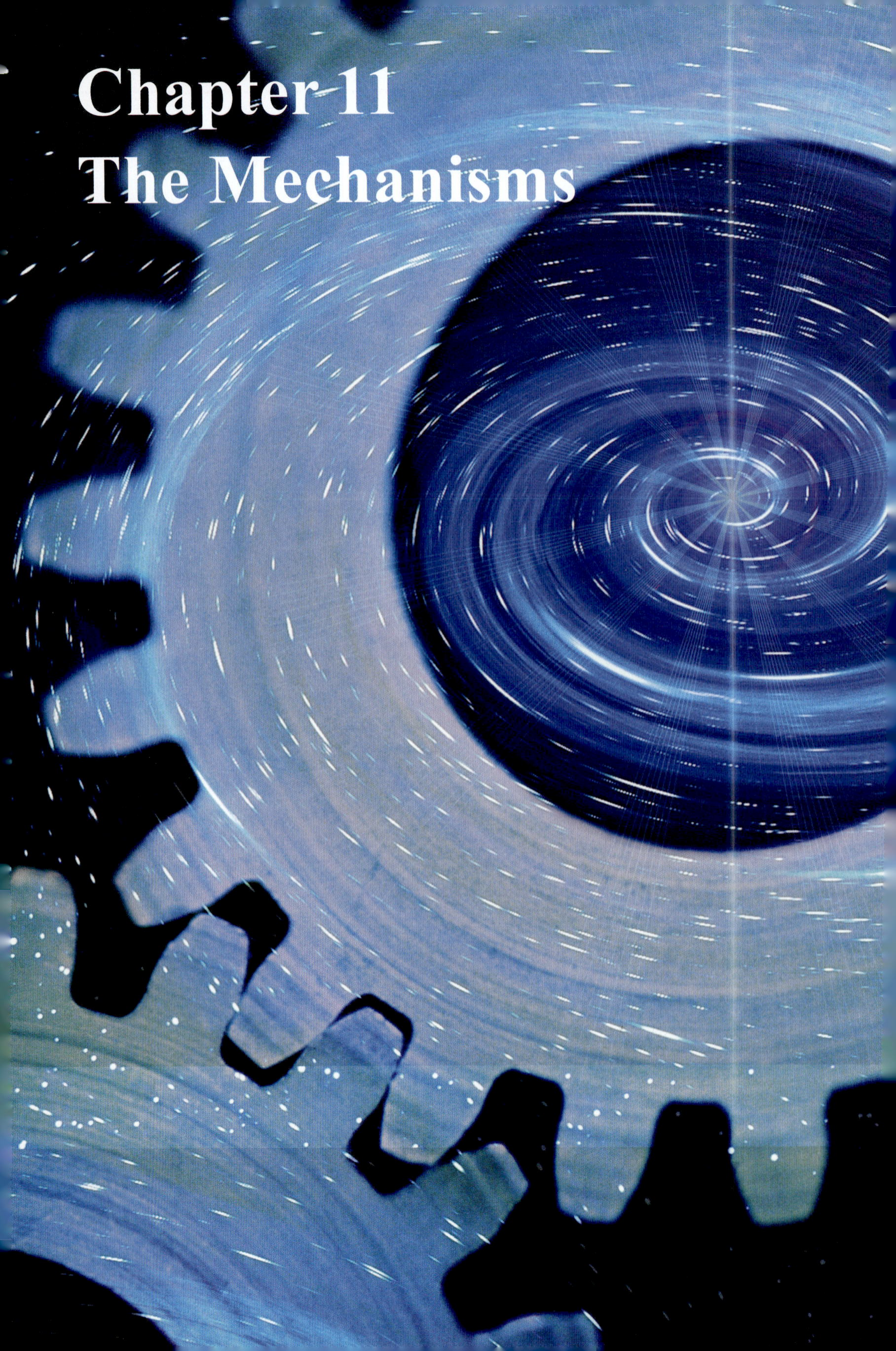

11.1 Are the biostimulative effects laser specific?

All forms of light affect the living organism. It has been shown that white light in certain doses influences seasonal depression conditions [240], see chapter 11.1.6 “Bright Light Phototherapy” on page 345 and that it shows stimulating effect on collagen production in skin that can be used for treatment of wrinkles. It is essential to clarify whether or not the biological effects obtained with laser therapy will appear only if the light source is a laser - that is, if the effects are laser specific. This is not just of theoretical interest. If one could just as well use a light bulb with a polarisation filter, so called Visible Incoherent Polarised light (VIP) - or ordinary Light Emitting Diodes (LED) of a certain colour or infrared light (such as in remote controls) - it would be considerably less expensive to manufacture therapeutic instruments. Some producers of therapeutic instruments claim that treatment with LEDs is as effective as laser treatment. Some producers even claim that LEDs are more efficient than lasers. They often make references to laser research in their marketing, obviously due to lack of support for LED effects.

We will discuss this problem closely in this chapter and the reader will, hopefully, feel more enlightened on the subject after having read this part of the book.

Furthermore, we will try to look into the mechanisms behind the healing laser light. But first we will take a look at the arguments advanced by some "non-believers".

11.1.1 Is it possible to prove that laser therapy doesn't work?

New knowledge and treatment modalities within medicine have not always been well received. When Louis Pasteur claimed that there are small microscopic beings that make meat decay, his contemporary colleagues scorned him. "But," said he, "have a look for yourselves in my microscope!" His colleagues laughed and said they would certainly not do that.

It is an interesting phenomenon that physicists have entered the debate in an attempt to prove that laser therapy just cannot work. As an example of this, we have chosen to discuss an article by King [12] who, like Greguss [233, 234, 235] before him, maintains that therapeutic lasers cannot work because it would be contrary to the laws of physics. King and Greguss claim that:

(A) In terms of their biological effect, lasers may just as well be replaced by a "normal light" with the same optical characteristics, due to the laser light's loss of coherence through scattering in tissue, and
(B) Laser light can have no medical effect, due to its minimal penetration in tissue.

We consider this to be a mistake, on the basis of the following:

Firstly: There have been quite a number of studies conducted on both people and laboratory animals [13, 14, 15, 16, 17, 158, 204, 205, 253, 332,

426, 493, 511, 659, 750, 851, 940, 1077, 1105, 1233] - even blind studies - in which the effect of laser light was compared with the effect of light from other sources, such as LED's. A significant effect was observed with lasers, which was not achieved with the other, less narrow-band light sources. Conclusion: Either all the investigators who conducted this research were mistaken, or the effects are specific to laser light.

Secondly: The coherence of laser light is not lost in tissue due to the phenomenon of scattering. Light is neither coherent nor incoherent but is more or less coherent (see the term "coherence" as explained above).

Thirdly: There is no "normal light" with the same optical properties as a laser, although if one did exist, it would of course produce the same biological effects as a laser.

Fourthly: The penetration of light into tissue is not minimal. This will be discussed later. (See chapter 11.1.5 “How deep does light penetrate into tissue?” on page 343.)

11.1.2 Comparisons between coherent and non-coherent light

In the literature there is good support for the hypothesis that at least some of the biostimulative effects ***in vivo*** are laser specific. In fact, we have not yet found even one single study indicating that non-coherent light is as efficient as coherent light. This does not mean that non-coherent light is not useful for therapy, only that it is less efficient and probably mainly useful on superficial structures.

Literature:

Bihari [13] treated three groups of patients with long-standing crural ulcers with HeNe, HeNe/GaAs and non-coherent unpolarised red light, respectively. Groups 1 and 2 demonstrated excellent healing, with group 2 slightly better than group 1, compared to group 3, which had a low effective percentage.

Kubota [14] found that a 830 nm GaAlAs laser increased flap survival area in a rat model. Laser treated flaps had better perfusion, a greater number of larger blood vessels and significantly enhanced flow rates. There was no difference between control and LED 840 nm groups.

Berki [15] used a HeNe laser to stimulate activation of cells in vitro. These effects (increased phagocytic activity, immunoglobulin secretion) were not seen when irradiating the cell cultures with normal monochromatic light of the same wavelength and doses.

Muldiyarov [16] used a HeNe laser on arthritis in rats and found that the laser exerted an evident therapeutic effect. Analysis of the cases where the rats were treated with ordinary red light revealed no essential differences from the control group.

Haina [17] compared the effects of HeNe-laser and incoherent light of the same wavelength. Experimental wounds were punched out in the muscle fascias of 249 Wistar rats. In the HeNe groups, the granulation tissue increased 13% at 0.5 J/cm^2 and 22% at 1.5 J/cm^2. The increase in the incoherent group was less than 10%.

Rochkind [158] compared five different wavelengths, giving a single transcutaneous irradiation to injured peripheral nerves. HeNe laser prevented the drop in functional activity following crush injury. 830 nm laser was less effective, 660 nm incoherent light was even less effective, and 880 and 950 nm incoherent light was completely ineffective.

Laakso [253] studied the relationship between laser therapy and opioids. In a double blind study, 56 selected patients with chronic pain conditions were treated with 820 nm laser therapy 25 mW, 670 nm laser therapy 10 mW, or 660 nm LED 9.5 mW. ACTH and ß-endorphin levels were significantly elevated in the laser therapy groups but not in the LED group.

Pöntinen [332] compared the effect of laser light (633 and 670 nm) and light from a LED-source (with 660 nm wavelength) on head skin blood flow in 10 healthy men, using laser doppler technology. Doses were from 0.1 to 1.36 J/cm^2. Skin blood flow was measured before, immediately after and 30 minutes after each treatment session at 4 sites on the scalp. The conclusion was that 670 nm laser induced a temporary vasodilatation and increased blood flow when the dose given was in the range of 0.12 - 0.36 J/cm^2. The non-coherent visible monochromatic irradiation with doses between 0.68 and 1.36 J/cm^2 decreased blood flow for at least 30 minutes after irradiation.

Lederer [426] found that "irradiation with coherent HeNe laser light affected leukocytes in migration inhibition assays. Incoherent light of the same wavelength and power density showed no influence."

Rosner [493] evaluated the ability of HeNe laser to delay posttraumatic optical nerve degeneration in rats. The optical nerve was crushed and irradiated through the eye. Interestingly enough, irradiation immediately before the injury was as effective as irradiation beginning soon after it. Non-coherent infrared light was ineffective or had an adverse effect. However, the non-coherent light had a wavelength of 904 nm, which makes comparisons difficult.

Nicola [511] developed a technique of causing highly reproducible inflammatory lesions on the skin of rats. HeNe laser with a dose of 1 J/cm^2 produced an acceleration of the healing process. Incoherent light of the same wavelength and dose was less favourable.

Onac [659] compared the effect of HeNe laser and monochromatic light at 618 nm. The intact skin of guinea pigs was irradiated with different doses. He not only compared the two different light sources but also compared them at different doses (from 0.63 J/cm^2 and up to 38.1 J/cm^2) and came to the following conclusion: Non-coherent monochromatic red light irradiation leads to tegument trophicity at 4.96 J/cm^2 (but less than a HeNe-laser); lower doses have no effect (the HeNe laser does) whereas higher doses cause focal epidermic hypertrophy. Thus, the therapeutic window seems to be narrower for monochromatic non-coherent light.

Nicola [750] investigated the role of polarisation and coherence of laser light on wound healing in rats. There were four groups of wounds:
#1 was treated with coherent and polarised HeNe laser light (633 nm).
#2 was treated with non-polarised, coherent HeNe laser light (633 nm).
#3 was treated with polarised, low degree coherent light (633 nm).
#4 was untreated and served as control.

After the fourth treatment, lesions #1 had healed completely; lesions #2 had not healed completely but showed a more advanced healing process than lesions #3. The lesions #4 showed a poor degree of cicatrisation as compared to lesions #1, #2 and #3.

One investigation that unexpectedly strengthens our hypothesis that most treatments in vivo are laser specific, was published by Zhou [825]. The study concerns PDT (Photo dynamic therapy) using three light sources: a) copper-vapour pumped-dye laser, b) HeNe laser, and c) non-coherent red light (filtered from a halogen lamp), when irradiating the liver in normal mice. The mice (each group containing 18 - 20 mice) received hematoporphyrin derivative in a dose of 10 mg/kg intravenously, 24 hours prior to light irradiation. The mice livers were directly irradiated with different types of red light at a dose of 5, 10, 25, 50, or 100 J/cm^2, respectively. Forty-eight hours later the mice were killed and the depth of liver necrosis was measured using a computerised image-analysis system. No necrosis was found in the control liver irradiated with 500 J/cm^2 alone. The depth of photodynamic necrosis showed a light dose-dependent response. The mean depth of necrosis of all groups was compared statistically. The Cu-dye laser showed the best effect, while the non-coherent light showed the poorest. There were significant differences between non-coherent light and laser-irradiated groups, but not between Cu-dye and HeNe laser groups. The results indicate that of the light sources examined, the Cu-dye laser is most suitable to photodynamic therapy (PDT) of tumours. However, the halogen lamp with a special filter device may still be occasionally used as a light source in PDT if needed.

In a wound healing study by Lowe [851], mouse skin was irradiated with 20 Gy X-ray irradiation. 72 hours later a wound was made on the dorsum and the area was treated with 890 monochromatic LED light three times weekly. There was no effect on the wound healing using 0.18 J/cm^2 or 0.54 J/cm^2 but an inhibiting effect at 1.45 J/cm^2.

In a study by Paolini [940], 99 patients with shoulder tendinitis were divided into three groups. One received HeNe laser irradiation, one LED 660 nm irradiation and one anti-inflammatory medication. 25 sessions with either laser or LED were given. The outcome of the laser group was better than the pharmacological group and much better than the LED group.

Antipa [1077] compared the effect of: 1) GaAlAs laser, 720 nm 3 mW, 2) non-coherent light at 750 nm, 9 mW, and 3) placebo irradiation. 74 patients with sciatic problems were treated. The positive results were 66.6%

for the laser group, 52% for the non-coherent group and 36.4% for the placebo group.

Simunovic [1105] compared the effects of 830 nm laser light with broadband, non-coherent, polarised light in the treatment of epicondylitis. Both groups of patients (n = 20) received 4 J/cm², 12 consecutive treatment sessions, excepting weekends. 40% of the laser treated patients recovered fully, while in the non-coherent group no patients recovered fully.

In a further study, Simunovic and Trobonjaca [1233] compared the efficiency of laser therapy on lateral epicondylitis (tennis elbow) in 120 patients with:

a) transcutaneous electro-neural stimulation (TENS),
b) visible, incoherent polarised light (VIP) and
c) placebo "treatment" with a non working laser unit.

The number or treatment sessions per patient was twelve. The laser dosage was 4 J/point and the VIP-light dosage was 4 J/cm². The results demonstrated that the laser therapy gave the highest percent of pain relief (>45% of lased patients reported 90-100% pain relief), TENS gave the second best pain relief. None of the patients in the VIP group reported 90-100% pain relief. The worst result was reported by the placebo group (<20% of average pain relief).

We wish to underline that the studies above do not indicate that non-coherent light therapy for suitable indications and with sufficient energy densities is inefficient. It only shows that whenever compared, coherent light has come out on top. But indeed, the effect of non-coherent light therapy has been verified [1074], even in double blind studies [433, 941, 1232]. However, in these studies, non-coherent light was not compared with coherent light.

11.1.2.1 Hode's hamburger

Hence, the literature gives no support to King's and Greguss' assumption that the coherence of laser light is lost when it penetrates tissue. We maintain that coherence is not lost.

It is, however, well known that the coherence length decreases in the event of diffuse reflection, but it does not drop to zero. We can firmly establish this by means of the following experiment, first demonstrated by Hode at The Ninth Congress of the International Society for Laser Surgery and Medicine in Los Angeles in 1991. Anyone with a HeNe laser can conduct this experiment.

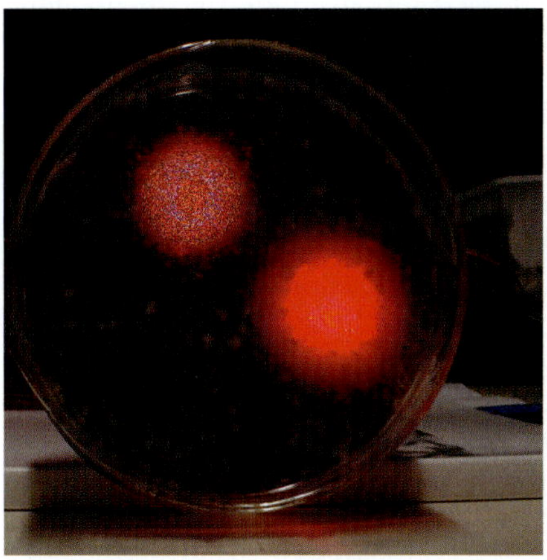

Figure 11.1 Hode's hamburger

1. Press newly minced fresh beef, e.g. raw hamburger meat, between two glass plates so that you have a 5 - 10 mm thick slab of minced beef.

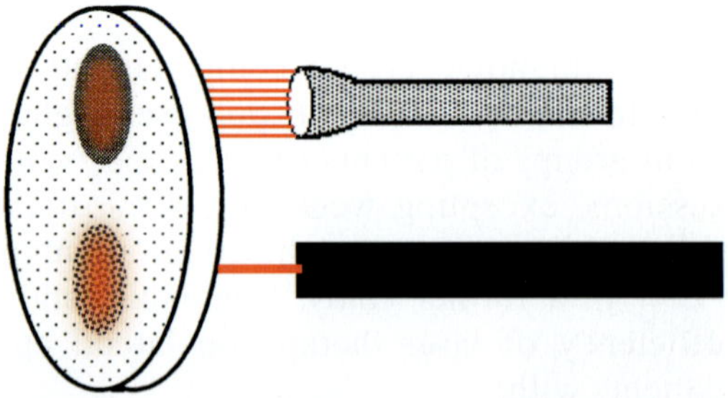

Figure 11.2 Set-up for Hode's hamburger experiment

2. Aim the light from a 5 - 10 mW HeNe or InGaAlP-laser (red visible light with a wavelength of 633 nm) at the glass plates with the minced beef slab as shown in the figure. You can see a red spot on the back of the minced beef where the light has penetrated.

3. Next, place a small penlight torch beside the laser and put its front end against the surface of the glass. The torch emits normal white light. This light also penetrates the minced beef and forms a light spot beside that caused by the laser. The spot from the penlight torch is also red, even though the torch emits white light. This is because the white light's blue, green and yellow colour components are absorbed, and only the red component penetrates.

4. Now study both the red light-spots on the back of the slab from a distance of a few metres. The laser light spot shows clear laser speckles which you can see if you slowly move your head. The spot from the torchlight has no laser speckles.

We can draw the following conclusions from this experiment:

A. Both light spots are red after their passage through the meat. This shows that red light has the best penetration of the visible light wavelengths. Measurements using instruments show that infrared radiation penetrates even better.

B. The coherence of the laser light does not disappear. The laser speckles can be clearly seen, and it is obvious that there is a difference between laser light and the light from a torch. This physical difference characterising the light after its passage through tissue can explain at least some of the research results mentioned above.

C. The HeNe laser beam is narrow and parallel (collimated) when it encounters the minced beef. After its passage through the meat, it is scattered considerably. If we use a laser with visible and highly divergent light (e.g. a diode laser) and place it close to the surface of the meat, we get the same light image on the back as with the collimated laser. The collimation therefore has no significance for the light image in tissue [429].

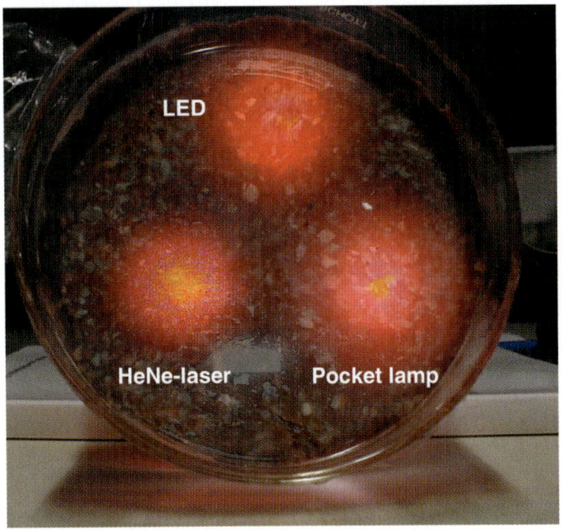

Figure 11.3 Extended set-up

It is easy to extend this experiment by including a red light LED. This gives the following result:

11.1.2.2 Hode's big burger

At the European Medical Laser Association 2nd International Meeting, Florence, October 28-31, 1999, Hode presented an extended version of the same experiment using four light sources - HeNe laser, InGaAlP diode laser (650 nm), a cluster of 7 red LEDs (660 nm) and a normal small pocket torch. Two of the four red light spots showed laser speckles and two of them did not - guess which one!

These nice and simple experiments can be performed by anyone who has a laser and a pocket light. Anyone can see the difference between the laser light and the non-coherent light after penetration of the tissue (meat). It is essential that one has a stable set-up so that movements do not distort the speckle pattern.

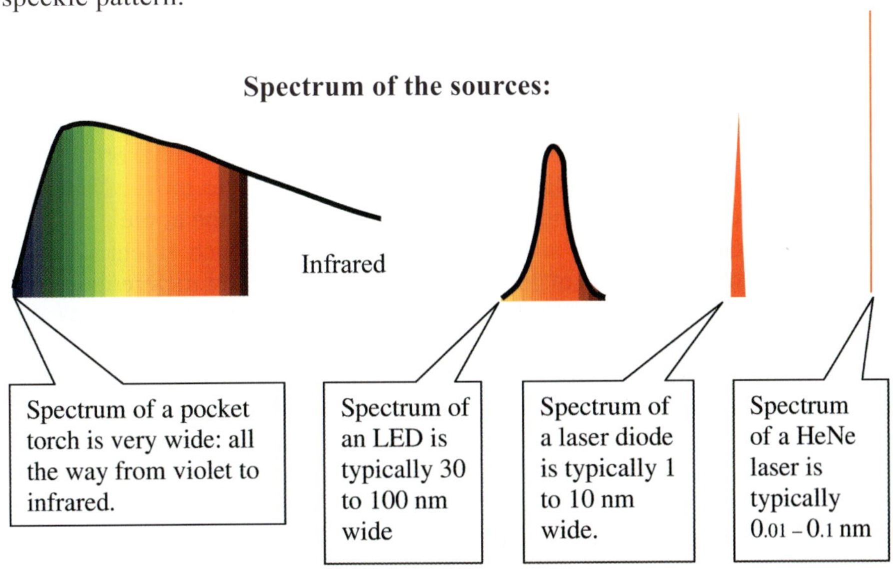

Figure 11.4 Different light sources have different spectra

Even though the laser diode has a much shorter coherence length than the HeNe-laser, the speckles are very pronounced in both laser spots. The LED has such a short coherence length that no speckles can be seen.The coherence length of a light source is more or less inversely proportional to its spectral bandwidth. This means that lamplight has a very short coherence length (in the order of nanometres) while a gas laser can have a coherence length of several metres.

We have noticed that in the treatment of ulcers, herpes and some other skin and mucous problems, a higher dose is needed when a diode laser is used than when a HeNe laser is used. This is most probably due to the difference in coherence length between those two sources.

11.1.3 Abrahamsson's apple

This is an other experiment showing that the coherence of laser light does not disappear when spread diffusely.

If we direct a narrow beam from a HeNe laser at an apple, we can see a halo with a diameter of 1-2 cm around the intense target point. This halo occurs because the laser light is spread and reflected in all directions in the tissue of the apple, and consequently, some of it is also, after scattering, reflected out of the apple. If we look at the halo, we also see laser speckles (virtual speckles), which shows that the laser light retains its coherence after its passage through the tissue of the apple. Furthermore, the coherence of the laser light is much greater than the coherence of light from a red LED, for example, which does not exhibit clear speckles when directed towards the apple. The distribution of the laser light inside the apple is not homogeneous but grainy, due to interference, i.e. it consists of a three-dimensional speckle structure (real speckles).

Abrahamsson, at The Swedish Royal Institute of Technology in Stockholm, observed these speckles through a microscope and was probably the first to notice that the speckles on the surface of an apple move. He could relate this movement to the movement within the cells of the apple.

The phenomenon has since been surveyed by French scientists [19], who studied the movement of the laser speckles and could differentiate two different forms of particle movement in the interior of the apple cells. As this is not possible with light sources other than laser, it is fairly obvious that there is a great difference in quality between laser light and incoherent light and that the coherence of laser light is not lost.

Kamikawa [359] shows in his article "Studies on low power laser therapy of pain" a picture of a finger that is transilluminated by a diode laser of 1 mW. The light from the laser passes through the finger and shows, on the opposite side, interference fringes. When the same experiment was done with an LED, no interference fringes appeared. This experiment also shows that coherence is not lost when laser light is diffusely scattered in tissue.

Enlarged real laser speckles recorded on a black and white film. Bright parts correspond to areas (volumes) with higher intensity than average.

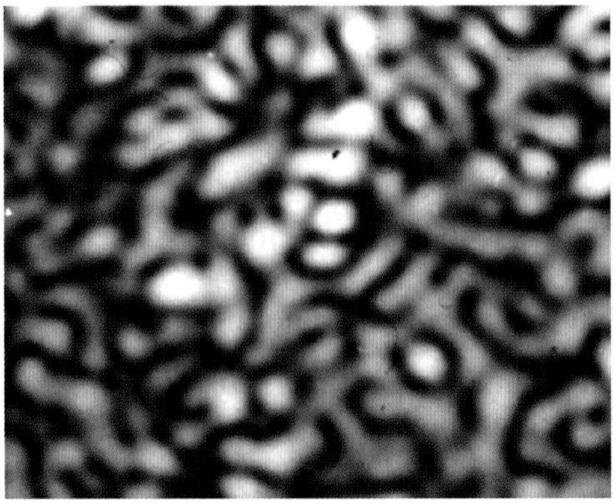

Figure 11.5 Enlarged real laser speckles
Photo: Lars Hode

11.1.4 Moonlight

King and Greguss also assert that, for example, the light from a HeNe laser (red visible light) only penetrates 1-2 millimetres into the skin and laser therapy can therefore have no effect, except for a very superficial one. They define the penetration as "the depth where the light intensity has dropped to 37% (=1/e of the intensity on the surface, where e = 2.71828...) of the intensity on the surface".

Svaasand [27] has tried to lead the way in proving that the reported effects of laser therapy on tissue would contradict the laws of physics. He has calculated that at the depth inside the body of, for example, a shoulder joint, laser treatment gives a light intensity equal to that of moonlight. This is probably correct. However, laser therapy is not a case of broadband moonlight, but of highly monochromatic and, at least partially, polarised, coherent laser light, which even at low levels can impart interference effects. And what light intensity does it have to be? Would perhaps starlight level be enough? In theory, one single photon can actually start a chain reaction.

Let us make a little calculation: A fully adapted human eye can see about 10^{-9} lux. This corresponds to about 1.5×10^{-17} watts of visible power or about 30 photons per second of energy through the pupil of an eye. This little energy flow can create a minute nerve signal.

In a dark room, a 10 mW HeNe-laser can transilluminate a hand. A GaAlAs laser (820 nm) has even better transmission but its longer wavelength cannot be seen by the naked eye. It has to be measured by instruments. 2 cm down in tissue, only between 0.1% and 0.01% of the incident power

BLT literature:	Our comments:
Rao [801]: Light treatment increases blood serotonin throughout the day. This increase is seen in all patients and healthy subjects after bright (2500 lux) as well as dim (50 lux) light. These results suggest that the influence of light is more pronounced on serotonin than melatonin metabolism. Treatment 2 hours daily.	Main influence on serotonin. This is also typical of laser therapy. It is surprising that the light intensity is not of greater importance. Maybe saturation is reached due to illumination of a large body area.
Rice [805] compared 2 weeks of light therapy with full spectrum white light with cool white light. Both treatment methods reduced depression scores, advanced the timing of the melatonin rhythm, and increased melatonin concentrations	Full spectrum white light also has a great deal of infrared radiation which cool light has not. Maybe the infrared part of the spectrum is of less importance. What about narrow band treatment or even laser light?
Wetterberg [819] writes "Light may be used to treat depression, sleep disorders, menstrual dysregulations and other illnesses with disturbed circadian and seasonal rhythms".	Treatment of menstrual dysregulations with laser therapy has succesfully done by Takac [143]
Bylesjö [787]: Three of the 4 women reduced their net weight (1.5-2.4 kg) and improved in mood. 1500 lux.	It was actually popular to treat overweight with laser therapy in Sweden. We don't know how successful these treatments were. Maybe it works …
Thalén [790]: Ninety patients with major depressive disorders were treated with a luminance of 350 cd/m² (approximately 1500 lux) at **eye level**. Depressed patients with a seasonal pattern improved significantly more than those with a non-seasonal pattern.	In this report, too, we can see that the author believes that the effects are due to retinal illumination. Spectrum, bandwidth, coherence, pulsing, different areas to treat, treatment interval, etc., remain to be investigated.
Lewy [807]: Morning light was more anti-depressant than evening light.	Thalén [790]: There were no significant dif-ferences between morning and evening BLT.
Kripke [818]: Light therapy can be combined with standard therapies for treating non-seasonal depressions and appears synergistic.	Laser therapy also acts synergistically with other therapies.

Table 11.2: BLT literature

Laser spectroscopy can be used for quantitative analysis of e.g. frozen skin biopsies for calcium, arsenic and gold. This technique has also found its application in forensic medicine. With the Laser Doppler Spectrometer, spermokhinezymetry can be performed.

Laser microscopy exists in many different forms, such as Laser Microscopic Masonic Analyzer (LAMMA) and Laser Fluorescent Microscopy.

Laser cytofluorometry utilises the argon laser for scanning single stained cells and has achieved utilisation in mass examination programs for Pap-smear determinations. The same technique is used in a cell sorting system that is now important in monoclonal antibody determination in hybridoma technology.

Lasers can also be used in laser particle size measurement techniques, and laser nephelometry for determination of immunoglobulin classes and autoantibodies such as rheumatoid factors.

Examples of other techniques are transillumination by lasers (diaphanography), laser retinoscopy and holography

Laser-based methods have also been used to study air pollution involving carcinogens in occupational exposures and for the detection of narcotic drugs.

Chapter 12
A guide for scientific work

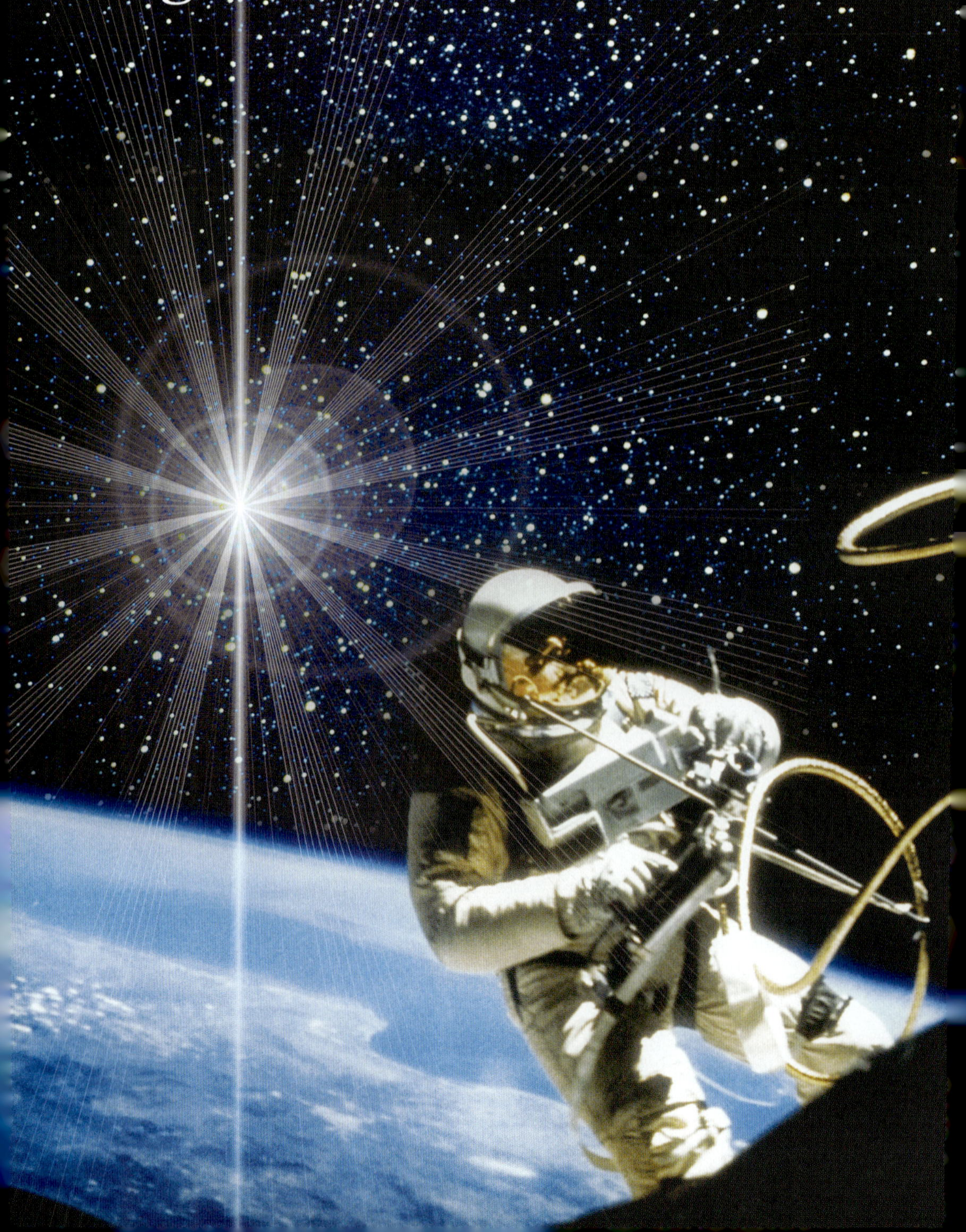

Designing a clinical trial is part science, part art. You need a sense of what works and the commitment to stick to it. The acceptance of a new method of medical treatment or medication must be based on good scientific research. In chapter 13 “The laser therapy literature” on page 379 in this book we will look at the laser therapy literature. We have found that many of the published articles are of low scientific value. However, this is not typical only of the positive studies. In the following chapter we suggest some guidelines for scientific work with laser therapy. Basically, laser therapy should be subject to the same standards of evaluation as other physical methods but must be combined with a knowledge of the special parameters of this method. Without this it will not become the valuable therapeutic tool in medicine that it has the potential to become. It is not uncommon to find a trial that is methodologically sound but not reproducible on the basis of the information supplied.

If you are going to perform a study and want to publish it, it is worth taking a look at how a study can be evaluated in a meta-analysis. Then you can allocate points to different criteria, such as the following, taken from the thesis by Lucas [1184].

A One point each if selection criteria are clearly described, restriction to a homogenous population with respect to diagnoses, duration of complaint, previous treatments and contra-indications for the laser treatment.

B Five points if randomisation procedure is described and is a procedure which excludes bias.

C Five points if smallest group is larger than 25 patients immediately following randomisation; ten points if larger than 50 patients and fifteen points if larger than 75 patients.

D Two points each if the study groups are comparable at baseline for (1) duration of complaint; (2) age; (3) baseline scores for outcomes measured; (4) recurrence status; (5) previous treatment of complaint.

E Five points if there are no dropouts after randomisation. Two points if there are dropouts, with the number of dropouts given for each study group. Three additional points if the reason for withdrawal after randomisation is given for each study group.

F Loss-to-follow up: 1 minus (the number of patients at the main moment of effect measurement / the number or patients at randomisation) x 100 %. One point if loss-to-follow up is less than 20 % in each group. Four points if it is less than 10 % in each group.

G Points are given to a description of the treatment. One point each for: (1) type of laser used; (2) wavelength and repetition rate [pulse frequency]; (3) duty cycle; (4) power; (5) irradiation [intensity]; (6) distance of probe

Chapter 13
The laser therapy literature

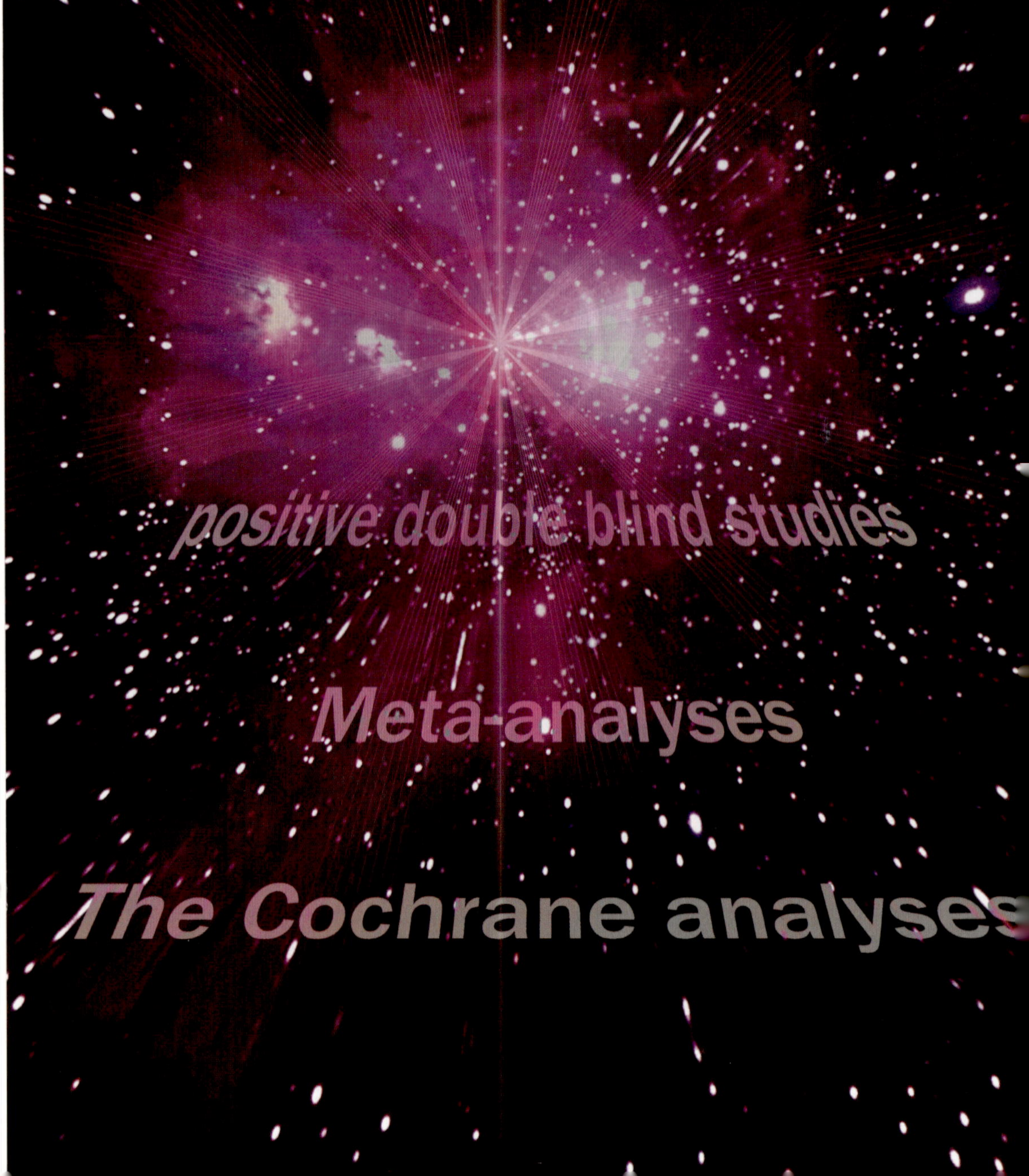

In this chapter we aim to discuss the laser therapy literature in more depth. Much more work should be done in the evaluation of the available literature, which consists of some 2500 studies. Since laser therapy is a fairly new treatment modality, many of the early studies were non-controlled and provided little information on the parameters used. Negative as well as positive studies must therefore be subjected to an objective analysis in the search for the optimal parameters. Some of the studies will have to be transferred to the wastebasket. The most striking general feature in the negative studies is the use of very low dosages. Similarly, most analyses of the literature are characterized by a lack of an evaluation of the connection between positive results and reasonable dosage on the one hand, and negative result and low dosage on the other hand. However, negative studies and poorly performed positive studies are not without interest. Negative studies, if performed correctly, are of great value. Positive studies may, even if poorly designed, stimulate further research in an interesting direction. In general, it is clear that the average methodological quality of the laser therapy literature is not very high. However, the quality is higher than for widely used methods such as ultrasound [1187].

13.1 The positive double blind studies

During the past 15 years the authors of this book have collected some 2000 studies. Among these, more than 100 positive double blind studies have been identified. All studies showing some positive effect of laser therapy have been regarded as positive, even if the effect has been low or only positive in one of several measured parameters. Two studies using a combination of laser and LED have been included (although this combination complicates evaluations), as well as a few laser acupuncture studies. In the following, some shortcomings of 100 selected (among 109) studies will be described. The studies are double blind but not always randomised. There are about 80 randomised studies, negative and positive together.

Many of these studies have been published in national or regional scientific magazines with a limited international circulation. In a Medline search, only 27 of the chosen 100 studies were found. It is obvious that anyone looking for laser therapy documentation on-line will have problems finding such studies. Further, Medline abstracts seldom give a full account of the laser parameters and a critical evaluation is rarely possible, whether negative or positive. In addition, some double blind titles actually found on Medline do not have an abstract at all. Some studies can be found in other on-line libraries (BIOSIS, Cambridge Scientific Abstracts, Excerpta Medica etc.), but these are often not free of charge or may only be available to the members or to a limited public.

43 studies have only been identified in the abstract form. They may have been published in a more extensive form but could not be found on Medline or elsewhere. Some studies are published in languages not known

by the authors (Russian/Japanese). If the report in such a study has an English abstract, it has been classified as “abstract” although a closer account of the study is actually published. Reports from SPIE proceedings are often detailed, but since they have not passed a regular referee system they have been classified as “abstracts”. 10 studies have been identified only by name through lists of references. Of the 100 selected references only 58 complete studies have been found and read in detail. 33 abstracts have been read and included in the analysis.

Negative as well as positive studies often lack an account of laser parameters. Each study in this analysis was given a mark for parameter account, using 5 as the top mark. To achieve a mark 5, the study must report all laser parameters and the laser output must have been independently measured. The information in glossy brochures is one thing, reality is another. The mark system, admittedly, becomes a bit arbitrary, but it is intended to give a general impression of the quality of parameter reporting. The average rating in the studied texts is 3.0. For the published studies the average is 3.6.

The size of the active and control groups varies from 10/10 to 522/146 respectively. The number as such is not very informative. An indication such as pain requires a large group while a smaller group is sufficient for more objectively measured indications such as mucositis.

Dose range is from 0.001 J/cm^2 to 48 J/cm^2. However, a meaningful comparison cannot be made, since a detailed account of the laser parameters and calculations is often lacking. Deeper lying targets have received higher doses to compensate for energy loss in tissue. Different wavelengths also influence the necessary dose level. Too often, either the dosage or the energy is missing in the specifications.

No less than 17 indications for laser therapy have been found in these 100 studies. While this supports the theory that laser therapy interacts with a multitude of bodily processes, some indications have only one or two supportive studies. 100 positive double blind studies on a single indication, like pain, would have made it much easier to establish credibility for the therapy as such.

The number of studies for each indication is as follows: pain 41, arthritis/rheumatism 17, wound healing 8, epicondylitis 6, nerve function 6, tendinitis 4, hypersensitive dentine 3, mucositis 3, post herpetic neuralgia 2, TMD 2, Herpes simplex 1, Sjögren’s syndrome 1, fibrositis 1, sinuitis 1, clonus 1, acupuncture 1, microcirculation 1 and trismus 1.

An evaluation of blinding procedures has not been made, nor an evaluation of the statistical quality of the studies. Such an analysis would add further criticism to many studies. As a general remark, though, it can be stated that double blind procedures with HeNe are problematic, since the typical speckle pattern is easily recognisable with the true lasers with visible wavelength.

Although the number of studies in the field of laser therapy is reasonably high and the number of positive double blind studies is more than 100,

[A45] Parker J, Dowdy D, Harkness E et al: The effects of laser therapy on tissue repair and pain control. A meta analysis of the literature. Proc. 3rd Congress of the World Ass for Laser Therapy, Athens, Greece, 2000, page 77.

[A46] Kaiser C et al: Estudio en doble ciego randomizado sobre la eficacia del HeNe en el tratamiento de la sinuitis maxilar aguda: en pacientes con exacerbación de una infección sinusal crónica. [Double blind randomised study on the effect of HeNe in the treatment of acute maxillary sinuitis: in patients with exacerbation of a chronic maxillary sinuitis]. Boletín CDL. 1986; 9: 15. Also in Av Odontoestomatol. 1987; 3 (2): 73-76.

[A47] Bjordal J M, Couppé C, Ljunggren A E: Low level laser for tendinopathy. Evidence of a dose-response pattern. Physical Therapy Reviews. 2001; 6: 91-99.

13.4 The Cochrane analyses – can they be improved?

The aim of the international Cochrane collaboration is to continuously evaluate new and old medical therapies. The basis for the systematic reviews is the recognition of Randomised Controlled Trials as the "gold standard" for scientific evaluation of small and moderate effects from treatment. A thorough search is made for the available literature and the most "qualified" studies are analysed. The purpose of the analysis is to find out whether or not there is any solid support for a specific medical treatment modality. Such analyses are published in medical journals and extended versions are quarterly updated in the Cochrane Library. Since the Cochrane reviews are influential, it is important that the persons performing them possess a thorough knowledge of all aspects of Low Level Laser Therapy. The aim of the present study is to "analyse the analyses".

Introduction

Three systematic reviews on the effectiveness of Laser Therapy have been published in the Cochrane Library. These reviews have evaluated the effect of Laser Therapy for Venous ulcers [B1] Osteoarthritis [B2] and Rheumatoid arthritis [B3]. However, the Cochrane style of reviewing has been criticised [B20] for not taking into account the variability of diagnoses, treatment procedures and dosages of the included trials. The impact of the Cochrane Library in the field of medicine is profound. It is therefore essential to "evaluate the evaluation", to find out whether or not these analyses can live up to the prestige of the Cochrane Library. The following text is a critical "analysis of the analyses".

1. Venous ulcers

Four trials are analysed: two comparing laser with placebo, one comparing laser with non-coherent light and one comparing laser with ultraviolet light. Two studies comparing laser with placebo were reported by the same investigators [B4, B5]. In the first report a 6 mW HeNe laser was used. 4 J/cm^2 was said to be given to the ulcers. Ulcer size ranged from 3-32 cm^2. Treatment technique was not stated. Regardless of technique, it would take between 36 minutes and 6 hours to achieve the stated dose per wound and session. Using a sweep technique with a focused beam, the power density would be around 0.15 W/cm^2. If a defocused beam were used to cover the entire largest wound (32 cm^2), energy density would be around 0.00019 W/cm^2, which is extremely low, lower than the energy density of the normal illumination in a medical clinic. A dose miscalculation is probable but the authors of the study have been reluctant to reveal the parameters used. In the absence of such parameters, this study cannot be properly evaluated, but very low power density is a probable reason for its negative results. In the second study [B5] on venous ulcer, GaAs was employed. 4 mW was used for 10 minutes on ulcers ranging from 4 to 52 cm^2, regardless of ulcer size. The 4 cm^2 wound would thus receive 0.6 J/cm^2 and the largest wound 0.046 J/cm^2, not the 1.96 J/cm^2 stated by the authors. Energy density as well as dose for larger wounds is thus low. Treatment technique is not indicated. The report states that: “the laser was held perpendicular to the surface of the wound”. This is not a sufficient description of the treatment method. There is a great difference between following the outer border of the wound (active healing area) and spreading the beam over the open wound area. The distance between diode and wound is not indicated.

In summary, the energy level said to be applied in these studies must be questioned. The Cochrane evaluators have not observed the essential contradiction between the actual dose and the dose indicated by the authors.Further, in one of the four studies(6) the laser wavelength and dose are not stated in the original paper. This makes an evaluation impossible.

2. Osteoarthritis

Five trials were included out of 142 potentially relevant articles. Six abstracts are awaiting assessment after the authors have been contacted for further details. In the meantime, some comments on the analysis follows:

Bülow [B7] (negative outcome) is a good study using a reasonable energy level (GaAlAs laser 22.5 J/session) for painful knee osteoarthritis. However, see discussion below about chosen outcome measurements.

Basford [B8](negative outcome) used HeNe laser 0.007 J per point for thumb arthritis. The dose used is virtually meaningless since it is too low.

Jensen [B9] (negative outcome) used GaAs laser, 0.2 J in total, for painful knee arthrosis. Here, too, the dose used is very low and below the dose levels that have been reported to be effective.

Stelian [B10](positive outcome) used GaAlAs laser around 11 J per session, twice daily, amounting to 22 J per knee per day, 10 consecutive days. This study has a dose that is acceptable even in the light of today's experience, although it was published as early as 1992. The outcome of this study stands in contrast to the rather similar study by Bülow. The dose is the same, and the number of sessions is almost the same (10/9). However, Bülow applied the treatment 2-4 times a week, Stelian twice daily.

Walker [B11] (positive outcome) is a classic positive study, but the use of a HeNe laser of less than 1 mW throws doubt on this study. In our opinion it should not be used as anything but a purely historical reference.

The crucial criticism of the evaluation of the studies above is that there is no discussion about dosage! On the Jadad quality scale (1-5), Basford is given 3 and Bülow 2. However, Basford used a non-significant dosage for a finger joint while Bülow has a reasonable dose for knee osteoarthritis. Johannsen (see Rheumatoid arthritis below) used a dose above the generally accepted dosage window. In retrospect, the Bülow trial has been criticised for overlooking a significant short-term effect of active laser treatment by only testing the statistical significance at follow-up. Stelian used 55 times more energy than Jensen for knee osteoarthritis! The Jadad quality scale is applied correctly to the studies. But without inclusion of the laser parameters in the scale, evaluation tends to become a "study design beauty contest" instead of an evaluation of therapeutical significance.

3. Rheumatoid arthritis

Eight of 191 articles met the inclusion criteria; five were Randomised Controlled Trials. Five further studies are waiting assessment pending answers from the authors.

Comments:

Johannsen [B13] (negative outcome) used 11.9 J GaAlAs laser per finger joint, which is a high dose, maybe too high.
Heussler [B14] (negative outcome) used 1.5 J GaAlAs laser per finger joint.
Walker [B15] (positive outcome) used less than 1 mW of HeNe laser. Although Johannsen used a dose 1700 times higher than Walker, both studies are "put in the same basket". A low/high dose evaluation is actually performed but the wide gap in dosages does not justify a subgroup analysis of merely two groups.
Hall [B16] and Goats [B17] used combined coherent and non-coherent light. Combined single wavelength coherent light and multi-wavelengths non-coherent light is a poorly studied area and there is no ground for postulating that they produce the same biological effects when used in various combinations or alone.
The meta analysis by Gam [B19] (one of the Cochrane co-authors) is referred to. This analysis did not find any effect of Laser Therapy for musculoskeletal pain. The re-evaluation of the same studies made by Bjordal [B21] found a clear effect when an analysis of the dosage and therapeutic tech-

niques was included. This latter meta-analysis is not mentioned. Critical comments on the Cochrane reviews are supposed to be continously included.

Conclusions

The evaluators of the Cochrane groups have been successful in finding many of the relevant studies in the literature. Several interesting observations have been made and a skilful analysis of the design parameters has been performed. Evaluation of effects is a universal problem for all empirically developed therapies, where consensus of a clearly defined optimal dose range and adequate treatment procedure is lacking. For clinicians practising laser therapy it is hard to understand why the reviewers have neglected some important factors, e.g. body area treated, size of area and dose. The methodology used seems to be that of drug studies. But drugs and laser therapy are quite different. Oral intake of a drug is the universal procedure. Laser therapy can be applied in several ways, such as local irradiation, trigger point irradiation, acupuncture irradiation and irradiation over peripheral nerves. All these methods must be evaluated separately.

The biggest problem has been the fact that most of the reviews have "put into the same basket" a variety of doses, energy densities and treatment procedures. New treatment methods are often subject to trials where clinicians include all their non-responding patients, and the early laser literature is no exception. Flaws in laser therapy studies are not uncommon [B21] . The laser literature includes about 100 positive and 40 negative double blind trials [B22] on a heterogeneous sample of more than 20 different diagnoses, which vary widely in pathology, tissue involved and prognosis. Added to this are all the inadequate treatment procedures and doses that have been employed in clinical laser therapy trials. Under such circumstances the majority of these trials will find no effect of active treatment. Therefore, we should be very careful when viewing all the trial results together to see if they add up to an effect significantly better than placebo. Future reviews are suggested to analyse the positive studies in order to find out what parameters seem to work. Subgroup analyses are of particular importance. Dosage analysis cannot be limited to the groups "high" and "low" because of the great variations in dosage. Neither can any wavelength be put into the "high" or "low" basket. 2 J HeNe for a finger joint may be "high" while 20 J HeNe for lumbar problem may be "low". GaAs requires lower doses than GaAlAs etc.

So what have these new Cochrane reviews brought us? Two distinct steps of progress can be identified. In the rheumatoid arthritis review, attempts have been made to evaluate effects separately for high and low dose. And secondly, they even give a (qualified) recommendation: "Low level laser therapy could be considered for treatment of rheumatoid arthritis for its short term effect and lack of side effects".

Future directions

Both laser researchers and reviewers have common responsibilities in enhancing our understanding of laser therapy The three existing Cochrane reviews on laser therapy have drawn some conclusions, to which we can comment that the literature on the evaluated indications is ambiguous, the average quality of the studies is not very high, and the number of relevant studies is rather low. It can therefore be postulated that there is still insufficient scientific support for the general use of Laser Therapy for the three indications reviewed by the Cochrane evaluators and that only moderate and short-term effects can be confirmed. However, the review methodology should include valid criteria for dose and target for laser irradiation (e.g. synovia, triggerpoints, acupuncture points, peripheral nerves, etc). Furthermore, the effect calculations could be performed for subgroups of different doses, treatment frequencies and laser types. There is also still room for improvement of the literature search. Further, reviewers must make their own dosage calculations, not taking the doses quoted in the studies for granted. Too many of the negative laser therapy studies contain serious flaws [B23], and such flaws must be firmly investigated when evaluating laser therapy studies.

References:

[B1] Flemming K, Cullum N: Laser Therapy for venous leg ulcers (Cochrane review). In: The Cochrane Library, 4, 2000.

[B2] Brosseau L, Welch V, Wells G et al: Low level laser therapy (Classes I, II and III) for treating Osteoarthritis. The Cochrane Library. Issue 4, 2000.

[B3] Brosseau L, Welch V, Wells G et al: Low level laser therapy (Classes I, II and III) for treating rheumatoid arthritis. The Cochrane Library. Issue 4, 2000.

[B4] Lundeberg T and Malm M: Low power HeNe laser treatment of venous leg ulcers. Annals of Plastic Surgery. 1991; 27: 537-539.

[B5] Malm M and Lundeberg T: Effect of low power gallium arsenide laser on healing of venous ulcers. Scandinavian Journal of Plastic Reconstruction and Hand Surgery. 1991; 25: 249-251.

[B6] Crous L and Malherbe C: Laser and ultraviolet light irradiation in the treatment of chronic ulcers. Physiotherapy. 1988; 44: 73-77.

[B7] Bülow P M, Jensen H and Danneskiold-Samsoe B: Low power GaAlAs laser treatment of painful osteoarthritis of the knee. Scandinavian Journal of Rehabilitation Medicine. 1994; 26: 155-159.

[B8] Basford JR, Sheffield C G, Mair S D, Ilstrup D M: Low-energy helium neon laser treatment of thumb osteoarthritis. Archive of Physical and Medical Rehabilitation. 1987; 68: 794-797.

[B9] Jensen H, Harreby M and Kjær J (1994): Infrared laser – effekt ved smertende knaearthrose? Ugeskrift for Laeger, 149: 3104-3106.

[B10] Stelian J, Gil I, Habot B et al: Improvement of pain and disability in elderly patients with degenerative osteoarthritis of the knee treated with narrow band light therapy. Journal of the American Geriatric Society. 1992; 40: 23-26.

[B11] Walker J: Relief from chronic pain by low power laser irradiation. Neuroscience Letters. 1983; 43: 339-344.

[B12] Marks R, de Palma F: Clinical efficacy of low power laser therapy in osteoarthritis. Physiotherapy Research International. 1999; 4 (2): 141-147.

[B13] Johannsen F, Hauschild B, Remvig L et al: Low energy laser therapy in rheumatoid arthritis. Scandinavian Journal of Rheumatology. 1994; 23: 145-147.

[B14] Heussler J K, Hinchey G, Margiotta E et al: A double blind randomised trial of low power laser treatment in rheumatoid arthritis. Annals of the Rheumatic Diseases. 1993; 52: 703-706.

[B15] Walker J, Akhanjee L K, Cooney M M et al: Laser therapy for pain of rheumatoid arthritis. Clinical Journal of Pain. 1987; 3: 54-59.

[B16] Hall J, Clarke AK, Elvins DM, Ring EFJ: Low level laser therapy is ineffective in the management of rheumatoid finger joints. British Journal of Rheumatology. 1994; 33: 142-147.

[B17] Goats G C, Flett E, Hunter J A, Sterling A: Low intensity laser and phototherapy for rheumatoid arthritis. Physiotherapy. 1996; 82 (5): 311-320.

[B18] Seichert N: Physiotherapy: Controlled trials and facts. In (Schlapbach P, Gerber NJ eds): Rheumatology. 1991; p. 205-217.

[B19] Gam A N, Thorsen H and Lonnberg F: The effect of low-level laser therapy on musculo-skeletal pain: a meta-analysis. Pain. 1993; 52: 63-66.

[B20] Bjordal J M, Greve G: "What may alter the conclusions of reviews?". Physical Therapy Reviews. 1998; 3: 121-132.

[B21] Tunér J, Hode L. It´s all in the parameters – a critical analysis of some well-known negative studies on low-level laser therapy. J Clin Lasers Med Surg. 1998; 16 (5): 245-248.

[B22] Tunér J: What is in the LLLT literature? In (Simunovic Z, ed): Lasers in Medicine and Dentistry, European Medical Laser Assn. 2000; pp 217-226. ISBN 953-6059-30-4.

13.5 Poor documentation – compared to what?

It is sometimes claimed that laser therapy has a rather poor scientific documentation. While this may be a valid point to some extent, it is suprisingly common for generally used treatment modalities to have a poor documentation without being questioned. It is interesting to compare the widely used ultrasound modality with laser therapy. In the book "Clinical electrotherapy – your guide to optimal treatment", Bjordal [1187] has compared the documentation found in the randomised studies on laser therapy and ultrasound in physiotherapy.

	Laser therapy	**Ultrasound**
Strong evidence of effect	Tendinopathy Osteoarthritis	None
Moderate evidence of effect	Myofascial trigger point syndrome	None
Weak evidence of effect	Rheumatoid arthritis Soft tissue injuries	Tendinopathy Soft tissue injuries Wounds

Table 13.12: Laser therapy - ultrasound

13.6 The Russian experience

A substantial part of the scientific laser therapy literature has been published by Russian researchers. Laser therapy was introduced very early in the former Soviet Union and many observations and discoveries have been made, not least the development of blood irradiation, see chapter 3.3.3.2.5 "Blood irradiation" on page 88 and irradiations through the urethra, rectum, oesophagus etc. There are several reasons for the fact that this experience has had rather a modest impact in the West and even in this book. One reason is the lack of scientific liberty that prevailed in the former Soviet Union. Another is the Russian language per se, which is not spoken by many western researchers. Even when English abstracts have been available, they have often been too brief for an evaluation of the study. Several studies report on the combined use of conventional and laser therapy. This may be a good clinical set-up, but studies do not always give information about the part played by the laser treatment as such. On the other hand it is claimed that blood irradiation increases microcirculation in pathologial tissues, thus improving the uptake and efficacy of traditional pharmaceuticals.

In recent years many Russian studies have been presented in English-language publications and in the proceedings of international congresses. The reports on the parameters are often incomplete and references are made to Russian studies, getting us back to the old language problem again.

The above may appear to present a rather negative opinion of the Russian literature. But that is not the case; it is only a description of some of the problems. Looking at things from the positive side, some of the very best scientific studies in the literature come from Russia and have for many years been published in English. The extensive research of the Tiina Karu group is one example of excellent research quality.

Even though there are shortcomings in the Russian literature, we can certainly state that this is also the case in the Western literature. And glancing through the Russian literature in the available abstract form, one can find a lot of innovative thinking. It is suggested that researchers find a concept of evaluating and publishing the vast Russian experience, to the benefit of everyone in the field of laser therapy. The lack of Russian research material in this book stems simply from our admitted ignorance.

The majority of the Russian studies are performed with HeNe or GaAs 890 nm. Blood irradiation can be performed in several ways:

- HeNe, usually 2-10 mW, is used intravenously for 30-60 minutes.
- HeNe or GaAs can be used to irradiate small volumes of blood extracorporally before reinfusing.
- GaAs irradiating transcutaneously at well vascularised areas.

In the following "menu" we present, as an appetiser and a fountain for inspiration, a number of indications found after a superficial search in the Russian/Ukranian language literature. The number of studies found within each indication is presented within brackets. * marks vascular irradiation directly into the blood or through the dermis.

An indication of particular interest is the rheological modification of blood through laser irradiation. Preliminary research indicates that laser-modified blood can be stored longer and can even be revitalised before use after storage. This could have an important impact on the blood donor situation. [987, 988, 989, 990, 998, 1013]

Interest in blood irradiation has spread to the West. The following study is an example:

Indication	Vascular	Studies
Acute calculous pyelonephritis	*	(1)
Acute pneumonia	*	(2)
Asthma		(6)
Bilateral destructive pneumonia	*	(1)
Biliary dyskinesia		(1)
Bronchical obstructive diseases	*	(1)
Climacterial disorders		(2)
Chronic cystitis and urethritis		(2)
Chronic glomerulonephritis		(1)
Chronic prostatitis		(1)
Circulatory encephalopathy	*	(1)
Diabetic angiopathies	*	(4)
Drug resistant forms of schizophrenia	*	(2)
Dystrophic diseases of the vulva		(1)
Epididymitis		(2)
Genital inflammation		(1)
Glaucoma		(1)
Hemorrhagic shock	*	(1)
Hepatitis		(1)
Ischemic heart conditions	*	(29)
Lung abscess	*	(1)
Mb Sluder		(1)
Nephritis	*	(1)
Occlusive vascular diseases	*	(1)
OPH gestosis	*	(1)
Pemphigus		(1)
Rheumatoid arthritis	*	(1)
Sinuitis		(3)
Trigeminal neuralgia		(1)
Tuberculosis		(11)
Trombophlebitis		(1)
Tourette's syndrome	*	(1)
Ulcerous colitis	(1)	

Table 13.13: Indication Russian/Ukranian language literature

Literature

Stadler [1031] irradiated human whole blood with 660 nm laser by using fluences between 0 and 5 J/cm^2. The lymphocytes were isolated after irradiation of the whole blood. As a control experiment, lymphocytes were first isolated and then irradiated with the same fluences. Lymphocyte proliferation was significantly higher in samples irradiated in the presence of whole blood compared with lymphocytes irradiated after isolation from whole blood. Free radical and lipid peroxide production also increased significantly when samples were irradiated in the presence of red blood cells. Thus, the reaction of light with haemoglobin seems to be one of the keys to biostimulation.

Further literature: [481, 670, 991-997, 1065]

13.7 The work of Tiina Karu

One of the most impressive scientists in the field of photobiology is Tiina Karu, head of the Laboratory of Laser Biology and Medicine at the Laser Technology Research Centre of the Russian Academy of Sciences, Troitsk, Moscow Region, Russian Federation. She has published or taken part in hundreds of investigations on light interaction with cells. Here follow her publications in this field (omitting all those in Russian, about 100 in all):

[C1] T.I. Karu, G.S. Kalendo, V.S. Letokhov: "Control of RNA synthesis rate in tumour cells HeLa by action of low-intensity visible light of copper laser". Lett. Il Nuovo Cimento 32, (2), 55-59, 1981.

[C2] T.I. Karu, P.G. Kryukov, V.S .Letokhov, Yu.A. Matveetz, V.A. Semchischen: "High quantum yield of photochemical reactions of protoporphyrin-IX induced by powerful ultrashort laser pulses". Applied Physics, 24, 245-247, 1981.

[C3] T.I. Karu, G.S. Kalendo, V.S. Letokhov, V.V. Lobko: "Biostimulation of HeLa cells by low intensity visible light". II Nuovo Cimento D, 1(6), 828-840, 1982.

[C4] T.I. Karu, O.A.Tiphlova, V.S. Letokhov, V.V.L obko: "Stimulation of E.coli growth by laser and incoherent red light". Il Nuovo Cimento D, 2(4), 1138-1144, 1983.

[C5] T.I. Karu, G.S. Kalendo, V.S. Letokhov, V.V. Lobko: "Different responses of proliferating and resting tumour cells to pulsed high repetition rate low-intensity laser light at 271 nm". Laser Chemistry, 1(3), 153-161, 1983.

[C6] T.I. Karu, G.S.Kalendo, V.S.Letokhov, V.V.Lobko: "Biostimulation of HeLa cells by low-intensity visible light. II. Stimulation of DNA and RNA synthesis in a wide spectral range". Il Nuovo Cimento D, 3(2), 308-318, 1984.

[C7] T.I. Karu, G.S.Kalendo, V.S.Letokhov, V.V.Lobko: "Biostimulation of HeLa cells by low intensity visible light. III. Stimulation of nucleic acid synthesis in plateau phase cells". Il Nuovo Cimento D, 3(2), 319-325, 1984.

[C8] T.I. Karu, O.A.Tiphlova, G.E.Fedoseyeva, G.S.Kalendo, V.S.Letokhov, V.V.Lobko, T.S.Lyapunova, N.A.Pomoshnikova, M.N.Meissel: "Biostimulating action of low-intensity monochromatic visible light: is it possible?", Laser Chemistry, 5(1), 19-25, 1984.

[C9] G.E. Fedoseyeva, T.I.Karu, V.S.Letokhov, V.V.Lobko, N.A.Pomoshnikova, T.S.Lyapunova, M.N.Meissel: "Effect of the HeNe laser radiation on the reproduction rate and protein synthesis of the yeasts". Laser Chemistry, 5(1), 27-33, 1984.

[C10] T.I. Karu, V.S.Letokhov: "Biological action of low-intensity monochromatic light in the visible range". In: Laser Photobiology and Photomedicine. Eds.S.Martellucci, A.N.Chester. Plenum Press., N.Y., 1985. pp.57-66.

[C11] T.I. Karu, V.S.Letokhov, V.V.Lobko: "Biostimulation of HeLa cells by low-intensity visible light. IV. Dichromatic irradiation". Il Nuovo Cimento D, 5(6), 483-496, 1985.

[C12] T.I. Karu: "Biological action of low-intensity visible monochromatic light and some medical applications of it". International Congress on Laser in Medicine and Surgery 26-28.06.85. Abstract Book, Ed.by G.Galletti, Monduzzi Editore, Bologna 1985, p.217.

[C13] T. Karu: "Biological action of low-intensity visible monochromatic light and some of its medical applications". In: Laser. Ed.by G.Galletti, Bologna: Monduzzi Editore, 1986, pp.25-29.

[C14] T.I. Karu: "Cell photosensitivity to low intensity visible monochromatic light". Abstr. of 1st European Congress on Photobiology, Grenoble, 1986, p.161.

[C15] N.P. Furzikov, T.I.Karu, V.S.Letokhov, A.A.Belyaev, S.E.Ragimov: "Main products of tissue destruction by XeCl laser radiation". 1st European Congress of Photobiology, (7-12 Sept., 1986), Grenoble, France. Abstract of papers, p.150, 1986.

[C16] T.I. Karu, O.A.Tiphlova, G.G.Lukpanova, I.M.Parkhomenko: "Effect of irradiation with monochromatic visible light on cAMP content in Chinese hamster fibroblasts". Il Nuovo Cimento D., 9(10), 1245-1252, 1987.

[C17] T.I .Karu: "Photobiology of low-power laser effects". Abstr. of First Symposium on Biological Effects, Hazard and Protection from Nonionizing Radiation in Outdoor Applications, 12-15.08.1987, Stockholm, p.7, 1987.

[C18] T.I. Karu: "Photobiological fundamentals of low-power laser therapy". IEEE J.Quantum Electronics, QE-23 (10) 1703-1717, 1987.

[C19] T.I. Karu, L.V.Pyatibrat, G.S.Kalendo: "Biostimulation of HeLa cells by low-intensity visible light. V. Stimulation of cell proliferation in vitro by HeNe laser radiation". Il Nuovo Cimento D. 9(12), 1485-1494, 1987.

[C20] T.I. Karu, O.A.Tiphlova: "Stimulation of E.coli WP2 growth by low-intensity visible light". Photochem. Photobiol., 45 Suppl p.95S, 1987.

[C21] N.K .Smolyaninova, G.E.Fedoseyeva, T.I.Karu, A.V.Zelenin: "Human lymphocyte chromatin changes following irradiation with HeNe laser". Abstr. of 2nd European Photobiol. Congress, 6-10.09.87, Padova, C-116, p.122, 1987.

[C22] N.P. Furzikov, T.I.Karu, V.S.Letokhov, A.A.Belyaev, S.E.Ragimov: "Relative efficiency and products of atherosclerotic plaque by pulsed laser radiation". Lasers in the Life Sci., 1(4), 265-274, 1987.

[C23] T.I. Karu, L.V.Pyatibrat, N.P.Furzikov: "Photosentized inactivation of HeLa cells by phtalocyanins". Abstr. of 2nd European Congress on Photobiology. 6-10.09.87., Padova, C-79, 1987.

[C24] T.I. Karu, G.S.Kalendo: "Response of plateau-phase HeLa cells to low-intensity pulsed and continuous-wave UV light near 270 nm". Abstr. of 2nd European Congress on Photobiology, 6-10.09.87, Padova, C-98, p.111, 1987.

[C25] O.A. Tiphlova, T.I.Karu, N.P.Furzikov: "Lethal and mutagenic action of XeCl laser radiation on E.coli". Abstr. of 2nd European Photobiol. Congress, 6-10.09.87, Padova, C-19, 1987.

[C26] T.I. Karu: "Molecular mechanism of the therapeutic effect of low-intensity laser radiation". Lasers in Life Sciences, 2(1), 53-74, 1988.

[C27] T.I. Karu: "Photobiological fundamentals of low-power laser therapy". Abstr. of International Conf. on Photodynamic Therapy and Medical Laser Applications, 19-21.07.88, London, Abstr. N- 282, 1988.

[C28] T.I. Karu "Photobiological basis of laser biostimulation". Proc. of 10th Intern.Conf. "IEEE Engineering in Medicine" 4-7.11.88, New Orleans, p.34-35, 1988.

[C29] T.I. Karu: "Fundamentals of low-power laser photomedicine". In: Laser Science and Technology; Eds. A.N.Chester, V.S.Letokhov, C.Martellucci, New York: Plenum Press, p.217-232, 1988.

[C30] G.E. Fedoseyeva, T.I.Karu, T.S.Lyapunova, N.A.Pomoshnikova, M.N.Meissel: "The activation of yeast metabolism with HeNe laser radiation. I.Protein synthesis in variations cultures". Lasers in the Life Sciences, 2(2), 137-146, 1988.

[C31] G.E. Fedoseyeva, T.I.Karu, T.S.Lyapunova, N.A.Pomoshnikova, M.N.Meissel: "The activation of yeast metabolism with HeNe laser radiation. II.Activity of enzymes of oxidative and phosphorous metabolism". Lasers in the Life Sciences, 2(2), 147-154, 1988.

[C32] T.I. Karu, G.E.Fedoseyeva, T.S.Lyapunova, N.A.Pomoshnikova, M.N.Meissel: "Activation of yeast metabolism with HeNe laser radiation". Photochem.Photobiol., 47 Suppl, p.14S, 1988.

[C33] O.A.Tiphlova, T.I.Karu: "Escherichia coli growth stimulation by low-intensity monochromatic visible light". Photochem.Photobiol., 47, 467-473, 1988.

[C34] G.E.Fedoseyeva, N.K.Smolyaninova, T.I.Karu, A.V.Zelenin: "Human lymphocyte chromatin changes following irradiation with a HeNe laser". Lasers in the Life Sciences, 2(3), 197-205, 1988.

[C35] O.A.Tiphlova, T.I.Karu, N.P.Furzikov: "Lethal and mutagenic action of XeCl laser radiation on E.coli". Lasers in the Life Sciences, 2(2), 155-159, 1988.

[C36] T.I.Karu, L.V.Pyatibrat, G.S.Kalendo: "Photosensitized inactivation of HeLa tumor cells by phtalocyanines". Abstr. on Intern. Congress on Photodynamics Therapy and Medical Laser Applications, 19-21.07.88, London, Abstr.116, 1988.

[C37] T.I. Karu: "Photobiology of low-power laser effects". Health Physics, 56(5), p.691-704, 1989.

[C38] T.I.Karu: “Photobiology of Low-Power Laser Therapy”. Chur, London, Paris, New York: Harwood Academic Publishers, 1989, 185 pages.

[C39] O.A. Tiphlova, T.I.Karu: "Role of primary photoacceptors in low-power laser effects: action of HeNe laser radiation on the bacteriophage T4-Escherichia coli interaction". Lasers in Surgery and Medicine, 9(1), 67-69, 1989.

[C40] T.I. Karu, T.P.Ryabykh, G.E.Fedoseyeva, N.I.Puchkova: "Induced by HeNe laser radiation respiratory burst on phagocytic cells". Lasers in Surgery and Medicine, 9(6), 585-588, 1989.

[C41] T.I. Karu: "Laser biostimulation: a photobiological phenomenon". J.Photochem. Photobiol., 3(4), 638-640, 1989.

[C42] T. Karu, I.Parkhomenko, G.Lukpanova: "Effect of irradiation with monochromatic visible light on cAMP content in Chinese hamster fibroblasts". Abstr. of 3rd Congress of the European Society for Photobiology, 27.08.-09.89., Budapest, p.146 (Abstr. C-70), 1989.

[C43] O.Tiphlova, T.Karu: "Effects of substrates and irradiation with monochromatic visible light on Escherichia coli division rate". Abstr. of 3rd Congress of the European Society for Photobiology, 27-08.-2.09.89., Budapest, p.300 (Abstr. P-121), 1989.

[C44] T.I. Karu: "Photobiological fundamentals of low-power laser therapy". Abstr. of 8th Congress of International Society for Laser Surgery and Medicine, Taipei, 8-11 Nov., 1989.

[C45] T. Karu: "Photobiochemistry of low-power laser therapy". In: Laseres y reacciones quimicas. Universidad Complutense de Madrid: El Escorial 1989, p.179-195.

[C46] O. Tiphlova, T.Karu: "Reduction by visible light on Escherichia coli respiratory chain acts upon the division of bacterial cells and infection of phage into host cell". Photochem.Photobiol., 51 Suppl p.1S (Abstr. SAM-A 2), 1990.

[C47] T. Karu, O.Tiphlova, M.Samokhina, C.Diamantopoulos, V.Sarantsev, V.Schveikin: "Effects of near infrared laser and superluminuous diode irradiation on Escherichia coli". IEEE J.Quantum Electr., QE-26(12), 2162-2165, 1990.

[C48] T. Karu: "Effects of visible radiation on cultured cells". Photochem. Photobiol., 52(6), 1089-1099, 1990.

[C49] T. Karu: "Irradiation with low-intensity laser light of lymphocytes and splenocytes". Programme and abstr. of First Meeting of the International Laser Therapy Association (Naha City, Okinawa, Japan), Oct.26-27, 1990, p.58.

[C50] T.I. Karu, O.A.Tiphlova: "Regulation of cellular metabolism with low-intensity monochromatic visible light". Proc. SPIE. 1990; Vol 1353: 68-78

[C51] T .Karu, G.Kalendo, L.Pyatibrat: "On the role of cells attachment and spreading in biostimulation effects". Lasers in the Life Sci., 3(3), 229-232, 1990.

[C52] T. Karu "Photostimulation". J.Photochem.Photobiol. B, 8, 120, 1990.

[C53] T.I. Karu: "Stimulation of metabolic processes by low-intensity visible light: a scientific basis for biostimulation". In: Laser Application in Biology and Medicine, Vol5,Ed.by M.Wolbarsht, Plenum Press, New York, pp.1-47, 1991.

[C54] N.K. Smolyaninova, T.I.Karu, G.E.Fedoseyeva, A.V.Zelenin: "Effect of HeNe laser irradiation on chromatin properties and nucleic acids synthesis of human blood lymphocytes". Biomedical Sciences, 2, 121-126, 1991.

[C55] T. Karu: "Effects of visible (laser) radiation on cultured cells". In: Laser Systems for Photobiology and Photomedicine, Eds. S.Martellucci, A.N.Chester. New York: Plenum Press. pp.89-113, 1991.

[C56] E.V. Kutomkina, T.I.Karu, H.S.Mushegian, V.I.Duda: "He-Ne laser induced germination of endospores of Anaerobacter polyendosporus". Lasers in the Life Sciences , 4(3) 147-152, 1991.

[C57] T. Karu, N.Smolyaninova, A.Zelenin: "Long-term and short-term responses of human lymphocytes to HeNe laser radiation". Lasers in the Life Sciences, 4(3), 167-178, 1991.

[C58] O. Tiphlova, T.Karu: "Action of low-intensity laser radiation on Escherichia coli". CRC Critical Reviews in Biomedical Engineering, 18(6), 387-412, 1991.

[C59] O. Tiphlova, T.Karu: "Dependence of Escherichia coli growth rate on irradiation with HeNe laser and growth substrates". Lasers in the Life Sci., 4(3), 161-166,1991.

[C60] T. Karu: "Low-intensity laser light action upon fibroblasts and lymphocytes". In: Progress in Laser Therapy. Ed. by T.Ohshiro, R.G.Calderhead; J.Wiley and Sons: Chichester, New York, Brisbane, Toronto, Singapore, 1991, pp.175-180.

[C61] T. Karu: "Photobiological fundamentals of low-power laser therapy". Abstract of European Quantum Electronics Conference and 10th National Quantum Electronics Conference, 27-30 Aug., 1991, Edinburgh, Technical Digest, p.208.

[C62] T.I. Karu, O.A.Tiphlova, Yu.A.Matveyets, A.P.Yartsev, V.S.Letokhov: "Comparison of the effects of visible femtosecond laser pulses and continuous wave laser radiation of low average intensity on the clonogenicity of Escherichia coli". J.Photochem. Photobiol. B: Biol., 10, 339-344, 1991.

[C63] T. Karu, E.Kutomkina, P.Balaban, V.Letokhov, R.Esenaliev, N.Ovcharenko, A.Oraevsky: "Stimulation of single identifiable neurons of Helix pomatia with HeNe laser radiation". Photochem.Photobiol., 53 Suppl, 112S, 1991.

[C64] T.I.Karu, N.K.Smolyaninova, A.V.Zelenin: "Irradiation of human lymphocytes with HeNe laser. I. Increase the blasttransformation caused by phytohemagglutinin". Laser and Technology, 1(2), 51-54, 1991.

[C65] T.I.Karu, N.K.Smolyaninova, A.V.Zelenin: "Irradiation of human lymphocytes with HeNe laser. II. Absence of expression of interleukin-2 receptors". Laser and Technology, 1(3), 99-101, 1991.

[C66] V.M.Manteifel, T.I.Karu: "Ultrastructural changes in human lymphocytes under HeNe laser radiation". Lasers in the Life Sciences, 4(4), 235-248, 1992.

[C67] P.Balaban, R.Esenaliev, T.Karu, E.Kutomkina, V.Letokhov, A.Oraevsky, N.Ovcharenko: "He-Ne laser irradiation of single identified neurons". Lasers in Surgery and Medicine, 12(3), 329-337, 1992.

[C68] T. Karu: "Derepression of the genome after irradiation of human lymphocytes with HeNe laser". Laser Therapy, 4(1), 5-24, 1992.

[C69] T. Karu, N.Smolyaninova, A.Zelenin: "Irradiation of human lymphocytes with HeNe laser increases the blast transformation caused by phytohemagglutinin". Chinese Journal of Lasers, 1(1), 89-92, 1992.

[C70] T. Karu, O. Tiphlova, Yu. Matveyets, A. Yartsev, V. Letokhov: "Local pulsed heating of light-absorbing microregions as a possible mechanism of low-power laser effects". Photochem. Photobiol., 55 Suppl, p.38S-39S, 1992.

[C71] V. Manteifel, T. Karu: "Ultrastructural changes in human lymphocytes under HeNe laser radiation". Lasers Surg. Medicine, Suppl 4, p.10 (Abst. No 32), 1992.

[C72] T. Karu: "Derepression of the genome after irradiation of human lymphocytes with HeNe laser". Abstracts of International Conference "Photodynamic Therapy and Medical Laser Applications", Milan, 25th-27th June 1992.

[C73] T.I. Karu, T.N.Andreichuk, T.P. Ryabykh: "Correlation between composition of spleen and changes in chemiluminescence of the splenocytes after diode laser irradiation". Absrtracts of International Conference "Photodynamic Therapy and Medical Laser Applications", Milan, 25th-27th June 1992.

[C74] T. Karu: "Fundamentals of interaction of visible and near infrared low-intensity laser radiation with cells". Abstract Book of 3rd World Congress of International Society for Low Power Laser Applications in Medicine, Bologna, 9th-13th September, 1992. Ed.by G. Galletti, L. Bolognani, G. Ussia. Monduzzi Editore, Bologna, 1992, p. 61.

[C75] T. Karu: "Local pulsed heating of absorbing chromophores as a possible primary mechanism of low-power laser effects". Abstract Book 3rd World Congress of International Society for Low-Power Laser Applications in Medicine, Bologna, 9th-12th September, 1992. Ed.by G. Galletti, L. Bolognani. Monduzzi Editore, Bologna, 1992, p.69.

[C76] V.M. Manteifel, T.I. Karu: "Ultrastructural changes in human lymphocytes under HeNe laser radiation". Abstract Book of 3rd World Congress of International Society for Low-Power Laser Applications in Medicine, Bologna, 9th-12th September, 1992. Ed.by G. Galletti, L. Bolognani, G. Ussia. Monduzzi. Editore, 1992, p.72.

[C77] T. Karu, T. Andreichuk, T. Ryabykh: "Correlation between cellular composition of spleen and changes in chemiluminescence of the splenocytes after diode laser irradiation". In: Photodynamic Therapy and Biomedical Lasers. Ed. by Spinelli, M. Dal Fante, R. Marchesini, Elsevier, Amsterdam, 1992, pp. 175-180.

[C78] T. Karu: "Should a PDT protocol certainly contain an experiment "light only?" " J.Photochem. Photobiol.: B, 16 (3-4), 385-387, 1992.

[C79] T. Karu: "Fundamentals of interaction of visible and near infrared low-intensity laser radiation with cells." In: Laser Application in Medicine and Surgery. Ed.by G. Galletti, L. Bolognani, G. Ussia. Monduzzi Editore: Bologna, 1992, pp.203-212.

[C80] T. Karu: "Local pulsed heating of absorbing chromophores as a possible primary mechanism of low-power laser effects". In: Laser Applications in Medicine and Surgery. Ed.by G. Galletti, L Bolognani, G. Ussia, Monduzzi Editore: Bologna, 1992, pp. 253-258.

[C81] T. Karu, L. Pyatibrat, G. Kalendo, N. Serebryakov: "Changes in ATP level of HeLa cells cultured in vitro after HeNe laser irradiation". Abstracts of 2nd International Congress of ILTA, London, 18th-20th September, 1992, p.49.

[C82] T. Karu: "Specificity of laser activation of neurons and immune system components". Abstracts of 2nd International Congress of ILTA, London, 18th-20th September, 1992, p.48.

[C83] T.Karu, T.Andreichuk, T.Ryabykh: "Changes in oxidative metabolism of murine spleen following diode laser (660-950nm) irradiation: effect of cellular composition and radiation parameters". Lasers Surg. Medicine, 13(4) 453-462, 1993.

[C84] T.Karu: "Can cellular responses to continuous-wave and pulsed UV radiation differ?". In: Environmental UV Photobiology, Ed. by A.R.Young L.O.Bjorn, J.Moan, and W.Nultsch, Plenum Publ., New York, 1993, pp. 203-232.

[C85] T.Karu, T.Andreichuk, T.Ryabykh: "Suppression of human blood chemiluminescence by diode laser radiation at wavelength 660, 820, 880 or 950 nm". Laser Therapy, 5 (3), 103-109,1993.

[C86] T.I.Karu, E.V.Kutomkina, N.A.Pomoshnikova: "The activation of yeast metabolism with HeNe laser radiation. III. Protein synthesis in Saccharomycodes ludwigii grown in aerobic and anaerobic conditions". Lasers in the Life Sciences, 5 (4), 259-266, 1993.

[C87] T.I.Karu. T.S.Lyapunova, N.A.Pomoshnikova: "The activation of yeast metabolism with HeNe laser radiation. IV. Relationship between the activity of catalase and stimulation of protein synthesis". Lasers in the Life Sciences, 5 (4), 251-258, 1993.

[C88] T.I.Karu: " Photobiological fundamentals of low-power laser therapy". Abstr. of 2nd Intern. Conference on Lasers and their Applications, 23-26 Aug. 1993, Tehran, Tehran: Atomic Energy Org. of Iran, 1993, p.117.

[C89] T.Karu: "Two-quantum photodecomposition of photoporphyrin IX can offer a new approach to photomedicine". Photodermatology, Photoimmunology and Photomedicine, December,1993.

[C90] T.Karu: "Photostimulation (Laser biostimulation)". J.Photochem. Photobiol., B: Biology, 22 (1), 85-86,1994.

[C91] T.Karu, V.Letokhov: "Possible benefits of two-quantum excitation in ALA-PDT?" J. Photochem. Photobiol., B: Biology, 23 (2-3), 261-262, 1994.

[C92] V.M.Manteifel, T.N.Andreichuk, T.I.Karu: "Influence of HeNe laser radiation and phytohemagglutinin on the ultrastructure of chromatin of human lymphocytes". Laser in the Life Sciences, 6 (1), 1-8, 1994.

[C93] T.Karu, L.Pyatibrat, G.Kalendo: "Irradiation with HeNe laser can influence the cytotoxic response of HeLa cells to ionizing radiation". Int. J. Radiation Biology, 65 (6), 691-697, 1994.

[C94] T.Karu, O.Tiphlova, R.Esenaliev, V.Letokhov "Two different mechanisms of low-intensity laser photobiological effects on Escherichia coli". J. Photochem. Photobiol. B: Biology, 24 (3), 155-161, 1994.

[C95] T.Karu: "Comparison between one and two-quantum photodecomposition of protoporphyrin, an endogenous photosensitizer induced by exogenous treatment with 5-aminolevulinic acid".Laser Surg. Medicine, Suppl 6, p. 42 (abstr. N= 221), 1994.

[C96] T.Karu, A.Kurchikov, V.Letokhov, V.Mokh: "Patch-clamp study of action of HeNe laser irradiation on ionic currents in cell membrane." Photochem. Photobiol. 53 (Special Issue), p. 33S, 1994 (abstr. SPM-H24).

[C97] V.Manteifel, L.Bakeeva, T.Karu: "Ultrastructural changes in mitochondria of human lymphocytes after irradiation with HeNe laser: Formation of giant mitochondria". Laser Therapy, 6 (1), 20-21, 1994.

[C98] T.Karu, L.Pyatibrat, R.Esenaliev: "Irradiation with monochromatic visible (laser) light increases cells adhesion: action spectrum". Laser Therapy, 6, 19, 1994.

[C99] T.Karu: "Action of pulsed visible and near IR laser irradiation on oxidative metabolism of cells evaluated by chemiluminescence measurements". Laser Therapy, 6, 18, 1994.

[C100] T.Karu, L.Pyatibrat, G.Kalendo: "Irradiation with HeNe laser increases ATP level in cells cultivated in vitro". J. Photochem. Photobiology B: Biology, 27(3), 219-223,1995.

[C101] T.Karu: "Interaction of monochromatic visible light and near infrared radiation with cells: currently discussed mechanisms". "Laser-Tissue Interaction VI". Ed. by S.L.Jacques, A. Katzir. Proc SPIE. 1995; Vol 2391: 576-586..

[C102] T.I.Karu, T.N.Andreichuk, T.P.Ryabykh: "On the action of semiconductor laser radiation (820 nm) on the chemiluminescence of blood of clinically healthy humans". Lasers in the Life Sciences, 6(4), 277-282, 1995.

[C103] T.Karu, L.Pyatibrat, G.Kalendo: "Increase in adhesion of HeLa cells after irradiation with monochromatic visible and near infrared (laser) light: time and wavelength dependences". Lasers in Surgery and Medicine, Suppl 7, p.73, 1995.

[C104] T.P. Ryabykh, T.I. Karu,T.A.Sidorova, Ya.V.Dobrynin: "The evaluation of sensitivity of blast cells in patients with hemoblastoses to antitumor drugs and low-intensity laser radiation by chemiluminescence test". Trk Onkologii Dergisi (Turkish Journal of Onkology), 10 (2), 103, 1995.

[C105] T. Karu: "Stimulation of cellular metabolism by monochromatic visible and near infrared radiation". Book of Abstracts of 6th Congress of the European Society of Photobiology (3-8 Sept. 1995, Cambridge, U.K.), 1995, p.18 (abstract IV-25/01).

[C106] T. Karu: "Pros and cons of low power laser effects". Abstract Book of European Biomedical Optics Week Bios Europe '95 (12-16 Sept. 1995, Barcelona, Spain), 1995, p.178 (abstract 2630-09).

[C107] T. Ryabykh, T. Karu: "Action of pulsed visible and near IR laser radiation on oxidative metabolism of cells evaluated by chemiluminescence measurement". Abstract Book of European Biomedical Optics Week Bios Europe '95 (12-16 Sept. 1995, Barcelona, Spain), 1995, p.179 (abstract 2630-13).

[C108] T. Ryabykh, T. Karu: "Action of pulsed visible and near IR laser radiation on oxidative metabolism of cells evaluated by chemiluminescence measurement". In: Effects of Low Power Light on Biological Systems, T.I.Karu, A.R.Young, eds. Proc SPIE. 1995; Vol 2630: 12-22.

[C109] T. Karu: "Mechanisms of interaction of monochromatic visible light with cells", In: Effects of Low Power Light on Biological Systems, T.I.Karu, A.R.Young, eds., Proc SPIE V.2630, pp. 2-9, 1995.

[C110] T.I.Karu, L.V.Pyatibrat, G.S.Kalendo, R.O.Esenaliev: "Effects of monochromatic low-intensity light and laser irradiation on adhesion of HeLa cells in vitro". Lasers in Surgery and Medicine, 18(2), 171-177, 1996.

[C111] T.Karu: "Activation of metabolism of nonphotosynthesizing microorganisms with monochromatic visible (laser) light:A critical review". Lasers in the Life Sciences, 7(1), 11-34, 1996.

[C112] T.I.Karu, T.P.Ryabykh, T.A.Sidorova, Ya.V.Dobrynin: "The use of a chemiluminescence test to evaluate the sensitivity of blast cells in patients with hemoblastoses to antitumor agents and low-intensity laser radiation". Lasers in the Life Sciences, 7(1), 1-10, 1996.

[C113] T.Karu, A.Kurchikov, V.Letokhov, V.Mok: "He-Ne laser radiation influences single-channel ionic currents through cell membranes: a patch-clamp study". Lasers in the Life Sciences, 7(1), 35-48,1996.

[C114] T. Karu: "Biophysical basis of low-power laser effects". In: Laser Chemistry, Biophysics, and Biomedicine, V.N. Zadkov, ed. Proc SPIE V. 2802, pp. 142-151, 1996.

[C115] T.I. Karu, T.P.Ryabykh, S.N.Antonov: "Different sensitivity of cells from tumor-bearing organisms to countinuous-wave and pulsed laser radiation, 632.8 nm, evaluated by chemiluminescence test. I. Comparison of responses of murine splenocytes: intact mice and mice with transplanted leukemia EL-4". Lasers in the Life Sciences, 7(2), 91-98, 1996.

[C116] T.I. Karu, T.P.Ryabykh, S.N.Antonov: "Different sensitivity of cells from tumor-bearing organisms to countinuous-wave and pulsed laser radiation ,632.8 nm, evaluated by chemiluminescence test. II. Comparison of responses of human blood: healthy persons and patients with colon cancer". Lasers in the Life Sciences, 7(2), 99-106, 1996.

[C117] L.N.Shliakhova, A.V.Itkes, V.M.Manteifel, T.I.Karu: "Expression of c-myc gene in irradiated at 670 nm human lympocytes. A preliminary report". Lasers in the Life Sciences, 7(2), 107-114, 1996.

[C118] T. Karu, T.Ryabykh, T.Sidorova, Y.Dobrynin: "Evaluation of individual sensitivity of blast cells in patents with hemoblastoses to antitumor agents and low-intensity laser radiation." Laser Therapy, 8 (1), 75-76, 1996.

[C119] L.Shliakhova, A.Itkes, T.Karu: "Accumulation of preliminary terminated proto-oncogene c-myc RNA in irradiated at 670 nm human lymphocytes." Laser Therapy, 8(1), 76, 1996.

[C120] T.Karu: "Interaction of monochromatic visible (laser) light and near infrared radiation with cells." Laser Therapy, 8(1), 14-15, 1996.

[C121] T.Karu: "Derepression of genome and alteration of DNA template activity in nonproliferating cells by means of UV and visible laser radiation In: Biological Optical Instrumentation and Laser-Assisted Biotechnology. Ed. by A.M.Verga Scheggi, S.Martellucci, A.N. Chester and R. Pratesi. Dordrecht, Boston, London: Kluwer Acad. Publ. 1996, pp. 45-62.

[C122] L. Shliakhova, A.Itkes, T.Karu: "Accumulation of preliminary terminated proto-oncogene c-myc RNA in irradiated at 670 nm human lymphocytes." Photochem. Photobiol. 63, Special Issue, May 1996, p.24S (abstr. SPM-F7).

[C123] T. Karu: "Biophysical basis of low-power laser effects." In: Biological Effects of Light. Ed. by M.F. Holick and E.G. Jung. Berlin, New York: Walter de Gruyter, pp. 246-248, 1996.

[C124] T. Karu, L.Pyatibrat, G.Kalendo: "Irradiation with HeNe laser can influence the cytotoxic response of HeLa cells to ionizing radiation." Abstracts of 12th International Congress on Photobiology (Vienna, Sept. 1-6, 1996), p. 240 (abstr. 0176).

[C125] T.I. Karu, T.P.Ryabykh, S.N.Antonov: "Different sensitivity of cells from tumor-bearing organisms to countinuous-wave and pulsed laser radiation, 632.8 nm, evaluated by chemiluminescence test." Abstracts of 12th International Congress on Photobiology (Vienna, Sept. 1-6, 1996), p. 241 (abstr. 0178).

[C126] T.I. Karu, T.P.Ryabykh, S.N.Antonov, V.S. Letokhov: "Different sensitivity of cells from tumor-bearing organisms to countinuous-wave and pulsed laser radiation, 632.8 nm, evaluated by chemiluminescence test." Abstract Book of European Biomedical Optics Week BIOS Europe'96 (Sept. 7-10, 1996, Vienna), p. 91 (abstr. 2929-01).

[C127] V. Manteifel, L.Bakeeva, T. Karu: "Ultrastructural changes in chondriome of human lymphocytes after irradiation with HeNe laser: appearance of giant mitochondria". Abstract Book of European Biomedical Optics Week BIOS Europe '96 (Sept. 7-10, 1996, Vienna), p. 92 (abstr. 2929-04).

[C128] T. Karu, L.Pyatibrat, G.Kalendo: "Irradiation with HeNe laser can influence the cytotoxic response of HeLa cells to ionizing radiation." Abstract Book of European Biomedical Optics Week BIOS Europe'96 (Sept. 7-10, 1996, Vienna), p. 92 (abstr. 2929-06).

[C129] T.I. Karu, T.P.Ryabykh, S.N.Antonov: "Different sensitivity of cells from tumor-bearing organisms to countinuous-wave and pulsed laser radiation, 632.8 nm, evaluated by chemiluminescence test". In: Effects of Low-Power Light on biological Systems II, G.Jori, T.I.Karu, eds., Proc SPIE Vol 2929, pp. 2-11, 1996.

[C130] V. Manteifel, L.Bakeeva, T. Karu: "Ultrastructural changes in chondriome of human lymhocytes after irradiation with HeNe laser: appearance of giant mitochondria". In: Effects of Low-Power Light on biological Systems II, G.Jori, T.I.Karu, eds., Proc SPIE Vol 2929, pp. 18-26, 1996.

[C131] T.I .Karu, L.Pyatibrat, G.Kalendo: "Irradiation with HeNe laser can influence the cytotoxic response of HeLa cells to ionizing radiation." In: Effects of Low-Power Light on biological Systems II, G.Jori, T.I.Karu, eds., Proc SPIE Vol 2929, pp. 38-46, 1996.

[C132] V. Manteifel, L.Bakeeva, T. Karu: "Ultrastructural changes in chondriome of human lymhocytes after irradiation with HeNe laser: appearance of giant mitochondria". Journal of Photochemistry and Photobiology, B: Biology. 38 (1), 25-30, 1997.

[C133] T.I. Karu, T.P.Ryabykh, V.S.Letokhov: "Different sensitivity of cells from tumor-bearing organisms to countinuous-wave and pulsed laser radiation, 632.8 nm, evaluated by chemiluminescence test. III. Effect of dark period between pulses." Lasers in the Life Sciences, 7 (3), 141-156, 1997.

[C134] T. Karu, L. Pyatibrat, T.Ryabykh: "Nonmonotonic behavior of the dose dependence of the radiation effect on cells in vitro exposed to pulsed laser radiation at 820 nm." Lasers in Surgery and Medicine, Suppl 9, p. 6, 1997 (abstr. 23).

[C135] T. Karu: "Photobiological mechanisms of cells photostimulation". Abstracts of 7th Congress of the European Society for Photobiology, Stresa, Italy, 8-13 Sept. 1997, p. 31 (abstr. S76).

[C136] T. Karu, N. Afanasyeva, S. Kolyakov, L.Pyatibrat: "Changes in absorption (500-860 nm) of cell monolayer under irradiation with semiconductor lasers at 670 or 820 nm". Abstract Book of BIOS Europe'97 (The European Biomedical Optics Week), 4-8 Sept. 1997, San Remo, Italy, p. 94 (abstr. 3198-01).

[C137] T. Karu, A. Kurchikov, V. Letokhov, V. Mokh: "He-Ne laser radiation influences single channel ionic currents through cell membranes: a patch-clamp study". Abstract Book of BIOS Europe'97 (The European Biomedical Optics Week), 4-8 Sept. 1997, San Remo, Italy, p.97 (abstr. 3198-05).

[C138] T.I. Karu, L.V. Pyatibrat, T.P. Ryabykh: "Nonmonotonic behavior of the dose dependence of the radiation effect on cells in vitro exposed to pulsed laser radiation at 820 nm." Lasers in Surgery and Medicine, 21(5), 485-492 ,1997.

[C139] T. Karu: "Photobiological fundamentals of low-power laser therapy." Proc. of 1st International Congress Laser and Health '97 (Nov. 11-16, 1997, Limassol, Cyprus), pp. 207-210.

[C140] T.I. Karu, T.P.Ryabykh, S.N. Antonov, V.S.Letokhov: "Different sensitivity of cells from tumor-bearing organisms to countinuous-wave and pulsed laser radiation (632.8 nm) evaluated by chemiluminescence test." Internet Journal of Science.

[C141] T. Karu, N. Afanasyeva, S. Kolyakov, L. Pyatibrat: "Changes in absorption (500-860 nm) of cell monolayer under irradiation with semiconductor lasers at 670 or 820 nm". In: Effect of Low Power Light on Biological Systems III, G.Bottiroli, T.Karu, R.Lubart, eds. Proc SPIE Vol 3198, pp 2-11, 1997.

[C142] T. Karu, A. Kurchikov, V. Letokhov, V. Mokh: "He-Ne laser radiation influences single channel ionic currents through cell membranes: a patch-clamp study". In: Effect of Low Power Light on Biological Systems III, G.Bottiroli, T.Karu, R.Lubart, eds. Proc SPIE Vol 3198, pp 57-66, 1997.

[C143] T. : "Low-power laser effects". In: Lasers in Medicine, Ed. by R.Waynant and P.Pettit, New York: Plenum Publ. Co, 1998, Ch.9 (in press).

[C144] T. Karu "The Science of Low Power Laser Therapy." Harwood Acad. Publ., London, 1998.

[C145] V. Manteifel, T.Karu: "Activation of chromatin in T-lymphocytes nuclei under the HeNe laser radiation." Lasers in the Life Sciences, in press.

[C146] T. Karu: "Basics of the action of monochromatic visible and near IR (laser) radiation on cells." In: Proceedings of 2nd International Conference on Bioelectromagnetism. (15-18 Febr. 1998, Melbourne). Ed. by B. Lithgow and J. Cosic. IEEE, 1997, pp. 125-126.

Tiina I. Karu received the diploma in physical chemistry from Tartu University, Tartu, Estonia, in 1970, the Ph.D. degree in photochemistry and chemical carcinogenesis from the National Cancer Research Center, Moscow,

U.S.S.R., in 1974, and the Doc.Sci. in biophysics from the U.S.S.R. Acadamy of Science, Leningrad, in 1990. Over the last 20 years, her main scientific interests have been in the field of laser light-tissue interactions. She has authored two books (Photobiology of Low Power Laser Therapy, 1989 and The Science of Low Power Laser Therapy, 1998) and approximately 200 papers. Since 1980, she has been the Head of the Laboratory of Laser Biology and Medicine, Laser Technology Research Center, Institute of Laser and Informatic Technologies, Russian Academy of Sciences, Moscow, Russia.

13.8 English language books on laser therapy:

1 Wolbarsht M L. (1977). Laser Applications in Medicine and Biology. Vol 3. 4.3. ISBN 0-306-37163-4 (v. 3). Plenum Press. New York, USA.

2 LASER. (1986). Proceedings of the International Congress on Laser in Medicine and Surgery. Bologna June 26-28, 1985. Edited by G. Galletti. Monduzzi Editore S.p.A, via Ferrarese 119/2, IT-40128 Bologna, Italy.

3 Ohshiro T. and Calderhead R G. (1988): Low Level Laser Therapy: A Practical Introduction. ISBN 0-471-91956-X. John Wiley & Sons, Chichester, England.

4 Colls J. Laser Therapy Today. 84-398-6137-0.

5 Kert J, Rose L. (1989). Clinical Laser Therapy. ISBN 87-983204-1-6. Scandinavian Medical Laser Technology, Copenhagen, Denmark.

6 Karu T. (1989). Photobiology of Low-Power Laser Therapy (Laser Science and Technology. ISBN: 3718649705. Harwood Academic Publ.

7 Goldman L. (1991): Laser Non-Surgical Medicine: New Challenges for an Old Application. ISBN 87762-792-4. Technomic Publishing Co, USA.

8 Wolbarsht M L. (1991). Laser Applications in Medicine and Biology. Vol 5. (See espec. chapter 1). ISBN 0-306-43753-8 (v. 5). Plenum Press. NY, USA.

9 Ohshiro T. (1991). Low Reactive-Level Laser Therapy: Practical Application. ISBN 0-471-92845-3. John Wiley & Sons, Chichester, England.

10 Ohshiro T, Calderhead R G. (1991). Progress in Laser Therapy. Selected Papers from the October 1990 ILTA Congress. ISBN 0-471-93154-3. John Wiley & Sons, Chichester, England.

11 Galletti G. (1992). Laser Applications in Medicine and Surgery. Monduzzi Editore S.p.A, via Ferrarese 119/2, IT-40128 Bologna, Italy.

12 Pöntinen P. (1992). Low level laser therapy as a medical treatment modality. ISBN 951-96632-0-7. Art Urpo Ltd, Tampere, Finland. www.prima-books.com.

13 Baxter G D. (1994). Therapeutic Lasers. Theory and practice. ISBN 0-443-04393-0. Churchill Livingstone, England.

14 Hajder D. (1994). Acupuncture and Lasers. 2nd ed. ISBN 86-81979-17-6. DaDa, Sredacka 11, Belgrad, Yugoslavia.

15 Tunér J, Hode L (1996). Laser Therapy in dentistry and medicine. ISBN SE 91-630-4078-6. Prima Books of Sweden.

16 van Breugel H. (1997). Laser Therapy in medical practice. ISBN 90-6523-048-3. Van den Boogaard Publishing, Oisterwijk, The Netherlands.

17 Karu T. (1998). The science of low power laser therapy. ISBN 90-5699-108-6. The Gordon and Breach Publishing Group.

18 Brugnera Junior A, Luiz B Pinheiro A. (1998). Lasers na Odontologia Moderna. ISBN 85-86266-09-4. Pancast Editora, São Paulo, Brazil.

19 Tunér J, Hode L. Low Level Laser Therapy, clinical practice and scientifick background. (1999). Prima Books in Sweden. ISBN 91-630-7616-0.

20 Lasers in Medicine and Dentistry. Basic science and up-to-date clinical application of low energy-level laser therapy, laser therapy. (2000): Ed: Simunovic Z. Laxxus AG, Freienbach, Switzerland. ISBN 953-6059-30-4.

21 Bjordal J M, Johnson M I, Couppè C. (2001). Clinical Electrotherapy. Your guide to optimal treatment. Høyskoleforlaget. Norwegian Academic Press. ISBN 82-7634-320-1.

13.9 Books in other languages, with ISBN.

Colls J. La Terapía Láser Hoy. 84-398-1811-4.

Trelles M A. Láser para la salud y la estética. 85667-02-6.

Trelles M A. Soft Láser Terapía. 84-300-7068-0.

Matura L. Lasertherapia - esperienze cliniche riabilative. 88-7449-137-9.

Longo L. Terapia Laser. 88-03-00185-9.

Fornezza U. (1986). Il laser in terapia e chirurgia - principi teorici e applicativi (Lasers in therapy and surgery. Theoretical and practical principles). English and Italian text. ISBN 88-85037-99-2. Cortina International, Verona, Italy de Cuyper H. Het Gebruik van Laser in de Fysiotherapie. 90-352-1008-5.

Danhof G. (1994). Lasertherapie in de tandheelkundige praktijk. (in Dutch) ISBN 90-6523-08-0. Uitgeverij Stubeg bv, Hoogezand, The Netherlands.

Popp F A. Biologie des Lichtes. 3-489-61734-7.

Bahn, Klima, Bischko. Laser und. Infratorstrahlen in der Akupunktur. 3-7760-0962-4.

Lievens P C. Laser-Thérapie. Théorie et applications pratiques. 2-87671-037-4.

Redureaux D. Le Laser. Application en physiothérapie. 2-224-01100-8.

Nogier R. Précis Pratique de Laserthérapie en Odontostomatologie.

Coche P. (1985). L'energie douce face à la doleur. ISBN 2-905692-00-6. Ateim, 8, rue Reyer, Toulouse, France.

Pöntinen P. Laser in der Akupunktur. 3-7773- 1019-0.

Danhof G. Lasertherapie in der Sportmedizin und Orthopädie. 3-921988-52-7.

Ambronn G. Laser- under Magnetfeld-terapie in der Tiermedizin. 3-334-60855-7.

Iliev E. (1988). Soft-laser in der Dermatologie. Edition Svesa, München, Germany. ISBN 3-927406-00-7.

Elias J. Akupunktur und Lasertherapie für die Praxis. 3925367-53-5.

Koebner K. LASER - von tödlichen zum heilenden Strahl. 3-921608-59-7.

Danhof G. (1991). Lasertherapie in der Allgemeinmedizin. WBV Biologisch-Medizinische Verlagsgesellschaft mbH & Co KG. DE-7060 Schorndorf, Germany. ISBN 3-921988-50-0

Danhof G. (1995). Lasertherapie in der Zahnheilkunde. ISBN-3-921988-54-3. WBV Biologisch-Medizinische Verlagsgesellschaft Schorndorf.

Pöntinen P. (1988). LASER Lääketieteellisenä hoitomuotona.ISBN 952-90050-9-1. Invarmex OY, Finland.

Kert J, Rose L. (1989). Klinisk laserbehandling.ISBN 87-983204-0-8. Scandinavian Medical Laser Technology. Copenhagen, Denmark.

Pöntinen P. (1991). Lågeffektslasern som medicinsk vårdform. 91-7736-267-4. Prima Books, Sweden.

Tunér J, Hode L. (1995). Lågeffektslaser inom odontologin. ISBN 91-971969-1-6. Swedish Laser-Medical Society, Stockholm, Sweden.

Tunér J, Hode L, Diklic S. (1996). Osnove primene lasera u medicini. Irradia DOO, Gavrila Principa 53, Sremska Kamenica, Yugoslavia.

13.10 Laser journals

Laser Therapy - an International Journal of Low Level Laser Therapy and Photobioactivation. Official Journal of WALT, The World Association for Laser Therapy. www.walt.nu.

Lasers in Surgery and Medicine. The American Society for Laser Medicine and Surgery. Wiley-Liss, Inc. New York, NY 10158, USA. Occasional laser therapy reports. www.aslms.org

Journal of Clinical Laser Medicine & Surgery. Mary Ann Liebert, Inc., NY, USA. Official publication of International Society for Laser Surgery and Medicine, Academy of Laser Dentistry and International Society for Lasers in Dentistry. Occasional laser therapy studies. www.liebertpub.com/lms

Medical Laser Applications. Urban Fischer Verlag, Berlin, Germany. Occasional laser therapy studies. www.urbanfischer.de.

SPIE - The International Society of Optical Engineering, Bellingham, WA, USA. Large numbers of proceedings reports from conferences, several on medical laser applications. www.spie.org

Laser Partner. Official journal of the Czech Society for the Use of Laser in Medicine. www.laserpartner.org

Laser & Technology. Journal of the European Medical Laser Association. www.emla-laser.com

Chapter 14
References - Abbreviations

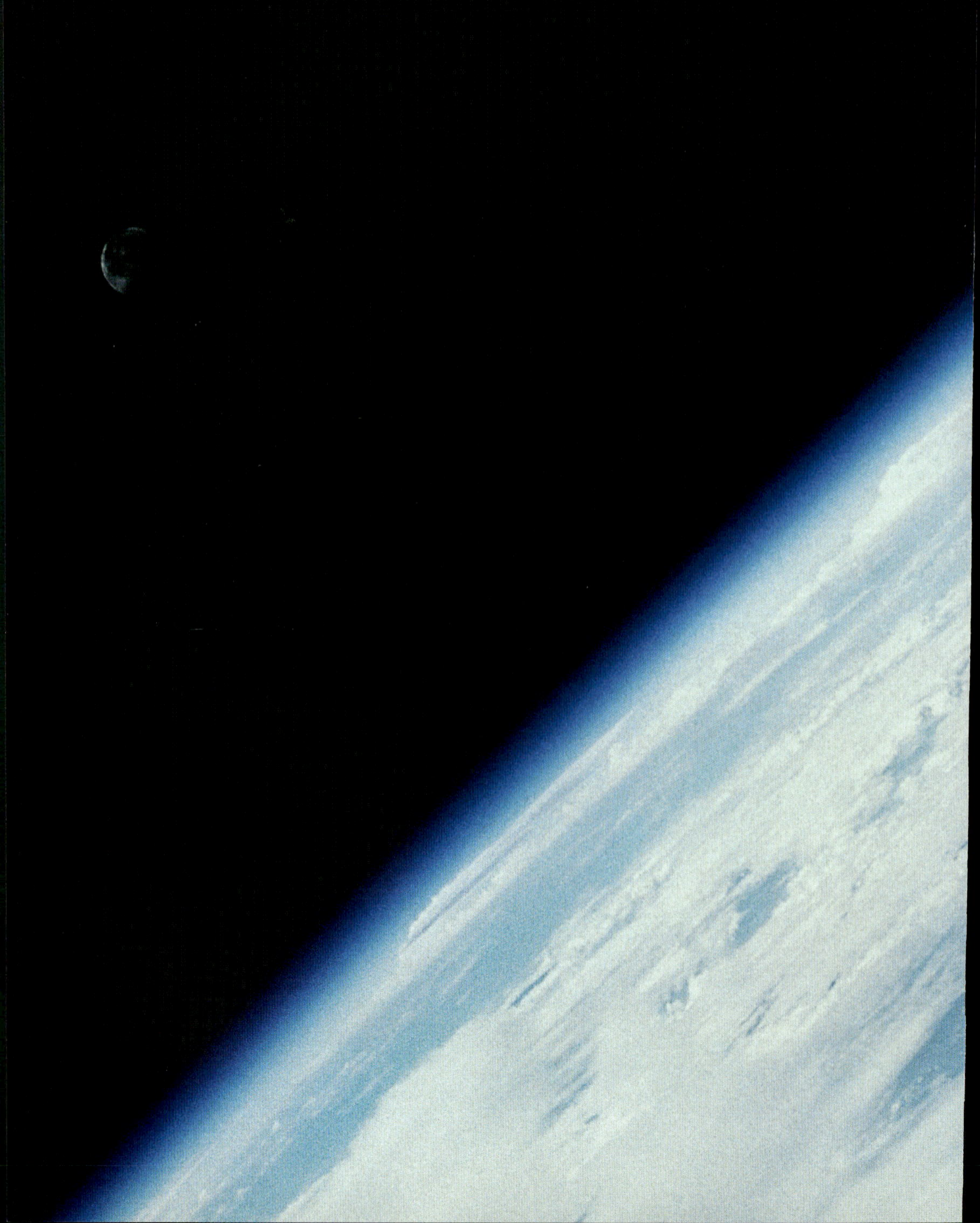

14.1 Numeric references referred to in the book.

[1] Dima F V et al. Doserelated immunological and morphological changes observed in rats with Walker-256 carcinosarcoma after photodynamic therapy: a controlled study. Laser Therapy. 1991; 3 (3): 159-168.

[2] Skobelkin O K et al. Preoperative activation of the immune system by low reactive level laser therapy (laser therapy) in oncologic patient: A preliminary report. Laser Therapy. 1991; 3 (4): 169-176.

[3] Mikhailov V A et al. Investigations on the influence of Low Level Diode Laser irradiation of the growth of experimental tumors. Laser Therapy. 1993; 5 (1): 33-38.

[4] Steinlechner C, Dyson M. The effect of low level laser therapy on the proliferation of keratinocytes. Laser Therapy; 1993; 5 (2): 65-74.

[5] Dyson M, Young S. Effect of Laser Therapy on Wound Contraction and Cellularity in Mice. Lasers in Medical Science. 1986; (1): 125-.

[6] Pedrola M et al. Acute cervical pain relieved with gallium arsenurio (GaAs) laser irradiation. A double blind study. Lasers in Surgery and Medicine.1995, suppl 7, p 10.

[7] Walsh D et al. The effect of low intensity laser irradiation upon conduction and skin temperature in the superficial radial nerve. Double blind placebo controlled investigation using experimental ischaemic pain. Proc. Second Meeting of the International Laser Therapy Association, London Sept 1992.

[8] Abergel P et al. Control of connective tissue metabolism by lasers: Recent developments and future prospects. J Am Acad Dermatol. 1984; 11: 1142-1150.

[9] Saldo I et al. Effects of GaAs-laser combined with radiotherapy on murine sarcoma depends on tumor size. Lasers in Surgery and Medicine. 1989; Suppl. 1:40.

[10] Mester E. et al. Untersuchungen über die hemmende bzw. fördernde Wirkung der Laserstrahlen. Arch Klin Chir. 1968; 322: 1022-.

[11] Mester Andrew, Mester Adam. Scientific background of laser biostimulation. LASER. Journ Eur Med Laser Ass. 1988; 1 (1): 23-.

[12] King P. Low Level Laser Therapy: A Review. Lasers in Medical Science. 1989; 4: 141-.

[13] Bihari I, Mester A. The biostimulative effect of low level laser therapy of long-standing crural ulcer using Helium Neon laser, Helium Neon plus infrared lasers and noncoherent light: Preliminary report of a ran-domized double blind comparative study. Laser Therapy. 1989; 1 (2): 97-102.

[14] Kubota J, Ohshiro T. The effects of diode laser low reactive-level laser therapy (laser therapy) on flap survival in a rat model. Laser Therapy. 1989; 1 (3): 127-134.

[15] Berki T et al. Biological Effect of Low-power Helium-Neon (HeNe) Laser Irradiation. Lasers in Medical Science. 1988; 3: 35-.

[16] Muldiyarov P et al. Effect of Monochromatic Helium-Neon Laser Red Light on the Morphology of Zymosan Arthritis in Rats. Biull Eksp Biol Med. 1983; 1: 55-.

[17] Haina D et al. Animal Experiments on Light-Induced Woundhealing. Biophysica, Berlin. 1973; 35 (3): 227-230.

[18] Calderhead G. Meeting report: Proc Ninth Congress of the International Society for Laser Surgery and Medicine, Anaheim, California, USA: 2-6 November 1991. Laser Therapy. 1992; 4 (1): 43.

[19] Oulamara A et al. Biological activity measurement on botanical specimen surfaces using a temporal decorrelation effect of laser speckle. Journal of Modern Optics. 1989; 36 (2): 165-.

[20] Cherry R. Measurement of Protein Rotational Diffusion in Membranes by Flash Photolysis. Methods in Enzymology. 1978; (54): 47-.

[21] Lubart R, Wollman Y, Friedman H, Rochkind S, Laulicht I. Effects of visible and near-infrared lasers on cell cultures. J. Photochem. Photobiol. B. 1992; 12: 305-310.

[22] Karu T. Photobiological Fundamentals of Low Power Laser Therapy. IEEE Journal of Quantum Electronics. 1987; 23 (10): 1703-.

[23] Mester E et al. Auswirkungen direkter Laserbestrahlung auf menschliche Lymphozyten. Arch Dermatol Res. 1978; 5: 31-.

[24] Dougherty T J. Therapy and detection of malignant tumors. Photochem Photobio. 1987; 45: 879-.

[25] Dougherty T J. Photodynamic therapy. In: Innovations in Radiation Oncology. Withers H, Peters L, eds. Berlin/Heidelberg, Springer-Verlag, 1988, p. 175.

[26] Bossy J et al. In Vitro Survey of Low Energy Laser Beam Penetration in Compact Bone. Faculté de Médecine et CHRU de Nimes, BP 26, 3000 Nimes, France (1985).

[27] Svaasand L. Biostimulering med lav-intensitetslasere. Fysikk eller metafysikk? ["Biostimulation with low intensity laser: Physics o or metaphysics?"] (in Norwegian) Nordisk Medicin. 1990; 103 (3): 72- .

[28] Derr V E et al. Free radical occurrence in some laser-irradiated biologic materials. Federal Proc. 1965; 24 (No 1, Suppl 14): 99-103.

[29] Lubart R et al. A possible Mechanism of Low Level Laser - Living Cell Interaction. Laser Therapy. 1990; 2 (2): 65-68.

[30] Kudoh Ch et al. Effects of 830 nm Gallium Aluminium Arsenide Diode Laser Radiation on Rat Saphenous Nerve Sodium-Potassium-Adenosine Triphosphatase Activity: A Possible Pain Attenuation Mechanism Examined. Laser Therapy. 1989; 1 (2): 63-67.

[31] Nasu F, Tomiyasu K, Inomata K, Calderhead R G. Cytochemical Effects of GaAlAs Diode Laser Radiation on Rat Saphenous Artery Calcium Ion Dependent Adenosine Triphosphatase Activity. Laser Therapy. 1989; 1 (2): 89-92.

[32] Rochkind S, Nissan M, Razon N et al. Electrophysiological Effect of HeNe Laser on Normal and Injured Sciatic Nerve in the Rat. Acta Neurochir. (Vienna). 1986; 83: 125-130.

[33] Karu T et al. Biostimulation of HeLa-cells by low-Intensity Visible Light. Nuovo Cimento. 1982; 1D (6): 828-.

[34] Mester E et al. The Biostimulating Effect of Laser Beam. Proc from Laser - 81, Opto-Elektronik, Munich 1981.

[35] Kovács I et al. Laser-Induced Stimulation of the Vascularization of the Healing Wound. Separatum Experientia. 1974; 30: 341-.

[36] Lederer H et al. Influence of Light on Human Immunocompetent Cells In Vitro. Proc of Laser -81, Opto-Elektronik. Munich, 1981.

[37] Pourreau-Schneider N et al. Helium-Neon Laser Treatment Transforms Fibroblasts into Myofibroblasts. Am J Pathol. 1990; 137: 171-.

[38] Walker J. Relief from Chronic Pain by Low Power Laser Irradiation. Neuroscience Letters. 1983; 43: 339-344.

[39] Rochkind S et al. Systemic Effects of Low-Power Laser Irradiation on the Peripheral and Central Nervous System, Cutaneous Wounds and Burns. Lasers in Surgery and Medicine. 1989; 9: 174-.

[40] Montesinos M. et al. Experimental Effects of Low Power Laser in Encephalin and Endorphin Synthesis. LASER. Journ Eur Med Laser Ass. 1988; 1 (3): 2-7.

[41] Anneroth G, Hall G, Rydén H, Zetterqvist L. The effect of Low-energy infrared laser radiation on woundhealing in rats. Brit J Oral & Max Surg. 1988; 26: 12-17.

[42] Rydén H, Persson L Preber H, Bergström J. Effect of low-energy laser on gingival inflammation. Swedish Dent J. 1990; 14: 47-

[43] Hedner E. Herpes simplex virus type 1 and intraoral wound healing (In Swedish). J of the S D A, 1994, 1: 8-10.

[44] Tamachi Y. Enhancement of antitumor chemotherapy effect by low level laser irradiation. Tokyo Medical College Newsletter; 1991: 888-893.

[45] Lundeberg T, Hode L, Zhou J. A comparative study of the pain-relieving effect of laser treatment and acupuncture. Acta Physiol Scand. 1987; 131: 161-.

[46] Pourreau-Schnedier N et al. Soft-Laser Therapy for Iatrogenic Mucositis in Cancer Patients Receiving High-Dose Fluorouacil: A preliminary report. J Nat Cancer Inst. 1992; 5 84): 358-.

[47] Ciais G et al. La laserthérapie dans la prévention et la traitement des mucities liées à la chimothérapie anticancéreuse. Bull Cancer. 1992; 79: 183-.

[48] Sapiera D et al. Demonstration of elevated type I and type III procollagen mRNA levels in cutaneous wounds treated with helium-neon laser. Biochem Biophys Res Com. l986; 3(138): 1123-1128.

[49] Hatano Y. Lasers in the diagnosis of the TMJ problems. In: Lasers in dentistry. Eds. Yamamoto Y et al. 1989; p. 169-172. Elsevier Science Publishing B.V, Amsterdam

[50] Braverman B et al. Effect of Helium-Neon and Infrared Laser Irrradiation on Wound Healing in Rabbits. Lasers in Surgery and Medicin; 1989; 9: 50-.

[51] David L, Abergel P. Laser for cosmetic surgery. Lasers in Surgery and Medicine. 1989; Suppl 1: 32.

[52] Nara Y et al. Stimulative effect of HeNe laser irradiation on cultured fibroblasts derived from human dental pulp. Lasers in the Life Sciences. 1992; 4 (4): 249-.

[53] Shiroto C et al. Retrospective study of diode laser therapy for pain attenuation in 3635 patients: Detailed analysis by questionnaire. Laser Therapy. 1989; 1(1): 41-.

[54] Mizokami T et al. Effect of diode laser for pain: A clinical study on different pain types. Laser Therapy. 1990; 2 (4): 171-.

[55] Hansen H, Thorøe U. Low power laser biostimulation of chronic orofacial pain. A double-blind placebo controlled cross-over study in 40 patients. Pain. 1990; 43: 169-.

[56] Maricic B et al. Analgetic effect of laser in dental therapy. Acta Stomat Croat. 1987; 21 (4): 291-.

[57] Moore K et al. Double blind crossover trial of low level laser therapy in the treatment of post herpetic neuralgia. Laser Therapy. 1988; (pilot issue): 7-10.

[58] McKibbin L et al. Treatment of post herpetic neuralgia using a 904 nm (infrared) low energy laser: A clinical study. Laser Therapy. 1991; 3 (1): 35-40.

[59] Hong J N, Kim T H, Lim S D. Clinical trial of low reactive-level laser therapy in 20 patients with postherpetic neuralgia. Laser Therapy. 1990; 2 (4): 167-170.

[60] Hachenberger I. Laserstrahlen bei Herpeserkrankungen. Ärztliche Kosmetologie. 1981; 11: 142-.

[61] von Ahlften U et al. Erfahrungen bei der Behandlung aphtöser und herpetiformer Mundschleimhauterkrankungen mit einem neuen Infrarotlaser. Die Quintessenz. 1987; 5: 927-.

[62] Abergel P. Laser treatment of acne scars. Lasers in Surgery and Medicine. 1992; Suppl 4: 70.

[63] Herman J, Khosla R. Nd:YAG laser modulation of synovial tissue metabolism. Clinic Exp Rheumatol. 1989; 7: 505-512.

[64] Guang Hua Wang et al. A study on the analgesic effect of low power HeNe-laser and its mechanism by electrophysiological means. In: Lasers in Dentistry. Excerpta Medica. Elsevier Science Publishers, Amsterdam. 1989: p. 277.

[65] Kaihøj P. Low Level Lasers Effekt på Følsomme Tandhalse - en klinisk pilottest. ["The Effect of Low Level Lasers on Sensitive Toothnecks - a Clinical Pilot Study"] (In Danish). Odont Pract. 1991; 6 (2): 229-.

[66] Wakabayashi H et al. Treatment of dentine hypersensitivity by GaAlAs soft laser irradiation. J Dent Research. 1988; 67: 182-.

[67] Kami T et al. Effect of low-powered diode lasers on flap survival. Ann Plast Surgery. 1985; 14 (3): 278-.

[68] Riendeau F. An in vivo study of the effects of Helium-Neon laser on the breaking force and histological characteristics of wound. Proc Int Congr of Lasers in Dentistry, Tokyo, August 5-6. 1988: p 20.

[69] Soudry M et al. Action d' un laser hélium-néon sur la croissance cellulaire: étude in vitro sur fibro-blastes gingivaux humains. J Biol Buccale. 1988; 16: 129.

[70] Chomette G et al. Effet du soft-laser sur le tissu conjunctif gingival. I - Effet sur les fibroblastes. Étude d'histoenzymologie et de microscopie eléctronique. J Biol Buccale. 1987; 15: 45-.

[71] Chomette G et al. Effet du soft-laser sur le tissu conjunctif gingival. II - Effet sur la cicatrisation. Étude en microscopie optique, histoenzymologie et microscopie électronique. J Biol Buccale. 1987; 15: 57-.

[72] Gretzinger H et al. An in vivo study of the effect of helium-neon laser on human fibroblast migration. Proc Int Congr of Lasers in Dentistry, Tokyo, August 5-6. 1988: p 23.

[73] Mousques T. Étude en double aveugle des effets du traitment unilateral au laser hélium-néon lors de chirurgies parodontales biláterales simultanés. Quest Odontostomatol. 1986; 11: 245-.

[74] Enwemeka C. Laser biostimulation of healing wounds: specific effects and mechanisms of action. J Orthop Sports Physical Therapy. 1988; 9: 333-.

[75] Loevschall H et al. Low Level Laser Irradiation of Human Oral Mucosa Fibroblast in Vitro in Cultures of Human Oral Fibroblasts. Lasers in Surgery and Medicine. 1994; 14: 347-.

[76] Loevschall H et al. Effect of Low Level Diode Laser Effect in Cultures of Human Oral Mucosa. Proc. Second Meeting of the Intern Laser Therapy Association, London, Sept 1992, p 55.

[77] Iwase T et al. Inhibitory effect of HeNe laser on dental plaque deposition in hamsters. J Periodont Research. 1989; 24: 282-.

[78] Schenk P et al. Elektronenmikroskopische Untersuchungen von oralen Schleimhautepithelien nach Bestrahlung mit dem Helium-Neon-Laser. Dtsch Z Mund Kiefer Gesichts Chir. 1985; 9: 278-.

[79] Wafa F et al. A clinical study of laser therapy in fixed prosthodontic pain control after tooth preparation to receive a crown. 1990; 2 (2): 83-88.

[80] Gomi A et al. A clinical study of soft Laser 632 Helium Neon low energy medical laser. 2nd report. The effects in the relieving the pain of hypersensitive dentine and the pain during seating inlay. Aichi Gukuin J Dent Sci. 1986; 24 (3): 390-.

[81] Harazaki M, Isshiki Y. Soft laser irradiation effects on pain reduction in orthodontic treatment. Bull Tokyo Dent Coll. 1997; 38 (4): 291-295.

[82] Haimovici N et al. Clinical use of antiinflammatory action of the laser in activated osteoarthritis of small peripheral joints. LASER. Journ Eur Med Laser Ass. 1988; 1 (2): 4-.

[83] Walker J et al. Laser Therapy for pain of Rheumatoid Arthritis. The Clinical Journal of Pain. 1987; 3 (53): 54-59.

[84] Carrillo J, Calatayud J, Manso F J et al. A randomized double-blind clinical trial on the effectiveness of helium-neon laser in the prevention of pain, swelling and trismus after removal of impacted third molars. Int Dent Journal. 1990; 40: 31-36.

[85] Hansson T. Infrared laser in the treatment of craniomandibular disorders, arthrogenous pain. J Prosthetic Dentistry. 1989; 61: 614-617.

[86] Nagasawa A et al. Fundamental studies in reactive histological changes in pulp tissue of lased teeth. J Jap Soc Laser Med Surg. 1989.

[87] Yaakobi T et al. Promotion of bone repair in the cortical bone of the tibia in rats by low energy laser (He-Ne) irradiation. Calcif Tissue Int. 1996; 59 (4): 297-300.

[88] Midamba E D, Haanaes H. Effect of low level laser therapy (laser therapy) on inferior alveolar, mental and lingual nerves after traumatic injury in 15 patients. A pilot study. Laser Therapy. 1993; 5 (2): 89-94.

[89] Walker J B, Akhanjee L K. Laser-induced somatosensory evoked potentials: evidence of photosensitivity in peripheral nerves. Brain Research. 1985; 344: 281-285.

[90] Tsai J-C, Kao M-C. The Biological Effects of Incident Low Power Density Laser Irradiation on Cultivated Rat Glial and Glioma Cells. Laser Therapy. 1989; 1 (4): 191-202.

[91] Asanami S, Shiba H, Ohtaishi M et al. The Activatory Effect of HeNe laser therapy Irradiation of Hydroxy-apatite Implants in the Rabbit Mandibular Bone. Laser Therapy. 1993; 5 (1): 29-32.

[92] Lievens P. Effects of Laser Treatment on the Lymphatic System and Wound Healing. LASER. Journ Eur Med Laser Ass. 1988; 1 (2): 12-.

[93] Røynesdal A et al. The effect of soft-laser application on postoperative pain and swelling. A double-blind, cross-over study. J Oral Maxillofac Surg. 1993; 22: 242-245.

[94] Zhang D, Zhou Y, Xiao B, Li G. The effect of postoperative irradiation with low incident levels of CO2 laser irradiation on skin flap survival and the possible mechanisms. Laser Therapy. 1992; 4 (2): 75-80.

[95] Kiyoizumi T. Low Level Diode Laser Treatment for Hematomas under Grafted Skin and its Photobiological Mechanisms. Keio J Med. 1988; 37: 415-.

[96] Honmura A et al. Anti-inflammatory effects of GaAlAs diode laser irradiation on carrageenin-induced inflammation in rats. Lasers in Surgery and Medicine 1992; 12: 441-.

[97] Palmgren N, Jensen G F, Kaae K et al. Low-Power Laser Therapy in Rheumatoid Arthritis. Lasers in Medical Science. 1989; 4: 193-196.

[98] Asada K, Yutani Y, Shimazu A. Diode Laser Therapy for Rheumatoid Arthritis: A Clinical Evaluation of 102 Joints Treated with Low Reactive-level Laser Therapy (laser therapy). Laser Therapy. 1989; 1 (3): 147-152.

[99] Oyamada Y et al. Trials in treatment of RA-related diseases by HeNe-laser. Surg Med Lasers. 1989; 2: 18-.

[100] Trelles M A, Rigau J, Sala P et al. Infrared Diode Laser in Low Reactive-Level Laser Therapy (laser therapy) for Knee Osteoarthroses. Laser Therapy. 1991; 3 (4): 149-154.

[101] Kim K S, Hun L D, Kun K S. Effects of Low Incident Energy Levels of Infrared Laser Irradiation on the Proliferation of Streptococcus Mutans. Laser Therapy. 1992; 4 (2): 81-86.

[102] Gilioli G et al. Studio ultrastrutturale di colture cellulari "vero" infettate con virus Herpes Simplex e sottoposte all'azione Laser. Int Congress on Laser Med and Surg, Bologna June 1985, p 207. Monduzzi Editore S.p.A, Bologna, Italy. Also in: Medical Laser Report 1985; 3: 28-31.

[103] Moustsen P et al. Laserbehandling af bihulebetændelse i almen lægepraxis vurderet ved en dobbelt-blind kontrolleret undersøgelse. [Laser Treatment of Sinuitis in General Medical Praxis Evaluated in a Double Blind Study] (In Danish). Ugeskrift Læger. 1991; 153 (32): 2232-.

[145] Schindl L, Kainz A, Kern H. Effect of Low Level Laser Irradiation on Indolent Ulcers Caused by Bürgers Disease. Laser Therapy. 1992; 4 (1): 25-32.

[146] Uchida K et al. Treatment of chronic prostatitis and prostatodynia with low reactive laser. Laser Therapy. (ILTA Okinawa Congr Abstr Issue) 1990; 2 (1): 36.

[147] Popova M et al. [Effect of Helium-Neon laser beam in regeneration of irradiated transplanted skeletal muscle]. Biull Exp Biol Med. 1978; 80: 333. (Russian with English abstract.)

[148] Asencio-Arana F et al. Endoscopic Enhancement of the Healing of High-Risk Colon Anastomoses by Low-Power Helium-Neon Laser. Dis Colon Rectum. 1992; 35: 568-.

[149] Dimitriadis V et al. Effect of HeNe Laser on the Midgut Cells of Drosophila Auraria Larvae and its Correlation with Acupuncture. Acup & Electro-Therap Res. Int J. 1985; 10: 67-.

[150] Abergel P et al. Non Thermal Effects of Nd:YAG Laser on the Biological Functions of the Human Skin Fibroblasts in Culture. Lasers in Surgery and Medicine. 1984; 3: 379-.

[151] Herman J et al. In vitro Effects of Nd:YAG Laser Radiation on Cartilage Metabolism. J Rheum. 1988; 15: 1818-.

[152] Goldman J, Chiapella J, Bass N et al. Laser Therapy of Rheumatoid Arthritis. Surgery and Medicine. 1980; 1: 93-100.

[153] Loevscall H. The Application of Low Level Laser in Dentistry - A Critical Review. Dept of Oral Pathology, Royal Dental College, Aarhus University, Vennelyst Boulevard, DK-8000 Aarhus C, Denmark. 1992.

[154] Saperia D et al. Demonstration of elevated type I and type III laser. Biochem and Biophys Res Communic. 1986; 138: 3-.

[155] Clokie C et al. The effects of helium-neon laser on postsurgical discomfort: A pilot study. Canadian Dent Ass Journal. 1991; 7 (57): 584-586.

[156] Bernal, G. Helium Neon and Diode Laser Therapy is an effective adjunctive therapy for facial paralysis. Laser Therapy. 1993; 5 (2): 79-87

[157] Maier M, Haina D, Landthaler M. Effect of Low Energy Laser on the Growth and Regeneration of Capillaries. Lasers in Medical Sciences. 1990; 5: 381-.

[158] Rochkind S, Nissan M, Lubart A. A single Transcutaneous Light Irradiation to Injured Peripheral Nerve: Comparative Study with Five Different Wavelengths. Lasers in Medical Sciences. 1989; 4: 259-.

[159] Parrado C et al. Quantitative study of the Morphlogical Changes in the Thyroid Gland Following IR Laser Radiation. Lasers in Med Sciences. 1990; 5: 77-.

[160] Ben Hatit Y. The Nd:YAG Laser in Dentistry. LASER. Journ Eur Med Laser Ass. 1991; 4 (1-2): 17-20.

[161] Mokhtar B et al. A double blind placebo controlled investigation of the hypoalgesic effects of low intensity laser irradiation of the cervical roots using experimental ischaemic pain. ILTA Congress, London l992, abstracts p 61

[162] Mokhtar B et al. The possible significance of pulse repetition rate in laser-mediated analgesia: a double blind placebo controlled investigation using experimental ischaemic pain. ILTA Congress, London l992, abstracts p 62.

[163] Taube S, Piironen J, Ylipaavalniemi P. Helium-neon laser therapy in the prevention of postoperative swelling and pain after wisdom tooth extraction. Proc Finn Dent Soc 1990; 86: 23-27.

[164] Kim K et al. Study on the effect of low power laser irradiation in treating gingival inflammation. Clinical, microbiological, histological study. J Korean Acad Oral Med. l987; 12: 5-16.

[165] Kim K et al. An experimental study on the effects of low power density laser (GaAs) on the wound healing of rat tongue and skin. J Korean Acad Oral Med. 1985; 10: 91-104.

[166] Armino L, Longo L. Effects of laser treatment on vulvar dystrophy. LASER. Journ Eur Med Laser Ass.; 1991:4 (1-2):10-.

[167] Porteder H. Einsatz des Helium-Neon-Lasers zur Förderung der Wundheilung. Z Stomat. 1983; 80: 333-339.

[168] Horch H et al. Erfahrungen mit der Laserbehandlung oberflächlicher Mundschleimhauterkrankungen. Dtsch Z Mund-, Kiefer- u Gesichtschir. 1983; 7:31-35

[169] Kopf K et al. Endothelregeneration nach Laserbestrahlung - tierexperimentelle Untersuchungen an Kaninchen. Fortschr Kiefer u Gesichtschir. 1983; 28:140-142.

[170] Senda A , Gomi A et al. A clinical study of Soft Laser 632, a Helium-Neon low energy medical laser. 1st report. The effect in releiving pain just after irradiation. Aichi-Gakuin J Dent Sci. 1985; 23 (4): 773-780.

[171] Lutsyk L et al. [Use of a helium-neon laser in the combined treatment of oral mucosa diseases in children]. Stomatologiia (Mosk). 1981; 60 (6): 15-.

[172] Luomanen M. A comparative study of healing of laser and scalpel incision wounds in rat oral mucosa. Scand J Dent Res. 1987; 95: 65-.

[173] Hatit B Y, Lammens J P. Laser therapy with 10600 nm defocused CO2 laser. Laser Therapy. 1992; 4 (4):175-178.

[174] Longo L, Tamburini A, Monti A et al.. Treatment with 904 nm and 10600 nm laser of acute lumbago - double blind control. LASER. Journ Eur Med Laser Ass. 1991; 3 (1): 16-19.

[175] Bahn J. Biostimulation laser: reality and perspectives. LASER. Journ Eur Med Laser Ass.; 1988:1 (1):17-.

[176] Kats A et al. [Use of laser in nonspecific inflammatory processes of the temporomnadibular joint]. Stomatologiia (Mosk). 1983; 62: 42-45.

[177] Kim, Ki-Suk and Kim, Young-Ku. Comparative study of the clinical effects of splint, laser acupuncture and laser therapy for temporomandibular disorders. J Dental College, Seoul Nat Univ. 1988: 1 (12):195-.

[178] Lee P, Kim Kibeom and Kim Ki-Suk. Effects of low incident energy levels of infrared laser irradiation on helaing of infected open skin wounds in rats. Laser Therapy 1993; 5 (2): 59-.

[179] Lomnitski I, Bibiashevski E V. [Substantiation of the optimal exposure to monochromatic red light for stimulating osteogenesis]. Stomatologiia (Rus). 1982; 2 (61):14-.

[180] Karu T, Andreichuck T, Ryabykh T. Supression of human blood chemi-luminescence by diode laser irradiation at wavelengths 660, 820, 880 or 950 nm. Laser Therapy. 1993; 5 (2): 103-.

[181] Shefer G, Halevy O, Cullen M, Oron U. Low level laser irradaition shows no histopathological effects on myogenic satellite cells in tissue culture. Laser Therapy. 1999; 11 (3): 114-118.

[182] Yarita T et al. Effect of low power laser on gingival microcirculation. Proc. X Internat Congress Int Soc Laser Surgery and Medicine, Bangkok 1993, p 235.

[183] Iijima K et al. Evaluation of Analgesic Effect of Low Power HeNe laser on Postherpetic Neuralgia Using VAS and Modified McGill Pain Questionaire. 1992. J Clin Laser Med Surg 1991. 2 (9):121-.

[184] Iijima K et al. [Evaluation of analgesic effect of low-power laser for outpatients in pain clinic]. J Jpn Soc Med Lasers. 1988; 9: 3-10 (Japanese).

[185] Obata J et al. Evaluation of acute pain-relief effects of low power laser therapy on rheumatoid arthritis by thermography. Laser Therapy. 1990; 2 (1): 28-

[186] Murakami F, Kemmotsu O, Kawano Y et al.. Diode low reactive level laser therapy and stellate ganglion block compared in the treatment of facial paralysis. Laser Therapy, 1993; 5 (3):131-135.

[187] Wu Wen-hsien, Ponnudurai R, Katz J et al. Failure to confirm report of light-evoked response of peripheral nerve to low power helium-neon laser light stimulus. Brain Research. 1987; 407-408.

[188] Honmura A et al. Analgesic Effect of Ga-Al-As Diode Laser Irradiation on Hyperalgesia in Carrageenin-Induced Inflammation. Lasers in Surgery and Medicine. 1993; 13: 463-.

[189] Taguchi T et al. Thermographic Changes Following Laser Irradiation for Pain Relief. J Clin Laser Med Surg. 1991; 9 (2): 143-.

[190] Wakabayashi H et al. Effect of Irradiation by Semiconductor Laser on Responses Evoked in Trigeminal Caudal Neurons by Tooth Pulp Stimulation. Lasers in Surgery and Medicine. 1993; 13: 605-.

[191] Walker J B et al. Laser Therapy for pain of trigeminal neuralgia. Pain 1987; 29: 585-.

[192] Yu I. Low Power Laser Therapy for carpal tunnel syndrome.Proc X Internat Congress Int Soc Laser Surg Med, Bangkok 1993, p. 197.

[193] Walker J B et al. Laser therapy for pain of rheumatoid arthritis. Lasers in Surgery and Medicine.1986; 6: 171-.

[194] Avila R et al. Histological effects of HeNe laser on chick embryo. Proc X Internat Congress Int Soc Laser Surg Med, Bangkok 1993, p. 164.

[195] England S, Farrell A J, Coppock J S.. Low power laser therapy of shoulder tendonitis. Scand J Rheumatology. 1989; 18 (6): 427-431.

[196] Dong-Sheng Zhan et al. The effect of postoperative irradiation of Low Level CO2 laser on the skin flap survival and its mechanism. Laser Therapy, (ILTA Okinawa Congr Abstr Issue). 1990; 2 (1): 36.

[197] Wasserman I, Rabau M Y, Shoshan S. Collagen metabolism in lowpower CO2 laser welded intesitinal anastomosis in rats. Proc Ninth Congress of the International Society for Laser Surgery and Medicine, Anaheim, Cal., 2-6 November 1991.

[198] Korytny D.L. [Use of Helium-Neon laser in therapeutic stomatology]. Stomatologiia (Mosk). 1978; 57 (5): 5-21.

[199] Gärtner C. Analgesy by low power laser (LPL): a controlled double blind study in ankylosing spondarthritis (SPA). Lasers in Surgery and Medicine. 1989; Suppl 1: 30.

[200] Gáspar L et al. Oral lesions induced by scalpel, electrocautery and CO2 laser compared with light scanning and electron microscopy. J Clin Laser Med Surg October 199; ;9: 349-.

[201] Kayano T. Effect of Er:YAG laser irradiation on human extracted teeth. J Clinical Laser Med Surg 1991; 9 (2): 147-.

[202] Kawamura M et al. Effect of Nd:YAG and diode laser irradiation on periodontal wound healing. Innov. Techn. Biol. Med. 1990; 11 (1) :113-.

[203] Kim, Dong-Won. The healing effects of low power density laser to the experimental periodontitis; histopathologic study. Thesis for M.S., Dept. of Dentistry, Dankook University, Korea. Advisor: Prof. Chung, Chin-Hyung. 1993.

[204] Kana J, Hutschenreiter G, Haina D, Waidelich W. Effect of low-power density laser radiation on healing of open skin wounds in rats. Arch Surg. 1981; 116: 293-296.

[205] Shiroto C et al. Effects of diode laser radiation in vitro on activity of human neutrofils. Laser Therapy. 1989; 1 (3): 135-.

[206] Bezuur N J, Hansson T L. The effect of therapeutic laser treatment in patient with cranomandibular disorders. J Cranomandib Disorders. 1988; 2: 83-86.

[207] Midamba E D, Haanaes H R. Low reactive-level 830 nm GaAlAs diode laser therapy (laser therapy) successfully accelerates regeneration of peripheral nerves in human. Laser Therapy, 1993; 5 (3): 125-130.

[208] Haker E, Lundeberg T. Is Low-Energy Laser Treatment Effective in Lateral Epicondylalgia? J Pain Symptom Managment. 1991; 6 (4): 241-.

[209] Ruffolo P et al. Impiego della Laser-terapia nelle leucoplachie del cavo orale. Int Congress on Laser Med and Surg, Bologna June 1985, p. 279. Monduzzi Editore S.p.A., Bologna, Italy.

[210] Obata J, Yanse M. Evaluation of the effects of low power laser therapy on rheumatoid arthritis joints by roentgenographic survey. Laser Bologna '92, p. 41. Monduzzi Editore S.p.A., Bologna, Italy.

[211] Parascandolo S et al. Azione della Laser-terapia nella nevralgia essenziale del trigemino. Int Congress on Laser in Med and Surg, Bologna June 1985, p 317. Monduzzi Editore S.p.A., Bologna, Italy.

[212] Cassese M et al. Laser-terapia nelle sindromi algico-disfunzionali delle articolazioni temoporo-mandibolari. Int Congress on Laser in Med and Surg, Bologna June 1985, p 337. Monduzzi Editore S.p.A, Bologna, Italy

[213] Kusakari H, Orikasa N, Tani H. Effects of low power laser on wound healing of gingiva and bone. Laser Bologna '92, p. 49-55. Monduzzi Editore S.p.A., Bologna, Italy.

[214] Konchugova T V et al. The enhancement of immune supression by local laser irradiation in rats exposed to cyclophosphane. Eksp Klin Farm. 1993; 56 (2): 42-.

[215] Abe M et al. Role of 830 nm low reactive level laser on the growth of an implanted glioma in mice. Keio J Med 1993; 42 (4): 177-179

[216] Fernando S et al. A randomised double blind comparative study of low level laser therapy following surgical extraction of lower third molar. Br J Oral Maxillofac Surg 1993; 31(3): 170-.

[217] Shiroto C. Clinical results of pain relief with low lever laser therapy. Laser Bologna '92, p. 25. Monduzzi Editore S.p.A., Bologna, Italy.

[218] Kaneko M et al. The application of Nd:YAG laser for low energy laser therapy in the intraoral region. Laser in Dentistry. Proceedings of the Intern Congr of Lasers in Dentistry, Tokyo, August 1988. p 131-136. Excerpta Medica, Elsevier Science Publishers, Amsterdam.

[219] Castro D J, Abergel R P, Johnston K et al. Wound healing: biological effects of Nd:YAG laser on collagen metabolism in pig skin in comparison to thermal burn. Ann Plast Surg 1983; 11: 131-.

[220] Castro D J, Abergel R P, Meweker C et al. Effects of the Nd:YAG laser on DNA synthesis and collagen production in human skin fibroblast cultures. Ann Plast Surg. 1983; 1 (3): 214-222.

[221] Boussignac G et al. Thermal effects of semiconductor lasers in men. Proc 6th Congress of The Internat Soc for Lasers in Surgery and Medicine. 1985; 77.

[222] Manne J. Le laser arséniure de gallium 6 watts, étude clinique en odonto-stomatologie. Le Chirurgien Dent de France 1985; 284: 15-.

[223] Donko Z. Possible ab-initio explanation of laser "biostimulation" effects. Laser Applications in Medicine and Surgery. G. Galletti et al, Eds.: Proc 3rd World Congr - Int Soc Low Power Laser Appl in Medicine.: 1992: 57. Monduzzi Editore S.p.A., Bologna.

[224] Spanner D C. The active transport of water under temperature gradient. Symp. Soc. Exp. Biol. 1954; 8: 76-.

[225] Hort O, Vanpel T. Die verteilung von Na+ und K+ unter dem Einfluss von Temperaturgradienten. Pflügers Arch. 1971; 323: 158-.

[226] Lögdberg-Andersson M, Mützell S, Hazel Å. Low Level Laser Treatment of Tendonitis and Myofascial Pains - a Randomized, Double-Blind Study. Laser Therapy. 1997; 9 (3): 79-86.

[227] Plog F. Biophysical application of the laser beam. 1980. In Koebner H K: Lasers in Medicine. John Wiley, New York.

[228] van Breugel H. et al. Power Density and Exposure Time of HeNe Laser Irradiation Are More Important Than Total Energy Dose in Photo-Biomodulation of Human Fibroblasts in Vitro. Lasers in Surgery and Medicine. 1992; 12: 528-.

[229] Nivbrant B, Friberg S. Therapeutic Laser Treatment in Gonarthroses. Acta Orthop Scand. 1989; 60 (suppl 231): 33.

[230] Lundeberg T, Haker E, Thomas M. Effect of laser versus placebo in tennis elbow. Scand J of Rehab Med. 1987; 19: 135-.

[231] Haker E, Lundeberg T. Laser treatment applied to acupuncture points in lateral humeral epicondylalgia. A double-blind study. Pain. 1990; 43: 243-.

[232] Sasaki K, Calderhead R G, Chin I, Inomata K. To examine the adverse photothermal effects of extended dosage laser therapy in vivo on the skin and subcutaneous tissue in the rat model. Laser Therapy. 1992; 4 (2): 69-74.

[233] Greguss P. Biostimulation of tissue by laser radiation. Lasers and Medicine. 1989; 1353: 79-.

[234] Greguss P. Interaction of optical radiation with living matter. Optics and Laser Technology. 1985; 3: 151-.

[235] Greguss P. Letter to the editor. Biological effects of low power laser radiation. Optics and Laser Technology. 1985; 3: 161.

[236] Rossman J A. Current research using the CO2 laser in guided tissue regeneration: animal studies. Proc Second Annual Advanced Application Seminar. Luxar Corp, USA., 1993.

[237] Israel M. Current research using the CO2 laser in guided tissue regeneration. Clinical studies. Proc Second Annual Advanced Application Seminar. Luxar Corp, USA. 1993.

[238] Takashi K. Clinical evaluation of a GaAlAs semiconductor unilaser irradiation on solitary aphta erosion and hypersensitive dentine. Shikwa Gauko. 1987; 87 (2): 295-.

[239] Landthaler M et al. Behandlung von Zoster, postzosterischen Schmerzen und Herpes simplex recidivans in loco mit Laser-Licht. Fortschr. Med. 1983; 101 (22): 1039-.

[240] Beck-Friis J, Borg G, Wetterberg L. Rebound increase of nocturnal melatonin levels following evening suppression by bright light exposure in healthy men: relationship to cortisol levels and morning exposure. In: The Medical and Biological Effects of Light. Wurtman RJ, ed. Ann. NY Acad Sci. 1985; 453: 371-375.

[241] Sasaki K, Ohshiro T. Role of Low Reactive-Level Laser Therapy (laser therapy) in the Treatment of Aquired and Cicatricial Vitiligo. Laser Therapy. 1989; 1 (3): 141-146.

[242] Gudmundsen J, Vikne J. Laserbehandling av epicondylitis humeri og rotatorcuffsyndrom. Dobbelt blindstudie - 200 pasienter. Telemark Sentralsjukehus, Norge. ["Laser Treatment of Epicondylitis Humeri and Rotator Cuff Syndrome. A Double-Blind Study - 200 Patients."] (In Norwegian.) Norsk Tidskrift for Idrettsme-disin 1987; 2: 6-.

[243] Juri H et al. Effects of Nd:YAG laser radiation on PGE_2 level in experimental arthtitis. Proc X Internat Congr Soc Lasers in Surgery and Medicine, Bangkok 1993, p. 314.

[244] Lopez V J. El láser en el tratiamento de las disfunciones de ATM. Revista de Actualidad de Odon-toestomatologica Española. 1986; (Jun): 35-.

[245] Calderhead R G, Inomata K. A study of the possible haemorrhagic effects of extended infrared diode laser irradiation on encapsulated and exposed synovial membrane articular tissue in the rat. Laser Therapy. 1992; 4 (2): 65-74.

[246] Vizi E, Mester E, Tisza S, Mester A. Acetylcholine releasing effect of laser irradiation on Auerbach's plexus in guinea-pig ileum. J. Neural Transmission. 1977; 40: 305-.

[247] Mizokami T, Aoki K, Iwabuchi S et al. Laser therapy (Low Reactive Level Laser Therapy) - a clinical study: relationship between pain attenuation and the serotonergic mechanism. Laser Therapy. 1993; 5 (4): 165-168.

[248] Ataka I et al. Studies of Nd:YAG Low Power Laser Irradiation on Stellate Ganglion. Lasers in Dentistry. 1989; page 271. Elsevier Science Publisher B.V. Amsterdam.

[249] Meyers A, Joyce J, Cohen J. Effects of low-watt Helium Neon laser radiation on human lymphocyte cultures. Lasers in Surgery and Medicine. 1987; 6: 540-.

[250] Lievens P. The Influence of Laser Irradiation on the Motricity of Lymphatical System and on the Wound Healing Process. Proc Int Congr on Laser in Med and Surg. Bologna, June 26-28, 1985; p. 171.

[251] Karu T, Tiphlova O. Stimulation of E. Coli growth by laser and incoherent red light. Nuovo Cimento. 1983; 2 (4): 1138-.

[252] Lubart R, Friedmann H, Peled I, Grossman N. Light effect on fibroblast proliferation. Laser Therapy. 1993; 5 (2): 55-58.

[253] Laakso E L, Cramond T, Richardson C, Galligan J P. Plasma ACTH and ß-endorphin levels in response to low level laser therapy for myofascial trigger points. Laser Therapy. 1994; (6) 3: 133-142.

[254] Mester E, Mester A F, Mester A. The biomedical effects of laser application. Lasers in Surgery and Medicine. 1985; 5: 31-39.

[255] Toya S, Motegi M, Inomata K, Ohshiro T. Report on a computer-randomized double blind clinical trial to determine the effectiveness of the GaAlAs (830 nm) diode laser for pain attenuation in selected pain. Laser Therapy 1994; 6 (3): 143-148.

[256] Klima H. Effect of Weak Laser Light and Oxygen Activation in Open Biological Systems. LASER - Journ Eur Med Laser Ass. 1988; 1 (No 2): 16-.

[257] Gaudel Y et al. Pico second study of free radical reactions in organized assemblies: Kinetics of univalent reduction of b -NAD+. Laboratoire d'Optique Appliquee INSERM U275. École Polytechnique-ENSTA, Palaiseau. p 219-.

[258] Chen Ji-wei, Zhou Yo-cheng. Effect of low level carbon dioxide laser radiation on biochemical metabolism of rabbit mandibular bone callus. Laser Therapy. 1989; 1 (2): 83-88.

[259] Parshad R, Sanford K. Proliferative response of human diploid fibroblasts to intermittent light exposure. J Cell Physiol. 1977; 92: 481-.

[260] Iilima K, Shimoyama N, Shimoyama M, Mizuguchi T. Red and green low-powered HeNe lasers protect human erythrocytes from hypotonic hemolysis. J Clin Laser Med Surg. 1991; 9: 385-.

[261] Labbe R, Skogerboe K, Davis H, Rettmer R. Laser photobioactivation mechanisms: In vitro studies using ascorbic acid uptake and hydroxyproline formation as bio-chemical markers of irradiation response. Lasers in Surgery and Medicine. 1990; 10: 201-.

[262] Trelles M A, Mayayo E. Mast cells are implicated in low power laser effect on tissue. A preliminary study. Lasers in Medical Science. 1992; 7: 73-.

[263] Mayayo E, Trelles M A, Calderhead R, Santafe M, Tomas J, Rigau J. Short term ultrastructural changes in soft tissue (Endomysium) after laser therapy Helium-Neon laser treatment. Laser Therapy. 1989; 1 (3): 119-126.

[264] Dyson M. Cellular and subcellular aspects of low level laser therapy. Progress in Laser Therapy. Eds. T. Ohshiro and R.G. Calderhead, John Wiley & Sons, England. 1991, p. 221

[265] Kubasova T, Kovács L, Somosy Z, Unk P, Kókai A. Biological effect of HeNe laser: Investigations on functional and micromorphological alterations of cell membranes, in vitro. Lasers in Surgery and Medicine. 1984; 4: 381-.

[266] Martin J L, Migus A, Poyart C, Lecarpentier Y, Antonetti A. Ultra-fast events in biological systems. Laboratoire d'Optique Appliquee INSERM U275. Ecole Polytechnique-ENSTA, Palaiseau, France. p. 218.

[267] Karu T. Photobiology of low-power laser effects. Health Physics. 1989; 56 (5): 691-704.

[268] Boulton M et al. HeNe-Laser Stimulation of Human Fibroblasts and Attachment in vitro. Lasers in Life Sciences. 1986; 1 (2): 125-.

[269] Vulliez C et al. Éffet du Laser Infra Rouge a Diode sur le Tissue Conjuctif. Innov. Tech Biol. Med. 1990; 11 (1): 143-.

[270] Trelles M A, Mayayo E, Miro L, Rigau J, Baudin G, Calderhead G. The action of low reactive level laser therapy (laser therapy) on mast cells. Laser Therapy. 1989; 1: 27-30.

[271] el Sayed S et al. The Effect of Low Level Laser Irradiation on Mast Cell Degranulation. Proc 7th Ann Meeting of Am Soc Laser Med Surg 1987.

[272] Fenyö M et al. Theoretical and experimental basis of biostimulation by laser irradiation. Optics and Laser Technology. 1984: No 4: 209-.

[273] Ohta A, Abergel P, Uitto J. Laser modulation of human immune system: Inhibition of lymphocyte proliferation by a gallium-arsenide laser at low energy. Lasers in Surgery and Medicine. 1987; 7: 199-.

[274] Zheng H, Qin J, Xin H, Xin S. The activation action of low level Helium Neon laser radiation on macrophages in the mouse model. Laser Therapy. 1992; 4 (2): 55-58.

[275] Karu T. Low Intensity Laser Light Action Upon Fibroblast and Lymphocytes. Progress in Laser Therapy, Eds. T. Ohshiro and R.G. Calderhead, John Wiley & Sons, England. 1991 p. 175.

[276] Weiss N, Oron U. Enhancement of muscle regeneration in the rat gastrocnemius muscle by low energy laser irradiation. Anat Embryol. 1992; 186: 497-503.

[277] Bibikova A, Oron U. Attenuation of the process of muscle regeneration in the toad gastrocnemius muscle by low energy laser irradiation. Lasers in Surgery and Medicine. 1994; 14: 355-361.

[278] Hall G, Anneroth G, Schennings T et al. Effect of low level energy laser irradiation on wound healing. An experimental study in rats. Swed Dent J. 1994; 18: 29-34.

[279] Kats A G et al. [Remote results of the complex treatment of chronic sialadenitis with the use of helium-neon lasers.] Vestnik Khirurgii Imeni i-i- Grekova. 1985; 135: 39-42.

[280] Morselli M et al. Effects of very low energy-density treatment of joint pain by CO2 laser. Lasers in Surgery and Medicine. 1985; 5:150-.

[281] Baxter G D et al. Low level laser therapy: Current clinical practice in Northern Ireland. Physiotherapy 1991; 3: 171-178.

[282] Iijima K et al. Treatment of low power laser in pain relief from herpetic and postherpetic neuralgia. Proc X Congress Int Soc Laser Surg and Med, Bangkok Nov 12-17, 1993: p 98.

[283] Kim K-S, Kim S-K, Lee P-Y et al. Effects of low incident energy levels of infrared laser irradiation on the proliferation of candida albicans. Part 1: A long term study on the pulse types. Laser Therapy. 1994; 6 (3): 161-166.

[284] Ohshiro T. Treatment techniques to achieve superficial and intermediate laser therapy irradiation. Laser Therapy. 1989; 3 (1): 153-155.

[285] Hernández L C, Santisteban P, del Valle-Soto M E et al. Changes in mRNA of thyroglobulin, cytoskeleton of thyroid cells and thyroid hormone levels induced by IR-laser radiation. Laser Therapy. 1989; 1 (4): 203-208.

[286] Humzah M D, Diamantopoulos C, Dyson M. Multi-wavelength low reactive-level laser therapy (laser therapy) as an adjunct in malignant ulcers; case reports. Laser Therapy. 1993; 5 (4): 149-152.

[287] Yasuda, Kubota J, Ohshiro T. The effects of diode laser low reactive-level laser therapy (laser therapy) on musculocutaneous flaps. Laser Therapy. 1993; 5 (4): 159-163.

[288] Yoo C, Lee W K, Kemmotsu O. Efficacy of polarized light therapy for musculoskeletal pain. Laser Therapy. 1993; 5 (4): 153-157.

[289] Bliddal H et al. Soft laser therapy of rheumatoid arthritis. Scand J Rheuma. 1987; 16: 225-228.

[290] Siebert W et al. What is the efficacy of "soft" and "mid" lasers in therapy of tendinopathies? Arch Ortop and Traum Surg. 1987; 106: 358-363.

[291] Bolton P, Young S, Dyson M. Macrophage responsiveness to light therapy with varying power and energy densities. Laser Therapy. 1991; 3 (3): 105-112.

[292] Baxter G D. Therapeutic Lasers. 1994; p 148. Churchill Livingstone. ISBN 0-443-04393-0

[293] Tasaki et et al. Application of low power laser therapy in closed lock temporomandibular joint dysfunction. Lasers in Surgery and Medicine. 1992; Suppl 4: 84.

[294] Chernoff W G et al. Cutaneous Laser Surfacing. Operative Techniques in Otolaryngology - Head & Neck Surgery. 1994; 5: 281-284.

[295] Chernoff W G. Cutaneous Laser Resurfacing. Clinical Laser Monthly. December 1994.

[296] Bellina J H. Laser in gynecology. Excerpts from Leventhal, J.M. et al (eds.): Current Problems in Obstetrics and Gynecology. Year Book Medical Publishers, Inc., Chicago. 1981.

[297] Armino L, Fornari B, Longo L, Losito A. Laser therapy in post-episiotomic nevralgie. LASER. Journ Eur Med Laser Ass. 1988; 1 (1):7-10.

[298] Lievens P C. The effect of I.R laser irradiation on the vasomotricity of the lymphatic system. Lasers in Medical Science. 1991; 6: 189-191

[299] Lievens P C. The effect of a combined HeNe and I.R. laser treatment on the regeneration of the lymphatic system during the process of wound healing. Lasers in Medical Science. 1991; 6: 193-199.

[300] Labajos M et al. Effect of the irradiation of GaAs diode laser on intestinal absorption: in vitro and in vivo studies. Lasers in Medical Science. 1986; 1: 21-25.

[301] Miro L et al. Estudio capilaroscópico de la acción de un laser AsGa sobre la microcirculación. Investig Clínica Láser. 1984; 1/2: 9-14.

[302] Airaksinen O et al. Effects of HeNe-laser irradiation on the trigger points of patients with chronic muscle tension in the neck. Scand J of Acup & Electrotherapy. 1989; 4: 63-65.

[303] Zhong X et al. Correlation between endogenous opiate-like peptides and serotonin in laseracupuncture analgesia. Am J Acupunct. 1989; 17: 39-43.

[304] Calderhead R G. Simultaneous low reactive-level laser therapy in laser surgery: the "alpha-phenomenon" explained. In: Progesss in Laser Therapy. 1991. John Wiley & Sons. P. 209-213.

[305] Fine S, Klein E. Interaction of laser irradiation with biological systems. Fed Proc 1965; 24: 35-45.

[306] Olivier J, Plath P. Combined low power laser therapy and extracts of Gingo Biloba in a blind trial of treatment for tinnitus. Laser Therapy. 1993; 5 (3): 137-140.

[307] Galletti G. Low-Energy Density CO2 Laser as Deep Tissue Stimulator: A Comparative Study. J. Clin. Laser Medicine & Surg. 1991; 9: 179-

[308] Martin D et al. Effect of laser pulse repetition rate upon peripheral blood flow in human volunteers. Lasers in Surgery and Medicine. 1991; Suppl 3: 83.

[309] Ponnudurai R N et al. Hypoalgesic effect of laser photobiostimulation shown by rat tail flick test. Intern J Acup and Electrother Res; 1987; 12: 93-100.

[310] Ivanov A S et al. [Effect of Helium-Neon laser radiation on the course of temporomandibular joint arthritis and arthrosis]. Stomatologiia (Mosk). 1985; 64: 81-82.

[311] Jensen H et al. Is infra-red laser effective in painful arthrosis of the knee? (In Danish) Ugeskr Laeger 1987; 149: 3104-3106.

[312] Fursinn G et al. Effects of Nd:YAG laser irradiation on human cartilage cell metabolism. Proc of Laser-81, Opto-Elektronik. München 1981. Abstr 200.

[313] Airaksinen O et al. Effects of infra-red laser irradiation at the trigger points. Scand J of Acup & Electrotherapy. 1988; 3: 56-61.

[314] Atsumi K et al. Biostimulation effect of low-power energy diode laser for pain relief. Lasers in Surgery and Medicine. 1987; 7: 77-.

[315] Ceccherelli F et al. Diode laser in cervical myofascial pain: A double blind study versus placebo. The Clinical J Pain. 1989; 5: 301-304.

[316] Emmanoulidis O et al. CW IR low-power laser application significantly accelerates chronic pain relief rehabilitation of professional athletes. A double blind study. Lasers in Surgery and Medicine. 1986; 6: 173-.

[317] Kovács I, Mester E, Görög P. Stimulation of wound healing with laser beam in the rat. Experientia. 1974; 30: 1275-.

[318] Hopkins G O et al. Double blind cross over study of laser versus placebo in the treatment of tennis elbow. Proc Internat Congr in Laser, "Laser Bologna". 1985; p 210. Monduzzi Editore S.p.A., Bologna.

[319] Kamikawa K, Kyoto J. Double blind experiences with mid-Lasers in Japan. 1985. Int Congr on Lasers in Med and Surg, Bologna June 1985, 165-169. Moduzzi Editore S.p.A., Bologna

[320] Ohshiro T. To publish, or not to publish. Editorial. Laser Therapy. 1989; 1 (2): 61-62.

[321] Basford J R et al. Low-energy Helium Neon laser treatment of thumb osteoarthritis. Arch Phys Med Rehab. 1987; 68: 794-797.

[322] McAuley R et al. Soft laser: A treatment for osteoarthritis of the knee. Arch Phys Med Rehab. 1985; 66: 553-554 (abstract).

[323] Kemmotsu M D at al. Laser therapy for pain attenuation - the current experience in the pain clinic. In: Progress in Laser Therapy. 1991: 197-200. John Wiley & Sons, Chichester, Engl. ISBN 0-471-93154-3.

[324] Kreczi T, Klinger D A. A comparison of laser acupuncture versus placebo in radicular and pseudoradicular pain syndromes as recorded by subjective responses of patients. Acupunct Electrotherap Res. 1986; 11: 207-216.

[325] Lonauer G. Controlled double blind study on the efficacy of HeNe-laser beams versus HeNe- plus Infrared-laser beams in the therapy of activated osteoarthritis of finger joints. Clin Experim Rheuma. 1987; 5 (suppl 2): 39. Also in Lasers in Surgery and Medicine. 1986; 7: 172.

[326] Mach E S et al. Helium-Neon (Red Light) Therapy of Arthritis. Rhevmatologia, 1983; 3: 36-.

[327] Mester A. Biostimulative effect in wound healing by continous wave 820 nm laser diode double-blind randomized cross-over study. Lasers in Med Science, abstract issue July 1988.

[328] Henderson A R. Laser radiation hazards. Optics and Laser Technology, 1984; 2: 75-

[329] Moore K, Hira N, Broome I J, Cruikshank J A. The effect of infra-red diode laser irradiation on the duration and severity of postoperative pain. A double-blind trial. Laser Therapy. 1992; 4 (4): 145-150.

[330] Palmieri B. A double blind stratified cross over study of amateur tennis players suffering from tennis elbow using infrared laser therapy. Medical Laser Report. 1984; 1: 3-4.

[331] Soriano F. The analgesic effect of 904 nm gallium arsenide semiconductor low level laser therapy (laser therapy) on osteoarticular pain: a report on 938 irradiated patients. Laser Therapy. 1995; 7 (2): 75-80.

[332] Pöntinen P et al. Comparative effects of exposure to different light sources (He-Ne laser, InGaAl diode laser, a specific type of noncoherent LED) on skin blood flow for the head. Acupunct Electrother Res. 1996; 21 (2): 105-118.

[333] Scudds R A et al. A double-blind crossover study of the effectiveness of low-power gallium arsenide laser on the symptoms of fibrositis. Physiotherapy Canada. 1989; 41: (suppl 3) 2.

[334] Molina Soto J J, Moller I. La laserterapia como coadyuvante en el tratamiento de la A.R. (Artritis Reumatoidea). Bol. C.D.L. 1987; 14: 4-8.

[335] Taghawinejag M, Fricke R. Laser Therapie in der Behandlung kleiner Gelenke bei chronischer Polyarthritis. Z Phys Med Baln Med Klin. 1985; 14: 402-408.

[336] Tsurko V V, Muldiyarov P Y, Sigidin Y A. [Laser therapy of rheumatoid arthritis. A clinical and morphological study]. Terap Arkh. 1983; 55: 97-102. (in Russian).

[337] Walker J. Temporary suppression of clonus in humans by brief photo-stimulation. Brain Research. 1985; 340: 109-113.

[338] Mazo V. Transrectal laser therapy in prostatic problems' management.Proc. X Internat Congr Soc Laser Surgery and Medicine, Bangkok. 1993, p. 153.

[339] Garkavoy D V et al. Use of the Helium-Neon laser in the treatment of ulcer disease. Proc X. Internat Congr Soc Laser Surgery and Medicine, Bangkok 1993; p. 160.

[340] Vasilotta A. I.R. laser: a new therapy in rhino-sino-nasal bronchial syndrome with asthmatic component. Proc X. Internat Congr Soc Lasers in Surgery and Medicine, Bangkok 1993, p. 161.

[341] Kovács L. The stimulatory effect of laser on the physiological healing process of portio surface. Lasers in Surgery & Medicine 1981; 1 (3): 241-52

[342] Frugoni P. Shoulder calcified periarthritis recovery with low power laser therapy. Proc X Internat Congr Soc Lasers in Surgery and Medicine, Bangkok 1993, p. 200.

[343] Hall J et al. Low level laser therapy is ineffective in the management of rheumatoid arthritic finger joints. British J Rheumat. 1994; 33: 142-.

[344] Kipshidze N N et al. Treatment of acute myocardial infarction with a low-intensity Helium-Neon laser. Proc X Internat Congr Soc Lasers in Surgery and Medicine, Bangkok 1993, p. 309.

[345] Castronuovo G et al. The skin role during a low level laser therapy. Laser Bologna '92, p. 19. Monduzzi Editore S.p.A., Bologna, Italy.

[346] Kamikawa K et al. Essential mechanisms of low power laser effects. Laser Bologna '92, p. 11. Monduzzi Editore S.p.A., Bologna, Italy.

[347] Herbert K E et al. Effect of laser light at 820 nm on adeonsine nucleotide levels in human lympho-cytes. Lasers Life Sci. 1989; 3: 37.

[348] Verbruggen L A et al. Low-power laser therapy in chronic rheumatic diseases: Western and Soviet experiences. Phys Med Rehab. 1991; 1: 101-.

[349] Obata J et al. The pain relief of low energy laser irradiation on rheumatoid arthritis. Pain Clin. 1987; 8: 18-.

[350] Schindl L et al. Influence of low-power laser irradiation on "arthus phenomenon" induced in rabbit cornea. Laser Therapy. 1994; 6 (1): 23. (absatract)

[351] Palmgren N et al. Low Level Laser Therapy of infected abdominal wounds after surgery. Lasers in Surgery and Medicine. 1991; Suppl 3:11.

[352] Lievens P. Infrared lasertherapy and bedsores. Lasers in Surgery and Medicine. 1992; Suppl 4: 11.

[353] van Breugel H et al. Low energy HeNe laser irradiation effects proliferation and laminin production of rat Schwann cells in vitro. Lasers in Surgery and Medicine. 1991;Suppl 3:10.

[354] Mulligan S et al. The effect of low energy HeNe laser irradiation on the neurite elongation in vitro. Lasers in Surgery and Medicine. 1991; Suppl 3: 10.

[355] Ben-Dov N, Shefer G, Irintchev A et al. Low energy laser irradiation affects cell proliferation and differentiation in vitro. Biochemica and Biophysica Acta. 1999; 1448: 372-380.

[356] Rezvani M et al. Prevention of x-radiation induced dermal necrosis in pig skin by monochromatic light. Lasers in Surgery and Medicine. 1991; suppl 3: 11.

[357] Palma J et al. Blockade of inflammatory signals by laser radiation. Lasers in Surgery and Medicine. 1991; Suppl 3: 11.

[358] Tardivo J P et al. Effect of low power laser over cells infected by herpes simplex virus (HSV). Lasers in Surgery and Medicine. 1989; Suppl 1: 31.

[359] Kamikawa K. Studies on low power laser therapy of pain. Lasers in Dentistry. 1989; p. 29-38. Elsevier Science Publisher B.V. Amsterdam

[360] Vélez-Gonsalez M et al. Treatment of relapse in Herpes Simplex on labial & facial areas and of primary herpes simplex on genital areas and "area pudenda" with low power laser (HeNe) or Acyclovir administred orally. Proc SPIE. 1995; Vol 2630: 43-50.

[361] Khullar S M, Brodin P, Barkvoll P et al. Preliminary study of low-level laser for treatment of long-standing sensory aberrations in the inferior alveolar nerve. J Oral Maxillofac Surg. 1996; 54 (2): 2-7.

[362] Snyder-Mackler L, Bork C, Bourbon B et al. Effect of Helium-Neon Laser on Musculoskeletal Trigger Points. Physical Therapy. 1986; 66 (7): 1087-1090.

[363] Kalivradzhiyan E et al. Usage of low-intensity laser radiation for the treatment of the inflammatory processes of the oral cavity mucosa after applying removable plate dentures. Proc SPIE. 1995; Vol 1984: 225-230.

[364] Sokolova I et al. Low-intensity laser radiation in complex treatment of inflammatory diseases of parodontium. Proc SPIE.1995; Vol 1984: 234-237.

[365] Mamedova F M et al. Microbiological estimate of parodontitis laser therapy efficiency. Proc SPIE. 1995; Vol 1984: 247-249.

[366] Podolskaya E et al. Radiation damage of lips and its treatment by low-intensity laser irradiation. Proc SPIE. 1995; Vol 1984: 245-246.

[367] Kolomiyets L A et al. Mechanism of treatment effect of low-energy laser irradiation. Proc SPIE. 1996; Vol 2728: 63-67.

[368] Kozlov V et al. Lasers in diagnostics and treatment of microcirculation disorders under parodontitis. Proc SPIE. 1995; Vol 1984: 253-264.

[369] Ozawa Y et al. Stimulatory effects of low-power laser irradiation on bone formation in vitro. Proc SPIE. 1995; Vol 1984: 281-288.

[370] Shimizu N et al. Prospect of relieving pain due to tooth momement during orthodontic treatment utilizing a GaAlAs diode laser. Proc. SPIE.. 1995; Vol 1984: 275-280.

[371] Soldo I et al. Effects of GaAs laser combined with radiotherapy on murine sarcoma depends on tumor size. Lasers in Surgery and Medicine. 1989; Suppl 1: 40.

[372] Dima F V, Vasiliu V, Ionescu M D, Dima S V.Studies on some biological functions of macrophages activated by HeNe laser photodynamic treatment as compared to coryne-bacterium parvum and interferon activation. Laser Therapy. 1993; 5 (3): 117-124.

[373] Takaduma K. Possible application of the laser in immunobiology.Keio J Med. 1993; 42 (4): 180-182.

[374] Lubart R, Rochkind S, Sharon U, Nissan M. A light source for phototherapy. Laser Therapy. 1991; 3 (1): 15-18.

[375] Friedman H, Lubart R. Nonlinear photobiostimulation: the mechanisms of visible and infrared laser-induced stimulation and reduction of neural excitability and growth. Laser Therapy. 1993; 5 (1): 39-42.

[376] Friedman H, Lubart R. Towards an explanation of visible and infrared laser induced stimulation and damage of cell cultures. Laser Therapy. 1992; 4 (1): 39-42.

[377] Friedman H et al. A possible explanation of laser-induced stimulation and damage of cell cultures. J Photochem Photobiol B Biol. 1991; 11: 87-95.

[378] Passarella S et al. Increase in the ADP/ATP exchange in rat liver mitochondria irradiated in vitro by helium-neon laser. Biochem Biophys Res Commun. 1988; 156 (2): 978-986.

[379] Lukashevich I G. [HeNe laser in facial pain]. Stomatologiia. 1985; 64: 29-31.

[380] Roumeliotis D, Emmanouilidis O, Diamantopoulos C. C.W. 820nm 15mW 4J/cm2, laser diode application in sports injunes. A double blind study. Proc. Fifth Annual Congress, 28-30 January 1987. British Medical Laser Association.

[381] Malta J et al. The influences of Low Level Laser Therapy on Wound Healing after Palatinal Surgery in Beagle Dogs. EOS. 1990; 122: 82.

[382] Manteifel V, Andreichuk T, Karu T, Chelidze p, Zelenin A. Activation of transcription in lymphocytes after exposure to a HeNe laser. Mol.Biol. 1990; 24: 860-867.

[383] Manteifel V, Andreichuk T, Karu T. Reaction of the mitocondrial apparatus of the lymphocytes to irradiation by a HeNe laser and to the mitogen phytohema-glutinin. Mol.Biol. 1991; 25: 229-235.

[384] Lowe A, Baxter D, Walsh D, Allen J. Effect of low intensity laser (830 nm) irradiation on skin temperature and antidromic conduction latencies in the human median nerve: Relevance of radiant exposure. Lasers in Surgery and Medicine. 1994; 14: 40-46.

[385] Lowe A S, Baxter G D, Walsh D M et al. Low-intensity laser irradiation of the human median nerve: effect of energy density upon conduction and skin temperature. Abstracts 'London Laser 1992', Second Meeting of the International Laser Therapy Association, p. 56.

[386] Abergel P, Lyons R, Castel J, Dwyer R, Uitto J. Biostimulation of wound healing by laser: Experimental approaches in animal models and in fibroblast cultures. J.Dermatol. Surg. Oncol. 1987; 13: 127-133.

[387] Anders J, Borke R, Woolery S, Van De Merwe W. Low power laser irradiation alters the rate of regeneration of the rat facial nerve. Lasers in Surgery and Medicine. 1993; 13: 72-82.

[388] Bolton P A, Young S R, Dyson M. Macrophage responsiveness to light therapy. A dose response study. Laser Therapy. 1990; 2 (3): 101-106.

[389] Bolton P A, Dyson M, Young S R. The effect of polarised light on the release of growth factors from the U-937 macrophage-like cell line. Laser Therapy. 1992; 4 (1): 33-42.

[390] Bosatra M, Lucci A, Olliaro P, Quacci D, Sacchi S. In vitro fibroblast activation by laser irradiation at low energy. Dermatologica. 1984; 168: 157-162.

[391] de Braekt M M H et al. Effect of low level laser therapy of wound healing after palatal surgery in beagle dogs. Lasers in Surgery and Medicine.1991; 11: 462-.

[392] Fitz-Ritson D. Low energy laser therapy efficacy in the extension neck muscle recovery after whiplash injury. Lasers Surgery and Medicine. 1993; 13: 9-.

[393] Friedman S, Liu M, Dörscher-Kim J, Kim S. In situ testing of CO2 laser on dental pulp function: Effects on microcirculation. Lasers in Surgery and Medicine. 1991; 11: 325-330.

[394] Assia E, Rosner M, Belkin M, Solomon A, Schwartz M. Temporal parameters of low energy laser irradiation for optimal delay of post-traumatic degeneration of rat optic nerve. Brain Research. 1989; 476: 205-212.

[395] Berki T, Németh, Hegedüs J. Effect of low-power continous-wave HeNe laser irradiation on in vitro cultured lymphatic cell lines and macrophages. Stud Biophys. 1985; 105: 141-.

[396] Kaneps A, Hultgren B, Riebold T, Shires G. Laser therapy in the horse: Histopathologic response. Am J Vet Res. 1984; 45(3): 581-.

[397] Obata J et al. Clinical effects of total laser irradiation for the control of disease activity of chronic rheumatoid arthritis. Surgical and Medical Lasers. 1990; 3 (3): 140 (abstract).

[398] Sato K, Kaseno S, Takigawa C et al. A double blind assessment of low power laser therapy in the treatment of postherpetic neuralgia. Surgical and Medical Lasers. 1990; 3 (3): 134. (abstract)

[399] Filho W, Nogueira T et al. Effects of irradiation with a HeNe laser on the healing of the hard tissue. Surgical and Medical Lasers. 1989; 2-3 (2): 71-.

[400] Calderhead G. Watt's A Joule?: On the Importance of Accurate and Correct Reporting of Laser Parameters in Low Reactive-Laser Therapy and Photobioactivation Research: Laser Therapy 1991; 3 (4): 177-182.

[401] Cheetham M J, Young R S, Dyson M. Histological effects of 820 nm laser irradiation on the healthy growth plate of the rat. Laser Therapy 1992; 4 (2): 59-64.

[402] Ito A et al. Studies of Nd:YAG low power laser irradiation on stellate ganglion. In: Lasers in dentistry. Ed. H Yamamoto. 1989; p. 271. Elsevier Science Publishers B.V.

[403] Kato M et al. Clinical studies of low power density HeNe laser irradiation on stellate ganglion. Jpn J Oral Maxillofac Surg.1987; 33 (12): 1-11.

[404] Moore K. Laser therapy in post herpetic neuralgia. Laser Therapy. 1996; 8 (1): 48 (abstract)

[405] Inoue K et al. Suppressed tuberculine reaction in guinea pigs following laser irradiation. Lasers in Surgery and Medicine. 1989; 9: 271-275.

[406] Yamamoto H et al. Pain clinic. 1987; 8: 43-48. (In Japanese).

[407] Waylonis G W et al. Chronic myofascial pain: management by low-output helium-neon laser therapy. Arch Phys Med Rehab. 1988; 69: 1017-.

[408] Yaakov N, Bdolah A, Wollberg Z et al. Recovery from sarafotoxin-b induced cardiopathological effects in mice following low energy laser irradiation. Basic Research Cardiology. 2000; 95: 385-389.

[409] Escola R et al. Beitrag zur ultrastrukturellen Untersuchung von Zahnfleischbeweben mit dem Soft-Laser. Zahnarztpraxis. 83: 110-115.

[410] Kazmina S et al. Laser prophylaxis and treatment of primary caries. Proc. SPIE.Vol 984; 1994: 231-233.

[411] Chen M et al.. Application of a pain alleviating effect of low power laser irradiation to patients in orthodontic treatment. J Jpn Soc Laser Med. 1933; 14: 5-11 (in Japanese).

[412] Yoshida T et al. Pain reduction effect of soft laser in orthodontic therapy. Proc. Annual Meeting Jpn Orthodont Soc. 1992: 69-.

[413] Motomura K et al. Effects of various laser irradiation on callus formation after osteotomy. J Jpn Soc Laser Med. 1984; 4: 195-196.

[414] Yamada K. Biological effects of low power laser irradiation on clonal osteoblastic cells (MC3T3-E1). Nippon Seikeigeka Gakkai Zasshi (J Jpn Orthop Assn). 1991; 65: 787-799.

[415] Rigau J, Trelles M A. Effects of the 633 nm laser on the behaviour and morphology of primary fibroblast culture. Proc SPIE.Vol 2630. 1995: 38-42.

[416] Michels H. Erfahrungen mit dem HeNe Laser bei Herpes Erkrankungen. Proc. 7th Int Congr Laser 1985. Edit. W Waidelinch. 1986; 116-119. Springer-Verlag (Berlin).

[417] Brill G et al. Influence of HeNe laser irradiation on giant chromosomes. Proc.SPIE. Vol 2630. 1995; 51-59.

[418] Yamada H, Ogawa H. Comparative study of 60 mW diode laser therapy and 150 mW diode laser therapy in the treatment of postherpetic neutralgia. Laser Therapy. 1995; 7 (2): 71-74.

[419] Bolton P, Young S, Dyson M. The direct effect of 860 nm light on cell proliferation and on succinic dehydrogenase activity of human fibroblasts in vitro. Laser Therapy. 1995; 7 (2): 55-60.

[420] Glinkowski W, Rowinski J. Effect of low incident levels of infrared laser energy on the healing of experimental bone fractures. Laser Therapy. 1995; 7 (2): 67-70.

[421] Otsuka H, Numasawa R, Okubo K et al. Effects of helium-neon laser therapy on herpes zoster pain. Laser Therapy. 1995; 7 (1): 27-32.

[422] Calderhead G. Meeting report: International low power laser symposium, Vienna, Austria, October 7th-8th, 1994. Laser Therapy. 1995; 7 (1): 39.

[423] Otsuka K et al. Low reactive level laser therapy near the stellate ganglion for postherpetic facial pain. Jpn J Anaesthes. 1991; 41: 1809-1813. (Abstr. in English)

[424] Villaplana L A, Sarti M A, Trelles NM A et al. Changes in albino rat testicle interstitial cells after pituitary stimulation in vivo with HeNe laser. Laser Therapy. 1995; 7 (1): 19-22.

[425] Gomez-Villamandos R J. HeNe laser therapy by fibroendoscopy in the mucosa of the equine upper airway. Lasers in Surgery and Medicine. 1995; 16: 184-188.

[426] Oron U, Yaakobi T, Oron A et al. Low energy laser irradiation reduces formation of scar tissue following myocardial infarction in dogs. Circulation. 2001, in press.

[427] Mester A et al. Irradiation of arthritis with 820 and 830 nm diode lasers. Laser Therapy. 1996; 8 (1): 33. (Abstract).

[428] Lubart R et al. Photosensitized biostimulation of fibroblasts by low energy visible light. Laser Therapy. 1996; 8 (1): 16. (Abstract).

[429] Gürsoy B, Bradley P F. Penetration studies of low intensity laser therapy (laser therapy) wavelengths. Laser Therapy, 1996; 8 (1): 18. (Abstract).

[430] Yaakobi T, Oron U. Enhancement of bone repair in the rat tibia by low energy laser irradiation. Laser Therapy. 1996; 8 (1):19. (Abstract).

[431] Bibikova A, Oron U. Attenuation of the process of skeletal muscle regeneration by low energy laser irradiation. Laser Therapy. 1996; 8 (1): 19. (Abstract).

[432] Mrowiec J et al. Analgesic effect of low-power infrared laser radiation in rats. Proc SPIE. 1997; Vol 3198: 83-89.

[433] Neuman I, Finklestein Y, Lubart R. Low energy phototherapy in allergic rhinitis and nasal polyposis. Laser Therapy. 1996. 1: 37 (abstract).

[434] Götte S et al. Doppelblindstudie zur überprüfung der Wirksamkeit und Verträglichkeit einer niederenergetischen Lasertherapie bei Patienten mit aktiver Gonarthrose. Jaros Orthopädie. 1995. 1: 30-34

[477] Kleinman Y, Simmer S, Braksma Y et al. Low power laser therapy in pateints with diabetic foot ulcers: early and long term outcome. Laser Therapy. 1996; 8 (3): 205-208.

[478] Schindl L et al. Topical low power laser irradiation shows a systemic increase in blood flow in conditions of disturbed microcirculation. Laser Therapy. 1996; 8 (1): 58 (abstract).

[479] Kubota J, Ohshiro T. The effect of diode laser laser therapy on flap survival: measurement of flap microcirculation with the laser specle method. Laser Therapy. 1996; 8 (4): 241-246.

[480] Amir A et al. The influence of low energy Helium-Neon laser irradiation on the viability of skin flaps of the rat. Laser Therapy. 1996; 8 (1): 59 (abstract)

[481] Koukoui L M et al. The differential approach to the application of laser, ultraviolet and roentgenological auto-blood irradiation for the correction of homeostatis. Laser Therapy. 1996; 8 (1): 60 (abstract).

[482] Samoilova K A, Kukui L M . Photochemotherapy in clinical and veterinary medicine: therapeutic effects and mechanisms. Laser Therapy. 1996; 8 (1): 62 (abstract)

[483] Kirichuk V F et al. Influence of low power laser radiation on platlet aggregation in pathological stress. Laser Therapy. 1996; 8 (1): 63 (abstract)

[484] Peláez A et al. Growing cartilage after IR laser radiation - utlrastructural study. Proc SPIE. 1993;. Vol 2086: 356-364.

[485] Antipa C et al. Use of pulsed laser therapy (Ga-As) in combined treatment of posttraumatic swellings and some dermatological disorders. Proc SPIE. 1993; Vol. 2086: 371-377.

[486] Fagnoni V et al. Use of HeNe soft-laser in 32 cases of mouth aphtha. Laser Abstracts (Rivista Europea di Laser Terapia Medica e Chirurgia). 2 (2): 25-29.

[487] Smith R J et al. The effect of low-energy laser on skin-flap survival in the rate and porcine animal models. Plastic and Reconstruct Surg. 1992; 89 (2): 306-310.

[488] Kasai S et al. Effects of low-power laser irradiation on impulse conductions in anaesthetized rabbits. J Clin Laser Med Surg. 1996; 14 (3): 107-109.

[489] Ulrich M et al. Influence of laser light (830 nm) on the growth kinetics of rat rhabdomyosarcomas. University of Hamburg, Department of Accident Surgery. Part of M.D. thesis

[490] Longo L et al. Effects of diodes-laser silver Arsenide-Aluminium (Ga-Al-As) 904 nm on healing of experimental wounds. 1987. Lasers in Surgery and Medicine; 7: 444-447.

[491] Makk A, Pollera M. Multicenter study related to laser treatment of TMJ syndrom. Proc. Internat Congress LASERMED, Munich, 1995, p. 104.

[492] Lubart R et al. Changes in calcium transport in mammalian sperm mitochondria and plasma membrane due to 630 nm and 780 nm laser irradiation. Proc. LASERMED Munich 1995, p. 104

[493] Rosner M, Caplan M, Cohen S et al. Dose and temporal parameters in delaying injured optic nerve degeneration by low-energy laser irradiation. Lasers in Surgery and Medicine. 1993; 13 (6): 611-617.

[494] Hoffman B, Bär Th. Reaktionen der Hautoberflächentemperatur - ein Vergleich zwischen Verum- und Placebo-Laserstimulation am Akupunkturpunkt Di 4. Dtsch. Zschr. Akup. 1994; 37 (2): 28.

[495] Mayordomo M M et al. Laser in painful process of locomotor system: our experience. 1985. Proc. of Laser Bologna 1985. Monduzzi Editore, Bologna.

[496] Choi J et al. A comparison of electroacupuncture, transcutaneous electrical nerve stimulation and laser photobiostimulation on pain relief and glucocorticoid excretion. Int J Acupunct Electrotherp Res. 1986; 11: 45-51.

[497] Haina D et al. Temperature of the skin during application of softlaser. Laser in Medicine and Surgery. 1988; 4 (1): 26-29.

[498] T W Marín V. Experimental wound healing with coherent and non-coherent radiation. Laser & Technology. 1992; 2 (3): 121-134.

[499] Labajos M et al. ß-endorphine levels modification after GaAs and HeNe laser irradiation on the rabbit. Comparative study. Investigación clínica láser. 1988; 1-2: 6-8.

[500] Fructuoso F J G, Moset J M. Randomized double blind study on the biostimulatory effect of laser irradiation of the parotid gland in patients suffering of Sjögren syndrome. Invest y Clinica Laser. 1987; 1: 18-25. In Sp with E abstr. Also published in Centro Documentación Láser. 1987: 4 (13): 4-.

[501] Kotani H. Effects of low power laser stimulation on wound healing in rats. Lasermedizin - Laser in Med Surg. 1995; 11 (2): 25- .

[502] Rossetti V et al. Experimental studies on the in vivo effects of HeNe laser irradiation in rat brain. Lasermedizin - Laser in Med Surg. 1995; 11 (2): 24- .

[503] Glinkowski W et al. Sprained ankles treatment with use of laser therapy. Lasermedizin -Laser in Med Surg. 1995; 11 (2): 42-.

[504] Véles-Gonzáles M A. Absorción subcutaneo del salicilato de dietilamina tras la irradiación laser. Boletín CDL. 1987; 4 (12): 4-8.

[505] Juri H et al. Efectos del láser HeNe sobre las concentraciones de fibrinogeno en el plasma de ratas en lesiones tistulares. Boletín CDL. 1986; 10: 5-6.

[506] Padulles J et al. [Laser treatment of spinal pinching due to discal hernias in dogs]. Boletín CDL. 1986; 2: 11-14. (in Spanish)

[507] Kaiser C, Manso F, Zaragoza J R. Estúdio en doble ciego randomizado sobre la eficacia del HeNe en el tratamiento de la sinuitis maxilar aguda: en pacientes con exacerbación de una infección sinusal crónica. (Double blind randomized study on the effect of HeNe in the treatment of acute maxillary sinuitis: in patients with exacerbation of a chronic maxillary sinuitis). Boletín CDL. 1986; 9: 15-.

[508] van den Brande P. Effect of HeNe - IR laser on cutaneous microcirculation in vascular patients. Proc. Lasertherapy III, Vrije Universiteit Brussel, October 1987.

[509] Fagnoni V et al. Trattamento delle nevralgie trigeminali con laser di bassa potenza. Laser Abstracts. 1985; 2: 23-36

[510] Yamada K. Effect of low power laser irradiation on osteoblastic cell growth. Surgical and Medical Lasers. 1989; 2-3 (2): 67 (abstract)

[511] Nicola J H et al. The role of coherence in wound healing stimulation by non-thermal laser radiation. Surgical and Medical Lasers. 1989; 2-3 (2): 70 (abstract)

[512] Karu T. Mechanisms of interaction of monochromatic visible light with cells. Proc. SPIE. 1995; Vol 2630: 2-9

[513] Friedmann H, Lubart R. Competition between activayting and inhibitory processes in photobiology. Proc. SPIE. 1995; Vol 2630: 60-64.

[514] Martelli M R A. A clinico statistical investigation of laser effect in the treatment of pain and dysfunction of temporo-mandibular joint (T.M.J.). J Dental Proth. 1990; (18): 31-36.

[515] Marei M K. Effect of low-energy laser application in the treatment of denture-induced mucosal lesions. J Prosthet Dent. 1997; 77 (3): 256-264.

[516] Kim K-S, Kim J-K, Kim S-W et al. Effects of low level laser irradiation (LLLI) with 904 nm pulsed diode laser on osteoblasts: a controlled trial with the rat osteoblast model. Laser Therapy. 1996; 8 (4): 223-232.

[517] Popov B. [Trigeminal neuralgia with local laser irradiation and laserpuncture]. Stomatologiia Bulgaria. 1986; 68: 25-29.

[518] Ortutay J, Mester A. Laserstimulation therapy in the rehabilitation medicine. Proc. Laser Florence '97, 5th Congr EMLA, p. 22.

[519] Tsuchiya K et al. Diode laser irradiation selectively diminishes slow component of axonal volleys to dorsal roots from the saphenous nerve in the rat. Neuroscience Letters. 1993; 161: 65-68. Also: Tsuchiya K, Kawatani M, Takeshige C, et al.Laser irradiation abates neuronal responses to nociceptive stimulation of rat-paw skin.Brain Res Bull. 1994; 34 (4): 369-374

[520] Carney S A et al. The effect of light from a ruby laser on the metabolism of skin in tissue culture. Biochem Biophys Acta. 1967; 148: 525-530.

[521] Lievens P, Mohebbian M. The effect of IR-laser irradiation on the regeneration of muscle fibres. In: Laser Therapy in Dentistry and Medicine. Prima Books in Sweden AB. Eds Jan Tunér and Lars Hode. 1996, p. 164-179.

[522] Ozawa Y et al. Low-energy diode laser irradiation reduced plasminogen activator activity in human periodontal ligament cells. Lasers in Surgery and Medicine. 1997; 21: 456-463.

[523] Ohtsuka H et al. [Low recative-level laser therapy near the stellate ganglion for postherpetic facial neuralgia]. (in Japanese). Masui. 1992; 41 (11): 1809-1813.

[524] Petrek M et al. Immunomodulatory effects of laser therapy in the treatment of chronic tonsillitis. Acta Univ Palacki Olomuc Fac Med. 1991; 129: 119-126.

[525] Colvard M, Kuo P. Managing aphtous ulcers: laser treatment applied. J Am Dent Assoc. 1991; 122 (7): 51-53.

[526] Zubkova S T. The use of helium-neon laser radiation in the treatment of trophic disorders in patients with diabetes mellitus. Klin Khir. 1992; 3: 47-49. (in Russian with English abstract)

[527] Grubnik V V et al. Combined laser therapy of diabetic gangrene of the lower limbs. Klin Khir. 1994; 7: 20-22. (in Russian with English abstract)

[528] Yu W et al. Effects of photostimulation on wound healing in diabetic mice. Lasers in Surgery and Medicine. 1997; 20 (1): 56-63.

[529] el Sayed S O, Dyson M. Effect of laser pulse repetition rate and pulse duration on mast cell number and degranulation. Lasers in Surgery and Medicine. 1996; 19 (4): 433-437.

[530] Ibañez J C, Medico R O. [Laser therapy in temporomandibular dysfunction]. Rev Fac Odont Univ Nac (Córdoba). 1989; 17 (1-2): 21-30. (in Spanish)

[531] Howell R M et al. The use of low energy laser therapy to treat aphtous ulcers. Ann Dent. 1988; 47 (2): 16-18.

[532] Bertolucci L E, Grey T. Clinical analysis of Mid-laser versus placebo treatment of arthralgic TMJ degenerative joints. J Craniomandib Practice. 1995; 13 (1): 26-29.

[533] Buliakova N V. Regereration of the x-ray irradiated gastrocnemius muscle in old rats after stimulation. Biull Eksp Biol Med. 1989; 108 (7): 123-126. (in Russian with English abstract)

[534] Pekli F F, Kruchinina I L. [Physiological functions of the nose befroe and after laser treatment of acute and chronic maxillary sinusitis in children]. Vestn Otorinolaringol. 1988; (3): 53-55.

[535] Nissen L R et al. [Low-energy laser therapy in medial tibial stress syndrome]. Ugeskrift Læger. 1994; 156 (49): 7329-7331. (in Danish)

[536] Luger E J, Rochkind S et al. Effect of low-power laser irradiation on the mechanical properties of bone fracture healing in rats. Lasers in Surgery and Medicine. 1998; 22 (2): 97-102.

[537] Wollman Y et al. Low power laser irradiation enhances migration and neurite sprouting of cultured rat embryonal brain cells. Neurol Res. 1996; 18 (5); 467-470.

[538] Weintraub M I. Noninvasive laser neurolysis in carpal tunnel syndrome. Muscle Nerve. 1997; 20 (8): 1029-1031.

[539] Wong E et al. Successful management of female office workers with "repetitive stress injury" or "carpal tunnel syndrome" by a new treatment modality - application of low level laser. Int J Clin Pharmacol Ther. 1995; 33 (4): 208-211.

[540] King C E et al. Effect of helium-neon laser auriculotherapy on experimental pain threshold. Phys Ther. 1990; 70 (1): 24-30.

[541] Kruchinina I et al. Therapeutic effect of helium-neon laser on microcirculation of nasal mucosa in children with acute and chronic maxillary sinuitis as measured by conjuncti-val biomocroscopy. Vestn Otorino-laringol. 1991; 3: 26-30. (In Russian with English abstr)

[542] Kruchinina I et al. Effect of laser therapy on the local synthesis of class A immuno-glubulin in children with acute and chronic maxillary sinuitis. Vestn Otorinolaringol. 1988; 2: 19-21. (In Russian with English abstr)

[543] Pluzhnikov S M et al. Use of intracavitary low-energy laser therapy in the complex treatment of inflammatory diseases in the sphenoid sinus. Vest Otoringolaringol. 1986; 4: 72-73. (In Russian with English abstr)

[544] Toscani A, Bombelli G. [Laser therapy in post-extraction alveolitis]. Dent Cadmos. 1987; 55 (9): 73-74. (In Italian)

[545] Kim Jin Wang, Lee Joung Ok. Double blind cross-over clinical study of 830 nm diode laser and 5 years clinical experience of biostimulation in plastic surgery & aesthetic surgery in Asians. Lasers in Surgery and Medicine. 1998; Suppl 10: 59.

[546] Reddy G K et al. Laser photostimulation of collagen production in healing rabbit achilles tendons. Lasers in Medicine and Surgery. 1998;22: 281-287.

[547] Axelsen S M, Bjerno T. [Laser therapy of ankle sprain]. Ugeskr Læger. 1993; 155 (48): 3908-3911. (in Danish)

[548] Darrre E M et al. [Laser treatment of achilles tendonitis]. Ugeskr Læger.1994; 156 (45): 6680-6683. (in Danish)

[549] Winther A, Laserklinikken, Copenhagen, Denmark. 1997. Personal communication.

[550] Lievens P, Lippens E. The influence of low level infra red lastertherapy on the regen-eration of cartilage tissue. Lasers in Surgery and Medicine. 1998; Suppl 10: 5.

[551] Gruszka M et al. Effect of low energy laser therapy on herniated lumbar discs. Lasers in Surgery and Medicine. 1998; Suppl 10: 6.

[552] Schindl A et al. Low intensity laser irradiation improves skin circulation in patients with diabetic microangiopathy. Diabetes Care. 1998; 21 (4): 580-584.

[553] Skoric T et al. Laser biostimulation: application of the gallium-arsenide laser in the therapy of ulcus cruris. Lasers in Surgery and Medicine. 1998; Suppl 10: 7.

[554] Konstantinovic L et al. [Combined low-power laser therapy and local infiltration of corticosteroids in the treatment of radial-humeral epicondylitis.] Vojnosanit Pregl. 1997; 54 (5): 459-463. (in Croatian)

[555] Tulebaev R K et al. [Indicators of the activity of the immune system during laser ther-apy of vasomotor rhinitis]. Vestn. Otorinolaringol. 1989; 1: 46-49. (in Russian)

[556] Sugrue M E et al. The use of infrared laser therapy in the treatment of venous ulcer-ation. Ann Vasc Surg. 1990; 4 (2): 179-181.

[557] Rakcheev A P et al. [Experimental and clinical substantiation of laser therapy of wounds and throphic ulcers] Ortop Travmatol Protez. 1989; 10: 66-70. (in Russian with English abstract)

[558] Georgadze A K et al. [Treatment of non-healing wounds and trophic ulcers by low-intensity laser irradiation in an outpatient clinic] Khirurgiia (Mosk). 1990; 12: 93-96. (in Rus-sian)

[559] Soriano F. Venous leg ulcers healed with GaAs laser. Argentine experience. Proc Congr Int Soc Laser Surg Med, Bangkok 1993, p. 35.

[683] Ocaña-Quero J M et al. Biological effects of helium-neon (He-Ne) laser irradiation on acrosome reaction in bull sperm cells. J Photochem Photobiol. B - Biol. 1997; 40 (3): 294-298.

[684] Kovalev E V. [The effect of low-intensity laser irradiation on spermatogenesis in men]. Voprosy Kurortol, Fizioter Lechebnoi Fizicheskoi Kultury. 1990; (5): 33-36.

[685] Tsushima T et al. Effects of two-point linear polarised near-infrared irradiation in difficult temporomandibular joint disorders. Proc. 2nd Congress World Assn for Laser Therapy, Kansas City, September 1998; p. 29-30.

[686] Shiomi Y et al. Efficacy of transmeatal low power laser irradiation on tinnitus: a preliminary report. Auris Nasus Larynx. 1997; 24: 39-42.

[687] Shiomi Y et al. [Effect of low power laser irradiation on innear ear.] Pract Otol (Kyoto). 1994; 87: 1135-1140 (in Japanese)

[688] Palchun V T et al. Low-energy laser irradiation in the combined treatment of sensorineural hearing loss and Ménière's disease. Vestnik Otorinolaring. 1996; (1): 23-25 (in Russian).

[689] Ribari O et al. [Closure of tympanic perforations with low-energy HeNe laser irradiation]. Acta Chir Academ Scient Hungaricae. 1980; 21 (3): 229-238.

[690] Bykov V L et al. [Low-energy laser irradiation in the complex treatment of patients with ear diseases.] Voprosy Kurortologii, Fizioterapii i Lechebnoi Fizicheskoi Kultury. 1985; (2): 60-62. (in Russian)

[691] Hashimoto T, Kemmutso O, Otsuka H et al. Efficacy of laser irradiation on the area near the stellate ganglion is dose-dependent: a double-blind crossover placebo-controlled study. Laser Therapy. 1997; 9 (1): 7-12.

[692] Kemmotsu O et al. Laser therapy for pain attenuation. Proc. 2nd Congress World Assn for Laser Therapy, Kansas City, September 1998; p. 7-8.

[693] Wahl G, Bastianer S. Soft laser in postoperative care in dentoalveolar treatment. ZWR. 1991; 100 (8): 512-515.

[694] Tiukhin N S et al. [Laser therapy in patients with inflammatory pleural exudates]. Problemy Tuberkuleza. 1997; 4: 38-40. (in Russian)

[695] Sudoh A et al. Effect of low power laser irradiation on experimental tooth movement. J Dent Res 74 (IADR Abstracts). 1995; p. 457. abstr. 453.

[696] Hashieh I A et al. Helium-neon laser irradiation is not a stressful treatment: a study on heat-shock protein (HSP70) level. Lasers in Surgery and Medicine. 1997; 20 (4): 451-460.

[697] Kats A. [Treatment of erosive-ulcerative forms of lichen planus with low-energy laser irradiation]. Vestnik Khirurgii Imeni i - i - Grekova 1990 144 (4): 121-123.

[698] Velizhanina I A et al. [The laser therapy of hypertension patients in the initial stages.] Voprosy Kuror Fizioter Lecheb Fiziches Kult. 1998; 1: 9-11.

[699] Melnichenko E M et al [The clinico-experimental validation of the use of low-intensity laser radiation for the treatment of exacerbated recurrent herpetic stomatitis in children]. Stomatologiia. 1992; (2): 76-78.

[700] Sitnikov V P et al. [Use of helium-neon lasers in the treatment of postoperative wounds of the phar-ynx]. Vestnik Otorinolaringologii. 1989; (5): 46-49.

[701] Hubacek J et al. Lymphocyte reaction in the palatine tonsils after use of the HeNe laser. Ceskoslov Gastroenterol a Vyziva. 1983; 37 (8): 467-71.

[702] Ben-Dov N, Shefer G, Irinitchev A et al. Low energy laser irradiation affects satellite cell proliferation and differentiation in vitro. Biochem Biophys Acta. 1999; 1448: 372-380.

[703] Thorsen H. [Low energy laser treatment-effect in localized fibromyalgia in the neck and shoulder regions.] Ugeskrift for Laeger. 1991; 17; 153 (25):1801-1804. (in Danish).

[704] Sinev I V et al. [The local treatment of chemical burns of the esophagus via an endoscope by means of laser therapy and adhesive application.] Vestnik Khirurgii Imeni i - i - Grekova 1990; 145 (11): 62-64.

(705] Yamaguchi M et al. [Clinical study on the treatment of hypersensitive dentine by GaAlAs laser diode using the double blind test.] Aichi Gakuin Daigaku Shigakkai Shi - Aichi-Gakuin Journal of Dental Science 1990; 28 (2): 703-707. (In Japanese)

[706] Trelles M A, Rotinen S. He/Ne laser treatment of hemorrhoids. Acupuncture & Electro-Therapeutics Research. 1983; 8 (3-4): 289-295.

[707] Matouskova I. [Reaction of the palatal tonsils after the application of a HeNe laser]. Acta Universitatis Palackianae Olomucensis Facultatis Medicae. 1984;107: 315-320.

[708] Millson C E, Wilson M et al. The killing of Helicobacter pylori by low-power laser light in the presence of a photosensitiser. J Med Microbiol 1996; 44 (4): 245-252

[709] Simunovic Z, Trobonjaca T. Soft tissue injury during sport activities and traffic accidents - treatment woth low level laser therapy: a multicenter double blind, placebo controlled clinical study on 132 patients. Proc. IXX Annual Congress of ASLMS, Orlando, Florida. April 1999.

[710] Shesterina M V. [Effects of laser therapy on immunity in patients with bronchial asthma and pulmonary tuberculosis.] Probl Tuberk. 1994; 5: 23-26.

[711] Myrhaug H. [The theory of otosclerosis and Morbus Ménière (Labyrintine vertigo) being caused by the same mechanism: physical irritants, an otognathic syndrome.] Bergmanns Boktrykkeri A/S, Bergen, Norway. 1981. (In Norwegian)

[712] Mischenkin N V et al. [Effects of helium-neon laser energy on the tissues of the middle ear in the presence of biological fluids and drug solutions]. Vestn Otorinolaringol. 1990; 5: 18-21.

[713] Bogomilskii M R et al. [Effects of low-energy laser irradiation on the functional state of the acoustic analyzer.] Vestn Otorinolaringol. 1989; 2: 29-34.

[714] Dcabrowska E et al. [Intravital treatment of the pulp with simultaneous laser biostimulation] Rocz Akad Med Bialymst. 1997; 42 (1): 168-176. (in Polish)

[715] Bhagwanani N S et al. Low level nitrogen laser therapy in pulmonary tuberculosis. J Clin Laser Med Surg. 1996; 14 (1): 23-25.

[716] Agaev F F. [Endobronchial laser therapy in the surgery of tuberculosis]. Probl Tuberk. 1998; 1: 33-36.

[717] Kipshidze N N et al. Photoremodeling of arterial wall reduces restenosis after balloon angioplasty in an atherosclerotic rabbit model. J Am Coll Cardiol. 1998; 31 (5): 1152-1157.

[718] Barberis G et al. In vitro synthesis of prostaglandin E2 by synovial tissue after helium-neon laser radiation in rheumatoid arthritis. J Clin Laser Med Surg. 1996; 14 (4): 175-177.

[719] Ohno T. [Pain suppressive effects of low power laser irradiation. A quantitative analysis of substance P in the rat spinal dorsal root ganglion]. Nippon Ika Daigaku Zasshi. (J Jap Med School) 1997; 64 (5): 395-400. (in Japanese with English abstract))

[720] Gupta A K et al. The use of low-energy photon therapy in the treatment of leg ulcers - a preliminary report. J Dermatol Treat. 1997; 8 (2): 103-108.

[721] Nicolopoulos N, Dyson M et al. The use of laser surgery in the subtotal meniscectomy and the effect of low-level laser therapy on the healing potential of rabbit meniscus: an experimental study. Lasers Med Sci. 1996; 11 (2): 109-115.

[722] Karpen M. Low-level laser therapy in trials for urologiclal applications. J Clin Laser Med Surg. 1995; 13 (4): 293-294.

[723] Itoh T et al. The protective effect of low power HeNe laser against erythrocytic damage caused by artificial heart-lung machines. Hiroshima J Med Sci. 1996; 45 (1): 15-22.

[724] Barabash A G et al. [Experience in treating patients with lichen ruber planus by using a helium-neon laser]. Stomatologiia; 1995; 74 (1): 20-21.

[725] Reddy G K et al. Biochemistry and biomechanics of healing tendon: Part II. Effects of combined laser therapy and electrical stimulation. Med Sci Sports Exerc. 1998; 30 (6): 794-800.

[726] Gum S L et al. Combined ultrasound, electrical stimulation, and laser promote collagen synthesis with moderate changes in tendon biomechanics. Am J Phys Med Rehabil. 1997; 76 (4): 288-296.

[727] Karu T. Depression of the genome after irradiation of human lymphocytes with HeNe laser. Laser Therapy. 1992. 4 (1): 5-24

[728] Reznikov L L et al. Biomechanism of low-energy laser irradiation is similar to a general adaptive reaction. Proc. SPIE. 1994; Vol 2086: 380-449.

[729] Pavlova R N. et al. Soft-laser radiation bioeffect: is laser a physical adaptogen? Proc. SPIE. 1993; Vol 1922: 225-229

[730] Reznikov L L et al. Similarity between the mechanisms of soft-laser radiation and chemical adapto-gen action. Proc. SPIE. 1993; Vol 1883: 91-98.

[731] Funk J O et al. Helium-Neon laser irradiation induces effects on cytokine production at the protein and the mRNA level. Experimental Dermatology. 1993; 2: 75-83.

[732] Bjordal J M. Low level laser therapy in shoulder tendinitis/bursitis, epicondylalgia and ankle sprain. A critical review on clinical effects. Master thesis in Physiotherapy Science, Div Physiotherapy Science, Univiersity of Bergen, Norway. 1997.

[733] Mester E, Szende B, Tota J. Die Wirkung der Laser-Strahlen auf den Haarwuchs der Maus. Radiobiol. Radiother. 9: 621-626.

[734] Mester E et al. Effect of laser-rays on wound healing. Am J Surg. 1971; 122: 532-.

[735] Conlan M J et al. Biostimulation of wound healing low-energy laser irradiation. A review. J Clin Periodontol. 1996; 23 (5): 492-496.

[736] Saunders L. The efficiacy of low-level laser therapy in supraspinatus tendinitis. Clin Rehab. 1995; 9: 126-134.

[737] Vecchio P et al. A double-blind study of the effectiveness of low level laser treatment of rotator cuff tendinitis. Br J Rheum. 1993; 32: 740-742.

[738] Heussler J K et al. A double blind randomized trial of low power laser treatment in rheumatoid arthritis. Annals Rheum Diseases. 1993; 52: 703-706.

[739] Tabau C. Contributions from Midlaser in the treatment of lateral ankle sprain. Medical Laser Report. 1984; 1: 29-32.

[740] Bjordal J M, Greve G. What may alter the conclusions of reviews? Physical Therapy Reviews. 1998; 3: 121-132.

[741] Exner K. Sitzber. Akad. Wiss., Wien 76II, 522 (1877).

[742] Gabor D. Laser Speckle and Its Elimination. IBM Journal of Res., Sept. 1970.

[743] Hode L, Biedermann K. Observation of surface deformation in real time using laser speckles. Proc Conference in Physics, Lund, Sweden, June 12-14. 1972.

[744] Ragnarsson S-I. Vision Research. 1972; 12: 411

[745] Hode L. Elektronisk bildbehandling för speckelinterferometri i reell tid. Proj.1006. Institutet för Optisk Forskning, Kungl. Tekniska Högskolan. Oktober 1973. (in Swedish).

[746] Burch J M. Interferometry with Scattered Light. Optical Instruments and Techniques. J. Home, Dickson ed. (Reading Conf. 1969) p. 213. Oriel Press, New Castle upon Tyne 1970.

[747] Carniel R. The 780 laser and the CO2-laser in chronic achilles tendinitis: Different methods compared. Proc. 2nd Congress World Assn for Laser Therapy, Kansas City, Sept 1998; p. 40-42.

[748] Gaydess E et al. The effects of laser stimulation on cell and bacterial growth in a cell culture wound model. Proc. 2nd Congress World Assn for Laser Therapy, Kansas City, Sept 1998; p. 72-73.

[749] Ribeiro M S, Zezell D M, Fontenele J D et al. Incorporation of [3H]-Proline in the Dermis of Mice Following He-He Polarized Laser Radiation in the Wound Healing Process. A preliminary Study. Proc. 2nd Congress World Assn for Laser Therapy, Kansas City, Sept 1998; p. 13-15. Also: Histological study on wound healing in rats following He-Ne and GaAlAs laser irradiation. Proc. SPIE. 1998; Vol 3569: 50-55.

[750] Nicola J H, Nicola E M D, Simões M, Paschoal J R. Role of polarization and Coherence of Laser Light on Wound Healing. Laser Tissue Interaction V (1994), S.L. Jacques, ed., Proc SPIE. 1994; 2134A: 448-450.

[751] Ivanov A S et al. [The morphofunctional status of the synovial membrane of the temporomandibular joint under exposure to helium-neon laser]. Morfologia. 1996; 109 (3): 59-63.

[752] Lee G et al. New concepts in pain management in the application of low-power laser for relief of cervicothoracic pain syndromes. Am Heart J. 1996; 132 (6): 1329-1334.

[753] Klima H, Haas O, Roschger P. In Photon emission from Biological Systems (Ed. J. Slawinsky, B. Kochel), World Publishing House, Singapore, 1987.

[754] Skinner S M, Gage J P, Wilce P A, Shaw R M. A preliminary study of the effects of laser radiation on collagen metabolism in cell culture. Aust Dent J 1996; 41 (3):188-192

[755] Valiente-Zaldivar C et al. Laserterapía en la neuralgía trigeminal. Informa preliminar. Rev Cubana de Estomat. 1990; 2 (22): 166-171.

[756] Valiente-Zaldivar et al. Lasers en estomatología. Rev Cubana de Estomat. 1989: 26: 336-343.

[757] Machnikowski I et al. [Application of therapeutic laser in treatment of the selected chronic illnesses of the oral cavity]. Protet Stomatol. 1989; 39 (3): 147-150.

[758] Bernardini U D, Longo L. Terapia laser nella nevralgia del trigemino. Proc. Atti dell'VIII Congresso Nazionale A.I.S.D., Verona. 1985: 80-81.

[759] Fagnoni V et al. Studio sulla guarigione di ferite chirurgiche eseguite sulla mucosa orale di coniglio trattata con soft-Laser. Int Congress on Laser in Med and Surg, Bologna June 1985, p 269.

[760] Fagnoni V et al. Laser therapy in dentistry and stomatology. Observations on 200 cases treated, Medical Laser Report 1984; 1: 36-40.

[761] Fagnoni V et al. Considerazioni clinico terapeutiche sull'íeffetto della luce laser di bassa potenza nell Herpes Simple Labiale. Laser Abstracts. 1984; 1: 28-33.

[762] Fagnoni V, Fontolan D. Importanza della laser-terapia di bassa potenza per la riduzione dei tempi di guarigione dopo interventi di chirurgia parodontale. Laser Abstracts. 3 (2): 25-33.

[763] Fagnoni V et al. Il laser di bassa potenza come coadiuvante nella terapia della sindrome algico-dizfunzionale dell'íarticolazione temporo-mandibulare. Laser Abstracts. 1985; 3: 16-26.

[764] Fagnoni V et al. Study of behaviour of dental enamel in acid solution after treatment with fluorine combined with low power laser. Laser Abstracts. 2 (1): 30-34.

[765] Fagnoni V et al. Verifica sperimentale delle variazioni degli oppioidi endogeni plasmatici in pazienti affetti da nevralgie trigeminali e trattati con laser di bassa potenza. Laser Abstracts. 1985: 3 (2): 35-42.

[766] Fagnoni V et al. Studio sulla guarigione di ferite chirurgiche della mucosa di coniglio precedentemente irradiate con laser I.R. a dosaggi diversi. Laser Abstracts. 1985; 3: 32-37.

[767] Fagnoni V et al. Verifica sperimentale sulle variazioni termiche nella cavità pulpare di denti humani estratti, durante irraggiamento con laser di bassa potenza. Laser Abstracts, 1985; 3 : 27-31.

[768] Fagnoni V et al. Su di un caso di emangioma della mucosa orale trattato mediante irraggiamento con laser di bassa potenza. Minerva Stomatologica. 1983; 32 (5): 701-703.

[769] Antipa C et al. Pulsed-laser therapy (GA-As) in combined treatment of post-traumatic swellings and some dermatological disorders.In: Medical Applications of Lasers. Proc. SPIE.1994; Vol 2086: 371-377

[770] Johnson D et al. Low-level laser therapy for Peyronie's disease. Proc. SPIE.1995; Vol 2395: 108-110.

[771] Kapinosov I K et al. Reaction of lymphoid organs to laser radiation with different pulsation rates. Proc. SPIE.1996; Vol 2678: 530-533. (Optical Diagnostics of Living Cells and Biofluids)

[772] Kucerová H et al. Modulatory frequency of lasers in connection to laser beam therapeutic effect Proc. SPIE.1998; Vol: 191-195. (Lasers in Dentistry IV)

[773] Kucerová H. et al. Effect of laser modulatory frequency on the secretion of IgA and albumin levels after the extraction of human molars in the lower jaw. In: Progress in Biomedical Optics, Proc. of Low-power Light on Biological Systems. Proc SPIE.1997; Vol 3198: 98-101.

[774] Pavlova R N, Gomberg V G, Boiko, V N et al. Effects of low-energy laser isolation upon the development of postradiation syndrome. Proc. SPIE.1996; Vol 2769: 78-81. (Laser Optics '95: Biomedical Applications of Lasers)

[775] Antipa C et al. Low-energy laser treatment of rheumatic diseases: a long-term study Proc. SPIE.1995; Vol 2391: 658-662. (Laser-Tissue Interaction VI)

[776] Telfer J, Filonenko N, Salansky N M. Leg ulcer plastic surgery descent by laser therapy. Proc. SPIE.1994; Vol 2086:.258-263. (Medical Applications of Lasers)

[777] Marchesini R, Dasdia T, Melloni E, Rocca E. Effect of low-energy laser irradiation on colony formation capability in different human tumor cells in vitro. Lasers in Surgery and Medicine. 1989; 9 (1): 59-62.

[778] Burns T, Wilson M, Pearson G J Killing of cariogenic bacteria by light from a gallium aluminium arsenide diode laser. J Dent 1994; 22 (5): 273-278

[779] Gross A J, Jelkmann W. Helium-neon laser irradiation inhibits the growth of kidney epithelial cells in culture. Lasers in Surgery and Medicine. 1990;10 (1): 40-44

[780] Antipa C et al. Laser biostimulation (He-Ne and Ga-As) effects as compared to the conventional therapy in several pelvic inflammatory diseases. Proc. SPIE.1993; Vol 1879: 15-22 (Lasers in Urology, Gynecology, and General Surgery).

[781] Xu Yong-Qing et al. Experimental study of the effects of helium-neon laser radiation on repair of injured tendon. Proc. SPIE.1993; Vol 1616: 598-604. (International Conference on Photodynamic Therapy and Laser Medicine)

[782] Jarry G, Debray S, Perez J, Lefebvre J P, de Ficquelmont-Loizos M, Gaston A. In vivo transillumination of the hand using near infrared laser pulses and differential spectroscopy. J Biomed Eng 1989; 11 (4):293-299.

[783] Tsang D, Yew D T, Hui B S. Further studies on the effect of low-dose laser irradiation on cultured retinal pigment cells of the chick. Acta Anat (Basel) 1986;125 (1):10-13.

[784] Yu W, Naim J O, McGowan M, Ippolito K, Lanzafame R J. Photomodulation of oxidative metabolism and electron chain enzymes in rat liver mitochondria. Photochem Photobiol 1997; (6):866-871.

[785] Murphy P J, Campbell S S. Enhanced performance in elderly subjects following bright light treatment of sleep maintenance insomnia. J Sleep Res 1996 Sep;5 (3):165-72.

[786] Campbell S S, Murphy P J. Extraocular circadian phototransduction in humans. Science 1998; 279 (5349): 396-399.

[787] Bylesjö E I, Boman K, Wetterberg L. Obesity treated with phototherapy: four case studies. Int J Eat Disord 1996; (4): 443-446.

[788] Thalén BE, Kjellman BF, Mörkrid L, Wetterberg L. Melatonin in light treatment of patients with seasonal and nonseasonal depression. Acta Psychiatr Scand 1995; (4): 274-284.

[789] Wikner J, Andersson DE, Wetterberg L, Röjdmark S. Impaired melatonin secretion in patients with Wernicke-Korsakoff syndrome. J Intern Med. 1995; 237 (6): 571-575.

[790] Thalén B E, Kjellman B F, Mörkrid L, Wibom R, Wetterberg L. Light treatment in seasonal and nonseasonal depression. Acta Psychiatr Scand 1995; 91 (5): 352-360.

[791] Wetterberg L. Light and biological rhythms. Läkartidningen 1992; 89 (37): 2915-2918. (In Swedish)

[792] Wetterberg L. Light therapy of depression; basal and clinical aspects. Pharmacol Toxicol 1992;71 Suppl 1:96-106.

[793] Wetterberg L et al. Light therapy of depression. Läkartidningen. 1991; 30; 88 (5): 310-312. (In Swedish)

[794] Wetterberg L. The importance of light for health and well-being. Läkartidningen. 1991; 88 (5): 295-296. (In Swedish)

[795] Petterborg L J, Kjellman B F, Thalen B E, Wetterberg L. Effect of a 15 minute light pulse on nocturnal serum melatonin levels in human volunteers. J Pineal Res. 1991; 10 (1): 9-13.

[796] Wetterberg L. The significance of lighting for health and wellbeing. Nord Med. 1991;106 (3): 90-91.(in Swedish)

[797] Wetterberg L. Lighting. Nonvisual effects. Scand J Work Environ Health. 1990; 16 Suppl 1: 26-28.

[798] Wu J, Sanchez de la Pena S, Hallberg F et al. Chronosynergistic effects of lighting schedule-shift and cefodizime on plasmacy-toma growth and host survival time. Chronobiologia. 1988; 15 (1-2): 105-128.

[799] Wetterberg L. Melatonin and affective disorders. Ciba Found Symp 1985; 117: 253-265.

[800] Illnerova H, Vanecek J, Krecek J, Wetterberg L, Sääf J. Effect of one minute exposure to light at night on rat pineal serotonin N-acetyltransferase and melatonin. J Neurochem. 1979; 32 (2): 673-675.

[801] Rao M L, Muller-Oerlinghausen B etv al. The influence of pho-totherapy on serotonin and melatonin in non-seasonal depression. Pharmacopsychiatry 1990; 23 (3): 155-158.

[802] Partonen T, Vakkuri O, Lönnqvist J. Suppression of melatonin secretion by bright light in seasonal affective disorder. Biol Psychiatry. 1997; 42 (6): 509-513.

[803] Salinas E O, Hakim-Kreis C M et al. Hypersecretion of melatonin following diurnal exposure to bright light in seasonal affective disorder: preliminary results. Biol Psychiatry. 1992; 32 (5): 387-398.

[804] Checkley S A, Murphy D G, Abbas M et al. Melatonin rhythms in seasonal affective disorder. Br J Psychiatry. 1993;:163: 332-337.

[805] Rice J, Mayor J, Tucker H A, Bielski R J. Effect of light therapy on salivary melatonin in seasonal affective disorder. Psychiatry Res. 1995; 56 (3): 221-228.

[806] Rao M L, Muller-Oerlinghausen B, Mackert A et al. Blood serotonin, serum melatonin and light therapy in healthy subjects and in patients with nonseasonal depression. Acta Psy-chiatr Scand. 1992; 86 (2): 127-132.

[807] Lewy A J, Bauer V K, Cutler N L et al.. Morning vs evening light treatment of patients with winter depression. Arch Gen Psychiatry. 1998; 55 (10): 890-896.

[808] Deltito J A, Moline M et al. Effects of phototherapy on non-seasonal unipolar and bipolar depressive spectrum disorders. J Affect Disord. 1991; 23 (4): 231-237.

[809] Lam R W, Terman M, Wirz-Justice A Light therapy for depressive disorders: indications and efficacy. Mod Probl Pharmacopsychiatry. 1997; 25 :215-234

[810] Wirz-Justice A. Beginning to see the light. Arch Gen Psychiatry. 1998; 55 (10): 861-862. Review.

[811] Light therapy for winter depression. Health News. 1998; Nov 20; 4 (14): 6.

[812] Light therapy. Health News. 1998; 4 (3): 5.

[813] Tolle R. Psychotherapy of depressive disorders: on the theoretical background and its clinical relevance. Nervenarzt. 1997; 68 (7): 602-605.

[814] Avery D H. A turning point for seasonal affective disorder and light therapy research? Arch Gen Psychiatry. 1998; Oct;55 (10): 863-4. Review.

[815] Melges F T. Efficacy of therapies for depression. Am J Psychiatry. 1981; 138 (11): 1513.

[816] Haffmans J et al. Suicide after bright light treatment in seasonal affective disorder: a case report. J Clin Psychiatry. 1998; 59 (9): 478.

[817] Ash J B, Piazza E, Anderson J L. Light therapy in the clinical management of an eating-disordered ado-lescent with winter exacerbation. Int J Eat Disord. 1998;23 (1): 93-97.

[818] Kripke D F. Light treatment for nonseasonal depression: speed, efficacy, and combined treatment. J Affect Disord. 1998; 49 (2): 109-117.

[819] Wetterberg L. Light and biological rhythms. J Intern Med. 1994; Jan;235 (1):5-19.

[820] Grzesiak-Janas, Grazyna A A. Low-power-laser therapy in Costen's syndrome. Proc. SPIE.1996; Vol 2781. 1996: 126-128. (Lasers in Medicine)

[821] Strupinska E. Low-power-laser therapy used in tendon damage. Proc. SPIE.1996; Vol 2781: 177-183. (Lasers in Medicine)

[822] De Paula Eduardo C et al. Benefits of low-power lasers on oral soft tissue. Proc. SPIE.1996; Vol 2672: 27-33. (Lasers in Dentistry II)

[823] Gao Yun-Qing, Liu Song-Hao, Zhang You, Liu T C. 367 cases of CO2 laser therapy on facial acne. Proc. SPIE. 1996; Vol 2887: 60-62. (Lasers in Medicine and Dentistry: Diagnostics and Treatment)

[824] Nicola E M, Nicola H. Low-power CO2 laser in the treatment of chronic pharyngitis: a five-year experience. Proc. SPIE.1994; Vol 2128: 85-87. (Laser Surgery: Advanced Characterization, Therapeutics, and Systems IV)

[825] Zhou, Chuannong; Song, Xuyan; Deng, Jinsheng; Liang, Junlin; Zhang, Hua; Huang, Wenjia; Liu, Tao; Ha, Xian-Wen Photodynamic effect of copper-vapor pumped-dye laser, HeNe laser, and noncoherent red light to the liver in normal mice. Proc. SPIE.1993; Vol 1616: 239-245. (International Conference on Photodynamic Therapy and Laser Medicine, Jun-Heng Li; Ed.)

[826] Lerner L A. [Effectiveness of laser therapy in Bechterew's disease.] Terapevticheskii Arkhiv. 1988, 60(4):134-136.

[827] Wilson M et al. Bacteria in supragingival plaque samples can be killed by low-power laser light in the presence of a photosensitizer. J Appl Bacteriol 1995; 78(5): 569-574.

[828] Bisht D et al. Effect of low intensity laser radiation on healing of open skin wounds in rats. Indian J Medical Research. 1994; 100: 43-46.

[829] Kleinman Y et al. Low level laser therapy in patients with venous ulcers: early and long-term out-come. Laser Therapy. 1996; 8 (3): 205-208.

[830] Ito A, Kakami K, Matsushita H, Fukaya M. Effects of Nd:YAG low power laser irradiation on the ulnar nerve. Aichi Gakuin Dent Sci. 1989; 2: 1-8

[831] Matsushita H, Kakami K, Ito A et al. Effect on the action potential of the low power Nd:YAG laser as irradiated directly to the nerve. Aichi Gakuin Dent Sci. 1989; 2: 19-28

[832] Pyczek M, Sopala M, Dabrowski Z. Effect of low-energy laser power on the bone marrow of the rat. Folia Biol (Krakow) 1994; 42 (3-4): 151-156

[833] Efendiev A I et al. [Increasing the scar strength after preventive skin irradiation with low-intensity laser.] Klin Khir 1992; (1): 23-25.

[834] Iakovleva N E, Liapina L A, Novoderzhkina I S et al. [The effect of low-intensity laser radiation on the parameters of the blood anticoagulation system in the early postresuscitation period]. Anaesteziol Reanimatol. 1997 ; (4): 36-38.

[835] Jimbo K, Noda K, Suzuki K, Yoda K. Suppressive effects of low-power laser irradiation on bradykinin evoked action potentials in cultured murine dorsal root ganglion cells. Neurosci Lett. 1998; 240 (2): 93-96.

[836] van Rensburg S D, Wiltshire W A. The effect of soft laser irradiation on fluoride release of two fluoride-containing orthodontic bonding materials. J Dent Assoc S Afr. 1994; 49 (3): 127-131.

[837] Hicks M J et al. Root caries in vitro after low fluence argon laser and fluoride treatment. Compend Contin Educ Dent. 1997; 18 (6): 543-548.

[838] Hsu J et al. Combined effects of laser irradiation/solution fluoride ion on enamel demineralization. J Clin Laser Med Surg. 1998; 16 (2): 93-105.

[839] Shi K, Lu R, Xu X. Influence of low energy HeNe laser on the regeneration of peripheral nerves. Chung Kuo Hsiu Fu Chung Chien Wai Ko Tsa Chih. 1997; 11 (1): 14-8. (In Chinese)

[840] Mikhailov V A et al. The immunomodulating action of low-energy laser radiation in the treatment of bronchial asthma. Vopr Kurortol Fizioter Lech Fiz Kult. 1998; (4): 23-5.

[841] Okamoto H, Iwase T, Morioka T. Dye-mediated bactericidal efffect of HeNe laser irradiation on oral microorganisms. Lasers in Surgery and Medicine. 1992; 12 (4): 450-458.

[842] Wilson M, Pratten A. Lethal photosensitisation of Staphylococcus aureus in vitro: effect of growth phase, serum, and pre-irradiation time. Lasers Med Surg. 1995; 16 (3): 272-276.

[843] CRA Newsletter. 1997; 21 (4). Clinical Research Associates, Provo, Utah, USA.

[844] Walter Wintsch, Switzerland, personal communication

[845] Orchardson R, Whitters C J. Effect of HeNe and pulsed Nd:YAG laser irradiation on intradental nerve responses to mechanical stimulation of dentine. Lasers in Surgery and Medicine. 2000; 26: 241-249.

[846] Cassone M C, Lombard A, Rossetti V, Urciuoli R, Rolfo P M. Effect of in vivo HeNe laser irradiation on biogenic amine levels in rat brain. J Photochem Photobiol B 1993; 18 (2-3): 291-294

[847] Loginov A S, Sokolova G N, Trubitsyna I E et al. [Biogenic amines and cyclic nucleotides in the laser therapy of long-term nonhealing stomach ulcers]. Vrach Delo 1991; (1): 24-27. (In Russian)

[848] Loginov A S, Sokolova G N, Sokolova S V et al. [The content of biologically active substances in the margin of a stomach ulcer being treated with a copper-vapor laser]. Ter Arkh. 1991; 63 (8): 75-78. (In Russian)

[1119] Kim S-Y, Park J-S. The effect of low level laser therapy at the trigger points in masseter and other muscles. J Korean Acad. Oral Med. 1996; 21 (1): 1-3.

[1120] Ghamsari S M, Taguchi K, Abe N et al. Histopathological effect of low-level laser therapy on sutured wounds of the teat in diary cattle. Vet Quarterly. 1996; 18 (1): 17-21.

[1121] Ghamsari S M, Acorda J A, Taguchi K et al. Evaluation of wound healing of the teat with and without low level laser therapy in diary cattle by laser Doppler flowmetry in comparison with histopathology, tensiometry and hydroxyproline analysis. Br Vet J. 1996; 152 (5): 583-592.

[1122] Pankov O P. Low-level therapy in ophthalmology. In: Novel Laser Methods in Medicine and Biology. Eds. Prokhorov A M, Pustovoy V I, Kuzmin G P. Proc. SPIE. 1998; Vol 3829: 13-17.

[1123] Stein A, Kraicer P, Oron U. Effect of low energy (He-Ne) irradiation on embryo implantation rate in the rat. In: Proc. Low Power Light Effects in Biological Systems. Proc. SPIE. 1997; Vol. 3198: 24-30.

[1124] Kipshidze N, Nikolaychik V, Keelan M et al. Low-power helium:neon laser irradiation enhances pro-duction of vascular endothelian growth factor and promotes growth of endothelian cells in vitro. Lasers in Surgery and Medicine. 2001; 28: 355-364.

[1125] De Scheerder I, Wang K, Zhou X R et al. Intravascular low power red laser light as an adjunct to coronary stent implantation evaluated in a porcine coronary model. J Invas Cardiol. 1998; 10: 534-538.

[1126] Kaul U, Singh B, Sudan D et al. Red light laser therapy after coronary stenting: angiographic and clinical follow up study in humans. J Invas Cardiol. 1998; 10: 269-273.

[1127] Brugnera A. LLLT in treating dentinary hypersensibility: A histological study and clinical application. Proc. 2nd ENSOMA Congress, Houston, Texas, USA. 2001.

[1128] Pinheiro A. Biomodulatory effects of LLLT on bone regeneration. Proc. 2nd ENSOMA Congress, Houston, Texas, USA. 2001.

[1129] Siposan D, Lukacs A. Relative variation to received dose of some erythrocytic and leukocytic indices of human blood as a result of low.level laser radiation: An in vitro study. J Clin Laser Med Surg. 2001; 19 (2): 89-103.

[1130] Kolárová H, Ditrichová D, Wagner J. Penetration of the laser light into the skin in vitro. Lasers in Surgery and Medicine. 1999; 24: 231-235.

[1131] Rochkind S, Nissan M, Alon M et al. Effects of laser irradiation on the spinal cord for the regeneration of crushed peripheral nerve in rats. Lasers in Surgery and Medicine. 2001; 28 (3): 216-219.

[1132] Simunovic Z, Simunovic K. Status after multiple teeth extractions treatment with low level laser therapy: A randomised clinical study with control group. Lasers in Surgery and Medicine. 2001; Suppl 13: 11.

[1133] Campaña V, Moya M, Gavotto A et al. Effects of helium-neon laser on microcrystalline arthropaties. Lasers in Surgery and Medicine. 2001; Suppl 13: 11.

[1134] Simunovic Z, Trobonjaca T. Comparison between low level laser therapy and visible incoherent polarised light in the treatment of lateral epicondylitis - tennis elbow. A pilot clinical study on 20 patients. Lasers in Surgery and Medicine. 2001; Suppl 13: 9.

[1135] Yan Li, Timon Cheng-Yi Liu, Rui Duan. Effects of some anaesthetics on wound healing: laser biomodulation mechanisms. Lasers in Surgery and Medicine. 2001; Suppl 13: 9. Lasers in Surgery and Medicine.2001; Suppl 13: 9.

[1136] Schindl A, Merwald H, Schindl L. Low intensity laser irradiation stimulates endothelial cell proliferation in an vitro model of diabetic microangiopathy. Lasers in Surgery and Medicine. 2001; Suppl 13: 7.

[1137] Tay E J, Lee L I, Yee S, Loh H S. Laser-induced reduction of post-operative pain following third molar surgery. Lasers in Surgery and Medicine. 2001; Suppl 13: 17.

[1138] Rogvi Hansen B et al. Low level laser treatment of chondromalacia patellae. Int Orthopaedics. 1991; 15: 359-361.

[1139] Lewith G T, Machin D. A randomized trial to evaluate the effect of infrared stimulation of local trigger points, versus placebo, on the pain caused by cervical osteoarthrosis. Acupunct Electro-Ther Res, 1981; 6: 277-284.

[1140] Tenenbaum J. The epidemiology of nonsteroidal anti-inflammatory drugs. Can J Gastroenterol. 1999; 13: 119-122.

[1141] Zhuk N A, Levencho M V, Barinova S E. Laser therapy of chronic tuberculosis. 8th Internat Congr of the European Medical Laser Assoc., Moscow, Russia, May 23-26 2001. Book of Abstracts, p. 17.

[1142] Baumler W, Neff S, Landthaler M et al. Laser Assisted Hair Removal: Comparison of a Normal Mode Ruby Laser and a High Power Laser Diode. Abstract volume, Laser Florence. 14:th International Congress of Laser Medicine, pp 11, Florence 1999.

[1143] Williams R, Havoonjian H, Isagholian K et al.. A clinical study of hair removal using the long-pulsed ruby laser. Dermatol Surg. 1998; 24 (8): 837-842

[1144] Boss W K Jrc, Usal H, Thompson R C, Fiorillo M A. A comparison of the long-pulse and short-pulse Alexandrite laser hair removal systems. Ann Plast Surg 1999; 42 (4): 381-384.

[1145] Bjerring R, Clement M, Heckendorff L et al. Selective non-ablative wrinkle reduction by laser. J Cutan Laser Ther. 2000; 2: 9-15.

[1146] Goldberg D, Metzler C. Skin resurfacing utilizing a low-fluence Nd:YAG laser. J Cutan Laser Ther. 1999; 1: 23-27.

[1147] Goldberg D J. Non-ablative subsurface remodeling: clinical and histological evaluation of a 1320 nm Nd:YAG laser. J Cutan Laser Ther. 1999; 1: 153-157.

[1148] Lupton J R, Alster T S. Non-ablative cutaneous laser resurfacing using a 1.54 µm erbium-doped phosphate glass laser: a clinical and histologic analysis. Laser Surg Med 2001; 27-.

[1149] Yu W, Naim J O, Lanzafame R J. The effects of photo-irradiation on the secretion of TGF-a, PDGF and bFGF from fibroblasts in vitro (abstract). Lasers in Surgery and Medicine. 1994; 6: 8.

[1150] Giavelli S, Fava G, Castronuovo G et al. Low power laser in the treatment of knee osteoarthritis in geriatric patients. Laser & Technology. 1994; 4 (1/2): 39-48.

[1151] Lizarelli R F, Ciconelli K P, Braga C A, Berro R J. Low-powered laser therapy associated with oral implantology. Proc SPIE.1999; Vol 3593: 69-73, Lasers in Dentistry V, John D. Featherstone; Peter Rechmann; Daniel Fried; Eds.

[1152] Smith C F, Vangsness C T, Anderson T & Good W. Treatment of repetitive use carpal tunnel syndrome. Proc. SPIE.1995; Vol 2395: 658-661. Lasers in Surgery: Advanced Characterization, Therapeutics, and Systems V, R. Rox Anderson; Ed.

[1153] Petersen S L, Botes C, Olivier A, Guthrie A J. The effect of LLLT on wound healing in horses. Equine Vet J. 1999; 31 (3): 228-231.

[1154] Brosseau L et al. Low level laser therapy for osteoarthritis and rheumatoid arthritis: a metaanalysis. J Rheumatol. 2000; 27 (8): 1961-1969.

[1155] Timirgalef M J et al. [Laser therapy of the inflammatory diseases of the accessory nasal sinuses]. Vestn Otorin. 1985; 3: 56-60.

[1156] Watanabe H, Ishikawa I, Susuki M et al. Clinical assessment of the Erbium:YAG laser for soft tissue surgery and scaling. J Clin Laser Med Surg. 1996; 14 (2): 67-75.

[1157] Ando Y, Watanabe H, Ishikawa I. Bactericidal effect of Erbium YAG laser on periodontal bacteria. Lasers in Surgery and Medicine. 1996; 19: 190-200.

[1158] Rajaratuan S, Bolton P, Dyson M. Macrophage responsiveness to laser therapy with varying pulsing frequencies. Laser Therapy. 1994; 6 (2): 107-102.

[1159] Kumæ T, Arakawa H. In vitro effects of therapeutic laser on superoxide generation from rat alveolar macrophage. Laser Therapy. 1999; 11 (3): 119-129.

[1160] Enwemeka C. Quantum Biology of Laser Photostimulation (editorial). Laser Therapy. 1999; 11 (2): 52-53.

[1161] Enwemeka C, Rodriguez O, Gall N et al. Morphometries of collagen fibril populations in HeNe photostimulated tendons. J Clin Laser Med Surg. 1990; 47-52.

[1162] Tang J, Godlewski G, Rovy S et al. Morphologic changes in collagen fibers after 830 nm diode welding. Lasers in Surgery and Medicine. 1997; 21: 438-443.

[1163] Duan R, Liu C-Y, Li Y et al. Signal transduction pathways involved in low intensity He-Ne laser-induced respiratory burst in bovine neutrophils: a potential mechanism of low intensity laser biostimulation. Lasers in Surgery and Medicine. 2001; 29: 174-178.

[1164] Verdote-Robertson R, Munchua M M, Reddon J R. The use of low intensity laser therapy (LILT) for the treatment of open wounds in psychogeriatric patients: A pilot study. Physical and Occupational Therapy in Geriatrics. 2000, 18(2): 1-19.

[1165] Lagan K M, McDonough S M, Clements B A, Baxter G D. A case report of low intensity laser therapy (LILT) in the management of venous ulceration: potential effects of wound debridement upon efficacy. J Clin Laser Medicine & Surgery. 2000; 18 (1): 15-22.

[1166] Velizhanina I A, Gapon L I, Shabalina M S et al. [Efficiency of low-intensity laser radiation in essential hypertension]. Klinicheskaia Meditsina (Mosk). 2001; 79 (1): 41-44.

[1167] Damjanova J, Manolov V. Therapeutic influence on patients with epiconoylitis and myotendinitis of upper extremity by the means of low-intensity laser. Fizikalna Kurortna i Rekhabilitatsiona Meditsina. 2000; 39 (1): 15.

[1168] Baratto L, Capra R, Farinelli M et al. A new type of very low-power modulated laser: soft-tissue changes induced in osteoarthritic patients revealed by sonography. International Journal of Clinical Pharmacology Research. 2000; 20 (1-2): 13-16.

[1169] Ilich-Stoianovich O, Nasonov E L, Balabanova R M. [Effects of low-intensity infrared impulse laser therapy on inflammation activity markers in patients with rheumatoid arthritis]. Terapevticheskii Arkhiv. 2000; 72 (5): 32-34.

[1170] Özdemir F, Birtane M, Kokino S. The clinical efficacy of low-power laser therapy on pain and function in cervical osteoarthritis. Clinical Rheumatology. 2001; 20 (3): 181-184.

[1171] Guzzardella G A, Morrone G, Torricelli P et al. Assessment of low-power laser biostimulation on chon-dral lesions: an "in vivo" experimental study. Artificial Cells, Blood Substitutes, and Immobilization Biotechnology. 2000; 28 (5): 441-449.

[1172] Morrone G, Guzzardella G A, Torricelli P et al. Osteochondral lesion repair of the knee in the rabbit after low-power diode Ga-Al-As laser biostimulation: an experimental study. Artificial Cells, Blood Substitutes, and Immobilization Biotechnology. 2000; 28 (4): 321-336.

[1173] Itoh T, Murakami H, Orihashi K et al. Low power laser protects human erythrocytes in an in vitro model of artificial heart-lung machines. Artificial Organs. 2000; 24 (11): 870-873.

[1174] Manukhin I B, Matafonov V A, Mamedov F M. [The efficacy of the transcutaneous magnetic-laser irradiation of the blood in acute salpingo-oophoritis] Voprosy kurortologii, fizioterapii, i lechebnoi fizicheskoi kultury. 2000; (1): 32-35.

[1175] Idrisova L T, Enikeev D A, Vasileva T V. [The effect of intravenous laser irradiation of the blood on the brain bioelectrical activity in patients in the postcomatose period]. Vopr Kurortol-Fizioter-Lech-Fiz-Kult. 2000; (2): 28-31.

[1176] Balakirev S A, Gusev L I, Kazanova M et al. [Low-intensity laser therapy in pediatric oncology]. Voprosy Onkologii. 2000; 46 (4): 459-461.

[1177] Polosukhin V V. Ultrastructure of the blood and lymphatic capillaries of the respiratory tissue during inflammation and endobronchial laser therapy. Ultrastructural Pathology. 2000; 24 (3): 183-189.

[1178] Forney R, Mauro T. Using lasers in diabetic wound healing. Diabetes Technology & Therapeutics. 1999; 1 (2): 189-192.

[1179] Schindl A, Schindl M, Pernerstorfer-Schoen H, Schindl L. Low intensity laser therapy in wound healing - A review with special respect to diabetic angiopathies. Acta Chirurgica Austriaca. 2001; 33: 3-.

[1180] Grzesiak-Janas G, Janas A. Conservative closure of antro-oral communication stimulated with laser light. Journal of Clinical Laser Medicine and Surgery. 2001; 19 (4): 181-184.

[1181] Ueda Y, Shimizu N. Pulse irradiation of low-power laser stimulates bone nodule formation. Journal of Oral Science. 2001; 43 (1): 55-60.

[1182] Shamir M H, Rochkind-S, Sandbank-J, Alon-M. Double-blind randomized study evaluating regeneration of the rat transected sciatic nerve after suturing and postoperative low-power laser treatment. Journal of Reconstructive Microsurgery. 2001; 17 (2): 133-137.

[1183] Cho K-A, Park J-S, Ko M-Y. The effect of low level laser therapy on pressure threshold in patients with temporomandinular disorders. A double blind study. J Korean Acad Oral Med. 1999; 24 (3): 281-300.

[1184] Lucas C. Efficacy of low level laser treatment in the management of chronic wounds. Thesis. Hogeschool van Amsterdam, The Netherlands. 2001. ISBN 90-9015244-X.

[1185] Forney R, Mauro T. Using lasers in diabetic wound healing. Diabetes Technology & Therapeutics. 1999; 1 (2): 189-192.

[1186] Oliveira N M, Parizzotto N A, Salvini T F. GaAs (904-nm) laser radiation does not affect muscle regeneration in mouse skeletal muscle. Lasers in Surgery and Medicine. 1999; 25: 13-21.

[1187] Bjordal J M, Johnson M I, Couppè C. Clinical Electrotherapy. Your guide to optimal treatment. Hoyskoleforlaget. Norwegian Academic Press. 2001. ISBN 82-7634-320-1.

[1188] Krasheninnikoff M, Ellitsgaard B, Rogvi-Hansen B et al. No effect of low power laser in lateral epicondylitis. Scand J Rheum. 1994; 23: 260-263.

[1189] Papadopoulos E S, Smith R W, Cawley M I D. Low-level laser therapy does not aid the management of tennis elbow. Clinical Rehabilitation. 1996; 10: 9-11.

[1190] Spivak J M, Grande D A et al. The effect of low-level Nd:YAG laser energy on adult articular cartilage in vitro. Arthroscopy. 1992; 8 (1): 36-43.

[1191] Ebert, D W, Bertone A L. Effect of irradiation with low intensity diode laser on the metabolism of equine articular cartilage in vitro. Am J Vet Res. 1998; 59 (12): 1613-1618.

[1192] Ghamsari S M, Taguchi K et al. Evaluation of low level laser therapy on primary healing of experimentally induced full thickness wounds in diary cattle. Vet Surg. 199; 26 (2): 114-120.

[1193] Kim. K-S et al. Effects of low level laser irradiation with 904 nm pulsed diode laser on the extraction wound. J of Korean Academy of Oral Medicine. 1998; 23: 301-307.

[1194] Lee K-H, Kim K-S. Effects of low level laser irradiation on the ALP activity and calcified nodule formation of rat osteoblastic cell. J of Korean Academy of Oral Medicine. 1996; 21: 279-292.

[1195] Migliorati C, Massumoto C, de Paula Eduardo F et al. Low-energy laser therapy in oral mucositis. J Oral Laser Applications. 2001; 1 (2): 97-101.

[1196] Lubart R, Breitbart H, Sofer Y, Lavie R. He-Ne irradiation of human spermatozoa: enhancement in hamster egg penetration. Laser Therapy. 1999; 11 (4): 171-176.

[1197] Yaakov N, Ben-Haim S, Oron U. Low level laser irradiation reduces interstitial scarring in the isoproternol-induced hypertrohpic rat heart. Laser Therapy. 1999; 11 (4): 190-197.

[1098] Oron U, Yaakobi T, Oron A et al. Attenuation of the formation of scar tissue in rats and dogs post myocardial infarction by low energy laser irradiation. Lasers in Surgery and Medicine. 2001; 28: 1-7.

[1278] Meersman P. Laser pharmacology and achilles tendinopathy. Laser Therapy. 1999; 11 (3): 144-150.

[1279] Mochizuki O N, Kataoka Y, Cui Y et al. Effects of near-infra-red laser irradiation on adenosine triphosphate and adenosine diphosphate contents of rat brain tissue. Neuroscience Letters. 2002; 323 (3): 207-210.

[1280] Lindholm A C, Swensson U, de Mitri N,Collinder E. Clinical Effects of Betamethasone and Hyaluronan, and of Defocalized Carbon Dioxide Laser Treatment on Traumatic Arthritis in the Fetlock Joints of Horses. J Vet Med. 2002: 189 -194.

[1281] Gür A, Karakoc M, Nas Ket al. Effects of low power laser and low dose amitriptyline therapy on clinical symptoms and quality of life in fibromyalgia: a single-blind, placebo-controlled trial. Rheumatol Int. 2002; 22 (5): 188-193.

14.2 Alphabetical register of references

Abe M et al. Role of 830 nm low reactive level laser on the growth of an implanted glioma in mice. Keio J Med 1993; 42 (4): 177-179.

Abeles M, Marlowe S, Ingentio F. Treatment of osteoarthritis of the hand with low power laser. Arthritis Rheum. 1988; 28: 294. (abstract).

Abergel P et al. Non Thermal Effects of Nd:YAG Laser on the Biological Functions of the Human Skin Fibro-blasts in Culture. Lasers in Surgery and Medicine. 1984; 3: 379-.

Abergel P, Lyons R, Castel J, Dwyer R, Uitto J. Biostimulation of wound healing by laser: Experimental approaches in animal models and in fibroblast cultures. J Dermatol Surg Oncol. 1987; 13: 127-133.

Abergel P. et al. Control of connective tissue metabolism by lasers: Recent developments and future prospects. J Am Acad Dermatol. 1984; 11: 1142-.

Abergel P. Laser treatment of acne scars. Lasers in Surgery and Medicine. 1992; Suppl 4: 70.

Abramovici A, Roisman P, Hirsch et al. HeNe laser irradiation accelerate healing process of open gingival wounds in cats. In:Anderson RR, ed. Laser surgery: Advanced characterization, therapeutics, and systems. IV. Proc. SPIE Vol. 2128: 248-256.

Ad N, Uron U. The impact of low energy laser irradiation on infarct size in the rat following myocardial infarction. Intern J Cardiol (accepted for publication).

Agaev F F. [Andobronchial laser therapy in the surgery of tuberculosis]. Probl Tuberk. 1998; 1: 33-36.

Agambar L, Herbert K E. Scott D L. Low powered laser therapy for rheumatoid arthritis. Br J Rheum. 1992; 31 (suppl 2): 81.

Ailioaie C, Ailioaie L, Topoliceanu F. Self-organizing phenomena at membrane levels and LLLT of rhinitis. Proc. SPIE. 2000; Vol. 416: 309-315.

Ailioaie C, Lupusoru-Ailioaie L M. Beneficial effects of laser therapy in the early stagers of rheumatoid arthritis onset. Laser Therapy. 1999; 11 (2): 79-87.

Ailioaie L, Ailioaie C. Self-organizing phenomena at membrane level and low level laser therapy of rhinitis. In: A window on the laser medicine world. Longo L ed. Proc. SPIE.1999, Vol 4166: 309-315.

Ailioaie C, Ailioaie L. The treatment of bronchial asthma with low level laser in attack-free period of children. Proc. SPIE. 2000; Vol. 4166: 303-308.

Airaksinen O et al. Effects of HeNe-laser irradiation on the trigger points of patients with chronic muscle ten-sion in the neck. Scand J of Acup & Electrotherapy. 1989; 4: 63-65.

Airaksinen O, et al. Effects of infra-red laser irradiation at the trigger points. Scand J of Acup & Electrotherapy. 1988; 3: 56-61.

Akai M et al. Laser's effect on bone and cartilage change induced by joint immobilization: an experiment with animal model. Lasers in Surgery and Medicine. 1997; 21 (5): 480-484.

Allan R C, Stjernholm R L, Steele R H. Biochem. Biophys. Res. Commun. 1972; 47: 679-

Almeida-Lopes L et al. The use of low level laser therapy for wound healing: comparative study. Proc. 3rd Congr World Assn for Laser Therapy, Athens, Greece, May 2000, p. 118.

Almeida-Lopes L, Rigau J, Zángaro R et al. Comparison of the low level laser therapy effects on cultured human gingival fibroblast proliferation using different irradiance and same fluency. Lasers in Surgery and Medicine. 2001; 29: 179-184.

Alstergren P et al. Interleukin 1ß in the arthritic temporomandibular joint fluid and its relation to pain, mobility and anterior open bite. Swedish Dent J. 1998; 2: 247.

Al-Watban F. Stimulation and inhibtion effects of Kr. laser for wound management. Lasers in Surgery and Medicine. 1998; Suppl 10: 5.

Al-Watban F, Zhang X Y. Comparison of the effects of laser therapy on wound healing using different laser wavelengths. Laser Therapy. 1996; 8 (2): 127-136.

Al-Watban F, Zhang X Y. Comparison of wound healing process using argon and krypton lasers. J Clin Laser Med Surg. 1997; 15 (5): 209-215.

Al-Watban F. Laser therapy am the healthy rat model for wound healing research - is it a feasible idea? LaserWorld Guest editorial, No 10, 2000. www.laser.nu/lllt/lllt_editorial.htm.

Al-Watban F. Laser acceleration of open skin wound closure in rats and its dosimetric dependence. Laser Therapy. 1996; 8 (1): 27. (abstract).

Al-Watban F, Andres B L. Laser photons and pharmacological treatment in wound healing. Laser Therapy. 2000; 12: 3-11.

Amano A et al. Histological studies on the rheumatoid synovial membrane irradiated with a low energy laser. Lasers in Surgery and Medicine. 1994; 15 (3): 290-294.

Amano A. Histological Studies on the Rheumatoid Synovial Membrane Irradiated with a Low Energy Laser. Lasers in Surgery and Medicine. 1994; 15: 290-294.

Amaral A C et al. HeNe laser action in the regeneration of the tibialis anterior muscle of mice. Proc. 2nd Con-gress World Assn for Laser Therapy, Kansas City, September 1998; pp 18-19.

Amir A et al. The influence of low energy Helium-Neon laser irradiation on the viability of skin flaps of the rat. Laser Therapy. 1996; 8 (1): 59. (abstract)

Amorim J C F, Ribeiro M S, Groth E B. Gingival healing after gingivectomy procedure and low intensity laser irradiation. A clinical and biometrical study in anima nobile. Laser Med Surg Abstract issue, 2002: 20.

Anders J et al. Low power laser irradiation alters the rate of regeneration of the rat facial nerve. Lasers in Sur-gery and Medicine. 1993; 13: 72-82.

Andersen B.R., Brendzdel A.M,. Lint T.F. Infect. immun. 1977; 17: 62-.

Ando Y, Watanabe H, Ishikawa I. Bactericidal effect of Erbium YAG laser on periodontal bacteria. Lasers in Surgery and Medicine. 1996; 19: 190-200.

Anneroth G, Hall G, Rydén H, Zetterqvist L. The effect of Low-energy infrared laser radiation on woundheal-ing in rats. Brit J Oral & Max Surg. 1988; 26: 12-17.

Antikas T. Low Power Laser Treatment of Musculoskeletal Disorders and Body Measurements of the Equine Athlete. Proc. SPIE (Lasers in Medicine). 1989; Vol 1353: 92-.

Antikatzides T. G. Soft Laser Treatment of Muskuloskeletal and Other Disorders in the Equine Athlete. Equine Practice. 1986; 8 (2): 24-.

Antipa C et al. Laser biostimulation (Ne-He and Ga-As) effects as compared to the conventional therapy in several pelvic inflammatory diseases. Proc. SPIE.1993; Vol 1879: 15-22 (Lasers in Urology, Gynecology, and General Surgery).

Basko I:. A New Frontier: Laser Therapy. California Veter. 1983; 10: 17.

Baumler W, Neff S, Landthaler M et al. Laser Assisted Hair Removal: Comparison of a Normal Mode Ruby Laser and a High Power Laser Diode. Abstract volume, Laser Florence. 14:th International Congress of Laser Medicine, pp 11, Florence 1999.

Baxter G D et al. Low level laser therapy: Current clinical practice in Northern Ireland. Physiotherapy 1991; 3:171-178.

Baxter G D. Therapeutic Lasers. 1994; p 148. Churchill Livingstone.

Beckerman H et al. Efficacy of physiotherapy for musculoskeletal disorders: what can we learn from research? Br J Gen Pract. 1993; 43 (367): 73-77.

Beck-Friis J, Borg G, Wetterberg L: Rebound increase of nocturnal melatonin levels following evening suppression by bright light exposure in healthy men: relationship to cortisol levels and morning exposure. In: The Medical and Biological Effects of Light. Wurtman RJ, ed. Ann. NY Acad Sci. 1985; 453: 371-375.

Ben-Dov N, Shefer G, Irinitchev A et al. Low energy laser irradiation affects satellite cell proliferation and differentiation in vitro. Biochem Biophys Acta. 1999; 1448: 372-380.

Belkin M, Schwartz M. Evidence for the existence of low-energy laser bioeffects on the nervous system. Neurosurg Rev 1994;17 (1): 7-17.

Belkin M, Schwartz M. Ophthalmic effects of low-energy laser irradiation. Survey of Ophthalmology. 1994; 39 (2): 113-122.

Bellina J H. Laser in gynecology. Excerpts from Leventhal, J.M. et al (eds.): Current Problems in Obstetrics and Gynecology. Year Book Medical Publishers, Inc., Chicago. 1981.

Ben Hatit Y. The Nd:YAG Laser in Dentistry. LASER. Journ Eur Med Laser Ass. 1991; 4 (1-2): 17.

Ben Hatit B Y, Lammens J P. Laser therapy with 10600 nm defocused CO2 laser. Laser Therapy. 1992; 4 (4): 175-178.

Benedicenti B. Valoración radioimunológica del nivel de ß-endorfina en el líquido encefaloraquídeo antes y después de irradiar con laser 904 nm, en neuralgia del trigemino. Inv. Clin Láser. 1984; 1 (3): 7-12.

Bensadoun R-J, Franqiun J C, Ciais C et al. Low energy He/Ne laser in the prevention of radiation-induced mucositis: A multicenter phase III randomized study in patients with head and neck cancer. Support Care Cancer. 1999; 7 (4): 244-252.

Bensadoun R-J, Ciais G. Radioation- and chemotherapy-induced mucositis in oncology: results of multicenter phase III studies. J Oral Laser Applications. 2000; 2: 115-120.

Berki T, Németh, Hegedüs J. Effect of low-power continous-wave HeNe laser irradiation on in vitro cultured lymphatic cell lines and macrophages. Stud Biophys. 1985; 105: 141-

Berki T et al. Biological Effect of Low-power Helium-Neon (HeNe) Laser Irradiation. Lasers in Medical Science. 1988; 3: 35-.

Bernal G. Helium Neon and Diode Laser Therapy is an effective adjunctive therapy for facial paralysis. Laser Therapy. 1993; 5 (2): 79-87

Bernardini U D, Longo L. Terapia laser nella nevralgia del trigemino. Proc. Atti dell'í VIII Congresso Nazionale A.I.S.D., Verona. 1985: 80-81.

Bertolucci L E, Grey T. Clinical analysis of Mid-laser versus placebo treatment of arthralgic TMJ degenerative joints. J Craniomandib Practice. 1995; 13 (1): 26-29.

Beyer W et al. Light dosimetry and preliminary clinical results for low level laser therapy in cochlear dysfunction. Proc. Laser Florence '99.

Bezuur N J, Hansson T L. The effect of therapeutic laser treatment in patient with cranomandibular disorders. J Cranomandib Disorders. 1988; 2: 83-86.

Bhagwanani N S et al. Low level nitrogen laser therapy in pulmonary tuberculosis. J Clin Laser Med Surg. 1996; 14 (1): 23-25.

Bibikova A et al. Enhancement of angiogenesis in regenerating gastrocnemius muscle of the toad (Bufo viridis) by low-energy laser irradiation. Anatomy & Embryology. 1994; 190 (6): 597-602.

Bibikova A, Oron U. Attenuation of the process of skeletal muscle regeneration by low energy laser irradiation. Laser Therapy. 1996; 8 (1): 19. (abstract).

Bibokova A, Oron U. Attenuation of the process of muscle regeneration in the toad gastrocnemius muscle by low energy laser irradiation. Lasers in Surgery and Medicine. 1994; 14: 355-361.

Bibikova A, Oron U. Regeneration in denervated toad (Bufo viridis) gastrocnemius muscle and the promotion of the process by low energy laser irradiation. The Anatomical Record. 1995; 241: 123-128

Bihari I, Mester A. The biostimulative effect of low level laser therapy of long-standing crural ulcer using Helium Neon laser, Helium Neon plus infrared lasers and noncoherent light: Preliminary report of a randomized double blind comparative study. Laser Therapy. 1989; 1 (2): 97-102.

Bisht D et al. Effect of low intensity laser radiation on healing of open skin wounds in rats. Indian J Medical Research. 1994; 100: 43-46.

Bisht D, Mehrotra R, Singh P A et al. Effect of helium-neon laser on wound healing. Indian Journal of Experimental Biology. 1999; 37(2): 187-189.

Bjordal J M. Low level laser therapy in shoulder tendinitis/bursitis, epicondylalgia and ankle sprain. A critical review on clinical effects. Master thesis in Physiotherapy Science, Div Physiotherapy Science, University of Bergen, Norway. 1997.

Bjordal J M, Greve G. What may alter the conclusions of reviews? Physical Therapy Reviews. 1998; 3: 121-132.

Bjordal J M, Couppe C, Ljunggren A. Low level laser therapy for tendinopathies. Evidence of a dose-response pattern. Physical Therapy Reviews. 2001; 6 (2): 91-100.

Bjordal J M, Couppe C, Tunér J, Ljunggren A E. A systemic reviewof low level laser therapy with location-specific doses for pain from chronic joint disorders. Submitted for publication 2002

Bjorne A, Agerberg G. Reduction in sick leave and costs to society of patients with Ménière´s disease after treatment of temporomandibular and cervical spine disorders: A controlled 6-year cost-benefit study. Accepted for publication 2002.

Bjorne A, Agerberg G. Symptom relief after treatment of temporomandibular and cervical spine disorders in patients with Ménière´s disease: A 3-year follow-up. Accepted for publication 2002.

Bjorne A. Berven A, Agerberg G. Cervical signs and symptoms in patients with Ménière's disease: a controlled study. J Cranomandib Practice. 1998; 16 (3): 194-202.

Bjorne A, Agerberg G. Symptom relief after treatment of temporomandibular and cervical spine disorders in patients with Meniere´s disease - a 3-year follow-up. Accepted for publication 2002.

Blay A, Blay C C, Groth E B et al. Effects of visible NIR low intensity laser on implant osseointegration in vivo. Laser Med Surg Abstract issue, 2002: 11.

Bliddal H et al. Soft laser therapy of rheumatoid arthritis. Scand J Rheuma. 1987; 16: 225-228.

Boboreko B A. [Helium-neon laser irradaition in the therapy of urinary bladder and uretral tubercolosis]. Probl Tuberk. 1999; 6: 38-40.

Boerner E, Podbielska H, Nesterowicz M et al. Double-blind study on the efficacy of the lasertherapy. Proc. SPIE; Vol. 2929: 75

Bogomilskii M R et al. [Effects of low-energy laser irradiation on the functional state of the acoustic analyzer.] Vestn Otorinolaringol. 1989; 2: 29-34.

Bolton P A, Dyson M, Young S R. The effect of polarised light on the release of growth factors from the U-937 macrophage-like cell line. Laser Therapy. 1992; 4 (1): 33-42.

Bolton P A, Young S R, Dyson M.. Macrophage responsiveness to light therapy. A dose response study. Laser Therapy. 1990; 2 (3): 101-106.

Bolton P, Young S, Dyson M. The direct effect of 860 nm light on cell proliferation and on succinic dehydrogenase activity of human fibroblasts in vitro. Laser Therapy. 1995; 7 (2): 55-60.

Bolton P, Young S, Dyson M. Macrophage responsiveness to light therapy with varying power and energy densities. Laser Therapy. 1991; 3 (3): 105-112.

Bosatra M, Lucci A, Olliaro P et al. In vitro fibroblast activation by laser irradiation at low energy. Dermatologica. 1984; 168: 157-162.

Boss W K Jrc, Usal H, Thompson R C, Fiorillo M A. A comparison of the long-pulse and short-pulse Alexan-drite laser hair removal systems. Ann Plast Surg 1999; 42 (4): 381-384

Bossy J et al. In Vitro Survey of Low Energy Laser Beam Penetration in Compact Bone. Faculté de Médecine et CHRU de Nimes, BP 26, 3000 Nimes, France. (1985).

Boulton M et al. HeNe-Laser Stimulation of Human Fibroblasts and Attachment in vitro. Lasers in Life Sciences. 1986; 1 (2): 125-.

Bounkeo J M, Brannon W M, Dawes Jr K S et al. The efficacy of laser therapy in the treatment of wounds: a meta analysis of the literature. Proc. 3rd Congress of the World Ass for Laser Therapy, Athens, Greece, 2000, page 79. Submitted 2001.

Boussignac G et al. Thermal effects of semiconductor lasers in men. Proc 6th Congress of The Internat Soc for Lasers in Surgery and Medicine. 1985; 77.

Bradley F G, Reynolds P A. Low reactive level laser therapy in Oral and Maxillofacial Surgery. Review of 100 cases. Laser Therapy. 1994; 6 (1): 67. (abstract)

Bradley P F, Rebliini Z. Low intensity laser therapy (LILT) for temporomandibular joint pain: a clinical electromyographic and thermographic study. Laser Therapy. 1996; 8 (1): 47 (abstract)

Bradley P. Thermographic Evaluation of Response to Low Level Laser Acupuncture. Proc. Second Meeting of the International Laser Therapy Association, London Sept 1992. p 32.

Braverman B, McCarthy R, Ivankovich A D et al. Effect of Helium-Neon and Infrared Laser Irrradiation on Wound Healing in Rabbits. Lasers in Surgery and Medicine. 1989; 9: 50-58.

Brill A G, Brill G E, Shenkman B et al. Low power laser irradiation of blood inhibits platlet function: role of cyclic GMP. Proc. SPIE. 1998; Vol 3569: 4-11.

Brill G et al. Influence of HeNe laser irradiation on giant chromosomes. Proc.SPIE. 1995; Vol 2630: 51-59.

Brill G, Brill A. [Guanilate cyclase and nitric oxide synthetsase as possible primary acceptors of low level laser radiation energy]. J Laser Medicine. 1997; 39-42. (in Russian)

Bringman W. Lasertherapie beim chronischen Schultertrauma. DZA. 1998; 4: 109-120.

Brosseau L et al. Low level laser therapy for osteoarthritis and rheumatoid arthritis: a metaanalysis. J Rheumatol. 2000; 27 (8): 1961-1969.

Brosseau L, Welch V, Wells G et al. Low level laser therapy (classes I, II and III) for treating rheumatoid arthritis. In: The Cochrane Library. Issue 4, 2000. Oxford: Update Software.

Brosseau L, Welch V, Wells G et al. Low level laser therapy (classes I, II and III) for treating oesteoarthritis. In: The Cochrane Library. Issue 4, 2000. Oxford: Update Software.

Brugnera A et al. Clinical results evaluation of dentinary hypersensitivity patients treated with laser therapy. Proc. SPIE. 1999; Vol 3593: 66-68.

Brugnera A et al. Low-reactive level laser treatment in facial paralysis. In: Lasers in Dentistry VI. Ed Featherstone J D et al. Proc. SPIE. 2000; Vol 3910: 68-74.

Brugnera A. LLLT in treating dentinary hypersensibility: A histological study and clinical application. Proc. 2nd ENSOMA Congress, Houston, Texas, USA. 2001.

Brugnera Jr A et al. Low level laser therapy in treatment of lesions in the inferior alveolar and mental nerves. Proc. 3rd Congr World Assn for Laser Therapy, Athens, Greece, May 2000, p.126.

Brugnera Junior A, Garrini A E, Pinheiro A et al. Laser therapy in the treatment of dental hypersensitivity - a histologic study and clinical application. Laser Therapy. 2000; 12: 16-21

Bucek M et al. Morphology of epithelizing varicose ulcers following HeNe laser therapy. Acta Universitatis Palackianae Olomucensis Facultatis Medicae. 1991; 131: 303-316.

Buliakova N V et al. Effects of helium-neon laser on regeneration capacity of skeletal muscles of adult guinea pigs. Biull Eksp Biol Med. 1992; 113 (4): 411-414.

Buliakova N V. Regereration of the x-ray irradiated gastrocnemius muscle in old rats after stimulation. Biull Eksp Biol Med. 1989; 108 (7): 123-126. (in Russian with English abstract)

Bülow P M, Jensen H, Danneskiold-Samsoe B. Low power Ga-Al-As laser treatment of painful osteoarthritis of the knee. Scan J Rehan Med. 1994; 26: 155-159.

Burch J M. Interferometry with Scattered Light. Optical Instruments and Techniques. J. Home, Dickson ed. (Reading Conf. 1969) p. 213. Oriel Press, New Castle upon Tyne 1970.

Burns T, Wilson M, Pearson G J Killing of cariogenic bacteria by light from a gallium aluminium arsenide diode laser. J Dent. 1994; (5) :273-278.

Bykov V L et al. [Low-energy laser irradiation in the complex treatment of patients with ear diseases]. Voprosy Kurortologii, Fizioterapii i Lechebnoi Fizicheskoi Kultury. 1985; (2): 60-62. (in Russian)

Bylesjö EI, Boman K, Wetterberg L. Obesity treated with phototherapy: four case studies. Int J Eat Disord. 1996; (4): 443-46.

Byrnes K R, Waynant R W, Ilev I K et al. Cellular invasion following spinal cord lesion and low power laser irradiation. Laser Med Surg Abstract issue, 2002: 11.

Byrnes K R et al. Low power laser treatment of cutaneous wounds in psammamys obesus. Lasers in Surgery and Medicine. 2000; Supplement 12: 4.

Calderhead G. Meeting report: International low power laser symposium, Vienna, Austria, October 7th-8th, 1994. Laser Therapy. 1995; 7 (1): 39.

Calderhead G. Meeting report: Proc Ninth Congress of the International Society for Laser Surgery and Medicine, Anaheim, California, USA: 2-6 November 1991. Laser Therapy. 1992; 4: 43.

Calderhead G. Watt's A Joule?: On the Importance of Accurate and Correct Reporting of Laser Parameters in Low Reactive-Laser Therapy and Photobioactivation Research: Laser Therapy 1991; 3 (4): 177-182.

Calderhead R G, Inomata K. A study of the possible haemorrhagic effects of extended infrared diode laser irradiation on encapsulated and exposed synovial membrane articular tissue in the rat. Laser Therapy. 1992; 4 (2): 65-74.

Calderhead R G. Simultaneous low reactive-level laser therapy in laser surgery: the "alpha-phenomenon" explained. In: Progesss in Laser Therapy. 1991. John Wiley & Sons. P. 209-213.

Cambier D C et al. Low-level laser therapy: the experience in Flanders. Eur J Phys Med Rehab. 1997; 7: 102-105.

Campaña V, Moya M, Gavotto A et al. Effects of helium-neon laser on microcrystalline arthropaties. Lasers in Surgery and Medicine. 2001; Suppl 13: 11.

Campbell S S, Murphy P J. Extraocular circadian phototransduction in humans. Science 1998; 279 (5349): 396-399.

Carney S A et al. The effect of light from a ruby laser on the metabolism of skin in tissue culture. Biochem Biophys Acta. 1967; 148: 525-530.

Carniel R. The 780 laser and the CO2-laser in chronic achilles tendinitis: Different methods compared. Proc. 2nd Congress World Assn for Laser Therapy, Kansas City, Sept 1998; p. 40-42.

Carrillo J, Calatayud J, Manso F J et al. A randomized double-blind clinical trial on the effectiveness of helium-neon laser in the prevention of pain, swelling and trismus after removal of impacted third molars. Int Dent Journal. 1990; 40: 31-36.

Cassese M et al. Laser-terapia nelle sindromi algico-disfunzionali delle articolazioni temoporo-mandibolari. Int Congress on Laser in Med and Surg, Bologna June 1985, p 337. Monduzzi Editore S.p.A, Bologna, Italy.

Cassone MC, Lombard A, Rossetti V, Urciuoli R, Rolfo PM. Effect of in vivo HeNe laser irradiation on biogenic amine levels in rat brain. J Photochem Photobiol B 1993; 18 (2-3): 291-294.

Castro D J, Abergel R P, Johnston K et al. Wound healing: biological effects of Nd:YAG laser on collagen metabolism in pig skin in comparison to thermal burn. Ann Plast Surg 1983; 11: 131-.

Castro D J, Abergel R P, Meweker C et al. Effects of the Nd:YAG laser on DNA synthesis and collagen production in human skin fibroblast cultures. Ann Plast Surg. 1983; 1 (3): 214-222.

Castronuovo G. et al. The skin role during a low level laser therapy. Laser Bologna '92, p. 19. Monduzzi Editore S.p.A., Bologna, Italy.

Ceccherelli F et al. Diode laser in cervical myofascial pain: A double blind study versus placebo. The Clinical J Pain. 1989; 5: 301-304.

Changjun C et al. The Preoperative Period of the Veterinary Anaesthesia by Laser. Sichuan Agricultural College, Sichuan. Acupuncture Res. 1984; 9 (1):16.

Chavrier C et al. Immunohistochemical localization of type I, ,III and IV collagen in healthy human gingiva. J de Biologie Buccale. 1981; 9: 271-277.

Checkley S A, Murphy D G, Abbas M J et al.Melatonin rhythms in seasonal affective disorder. Br J Psychiatry. 1993;163: 332-337.

Cheetham M J, Young R S, Dyson M. Histological effects of 820 nm laser irradiation on the healthy growth plate of the rat. Laser Therapy 1992; 4 (2): 59-64.

Chen M et al. Application of a pain alleviating effect of low power laser irradiation to patients in orthodontic treatment. J Jpn Soc Laser Med. 1933; 14: 5-11. (in Japanese).

Chen, Ji-wei, Zhou, Yo-cheng. Effect of low level carbon dioxide laser radiation on biochemical metabolism of rabbit mandibular bone callus. Laser Therapy. 1989; 1 (2): 83-88.

Cheng ZY, Zhao CX, Zhang YH, et al. Superficial acupuncture combined with He-Ne laser radiation in the treatment of facial spasm. Int J Clin Acupunct 1991; 2 (1): 95-97.

Chernoff W G et al. Cutaneous Laser Surfacing. Operative Techniques in Otolaryngology - Head & Neck Surgery. 1994; 5: 281-284.

Chernoff W G. Cutaneous Laser Resurfacing. Clinical Laser Monthly. December 1994.

Cherry R. Measurement of Protein Rotational Diffusion in Membranes by Flash Photolysis. Methods in Enzymology. 1978; (54): 47-.

Chio C-C, Lin S-J, Kao M-C. Cytogenic effects of low level laser irradiation of human leukocytes. Laser Therapy. 1990; 2 (3): 111-116.

Chistov V B. [The effect of low-intensity radiation from a helium-neon laser on the alkaline phosphatase activity in an uncomplicated mandibular fracture and in traumatic osteomyelitis]. Stomatologiia 1989; 68 (6): 13-15.

Choi J et al. A comparison of electroacupuncture, transcutaneous electrical nerve stimulation and laser photo-biostimulation on pain relief and glucocorticoid excretion. Int J Acupunct Electrotherp Res. 1986; 11: 45-51.

Klima H. Effect of Weak Laser Light and Oxygen Activation in Open Biological Systems. LASER - Journ Eur Med Laser Ass. 1988; 1 (2): 16-.

Ko et al . Clinical evaluation of low level laser therapy on the trigger points. Proc. 7th Int Congr Lasers in Dentistry, ISLD, Brussels, Belgium, July 2000, abstr. 25.

Kobayashi M et al. Studies of the diode laser therapy on blood supply in the rat model. Proc. 2nd Congress World Assn for Laser Therapy, Kansas City, September 1998; p. 70-71.

Kólarová H et al. Effect of HeNe laser irradiation on phagocytic activity of leukocytes in vitro. Acta Universitatis Palackianae Olomucensis Facultatis Medicae. 1991; 129: 127-132.

Kolárova H et al. Penetration of the laser light into the skin in vitro. Lasers in Surg Med. 1999; 24: 231-235.

Kolárová H, Ditrichová D, Wagner J. Penetration of the laser light into the skin in vitro. Lasers in Surgery and Medicine. 1999; 24: 231-235.

Kolomiyets L A et al. Mechanism of treatment effect of low-energy laser irradiation. Proc SPIE. 1996; Vol 2728: 63-67.

Konchugova T V et al. The enhancement of immune supression by local laser irradiation in rats exposed to cyclophosphane. Eksp Klin Farm. 1993; 56 (2): 42-.

Kono A, Fujumasa I. The evaluation of pain therapy with low power laser: comparative study on thermography and double blind test. Thermologie Österreich. 1995: 5 (3): 112

Konstantinovic L et al. [Combined low-power laser therapy and local infiltration of corticosteroids in the treatment of radial-humeral epicondylitis.] Vojnosanit Pregl. 1997; 54 (5): 459-463. (in Croatian)

Kopf K et al: Endothelregeneration nach Laserbestrahlung - tierexperimentelle Untersuchungen an Kaninchen. Fortschr Kiefer u Gesichtschir. 1983; 28: 140-142.

Korochkin I M et al. [Clinico-biochemical parallels against background of traditional treament and laser therapy of patients with ischemic heart disease]. Ter Arkh. 1988; 60 (12): 40-44.

Korochkin I M et al.[Helium-neon laser therapy in multimodal treatment of acute pneumonia]. Sov Med. 1990; (3): 12-5.

Korochkin I M et al. [Helium-neon laser therapy in patients with ischemic heart disease]. Kardiologiia 1990; 30 (3): 24-28.

Korochkin I M et al. I[ntravenous laser therapy in multimodal treatment of acute pneumonia]. Sov Med. 1989; (7): 22-26.

Korolev Iu N, Panova L N, Geniatulina M S. [The correction of the subcellular postradiation changes in the hypothalamus and parathyroid gland by using low-intensity laser radiation. An experimental study]. Vopr Kurortol Fizioter Lech Fiz Kult. 2000; (3): 3-4.

Korytny D.L.[Use of Helium-Neon laser in therapeutic stomatology]. Stomatologiia (Mosk). 1978; 57 (5): 21-.

Kosilov K V. The treatment of neurogenic hyperreflexic bladder dysfunctions in girls with low-intensity laser radiation. Urologiia i Nefrologiia. 1995; 2: 16-19. (in Russian)

Koslov V I et al. The microcirculation of patients with arterial ischemia of the lower extremities during laser therapy. Fiziol Zh SSSR Im I M Sechenova. 1991; 77 (6): 55-67. (in Russian)

Kotani H. Effects of low power laser stimulation on wound healing in rats. Lasermedizin - Laser in Med Surg. 1995; 11 (2): 25- .

Koukoui L M et al. The differential approach to the application of laser, ultraviolet and roentgenological auto-blood irradiation for the correction of homeostatis. Laser Therapy. 1996; 8 (1): 60. (abstract).

Kovács I, Mester E, Görög P. Stimulation of wound healing with laser beam in the rat. Experientia. 1974; 30: 1275-.

Kovács I et al. Laser-Induced Stimulation of the Vascularization of the Healing Wound. Separatum Experientia. 1974; 30: 341-.

Kovács L. The stimulatory effect of laser on the physiological healing process of portio surface. Lasers in Surgery & Medicine 1981; 1 (3): 241-52

Kovalev E V. [The effect of low-intensity laser irradiation on spermatogenesis in men]. Voprosy Kurortol, Fizioter Lechebnoi Fizicheskoi Kultury. 1990; (5): 33-36.

Kovalev E V. The effect of low-intensity laser radiation on spermatogenesis in men. Vopr Kurortol Fizioter Lech Fiz Kult. 1990; (5): 33-36.

Kovalev M I. et al. [Prevention of lactation mastitis by the use of low-intensity laser irradiation]. Akush Ginekol (Mosk.). 1990; (2): 57-61.

Kozlov V et al. Lasers in diagnostics and treatment of microcirculation disorders under parodontitis. Proc SPIE. 1995; Vol 1984: 253-264.

Krasheninnikoff M, Ellitsgaard B, Rogvi-Hansen B et al. No effect of low power laser in lateral epicondylitis. Scand J Rheum. 1994; 23: 260-263.

Kramer J F, Sandrin M. Effects of Low-Power Laser and white light on sensory conduction rate of the superficial radial nerve. Physiotherapy Canada. 1993; 45 (3): 165-170.

Kreczi T, Klinger D A. A comparison of laser acupuncture versus placebo in radicular and pseudoradicular pain syndromes as recorded by subjective responses of patients. Acupunct Electrotherap Res. 1986; 11: 207-216.

Kripke DF. Light treatment for nonseasonal depression: speed, efficacy, and combined treatment. J Affect Disord. 1998; May;49 (2): 109-117.

Kruchinina I et al. Effect of laser therapy on the local synthesis of class A immunoglubulin in children with acute and chronic maxillary sinuitis. Vestn Otorinolaringol. 1988; 2: 19-21. (in Russian with English abstr)

Kruchinina I et al. Therapeutic effect of helium-neon laser on microcirculation of nasal mucosa in children with acute and chronic maxillary sinuitis as measured by conjunctival biomocroscopy. Vestn Otorinolaringol. 1991; 3: 26-30. (in Russian with English abstr)

Kubasova T, Kovács L, Somosy Z, Unk P, Kókai A. Biological effect of HeNe laser: Investigations on functional and micromorphological alterations of cell membranes, in vitro. Lasers in Surgery and Medicin. 1984; 4: 381.

Kubota J, Ohshiro T. The effect of diode laser laser therapy on flap survival: measurement of flap microcirculation with the laser specle method. Laser Therapy. 1996; 8 (4): 241-246.

Kubota J, Ohshiro T. The effects of diode laser low reactive-level laser therapy (laser therapy) on flap survival in a rat model. Laser Therapy. 1989; 1 (3): 127-134.

Kubota J. Treatment of skin ulcers with defocused diode laser therapy. Lasers in Surgery and Medicine. Suppl 13, 2001; p. 57.

Kucerová H J. et al. Effect of laser modulatory frequency on the secretion of IgA and albumin levels after the extraction of human molars in the lower jaw. In: Progress in Biomedical Optics, Proc. of Low-power Light on Biological Systems. Proc SPIE.1997; Vol 3198: 98-101.

Kucerová H et al. Modulatory frequency of lasers in connection to laser beam therapeutic effect Proc. SPIE.1998; Vol: 191-195 (Lasers in Dentistry IV)

Kucerová H, Dostálová T, Himmlová L et al. Low-level laser therapy after molar extraction. J Clin Laser Med Surg. 2000; 18 (6): 309-315.

Kudoh Ch et al. Effects of 830 nm Gallium Aluminium Arsenide Diode Laser Radiation on Rat Saphenous Nerve Sodium-Potassium-Adenosine Triphosphatase Activity: A Possible Pain Attenuation Mechanism Exam-ined. Laser Therapy. 1989; 1 (2): 63-67.

Kulikova N G. The effect of low-intensity infrared laser therapy on the endocrine function of patients with climacteric disorders. Vopr Kurortol Fizioter Lech Fiz Kult. 1996; 5: 25-26.

Kumæ T, Arakawa H. In vitro effects of therapeutic laser on superoxide generation from rat alveolar macrophage. Laser Therapy. 1999; 11 (3): 119-129.

Kunin A A, Bykov E I, Podolskaya E E et al. Clinical and morphological indications for laser treatment of patients with precancerous diseases of the oral cavity. Proc. SPIE. 1996; Vol 2929: 185-197.

Kunin A A. et al. Biological effects caused by low power laser light in the treatment of the dentition, parodontium and mucosa of the oral cavity and lip diseases. Proc. SPIE.1997. Vol 3198: 37-47.

Kunin S, Pankova Y, Oleinik T et al. The influence of low level lasers together with modern filling materials and bonding systems on mineral metabolism of hard tissues. Proc. European Conf Biomed Optics, Munich, Germany, June 2001, p. 18.

Kurland H D. Releif of low back pain with low-reactive laser acupuncture techniques. Aku. 1999; 27 (4) (abstract).

Kurumada F A study on the application of Ga-As semiconductor laser to endodontics. The effects of laser irradiation on the activation of inflammatory cells and the vital pulpotomy. Ohu Daigaku Shigakushi. 1990; 17 (3) :233-244.

Kusakari H, Orikasa N, Tani H. Effects of low power laser on wound healing of gingiva and bone. Laser Bologna '92, p. 49-55. Monduzzi Editore S.p.A., Bologna, Italy.

Kusakari H. The use of lasers to dental implant. Proc X Internat Congr Soc Lasers in Surgery and Medicine, Bangkok, 1993, p 332.

Laakso E L, Cramond T, Richardson C, Galligan J P. Plasma ACTH and ß-endorphin levels in response to low level laser therapy for myofascial trigger points. Laser Therapy. 1994; (3) 6: 133-142.

Laakso L. Richardson C. Cramond T. Quality of light - is laser necessary for effective photobiostimulation? Australian Journal of Physiotherapy. 1993; 39 (2): 87-92.

Labajos M et al. ß-endorphine levels modification after GaAs and HeNe laser irradiation on the rabbit. Comparative study. Investigación clínica láser. 1988; 1-2: 6-8.

Labajos M et al. Effect of the irradiation of GaAs diode laser on intestinal absorption: in vitro and in vivo studies. Lasers in Medical Science. 1986; 1: 21-25.

Labbe R et al. Laser photobioactivation mechanisms: in vitro studies using ascorbic acid uptake and hydroxyproline formation as biochemical markers of irradiation response. Lasers in Surgery and Medicin. 1990; 10: 201-207.

Labbe R, Skogerboe K, Davis H, Rettmer R: Laser photobioactivation mechanisms: In vitro studies using ascorbic acid uptake and hydroxyproline formation as bio-chemical markers of irradiation response. Lasers in Surgery and Medicine. 1990; 10: 201.

Ladalardo et al. The effect of diode laser in the treatment of paraesthesia due to surgical procedures. Proc. 7th Int Congr Lasers in Dentistry, ISLD, Brussels, Belgium, July 2000, abstr. 26.

Lagan K M, McDonough S M, Clements B A, Baxter G D. A case report of low intensity laser therapy (LILT) in the management of venous ulceration: potential effects of wound debridement upon efficacy. Journal of Clinical Laser Medicine & Surgery. 2000; 18 (1): 15-22.

Lam R W, Terman M, Wirz-Justice A. Light therapy for depressive disorders: indications and efficacy. Mod Probl Pharmacopsychiatry. 1997; 25: 215-234

Landau Z. Topical hyperbaric oxygen and low energy laser for the treatment of diabetic foot ulcer. Archives of Orthopaedic & Trauma surgery. 1998; 117 (3): 156-158.

Landthaler M et al. Behandlung von Zoster, postzosterischen Schmerzen und Herpes simplex recidivans in loco mit Laser-Licht. Fortschr. Med. 1983; 101 (22): 1039-.

Laor Y et al. The pathology of laser irradiation of the skin and body wall of the mouse. 1965; 47 (4): 643-662.

Lederer H et al. Influence of light on human immunocompetent cells in vitro. Proc. Laser Opto-Elektronik, Munich 1981.

Lee G et al. New concepts in pain management in the application of low-power laser for relief of cervicothoracic pain syndromes. Am Heart J. 1996; 132 (6): 1329-1334.

Lee P, Kim Kibeom and Kim Ki-Suk. Effects of low incident energy levels of infrared laser irradiation on helaing of infected open skin wounds in rats. Laser Therapy 1993; 5 (2): 59-.

Lee, Chang Woo and Kim, Ki Suk. Study on the Effect of Low Denisty Power Laser Radiation in Treating Gingival Inflammation. Clinical, Microbiological, Histological Study. J Korean Acad Oral Med 1987; 1 (12).

Lee K-H., Kim K-S. Effects of low level laser irradiation on the ALP activity and calcified nodule formation of rat osteoblastic cell. J of Korean Academy of Oral Medicine. 1996; 21: 279-292.

Leonid Reznikov, Personal communication, Dec 1998.

Lerner LA. Effectiveness of laser therapy in Bechterew's disease. Terapevticheskii Arkhiv. 1988, 60(4): 134-136. (in Russian)

Lewith G T, Machin D. A randomized trial to evaluate the effect of infrared stimulation of local trigger points, versus placebo, on the pain caused by cervical osteoarthrosis. Acupunct Electro-Ther Res, 1981; 6: 277-284.

Lewy AJ, Bauer VK, Cutler NL, Sack RL, Ahmed S, Thomas KH, Blood ML, Jackson JM. Morning vs evening light treatment of patients with winter depression. Arch Gen Psychiatry. 1998; 55 (10): 890-896.

Li X H. Laser in the Department of Traumatology. With a report of 60 cases of soft tissue injury. Laser Therapy. 1990; 2 (3): 119-122.

Lichtenstein D, Morag B. Low level laser therapy in ambulatory patients with venous stasis ulcers. Laser Therapy. 1999; 11 (2): 71-78.

Lichtenstein D, Morga B. Laser therapy in ambulatory patients with venous stasis ulcers. Proc. 2nd Congress World Assn for Laser Therapy, Kansas City, September 1998; p. 31-32.

Leichliter S G, Williams K, Whitehorse T et al. Low level laser therapy in the treatment of cervical strain in active duty military. Proc. 3rd Congr World Assn for Laser Therapy, Athens, Greece, May 2000.

Lievens P C. The effect of a combined HeNe and I.R. laser treatment on the regeneration of the lymphatic system during the process of wound healing. Lasers in Medical Science. 1991; 6: 193-199.

Lievens P C. The effect of I.R. laser irradiation on the vosomotricity of the lymphatic system. Lasers in Medical Science. 1991; 6: 189-191

Lievens P, Lippens E. The influence of low level infra red lastertherapy on the regeneration of cartilage tissue. Lasers in Surgery and Medicine. 1998; Suppl 10: 5.

Lievens P, Mohebbian M. The effect of IR-laser irradiation on the regeneration of muscle fibres. In: Laser Therapy in Dentistry and Medicine. Prima Books in Sweden AB. Eds Jan Tunér and Lars Hode. 1996, p. 164-179.

Lievens P. Effects of Laser Treatment on the Lymphatic System and Wound Healing. LASER. Journ Eur Med Laser Ass. 1988; 1 (2): 12.

Lievens P. Infrared lasertherapy and bedsores. Lasers in Surgery and Medicine. 1992; Suppl 4:11.

Lievens P. The Influence of Laser Irradiation on the Motricity of Lymphatical System and on the Wound Healing Process. Proc Int Congr on Laser in Med and Surg. Bologna, June 26-28, 1985; p. 171

Light therapy for winter depression. Health News. 1998; 4 (14): 6-.

Light therapy. Health News. 1998; Mar 10;4 (3): 5.

Lilge L, Tierney K, Nussbaum E. Low-level laser for wound healing: feasibility of wound dressing transillumination. J Clin Laser Med Surg. 2000; 18 (5): 235-240.

Lim, Hong Meng et al. A clinical investigation of the efficacy of low level laser therapy in reducing orthodontic postadjustment pain. Am J Orthod Dentofac Orthop. 1995; 108: 614-22.

Lindén L-Å . Enhanced curing of dental lasers. Swedish Dental J. 1997; 6: 242.

Lindholm A, de Mitri N, Swensson U. Clinical effect of non-fucuses CO2 laser on traumatic arthritis in horses. Lasers Med Surg. Supplement 12, 2000: 51.

Lindholm A C, Swensson U, de Mitri N,Collinder E. Clinical Effects of Betamethasone and Hyaluronan, and of Defocalized Carbon Dioxide Laser Treatment on Traumatic Arthritis in the Fetlock Joints of Horses. J Vet Med. 2002: 189 -194.

Litscher G et al. Specific effects of laserpuncture on the cerebral circulation. Lasers in Medical Science. 2000; 15 (1): 57-62.

Liu et al. The effectiveness of semiconductor laser in the treatment of post-endodontic filling pain. Proc. 7th Int Congr Lasers in Dentistry, ISLD, Brussels, Belgium, July 2000, abstr. 28.

Liu H-C, Lan W-H. The combined effectiveness of the semiconductor laser with Duraphat in the treatment of dentin hypersensitivity. J Clin Laser Med Surg. 1994; 12 (6): 315-319.

Lizarelli R F, Lamano-Carvalho T, Brentegani G. Histometrical evaluation of the healing of the dental alveolus in rats after irradiation with a low-powered GaAlAs laser. In Lasers in Dentistry V. Proceedings SPIE. 1999; Vol 3593: 49-56.

Lizarelli R F, Ciconelli K P, Braga C A, Berro R J. Low-powered laser therapy associated with oral implantology. Proc SPIE.1999; Vol 3593: 69-73, Lasers in Dentistry V, John D. Featherstone; Peter Rechmann; Daniel Fried; Eds.

Loevscall H. The Application of Low Level Laser in Dentistry - A Critical Review. Dept of Oral Pathology, Royal Dental College, Aarhus University, Vennelyst Boulevard, DK-8000 Aarhus C, Denmark. 1992.

Loevschall H et al. Effect of Low Level Diode Laser Effect in Cultures of Human Oral Mucosa. Proc. Second Meeting of the Intern Laser Therapy Association, London, Sept 1992, p 55.

Loevschall H et al. Low Level Laser Irradiation of Human Oral Mucosa Fibroblast in Vitro in Cultures of Human Oral Fibroblasts. Lasers in Surgery and Medicine. 1994; 14: 347-.

Lögdberg-Andersson M, Mützell S, Hazel Å. Low Level Laser Treatment of Tendonitis and Myofascial Pains - a Randomized, Double-Blind Study. Laser Therapy. 1997; 9 (3): 79-86.

Loginov A S, Sokolova G N, Sokolova S V et al. [The content of biologically active substances in the margin of a stomach ulcer being treated with a copper-vapor laser]. Ter Arkh. 1991; 63 (8): 75-78. (in Russian)

Loginov A S, Sokolova G N, Trubitsyna I E et al. [Biogenic amines and cyclic nucleotides in the laser therapy of long-term nonhealing stomach ulcers]. Vrach Delo 1991; (1): 24-27. (in Russian)

Lomnitski I, Bibiashevski E V. Substantiation of the optimal exposure to monochromatic red light for stimulating osteogenesis. Stomatologiia (Rus). 1982; 2 (61):14-.

Lomnitski I. The mechanism of stimulation of reparative osteogenesis with laser radiation. Stomatologiia (Mosk). 1983; 5: 18-20.

Lomnitski I. Clinical X-ray characteristics of the healing of mandibular fractures following the use of HeNe laser radiation. Stomatologiia (Mosk). 1985; 3: 38-40.

Lonauer G. Controlled double blind study on the efficacy of HeNe-laser beams versus HeNe-plus Infrared-laser beams in the therapy of activated osteoarthritis of finger joints. Clin Experim Rheuma. 1987; 5 (suppl 2): 39. Also in Lasers in Surgery and Medicine. 1986; 7: 172.p

Marchesini R, Dasdia T, Melloni E, Rocca E. Effect of low-energy laser irradiation on colony formation capability in different human tumor cells in vitro. Lasers in Surgery and Medicine. 1989; 9 (1): 59-62.

Marei M K. Effect of low-energy laser application in the treatment of denture-induced mucosal lesions. J Prosthet Dent. 1997; 77 (3): 256-264.

Maricic B et al. Analgetic effect of laser in dental therapy. Acta Stomat Croat. 1987; 21 (4): 291-.

Marino A, Giavelli S, Galanti A et al. Low level laser therapy of chronic wounds of geriatric patients: preliminary report. Laser & Technology. 1996; 6 (1/2): 41-47.

Marks, R, de Palma F. Clinical efficacy of low power laser therapy in osteoarthritis. Physiother Res Int. 1999; 4 (2): 141-157.

Martelli M R A. A clinico statistical investigation of laser effect in the treatment of pain and dysfunction of temporo-mandibular joint (T.M.J.). J Dental Proth. 1990; (18): 31-36.

Martin D et al. Effect of laser pulse repetition rate upon peripheral blood flow in human volunteers. Lasers in Surgery and Medicine. 1991; Suppl 3: 83.

Martin J L, Migus A, Poyart C et al. Ultra-fast events in biological systems. Laboratoire d'Optique Appliquee INSERM U275. Ecole Polytechnique-ENSTA, Palaiseau. p. 218.

Masse J-F et al. Effectiveness of soft laser treatment in periodontal surgery. Int Dent J. 1993; 43: 121-127.

Matouskova I. [Reaction of the palatal tonsils after the application of a HeNe laser]. Acta Universitatis Palackianae Olomucensis Facultatis Medicae. 1984;107: 315-320.

Matsushita H, Kakami K, Ito A et al. Effect on the action potential of the low power Nd:YAG laser as irradiated directly to the nerve. Aichi Gakuin Dent Sci. 1989; 2: 19-28.

Matulis A A, Vasilenkaitis V V, Raistensky I L et al. Laser therapy and laseracupuncture in rheomatoid arthritis, osteoarthritis deformans and psoriatric arthropathy. Ther Arkh. 1983; 55 (7): 92-97.

Mayayo E, Trelles M, Calderhead R, Santafe M, Tomas J, Rigau J. Short term ultrastructural changes in soft tissue (Endomysium) after laser therapy Helium-Neon laser treatment. Laser Therapy. 1989; 1 (3): 119-126

Mayordomo M M et al. Laser in painful process of locomotor system: our experience. 1985. Proc. of Laser Bologna 1985. Monduzzi Editore, Bologna.

Mazo V. Transrectal laser therapy in prostatic problems' management.Proc. X Internat Congr Soc Laser Surgery and Medicine, Bangkok. 1993, p. 153.

Mc Kibbin L. Low Level Laser Therapy in Veterinary Practice on Standardbred Horses. In: Low Level Laser Therapy. A Practical Introduction, Eds Ohshiro & Calderhead. John Wiley & Sons. 1988: 77-.

McAuley Ret al. Soft laser: A treatment for osteoarthritis of the knee. Arch Phys Med Rehab. 1985; 66: 553-554. (abstract).

McKibbin L et al. Treatment of post herpetic neuralgia using a 904 nm (infrared) low energy laser: A clinical study. Laser Therapy. 1991; 3 (1): 35-40.

McKibbin L, Paraschak D A. Study of the Effects of Lasering on Chronic Bowed Tendons at Whitney Hall Farm Limited, Canada. Lasers in Surgery and Medicine. 1983; 3: 55-.

McMeeken J, Stillman B. Perceptions of the clinical efficacy of laser therapy. Australian J Physiotherapy. 1993; 39 (2): 101-105.

McNamara D C, Rosenberg I, Jackson P A et al. Efficacy of arthroscopic surgery and midlaser treatment for chronic temporomandibular joint articular disc derangement following motor vehicle accident. Austr Den J. 1996; 41 (6): 377-387.

Medrado R A P, Pugliese L S, Reis S R A, Andreade Z A A. The influence of low level laser therapy on wound healing and its biological action upon myofibroblasts. Submitted for publication, 2002.

Meersman P. Laser pharmacology and achilles tendinopathy. Laser Therapy. 1999; 11 (3): 144-150.

Meier J-L, Kerkour K. Traitement laser de la tendinite. Méd et Hyg. 1988; 46: 907-911.

Melges F T. Efficacy of therapies for depression. Am J Psychiatry. 1981; 138 (11): 1513.

Melnichenko E M et al. [The clinico-experimental validation of the use of low-intensity laser radiation for the treatment of exacerbated recurrent herpetic stomatitis in children]. Stomatologiia. 1992; (2): 76-78.

Melo C A, Lima A L, Brasil I et al. Characterization of light penetration in rat tissues. J Clin Laser Med Surg. 201;19 (4): 175-179.

Mester A et al. Irradiation of arthritis with 820 and 830 nm diode lasers. Laser Therapy. 1996; 8 (1): 33. (Abstract).

Mester A, Ortutay J, Barabás K. Laser therapy in rheumatology. Abstracts of 7th Int Congr European Medical Laser Assn, Dubrovnik, Croatia 2000, p. 36.

Mester A. Biostimulative effect in wound healing by continous wave 820 nm laser diode double-blind randomized cross-over study. Lasers in Med Science, abstract issue July 1988.

Mester Andrew, Mester Adam. Scientific background of laser biostimulation. LASER. Journ Eur Med Laser Ass. 1988; 1 (1): 23-.

Mester E et al. Effect of laser-rays on wound healing. Am J Surg. 1971; 122: 532-.

Mester E, Mester A F, Mester A. The biomedical effects of laser application. Lasers in Surgery and Medicine. 1985; 5: 31-39.

Mester E, Szende B, Tota J. Die Wirkung der Laser-Strahlen auf den Haarwuchs der Maus. Radiobiol. Radiother. 9: 621-626.

Mester E. et al. Auswirkungen direkter Laserbestrahlung auf menschliche Lymphozyten. Arch Dermatol Res. 1978; 5: 31-

Mester E. et al. The Biostimulating Effect of Laser Beam. Proc from Laser - 81, Opto-Elektronik, Munich 1981.

Mester E. et al. Untersuchungen über die hemmende bzw. fördernde Wirkung der Laserstrahlen. Arch Klin Chir. 1968; 322: 1022-.

Meyers A, Joyce J, Cohen J. Effects of low-watt Helium Neon laser radiation on human lymphocyte cultures. Lasers in Surgery and Medicine. 1987; 6: 540-.

Mezawa S et al. The possible analgesic effect of soft-laser irradiation on heat nociceptors in the cat tounge. Ach Oral Biol. 1988; 33 (9): 693-.

Michels H. Erfahrungen mit dem HeNe Laser bei Herpes Erkrankungen. Proc. 7th Int Congr Laser 1985. Edit. W Waidelinch. 1986; 116-119. Springer-Verlag (Berlin).

Midamba E D, Haanaes H R. Low reactive-level 830 nm GaAlAs diode laser therapy (laser therapy) successfully accelerates regeneration of peripheral nerves in human. Laser Therapy, 1993; 5 (3): 125-130.

Midamba E D, Haanaes H. Effect of low level laser therapy (laser therapy) on inferior alveolar, mental and lingual nerves after traumatic injury in 15 patients. A pilot study. Laser Therapy.1993; 5 (2): 89-94.

Migliorati C, Massumoto C, de Paula Eduardo F et al. Low-energy laser therapy in oral mucositis. J Oral Laser Applications. 2001; 1 (2): 97.101-.

Mika T et al. [Infrared laser radiation in the treatment of low back pain syndrome]. Wiad Lek. 1990; 43 (11): 511-516. (in Polish)

Mikhailov V A et al. Results of treatment of the patients with IInd - IIIrd st. breast cancer by combination of low level laser therapy (laser therapy) and surgery -10-years experience. In: A window on the laser medicine world. Longo L ed. Proc. SPIE.1999; Vol 4166: 40-42.

Mikhailov V A et al. Results of treatments of patients with stomach cancer advanced form treated by combination of low level laser therapy (laser therapy) and other methods (10-years experience). In: A window on the laser medicine world. Longo L ed. Proc. SPIE. 1999; Vol 4166: 43-47.

Mikhailov V A et al. The immunomodulating action of low-energy laser radiation in the treatment of bronchial asthma. Vopr Kurortol Fizioter Lech Fiz Kult. 1998; (4): 23-25.

Mikhailov V A et al. Use of immunomodulative influence of low-level laser radiation in the treatment of an autoimmune thyroiditis. In: A window on the laser medicine world. Longo L ed. Proc. SPIE.1999, Vol 4166: 319-322.

Mikhailov V A et al. Investigations on the influence of Low Level Diode Laser irradiation of the growth of experimental tumors. Laser Therapy. 1993; 5 (1): 33-38.

Mikhailov V A, Denisov I N. Activation of the immune system by low level laser therapy (laser therapy) for treating patients with stomach cancer in advanced form. Laser & Technology. 1997; 7 (1): 31-44.

Mikhailova R I et al. The laser therapy and laser acupuncture of patients with chronic recurrent aphtous stomatitis. Stomatologiia (Moscow). 1992; 3-6: 27-28.

Miles V, Klein. Optics. John Wiley & Sons inc. New York. Chapter 10.3, page 507-520

Millson C E, Wilson M et al. The killing of Helicobacter pylori by low-power laser light in the presence of a photosensitiser. J Med Microbiol. 1996; 44 (4): 245-52.

Miloro M, Repasky M. Low-level laser effect on neurosensory recovery after sagittal ramus osteotomy. Oral surgery, oral medicine, oral pathology, oral radiology,and endodontics. 2000; 89 (1): 12-18.

Miro L et al. Estudio capilaroscópico de la acción de un laser AsGa sobre la microcirculación. Investig Clínica Láser. 1984; 1/2: 9-14.

Mirz F, Zachariae R, Andersen S E et al. The low-power laser in the treatment of tinnitus. Clin Otolaryngol 1999; 24: 346-354.

Mischenkin N V et al. [Effects of helium-neon laser energy on the tissues of the middle ear in the presence of biological fluids and drug solutions]. Vestn Otorinolaringol. 1990; 5: 18-21.

Miyagi K. Double-blind comparative study of the effect of low-energy laser irradiation to rheumatoid arthritis. In: Current awareness of Excerpts Medica. Amsterdam. Elsevier Science Publishers BV. 1989; 25: 315. Also: J Jap Assoc Physical Med Balneol & Climatol. 1989; 52 (3): 117-126.

Miyajima K, Yoshida K, Iwata T, et al. Effects of HeNe laser irradiation on gingival fibroblasts. Aichi-Gakuin Dent Sci. 1994; 7: 1-5.

Mizokami T et al. Effect of diode laser for pain: A clinical study on different pain types. Laser Therapy. 1990; 2 (4): 171.

Mizokami T, Aoki K, Iwabuchi S et al. Laser therapy (Low Reactive Level Laser Therapy) - a clinical study: relationship between pain attenuation and the serotonergic mechanism. Laser Therapy. 1993; 5 (4): 165-168.

Mochizuki O N, Kataoka Y, Cui Y et al. Effects of near-infra-red laser irradiation on adenosine triphosphate and adenosine diphosphate contents of rat brain tissue. Neuroscience letters.2002; 323 (3): 207-210.

Mochizuki O N, Kataoka Y, Cui Y et al. Effects of near-infra-red laser irradiation on adenosine triphosphate and adenosine diphosphate contents of rat brain tissue. Neuroscience Letters. 2002; 323 (3): 207-210.

Mokhtar B et al. A double blind placebo controlled investigation of the hypoalgesic effects of low intensity laser irradiation of the cervical roots using experimental ischaemic pain. ILTA Congress, London 1992, abstracts p 61.

Mokhtar B et al. The possible significance of pulse repetition rate in laser-mediated analgesia: a double blind placebo controlled investigation using experimental ischaemic pain. ILTA Congress, London 1992, abstracts p 62.

Molina Soto J J, Moller I. La laserterapía como coadyuvante en el tratamiento de la A.R. (Artritis Reumatoidea). Bol. C.D.L. 1987; 14: 4-8.

Monich V A, Malinovskaja S, Lockhmachova E et al. Effect of low-power luminescent irradiation on surgical and burn wounds of soft tissues. Proc. SPIE. 1996; Vol 2929: 58-62.

Monteiro Martins P P et al. P.P.M.M. implant system has osseointegration improved by laser therapy. Proc. 3rd Congr World Assn for Laser Therapy, Athens, Greece, May 2000, p. 124.

Montesinos M. et al. Experimental Effects of Low Power Laser in Encephalin and Endorphin Synthesis. LASER. Journ Eur Med Laser Ass. 1988; 1 (3): 2.

Moore K C. Postherpetic neuralgia as a complication of malignant disease and its treatment using a GaAlAs diode laser. Laser Therapy. 1996; 8 (1): 49 (abstract).

Moore K, Hira N, Kumar. Ohshiro. Double blind crossover trial of low level laser therapy in the treatment of post herpetic neuralgia. Laser Therapy. 1988; (pilot issue): 7-10.

Moore K, Hira N, Broome I J, Cruikshank J A. The effect of infra-red diode laser irradiation on the duration and severity of postoperative pain. A double-blind trial. Laser Therapy. 1992; 4 (4): 145-150.

Moore K. Laser therapy in post herpetic neuralgia. Laser Therapy. 1996; 8 (1): 48 (abstract)

Moritz A et al. Advantage of a pulsed CO2 laser in direct pulp capping. A long-term in vivo study.Lasers in Surgery and Medicine. 1998; 22: 288-293.

Moritz A et al. Irradiation of infected root canals with a diode laser in vivo: results of microbiological examinations. Lasers in Surgery and Medicine. 1997; 21: 221-226.

Moritz M D et al. The advantage of CO2 treated dental necks, in comparison with a standard method: Results from an in vitro study. J Clin Laser Med Surg. 1996; 14 (1): 27.

Morozova S V et al. [Possibilities of helium-neon lasers in olfactory disorders]. Vestn Otorinolaringol. 1995; 5: 35-36.

Morrone G et al. Muscular trauma treated with GaAlas diode laser: in vivo experimental study. Lasers in Medical Science. 1998; 13 (4): 293-298.

Morrone G, Guzzardella G A, Tigani D et al. Biostimulation of human chondrocytes with Ga-Al-As diode laser: 'In vitro' research. Artificial Cells, Blood Substitutes, and Immobilization Biotechnology. 2000; 28 (2):193-201.

Morrone G, Guzzardella G A, Torricelli P et al. Osteochondral lesion repair of the knee in the rabbit after low-power diode Ga-Al-As laser biostimulation: an experimental study. Artificial Cells, Blood Substitutes, and Immobilization Biotechnology. 2000; 28 (4): 321-336.

Morselli M et al. Effects of very low energy-density treatment of joint pain by CO2 laser. Lasers in Surgery and Medicine. 1985; 5:150-.

Morton A R, Fazio S M, Miller D. Efficacy of laser-acupuncture in the prevention of exercise-induced asthma. Ann Allergy 1993; 70 (4): 295-298.

Motomura K et al. Effects of various laser irradiation on callus formation after osteotomy. J Jpn Soc Laser Med. 1984; 4: 195-196.

Mousques T. Étude en double aveugle des effets du traitment unilateral au laser hélium-néon lors de chirurgies parodontales biláterales simultanés. [Double blind study on the effects of helium-neon laser in simultaneous bilateral periodontical surgery] Quest Odontostomatol. 1986; 11: 245-254

Mousques T: Étude en double aveugle des effets du hélium-néon en chirurgie parodontale [Double blind study on the effects of helium-neon laser in periodontal surgery]. Quest Odonto-Stomatol 1986; 11: 233-244.

Moustsen P et al. Laserbehandling af bihulebetændelse i almen lægepraxis vurderet ved en dobbeltblind kontrolleret undersøgelse. [Laser Treatment of Sinuitis in General Medical Praxis Evaluated in a Double Blind Study]. Ugeskrift Læger. 1991; 153 (32): 2232. (in Danish)

Mozgunov V N et al. [Method of treatment of common warts with low-energy laser irradiation.] Vestnik Dermatologii i Venerologii. 1985; (2): 55-56.

Mrowiec J et al. Analgesic effect of low-power infrared laser radiation in rats. Proc SPIE. 1997; Vol 3198: 83-89.

Mrowiec J et al. The antinociceptive effect of infrared laser radiation in experimental animals. Laser Therapy. 1996; 8 (1): 25 (abstract).

Muldiyarov P et al. Effect of Monochromatic Helium-Neon Laser Red Light on the Morphology of Zymosan Arthritis in Rats. Biull Eksp Biol Med. 1983; 1: 55-.

Mulligan S et al. The effect of low energy HeNe laser irradiation on the neurite elongation in vitro. Lasers in Surgery and Medicine. 1991; Suppl 3: 10.

Murakami F, Kemmotsu O, Kawano Y et al.. Diode low reactive level laser therapy and stellate ganglion block compared in the treatment of facial paralysis. Laser Therapy, 1993; 5 (3):131-135.

Murphy PJ, Campbell SS. Enhanced performance in elderly subjects following bright light treatment of sleep maintenance insomnia. J Sleep Res. 1996 ; (3): 165-72.

Myrhaug H. The theory of otosclerosis and Morbus Ménière (Labyrintine vertigo) being caused by the same mechanism: physical irritants, an otognathic syndrome. Bergmanns Boktrykkeri A/S, Bergen, Norway. 1981.

Naeser M A. Treatment of carpal tunnel syndrome: research and clinical studies with laser acupuncture and microamps TENS. Proc. 2nd Congress World Assn for Laser Therapy, Kansas City, September 1998; p. 145-146.

Nagasawa A et al. Fundamental studies in reactive histological changes in pulp tissue of lased teeth. J Jap Soc Laser Med Surg.

Nagasawa A, Negishi A, Kato K. Clinical Applications of laser therapy in Dental and oral Surgery in the Urawa Clinic. Laser Therapy. 1991; 3 (3): 119-122.

Nagasawa A. Application of laser therapy in Dentistry.In: Low-Reactive Laser Therapy - Practical Application. T. Ohshiro. John Wiley & Sons. 1991: 76-.

Nakashima T, Ueda H, Misawa H et al. Transmeatal low-power laser irradiation Nakashima T, Ueda H, Misawa H et al. Transmeatal low-power laser irradiation for tinnitus. Otology & Neurotology. 2002; 23 (3): 296-300.

Nara Y et al. Stimulative effect of HeNe laser irradiation on cultured fibroblasts derived from human dental pulp. Lasers in the Life Sciences. 1992; 4 (4): 249-.

Nasu F, Tomiyasu K, Inomata K, Calderhead R G. Cytochemical Effects of GaAlAs Diode Laser Radiation on Rat Saphenous Artery Calcium Ion Dependent Adenosine Triphosphatase Activity. Laser Therapy. 1989; 1 (2): 89-92.

Naveh N et al. Low-energy laser. a new measure for suppression of arachidonic acid metabolism in the optic nerve. J Neurosci Res. 1990; 26: 386-389

Nelson A J, Friedman M H. Somatosensory trigeminal evoked potential amplitudes following low level laser and sham irradiation over time. Laser Therapy. 2001; 13: 60-64.

Nelson R.D,. Mills E.L,. Simmons R.L. et al. Infect. Immun., 1976; 14: 29-.

Neuman I, Finklestein Y, Lubart R. Low energy phototherapy in allergic rhinitis and nasal polyposis. Laser Therapy. 1996. 1: 37 (abstract).

Nicola J H et al. The role of coherence in wound healing stimulation by non-thermal laser radiation. Surgical and Medical Lasers. 1989; 2-3 (2): 70 (abstract)

Nicola J H, Nicola E M D, Simões M, Paschoal J R. Role of polarization and Coherence of Laser Light on Wound Healing. Laser Tissue Interaction. V S.L. Jacques, ed. Proc SPIE.1994; Vol 2134A: 448-450.

Nicola E M, Nicola J H. Low-power CO2 laser in the treatment of chronic pharyngitis: a five-year experience. Proc. SPIE.1994; Vol 2128: 85-87. (Laser Surgery: Advanced Characterization, Therapeutics, and Systems IV)

Nicolau R A, Jorgetti V, Rigau J et al. Effect of low power laser Ga-Al-As (660 nm) in the bone tissue remodelation in mice. Proc. 4th Congress of the World Association for Laser Therapy, Tokyo, Japan, June 27-30. 2002; p. 127.

Nicolopoulos C et al. Clinical application of helium neon (632 nm) plus infrared diode laser GaAlAs (830 nm) and CO2 laser in the treatment of onychomycotic nails. Foot. 1999; 9 (4): 181-184.

Nicolopoulos N, Dyson M et al. [The use of laser surgery in the subtotal meniscectomy and the effect of low-level laser therapy on the healing potential of rabbit meniscus: an experimental study]. Lasers Med Sci. 1996; 11 (2): 109-115.

Nikitin A V, Karpukhina E P. The effect of endovascular laser therapy on the clinical course and on the mechanisms of antioxidant protection in brochical asthma patients. Ter Arkh. 1992; 64 (1): 62-64. (in Russian)

Nikitin A V, Kashin A V, Karpukhina EP. Correction of the antioxidant defence in patients with bronichial asthma by the method of intravascular laser irradiation. Probl Tuberk. 1993; 3: 46-47.

Nishida J, Satoh T, Satodate R et al. Histological evaluation of the effect of HeNe laser irradiation on the synovial membrane in rheumatoid arthritis. Jap J Rheumatol. 1990; 2: 251-260.

Nissan J, Binderman I. Effect of soft laser on bone healing of surgical defect in rat mandible. J Dent Res. 1993; 72 (4) :776, Abstract 53.

Nissen L R et al. [Low-energy laser therapy in medial tibial stress syndrome]. Ugeskrift Læger. 1994; 156 (49): 7329-7331. (in Danish)

Nivbrant B, Friberg S. Knee - Therapeutic Laser Treatment in Gonarthroses. Acta Orthop Scand. 1989; 60 (suppl 231): 33.

Noro S. Semi-conductor laser application for pain attenuation in the temporo-mandibular joint following facial contusion and facial fracture. Meeting report from the 1st Congr of the IALSM 1997. Laser Therapy. 1997; 9 (4): 184.

Numazawa R, Kemmotsu O, Otsuka H et al. The role of laser therapy in intensive pain management of postherpetic neuralgia. Laser Therapy. 1996; 8 (2): 143-148.

Nussbaum E et al. Comparison of ultrasound/ultraviolet-C and laser for treatment of pressure ulcers in patients with spinal cord injury. Phys Ther. 1994; 74: 812-823.

Nussbaum E L. Low-intensity laser therapy for benign fibrotic lumps in the breast following reduction mammaplasty. Physical Therapy. 1999; 79 (7): 691-698.

Oasevich I A, Shargorodskii A G. [Low-intensity infrared laser radiation in the diagnosis and combined treatment of acute nonspecific lymphadenitis of the face and neck in children] Infrakrasnoe nizkointensivnoe lazer-noe izluchenie v diagnostike i kompleksnom lechenii ostrogo nespetsificheskogo limfadenita litsa i shei u detei. Stomatologiia (Mosk). 1999; 78 (2): 28-30.

Obata J et al. Clinical effects of total laser irradiation for the control of disease activity of chronic rheumatoid arthritis. Surgical and Medical Lasers. 1990; 3 (3): 140. (abstract).

Obata J et al. Evaluation of acute pain-relief effects of low power laser therapy on rheumatoid arthritis by thermography. Laser Therapy. 1990; 2: 28-

Obata J et al. The pain relief of low energy laser irradiation on rheumatoid arthritis. Pain Clin. 1987; 8: 18-.

Obata J, Yanse M. Evaluation of the effects of low power laser therapy on rheumatoid arthritis joints by roentgenographic survey. Laser Bologna '92, p. 41. Monduzzi Editore S.p.A., Bologna, Italy

Ocaña-Quero J M et al. Biological effects of helium-neon (He-Ne) laser irradiation on acrosome reaction in bull sperm cells. J Photochem Photobiol. B - Biol. 1997; 40 (3): 294-298.

Ocaña-Quero J M et al. Helium-Neon (He-Ne) laser irradiation increases the incidence of unreduced bovine oocytes during the first meiotic division in vitro. Lasers in Medical Science. 1998; 13 (4): 260-264.

Odud A M, Potapenko P I. [The effectiveness of laser puncture in hypertension patients]. Vrach Delo. 1990; (6): 19-21. (in Russian)

Odud A M, Potapenko P I. [The use of laser puncture for managing hypertensive crises]. Vrach Delo. 1991; (7): 34-36. (in Russian).

Oezdemir F, Birtane M, Kokino S. The clinical efficacy of low-power laser therapy on pain and function in cervical osteoarthritis. Clinical Rheumatology. 2001; 20 (3): 181-184.

Ohbayashi E, Matsushima K, Hosoya S et al. Stimulatory effect of laser irradiation on calcified nodule formation in human dental fibroblasts. J Endod. 1999. 25; 1: 30-33.

Ohno T. Pain suppressive effect of low power laser irradiation. A quantitative analysis of substance P in the rat spinal dorșal root ganglion. Nippon Ika Daigaku Zasshi (J Nippon Med School). 1997; 64 (5): 395-400. (in Japanese with English abstract)

Ohshiro T etr al. The Japanese experience in sumo wrestling. Proc. II Congr Internat Assn for Laser and Sports Medicine. Rosario, Argentina. March 2000.

Ohshiro T. Fujii S, Sasaki K et al. Laser therapy as an adjunct treatment for severe female infertility - a preliminary report. Laser Therapy. 1999; 11 (2): 96-102.

Ohshiro T. To publish, or not to publish.Editorial. Laser Therapy. 1989; 1 (2): 61-62.

Ohshiro T. Treatment techniques to achieve superficial and intermediate laser therapy irradiation. Laser Therapy. 1989; 3 (1): 153-155.

Ohshiro T. Alleviating Sport-relating pain with the diode laser. J Jap Soc Laser Med Surg. 1985; 5 (3): 221-.

Ohta A, Abergel P, Uitto J. Laser modulation of human immune system: Inhibition of lymphocyte proliferation by a gallium-arsenide laser at low energy. Lasers in Surgery and Medicine. 1987; 7: 199-.

Ohtsuka H et al. Low recative-level laser therapy near the stellate ganglion for postherpetic facial neuralgia. (in Japanese). Masui. 1992; 41 (11): 1809-1813.

Okamoto H, Iwase T, Morioka T. Dye-mediated bactericidal efffect of HeNe laser irradiation on oral microorganisms. Lasers in Surgery and Medicine. 1992; 12 (4): 450-458.

Olban M, Wachowicz B, Koter M, et al. The biostimulatory effect of red laser irradiation on pig blood platelet function. Cell Biol Int. 1998: 22 (3): 245-248.

Oliveira N M, Parizzotto N A, Salvini T F. GaAs (904-nm) laser radiation does not affect muscle regeneration in mouse skeletal muscle. Lasers in Surgery and Medicine. 1999; 25: 13-21.

Olivier J, Plath P. Combined low power laser therapy and extracts of Gingo Biloba in a blind trial of treatment for tinnitus. Laser Therapy. 1993; 5 (3): 137-140.

Omura Y, Losco B M, Omura A K et al. Common factors contributing to intractable pain and medical problems with sufficient drug uptake in areas to be treated, and their pathologies and treatment. Acupunct Electrother Res. 1992; 17 (2): 107-

Onac I et al. Histological study regarding the effects of HeNe (632.8 nm) laser biostimu-lation upon the tegument of Cavia Cobaia as compared with that of monochromatic red light (618 nm). Proc. 2nd Congress World Assn for Laser Therapy, Kansas City, September 1998; p. 52-53.

Önal B et al. Preliminary report on the application of pulsed CO2 laser radiation on root canals with AgCl fibers: a scanning and transmission electron microscopic study. J Endodontics. 1993; 19 (6): 272-276.

Orchardson R, Whitters C J. Effect of HeNe and pulsed Nd:YAG laser irradiation on intradental nerve responses to mechanical stimulation of dentine. Lasers in Surgery and Medicine. 2000; 26: 241-249.

Oron U, Yaakobi T, Oron A et al. Attenuation of the formation of scar tissue in rats and dogs post myocardial infarction by low energy laser irradiation. Lasers in Surgery and Medicine. 2001; 28: 1-7.

Oron U, Yaakobi T, Oron A et al. Attenuation of infarct size in rats and dogs after myocardial infarction by low-energy laser irradiation. Lasers in Surgery and Medicine. 2001; 28 (3): 204-211.

Ortutay J, Koo E, Mester A. Psoriatic arthritis treatment with low power laser irradiation. A double blind clinical study. Lasermedizin - Laser in Med Surg. 1998; 13 (3-4): 140-.

Ortutay J, Mester A. Laserstimulation therapy in the rehabilitation medicine. Proc. Laser Florence '97, 5th Congr , p. 22.

Otsuka H, Numasawa R, Okubo K et al. Effects of helium-neon laser therapy on herpes zoster pain. Laser Therapy. 1995; 7 (1): 27-32.

Otsuka K et al. Low reactive level laser therapy near the stellate ganglion for postherpetic facial pain. Jpn J Anaesthes. 1991; 41: 1809-1813. in Japanese with abstract in English)

Oudoff HAF; van der Kuiji P. Inquiry about the application of low reactive level laser therapy in dental clinics in The Netherlands. Laser Therapy. 1996; 8 (1): 42. (abstract)

Oulamara A. et al. Biological activity measurement on botanical specimen surfaces using a temporal decorrelation effect of laser speckle. Journal of Modern Optics. 1989; 36 (2): 165-.

Oyamada Y et al. Trials in treatment of RA-related diseases by HeNe-laser. Surg Med Lasers. 1989; 2: 18-.

Oyamada Y et al. A double blind study of low power HeNe laser therapy in rheumatioid arthritis. In: Optoelectronics in Medicine. 1987; p 747-750. Springer Verlag, Berlin (abstract). Complete study in Boletín de CDL. 1988; 17: 8-12.

Ozawa Y et al. Low-energy diode laser irradiation reduced plasminogen activator activity in human periodontal ligament cells. Lasers in Surgery and Medicine. 1997; 21: 456-463.

Ozawa Y et al. Stimulatory effects of low-power laser irradiation on bone formation in vitro. Proc SPIE. 1995; Vol 1984: 281-288.

Ozawa Y, Shimizu N, Kariya G et al. Low-energy laser irradiation stimulates bone nodule formation at early stages of cell culture in rat calvarial cells . Bone. 1998; 22 (4): 347-354.

Padua L et al. Clinical outcome and neurophysiological results of low power laser irradiation in carpal tunnel syndrome. Lasers Med Sci. 1999; 14 (3); 196-202.

Padulles J et al. [Laser treatment of spinal pinching due to discal hernias in dogs]. Boletín CDL. 1986; 2: 11-14. (in Spanish)

Palchun V T et al. [Low-energy laser irradiation in the combined treatment of sensorineural hearing loss and Ménière's disease]. Vestnik Otorinolaring. 1996; (1): 23-25. (in Russian).

Paleev NR, Slinchenko O, Ilchenko VA et al. Influence of He-Ne laser blood irradiation on morphofunctional state of monocytes in asthmatic patients. In: Effects of low-power light on biological systems. Proce. SPIE. 1999; Vol 2630: 142-146.

Palma J et al. Blockade of inflammatory signals by laser radiation. Lasers in Surgery and Medcine. 1991; suppl 3: 11

Palmgren N et a. Low Level Laser Therapy of infected abdominal wounds after surgery. Lasers in Surgery and Medicine. 1991; Suppl 3:11.

Palmgren N, Jensen G F, Kaae K et al. Low-Power Laser Therapy in Rheumatoid Arthritis. Lasers in Medical Science. 1989; 4: 193-196.

Palmieri B A double blind stratified cross over study of amateur tennis players suffering from tennis elbow using infrared laser therapy. Medical Laser Report. 1984; 1: 3-14

Pankov O P. Low-level therapy in ophthalmology. In: Novel Laser Methods in Medicine and Biology. Eds. Prokhorov A M, Pustovoy V I, Kuzmin G P. Proc. SPIE. 1998; Vol 3829:13-17.

Paolini D, Paolini-Pisani L. Tratamiento de la lesion del tendón manguito de los rotadores con láser de baja potencia. Estúdio prospectivo. Proc. II Congr Internat Assn for Laser and Sports Medicine. Rosario, Argentina. March 2000.

Paolini L E et al. Tratamiento de la lesion Osgood-Schlatter con láser de baja potencia - estúdio prospectívo.Proc. II Congr Internat Assn for Laser and Sports Medicine. Rosario, Argentina. March 2000.

Paolini L E, Paolini D. Tratamiento de la parálisis de Bell con láser de baja potencia. Estúdio prospectivo. Proc. II Congr Internat Assn for Laser and Sports Medicine. Rosario, Argentina. March 2000.

Papadopoulos E S, Smith R W, Cawley M I D. Low-level laser therapy does not aid the management of tennis elbow. Clinical Rehabilitation. 1996; 10: 9-11.

Parascandalo S et al. Azione della Laser-terapia nella sindrome di Sluder: considerazioni clinico-etiopatogenetiche. Int Congress on Laser in Med and Surg, Bologna June 1985, p 325.

Parascandolo S et al. Azione della Laser-terapia nella nevralgia essenziale del trigemino. Int Congress on Laser in Med and Surg, Bologna June 1985, p 317. Monduzzi Editore S.p.A., Bologna, Italy.

Parizotto N A, Baranauskas V. Structural analysis of collagen fibrils after HeNe laser photostimulated regenerating rat tendon. Proc. 2nd Congress World Assn for Laser Therapy, Kansas City, September 1998; p. 66.

Parker J, Dowdy D, Harkness E et al. The effects of laser therapy on tissue repair and pain control. A meta analysis of the literature. Proc. 3rd Congress of the World Ass for Laser Therapy, Athens, Greece, 2000, page 77. Submitted Lasers in Surgery and Medicine 2001.

Parman E M. [Low-intensity laser radiation in combined treatment of urinary system tuberculosis]. Probl Tuberk. 1999; 6: 34-37.

Parrado C et al. Quantitative study of the Morphlogical Changes in the Thyroid Gland Following IR Laser Radiation. Lasers in Med Sciences. 1990; 5: 77-.

Parshad R, Sanford K. Proliferative response of human diploid fibroblasts to intermittent light exposure. J Cell Physiol. 1977; 92: 481-.

Partheniadis-Stumpf M, Maurer J, Mann W. Soflasertherapie in Kombination mit Tebonin i.v. bei Tinnitus. Laryngorhinootologie 1993; 72 (1): 28-31

Partonen T, Vakkuri O, Lönnqvist J. Suppression of melatonin secretion by bright light in seasonal affective disorder. Biol Psychiatry. 1997; Sep 15;42 (6): 509-513.

Paschaud Y et al. Effet du soft-laser sur la néofromation d´un pont dentinaire après coiffage pulpaire direct de dents humaines à l' hydroxyde de calcium. Rev Mens Suisse Odont-Stomatol. 1988; 98 (4): 345-.

Passarella S et al. Increase in the ADP/ATP exchange in rat liver mitochondria irradiated in vitro by helium-neon laser. Biochem Biophys Res Commun. 1988; 156 (2): 978-986.

Passarella S et al. Increase of proton electrochemical potential and ATP synthesis in rat liver mitochondria irradiated in vitro by helium-neon laser. FEBS Letters. 1984; 175 (1): 95-99.

Passeniouk A M, Mikhailov V A. Application of low-level laser therapy for the treatment of vaginitis. In: A window on the laser medical world. Longo L ed. Proc. SPIE. 1999; Vol 4166: 316-318.

Pastore D et al. Stimulation of ATP synthesis via oxidative phosphorylation in weak mitochondria irradiated with helium-neon laser. Biochem Mol Biol Int. 1996; 39 (1): 149-157.

Pavlova R N. et al. Soft-laser radiation bioeffect: is laser a physical adaptogen? Proc. SPIE. 1993; Vol 1922: 225-229.

Pavlova, R N.; Gomberg, V. G.; Boiko, V. N.; Pupkova, L. S.; Reznikov, Leonid L.; Dadali, V. A. Effects of low-energy laser isolation upon the development of postradiation syndrome. Proc. SPIE.1996; Vol 2769: 78-81. (Laser Optics '95: Biomedical Applications of Lasers)

Pedrola M et al. Acute cervical pain relieved with gallium arsenurio (GaAs) laser irradiation. A double blind study. Lasers in Surgery and Medicine. 1995, suppl 7, p 10.

Pekli F F, Kruchinina I L. [Physiological functions of the nose befroe and after laser treatment of acute and chronic maxillary sinusitis in children]. Vestn Otorinolaringol. 1988; (3): 53-55.

Peláez A et al. Growing cartilage after IR laser radiation - utlrastructural study. Proc SPIE. 1993;. Vol 2086: 356-364.

Perrin D, Jolivald J R, Triki H et al. Pathol Biol. 1997; 45 (1) : 24-27.

Petersen S L, Botes C, Olivier A, Guthrie A J. The effect of LLLT on wound healing in horses. Equine Vet J. 1999; 31 (3): 228-231.Petrek M et al. Immunomodulatory effects of laser therapy in the treatment of chronic tonsillitis. Acta Univ Palacki Olomuc Fac Med. 1991; 129: 119-126.

Petrischev N N, Leontjeva N V, Leontjeva T A. Influence of irradiation of helium-neon laser on microcirculation blood vessels. Proc. SPIE. 1996; Vol 2929: 198-.

Petterborg L J, Kjellman B F, Thalén B E, Wetterberg L. Effect of a 15 minute light pulse on nocturnal serum melatonin levels in human volunteers. J Pineal Res. 1991; 10 (1): 9-13.

Piller N B, Thelander A, Esterman A. The objective assessment of the effect of low level laser therapy on chronic secondary arm and leg lymphoedemas. Proc. 3rd Cong World Ass for Laser Therapy, Athens, Greece, May 2000, p. 78.

Piller N B, Thelander A. Treatment of chronic postmastectomy lymphoedema with low level laser therapy: A 2.5 year follow-up. Lymphology. 1998; 31: 74-86.

Pinheiro A L, Carneiro Nascimento S, De Barros Vieira A L et al. Effects of low-level laser therapy on malignant cells: In vitro study. J Clin Med Surg. 2002; 20 (1): 23-26.

Pinheiro A L et al. Low-level laser therapy in the management of disorders of the maxillofacial region. J Clin Laser Med Surg. 1997; 15 (4): 181-183.

Pinheiro A, Oliveira M G, Martins P P M et al. Biomodulatory effects of LLLT bone regeneration. Laser Therapy. 2001; 13: 73-79.

Plavnik L, Crosa M, Malberti A. Effect of low power laser radiation on guinea pig submandibular glands: a structural and biomechanical study. J Dent Res. 2000; 79 (5): 1010-.

Plog F. Biophysical application of the laser beam. 1980. In Koebner H.K: Lasers in Medicine. John Wiley, New York.

Pluzhnikov S M et al. Use of intracavitary low-energy laser therapy in the complex treatment of inflammatory diseases in the sphenoid sinus. Vest Otoringolaringol. 1986; 4: 72-73. (in Russian with English abstr)

Podelinskaia L V et al. Effects of low-intensity laser irradiation on several parameters of microcirculation in the bulbar conjunctiva of patients with scleroderma. Vestn Oftalmol. 1995; 111 (2): 10-12.

Podolskaya E et al. Radiation damage of lips and its treatment by low-intensity laser irradiation. Proc SPIE. 1995; Vol 1984: 245-246.

Polonskii A K, Kharlampovich S I, Maschanova D D et al. [Effect of laser irradiation on a dystrophic process in the liver due to x-ray irradiation]. Med Radiol. 1983; 28: 59-61.

Polosukhin V V. Ultrastructure of the blood and lymphatic capillaries of the respiratory tissue during inflammation and endobronchial laser therapy. Ultrastructural Pathology. 2000; 24 (3): 183-189.

Ponnudurai R N et al. Hypoalgesic effect of laser photobiostimulation shown by rat tail flick test. Intern J Acup and Electrother Res. 1987; 12: 93-100.

Pöntinen P et al. Comparative effects of exposure to different light sources (He-Ne laser, InGaAl diode laser, a specific type of noncoherent LED) on skin blood flow for the head. Acupunct Electrother Res. 1996; 21 (2): 105-118.

Popov B. Trigeminal neuralgia with local laser irradiation and laserpuncture. Stomatologiia Bulgaria. 1986; 68: 25-29.

Popova M et al. Effect of Helium-Neon laser beam in regeneration of irradiated transplanted skeletal muscle. Biull Exp Biol Med. 1978; 80: 333. (Russian with English abstract.)

Porteder H. Einsatz des Helium-Neon-Lasers zur Förderung der Wundheilung. Z Stomat. 1983: 80: 333-339.

Pothman R, Yeh H L. The effects of treatment with antibiotics, laser and acupuncture upon chronic maxillary sinusitis in children. Am J Chin Med. 1982; 10 (1-4): 555-558.

Pourreau-Schnedier N et al. Soft-Laser Therapy for Iatrogenic Mucositis in Cancer Patients Receiving High-Dose Fluorouacil: A preliminary report. J Nat Cancer Inst. 1992; 5 (84): 358-.

Pourreau-Schneider N et al. Helium-Neon Laser Treatment Transforms Fibroblasts into Myofibroblasts. Am J Pathol. 1990; 137: 171-.

Prochazka, Koci K. Non-invasive laser therapy of morbus perronie - induratio penis placstica. Abstracts of 7th Int Congr European Medical Laser Assn, Dubrovnik, Croatia 2000, p. 39.

Prochazka M, Tejnska R. Noninvasive laser in therapy of tinnitus. In: A window on the laser medicine world. Proc. SPIE.1999, Vol 4166: 222-223. Also: Laserpartner Journal; May 2001.

Prokofeva G L, Kravchenko E V, Mozherenkov V P. [Effects of low-intensity infrared laser irradiation on the eye An experimental study]. Vestn-Oftalmol. 1996; 112 (1): 31-32

Prokopova L V et al. Effect of intravascular laser therapy on rheologic properties of blood in children with bilateral destructive pneumonia. Klin Khir. 1992; (6): 7-9.

Pyczek M, Sopala M, Dabrowski Z. Effect of low-energy laser power on the bone marrow of the rat. Folia Biol (Krakow) 1994; 42 (3-4): 151-156

Radelli J, Cieslar G, Sieron A, Grzybek H. Influence of low-power laser radiation on carbohydrate metabolism and insulin-glycemic balance in experimental animals. Proc. SPIE. 1996, Vol 2929: 94-102.

Radelli, J et al. Metabolism and insulin-glycemic balance in rats. Laser Therapy. 1996; 8 (1): 26. (abstract).

Ragnarsson S-I. Vision Research. 1972; 12: 411

Rajab A A. A study on the effect of low intensity laser therapy on the osseointegration of hydroxylapatite implants. 1999. University of London PhD thesis.

Rajaratuan S, Bolton P, Dyson M. Macrophage responsiveness to laser therapy with varying pulsing frequencies. Laser Therapy. 1994; 6: 107-102.

Rakcheev A P et al. Experimental and clinical substantiation of laser therapy of wounds and throphic ulcers. Ortop Travmatol Protez. 1989; 10: 66-70. (in Russian with English abstract)

Rao M L, Muller-Oerlinghausen B, Mackert A et al. The influence of phototherapy on serotonin and melatonin in non-seasonal depression. Pharmacopsychiatry. 1990; 23 (3): 155-158.

Rao M L, Muller-Oerlinghausen B, Mackert A, Strebel B, Stieglitz RD, Volz HP. Blood serotonin, serum melatonin and light therapy in healthy subjects and in patients with nonseasonal depression. Acta Psychiatr Scand. 1992; 86 (2): 127-132.

Reddy G K et al. Biochemistry and biomechanics of healing tendon: Part II. Effects of combined laser therapy and electrical stimulation. Med Sci Sports Exerc. 1998; 30 (6): 794-800.

Reddy G K et al. Laser photostimulation of collagen production in healing rabbit achilles tendons. Lasers in Medicine and Surgery. 1998; 22: 281-287.

Reddy G K et al. The effects of laser stimulation on wound healing in diabetic rats. Proc. 2nd Congress World Assn for Laser Therapy, Kansas City, September 1998; p. 124-125.

Reddy K, Stehno-Bittel L, Enwemeka C. Laser photostimulation accelerates wound healing in diabetic rats. Wound Repair and Regeneration. 2001, 9 (3): 248-255.

Reznikov L L et al. Urol Nefrol. 1991; 2: 45-49.

Reznikov L L. et al. Biomechanism of low-energy laser irradiation is similar to a general adaptive reaction. Proc. SPIE. 1994; Vol 2086: 380-449

Reznikov L L et al. Similarity between the mechanisms of soft-laser radiation and chemical adaptogen action. Proc. SPIE. 1993; Vol 1883: 91-98

Rezvani M et al. Prevention of x-radiation induced dermal necrosis in pig skin by monochromatic light. Lasers in Surgery and Medicine. 1991; suppl 3: 11

Ribari O et al. Closure of tympanic perforations with low-energy HeNe laser irradiation. Acta Chir Academ Scient Hungaricae. 1980; 21 (3): 229-238.

Ribeiro M S, Zezell D M, Fontenele J D, Pellegrini C M R, Zorn T M T. Incorporation of [3H]-Proline in the Dermis of Mice Following He-He Polarized Laser Radiation in the Wound Healing Process. A preliminary Study. Proc. 2nd Congress World Assn for Laser Therapy, Kansas City, Sept 1998; p. 13-15. Also: Histological study on wound healing in rats following He-Ne and GaAlAs laser irradiation. Proc. SPIE. 1998; Vol 3569: 50-55.

Rice J, Mayor J, Tucker HA, Bielski RJ. Effect of light therapy on salivary melatonin in seasonal affective disorder. Psychiatry Res. 1995; 56 (3): 221-228.

Riendeau F. An in vivo study of the effects of Helium-Neon laser on the breaking force and histological characteristics of wound. Proc Int Congr of Lasers in Dentistry, Tokyo, August 5-6. 1988: 20.

Rigau J, Trelles M A. Effects of the 633 nm laser on the behaviour and morphology of primary fibroblast culture. Proc SPIE. 1995; Vol 2630: 38-42.

Robinson J F et al. Wound healing in porcine skin following low output carbon dioxide laser irradiation of the lesion. Annals Plastic Surgery. 1987; 18 (6): 449-505.

Rochkind S, Barr-Nea L, Bartal A et al. New method of treatment of severely injured sciatic nerve and spinal cord. An experimental study. Acta Neurochirurgica. 1988; Suppl 43: 91-93.

Rochkind S, Nissan M, Lubart A. A single Transcutaneous Light Irradiation to Injured Peripheral Nerve: Comparative Study with Five Different Wavelengths. Lasers in Medical Sciences. 1989; 4: 259-.

Rochkind S, Alon M, Drory V et al. Laser therapy as a new modality in the treatment of incomplete periph-eral nerve and brachial plexus injuries: prospective clinical double blind placebo-controlled randomized study. In: Abstract book of the Annual Meeting 2001, American Society for Peripheral Nerve, San Diego, California, USA, January 2001, p. 21

Rochkind S, Nissan M, Alon M et al. Effects of laser irradiation on the spinal cord for the regeneration of crushed peripheral nerve in rats. Lasers in Surgery and Medicine. 2001; 28 (3): 216-219.

Rochkind S, Rousso M, Nissan M et al. Systemic effects of low-power laser irradiation on the peripheral and central nervous system, cutaneous wounds and burns. Lasers in Surgery and Medicine. 1989; 9: 174-182.

Rochkind S, Nissan M, Razon N et al. Electrophysiological Effect of HeNe Laser on Normal and Injured Sciatic Nerve in the Rat. Acta Neurochir. (Vienna). 1986; 83: 125-130.

Rochkind S et al. Double-blind Randomized Study Using Neurotube and Laser Therapy in the Treatment of Complete Sciatic Nerve Injury of Rats. Proc. 2nd Congr World Assoc. for Laser Therapy, Kansas City, 1998.

Rochkind S et al. Systemic Effects of Low-Power Laser Irradiation on the Peripheral and Central Nervous System, Cutaneous Wounds and Burns. Lasers in Surgery and Medicine. 1989; 9: 174-.

Rodrigues M T J, Ribeiro M S, Groth E B et al. Evaluation of effects of laser therapy (wavelength=830 nm) on oral ulcertation induced by fixed orthodontic appliances. Laser Med Surg Abstract issue, 2002: 15.

Rogowski M, Menich S, Gindzienska E, Lazarczyk B. [Low-power laser in the treatment of tinnitus - a placebo-controlled study]. Laser niskoenergetyczny w leczeniu szumow usznychó-badania porownawcze z placebo. Otolaryngologia polska. Otolaryngol-Pol. 1999; 53 (3): 315-320

Rogvi Hansen B et al. Low level laser treatment of chondromalacia patellae. Int Orthopaedics. 1991; 15: 359-361.

Roig J, Fleites A, Bécquer R. Tratamiento del síndrome del túnel carpiano con láser HeNe e infrarojo. Evaluación clínica y electrofisiológica de los resultados.[Treatment of the carpal tunnel syndrome with HeNe and infrared laser. Clinical and electrophysical evaluation of the results]. Rev Cubana Ortop Traumatol. 1992; 6 (2): 139-143.

Rosen H S., Klebanoff S J. Federal Proceedings, 1976; 35: 1391.

Roshal L. Application of Low-Level Laser in Pediatry and Pediatric Surgery in the USSR. In: Progress in Laser Therapy. Editors: Ohshiro & Calderhead. John Wiley & Sons. 1991, p. 112.

Rosner M, Caplan M, Cohen S et al. Dose and temporal parameters in delaying injured optic nerve degeneration by low-energy laser irradiation. Lasers in Surgery and Medicine. 1993; 13 (6): 611-617.

Rossetti V et al. Experimental studies on the in vivo effects of HeNe laser irradiation in rat brain. Lasermedizin - Laser in Med Surg. 1995; 11 (2): 24 .

Rossman J A. Current research using the CO_2 laser in guided tissue regeneration: animal studies. Proc Second Annual Advanced Application Seminar. Luxar Corp, USA., 1993.

Roumeliotis D, Emmanouilidis O, Diamantopoulos C. C.W. 820nm 15mW 4J/cm^2, laser diode application in sports injunes. A double blind study. Proc. Fifth Annual Congress, 28-30 January 1987. British Medical Laser Association.

Røynesdal A et al. The effect of soft-laser application on postoperative pain and swelling. A double-blind, cross-over study. J Oral Maxillofac Surg. 1993; 22: 242-245.

Ruffolo P et al. Impiego della Laser-terapia nelle leucoplachie del cavo orale. Int Congress on Laser Med and Surg, Bologna June 1985, p. 279 Monduzzi Editore S.p.A., Bologna, Italy.

Ruiz I et al.. Histological and clinical responses of articular cartilage to low level laser therapy: Experimental study. Lasers in Medical Science, 1997. 12 (2): 117-121.

Ryabykh T, Karu T. Action of pulsed visible and near IR laser radiation on oxidative metabolism of cells evaluated by chemiluminescence measurement. Proc SPIE. 1995; Vol 2630: 12-21.

Rydén H, Persson L, Preber H, Bergström J. Effect of low-energy laser on gingival inflammation. Swedish Dent J. 1994; 18: 35-41.

Sagalovich E E. Secretory immunity changes in patients with acute and chronic herpetic stomatitis by laser therapy. Clin Immunol Immunopathol. 1995. 1 (7): 385-.

Saito K. Effects of 830 nm diode laser irradiation on superficial blood circulation in college sumo wrestlers. Meeting report from the 1st Congr of the IALSM 1997. Laser Therapy. 1997; 9 (4): 187.

Saito S, Shimizu N. Stimulatory effects of low-power laser irradiation on bone regeneration in midpalatal suture during expansion in the rat. Am J Ortod Dentofac Orthop. 1997; 11 (5): 525.

Sakihama I. Effect of a helium-neon laser on cutaneous inflammation. Karume Medical J. 1995; 52 (4): 299-305.

Sakurai Y; Yamaguchi M; Abiko Y. Inhibitory effect of low-level laser irradiation on LPS-stimulated prostaglandin E2 production and cyclooxygenase-2 in human gingival fibroblasts. Eur J Oral Sci. 2000; 108 (1): 29-34.

Saldo I et al. Effects of GaAs-laser combined with radiotherapy on murine sarcoma depends on tumor size. Lasers in Surgery and Medicine. 1989; Suppl 1: 40.

Salinas E O, Hakim-Kreis C M, Piketty M L et al. Hypersecretion of melatonin following diurnal exposure to bright light in seasonal affective disorder: preliminary results. Biol Psychiatry. 1992; Sep 1; 32 (5) : 387-398.

Samoilova K, Snopov S. A key role on whole circulating blood modification in therapeutic effects of ultraviolet and visible light. Proc. 2nd Congress World Assn for Laser Therapy, Kansas City, September 1998; p. 92-94.

Samoilova K A, Kukui L M. Photochemotherapy in clinical and veterinary medicine: therapeutic effects and mechanisms. Laser Therapy. 1996; 8 (1): 62. (abstract)

Sandford M A, Walsh L J. Thermal effects during desensitisation of teeth with gallium-aluminum-arsenide lasers. Periodontol 1994; 15 (1): 25-30.

Sanseverino N T M, Sanseverino C A M, Ribeiro M S et al. Clinical evaluation of the low intensity laser antialgic action of GaAlAs (wavelength=785 nm) in the treatment of the temporomandibular disorders. Laser Med Surg Abstract issue, 2002: 18.

Sant'Anna G R et al. Photodynamic therapy using low level laser as a disinfecting approach to carious dentine: in vivo microbiological study. Proc. 7th Int Congr Lasers in Dentistry, ISLD, Brussels, Belgium, July 2000, abstr. 43.

Sant'Anna G R, Duarte D A, Brugnera Jr A et al. Dye-assisted laser therapy as a disinfecting approach to caries dentine. In vivo microbiology study. Proc. 3rd Congr World Assn for Laser Therapy, Athens, Greece, May 2000, p. 62.

Santana-Black L A, Rodriguez-Santana E, Scott-Algara D et al. Short-term bioeffects of an infrared pulsed laser device on burned rat skin monitored by transverse relaxation times (TMR). Lasers in Surgery and Medicine. 2000; 27: 411-419.

Santoianni P et al. Inadequate effect of helium-neon laser on venous leg ulcers. Photodermatology. 1984; 1: 245-249.

Saperia D et al. Demonstration of elevated type I and type III laser. Biochem and Biophys Res Communic. 1986; 138: 3-.

Sapiera D et al. Demonstration of elevated type I and type III procollagen mRNA levels in cutaneous wounds treated with helium-neon laser. Biochem Biophys Res Com. l986; 3 (138): 1123-1128.

Sasaki K, Ohshiro T, Hoshino T. A preliminary double blind controlled study on free amino acid analysis in burn wounds in the mouse following 830 nm diode laser therapy. Laser Therapy. 1997; 9 (2): 59-66.

Sasaki K et al. Low level laser therapy (laser therapy) for thromboangitis obliterans. Proc. 2nd Congress World Association for Laser Therapy, Kansas City, USA, September 2-5 1998; p 95-96.

Sasaki K, Calderhead R G, Chin I, Inomata K. To examine the adverse photothermal effects of extended dosage laser therapy in vivo on the skin and subcutaneous tissue in the rat model. Laser Therapy. 1992; 2: 69-74.

Sasaki K, Ohshiro T. Role of Low Reactive-Level Laser Therapy (laser therapy) in the Treatment of Aquired and Cicatricial Vitiligo. Laser Therapy. 1989; 1 (3): 141-146.

Sato H. The effects of laser light on sperm motility and velocity in vitro. Andrologia. 1984; 16 (1): 23-25.

Sato K, Kaseno S, Takigawa C et al. A double blind assessment of low power laser therapy in the treatment of postherpetic neuralgia. Surgical and Medical Lasers. 1990; 3 (3): 134. (abstract)

Sattayut S, Bradley P F. Low intensity laser therapy (LILT) for TMD myofascial pain: results from a pilot study. 1998. Proc. 6th Int Congr Lasers in Dentistry. University of Utah Press. Ed: J Frame. ISBN 0-87480-606-2, p. 152-156.

Sattayut S, Hughes F, Bradley P. 820 nm gallium aluminium arsenide laser modulation of prostaglandin E2 production in interleukin-1 stimulated myoblasts. Laser Therapy. 1999; 11 (2): 88-95.

Sattayut S A study on the influence of low intensity laser therapy on painful temporomandibular disorders 1999;. University of London PhD thesis (prof. P Bradley).

Saunders L. The efficiacy of low-level laser therapy in supraspinatus tendinitis. Clin Rehab. 1995; 9: 126-134.

Schaffer M et al. Biomodulative effects induced by 805 nm laser light irradiation of normal and tumor cells. J Photochem Photobiol B:Biol. 1997; 40: 253-257.

Schaffer M et al. Magnetic resonance imaging (MRI) controlled outcome of side effects caused by ionizing radiation, treated with with 780-nm diode laser - preliminary results. J Photochemistry and Photobiology B: Biology. 2000; 59: 1-8.

Schaffer M et al. Mitotic rate of normal mouse fibroblast cells and human tumor cells after diode laser irradiation. Laser Therapy. 1996; 8 (1) 23. (abstract).

Schaffer M, Bonel H, Sroka-R et al. Effects of 780 nm diode laser irradiation on blood microcirculation: Preliminary findings on time-dependent T1-weighted contrast-enhanced magnetic resonance imaging (MRI). J Photochemistry and Photobiology B: Biology 2000; 54 (1): 55-60.

Schenk P et al. Elektronenmikroskopische Untersuchungen von oralen Schleimhautepithelien nach bestrahlung mit dem Helium-Neon-laser. Dtsch Z Mun Kiefer Gesischts Chir. 1985; 9: 278-.

Schindl A et al. Increased dermal neovascularization after low dose laser therapy of chronic radiation ulcer determined by a video measuring system. Proc. 2nd Congress World Assn for Laser Therapy, Kansas City, September 1998; p. 34.

Schindl A et al. Low intensity laser irradiation improves skin circulation in patients with diabetic microangiopathy. Diabetes Care. 1998; 21 (4): 580-584.

Schindl A et al. Low intensity laser irradiation in the treatment of recalcitrant radiation ulcers in patients with breast cancer - long term results of 3 cases. Photodermatol-Photoimmunol-Photomed. 2000; 16 (1): 34-37.

Schindl A, Merwald H, Schindl L. Low intensity laser irradiation stimulates endothelial cell proliferation in an vitro model of diabetic microangiopathy. Lasers in Surgery and Medicine. 2001; Suppl 13: 7.

Schindl A, Neuman R. Low-intensity laser therapy is an effective treatment for recurrent herpes simplex infection. Results from a randomized double-blind placebo controlled study. J Investigative Dermatology. 1999; 113 (2): 221-223.

Schindl A, Schindl L. Systemic increase in blood flow in conditions of disturbed microcirculation after low-power laser irradiation. Proc. SPIE. 1996, Vol 2929: 63-69.

Schindl L et al. Effects of low power laser-irradiation on differential blood count and body temperature in endotoxin-preimmunized rabbits. Life Sci. 1997; 60 (19): 1669-1677.

Schindl L et al. Topical low power laser irradiation shows a systemic increase in blood flow in conditions of disturbed microcirculation. Laser Therapy. 1996; 8 (1): 58. (abstract).

Schindl L et al. Influence of low-power laser irradiation on "arthus phenomenon" induced in rabbit cornea. Laser Therapy. 1994; 6 (1); 23. (abstract)

Schindl L, Kainz A, Kern H. Effect of Low Level Laser Irradiation on Indolent Ulcers Caused by Bürgers Disease. Laser Therapy. 1992; 4 (1): 25-32.

Schindl A, Schindl M, Pernerstorfer-Schön H et al. Low-intensity laser therapy: a review. J Invest Med. 2000; 48 (5): 312-326.

Schindl A, Schindl M, Pernerstorfer-Schoen H, Schindl L. Low intensity laser therapy in wound healing - A review with special respect to diabetic angiopathies. Acta Chirurgica Austriaca. 2001; 33: 3.

Schindl M, Schindl A, Polzleitner D et al. Healing of bone affections and gangrene with low-intensity laser irradiation in diabetic patiens suffering from foot infections. Forch Komplementarmed. 1998; 5: 244-247.

Schlager A et al. Laser stimulation of acupuncture point P6 reduces postoperative vomiting in children undergoing strabismus surgery. Br J Anaesth. 1998; 81 (4): 529-532

Schlager A, Kronberger P, Petschke F et al. Low-power laser light in the healing of burns: a comparison between two different wavelengths (635 nm and 690 nm) and a placebo group. Lasers in Surg Med. 2000; 27: 39-42.

Schultz R J, Krishnamurthy S, Thelmo W et al. Effects of varying intensities of laser energy on articular cartilage: A preliminary study. Lasers in Surgery and Medicine. 1985; 5: 557-588.

Schuster M A et al. [Treatment of vasomotor rhinitis, trigeminal neuralgia and Sluder's syndrome by helium-neon laser irradiation of the pterygopalatine ganglion]. Vest. Otorinolar. 1988; 4: 35-40.

Schwartz F et al. Effect of low energy laser irradiation on cytokines secretion from skeletal muscle cells - involvement of calcium in the process. Proc SPIE.1997. Vol 3198: 48-54.

Schwartz M et al. Effect of low-energy HeNe laser irradiation on posttraumatic degeneration of adult rabbit optic nerve. Lasers Sur Med. 1987; 7: 51-55.

Scudds R A et al. A double-blind crossover study of the effectiveness of low-power gallium arsenide laser on the symptoms of fibrositis. Physiotherapy Canada. 1989; 41: (suppl 3):2.

Senda A , Gomi A et al. A clinical study of Soft Laser 632, a Helium-Neon low energy medical laser. 1st report. The effect in releiving pain just after irradiation. Aichi-Gakuin J Dent Sci. 1985; 23 (4): 773-780.

Senda N, Ito K, Sugano N et al. Inhibitory effect of yellow He-Ne laser irradiation mediated by crystal violet solution on early plaque formation in human mouth. Lasers Med Sci. 2000; 15 (3): 174-180.

Sepp W, Haina D et al. Laserstrahlen in der Dermatologie- Der Deutsche Dermatologe. 1978; 11 (26): 557-575.

Severtsev A N et al. The preliminary results of the immunomodulatory effects of HeNe-laser irradiation in human mixed lymphocytes culture. Lasers in Surgery and Medicine, Suppl 5. 1993; 10.

Shamir M H, Rochkind S, Sandbank J, Alon M. .Double-blind randomized study evaluating regeneration of the rat transected sciatic nerve after suturing and postoperative low-power laser treatment. Journal of Reconstructive Microsurgery.2001; 17 (2): 133-137.

Shchepetkin I A The effect of He-Ne laser radiation on the chemiluminescence of human neutrophils. Radio-biologiia. 1993; 33 (3): 377-382.

Shear J B, Xu C, Webb W W. Multiphoton-excited visible emission by serotonin solutions. Photochem Photobiol 1997; 65 (6): 931-936.

Shefer G, Oron U, Irintchev A. Low energy laser irradiation activates specific signal transduction pathways in skeletal muscle cells. J Cell Physiol. 2001; 187: 73-80.

Shesterina M V. [Effects of laser therapy on immunity in patients with bronchial asthma and pulmonary tuberculosis.] Probl Tuberk. 1994; 5: 23-26.

Shi K, Lu R, Xu X. Influence of low energy HeNe laser on the regeneration of peripheral nerves. Chung Kuo Hsiu Fu Chung Chien Wai Ko Tsa Chih. 1997; 11 (1): 14-8. (in Chinese)

Shimizu N et al. Prospect of relieving pain due to tooth momement during orthodontic treatment utilizing a GaAlAs diode laser. Proc. SPIE. 1995; Vol 1984: 275-280.

Shimizu N, Yamaguchi M, Goseki T et al. Inhibition of prostaglandin E2 and interleukin 1-ß production by low-power laser irradiation in stretched human periodontal ligament cells. J Dent Res. 1995; 74 (7): 1382-1388.

Shiomi Y et al. Efficacy of transmeatal low power laser irradiation on tinnitus: a preliminary report. Auris Nasus Larynx. 1997; 24: 39-42.

Shiomi Y et al. [Effect of low power laser irradiation on innear ear.] Pract Otol (Kyoto). 1994; 87: 1135-1140 (in Japanese)

Shiroto C et al. Effects of diode laser radiation in vitro on activity of human neutrofils. Laser Therapy. 1989; 1 (3): 135-.

Shiroto C et al: Retrospective study of diode laser therapy for pain attenuation in 3635 patients: Detailed analysis by questionnaire. Laser Therapy. 1989; 1 (1): 41-.

Shiroto C. Clinical results of pain relief with low lever laser therapy. Laser Bologna '92, p. 25. Monduzzi Editore S.p.A., Bologna, Italy.

Shishkin S A. Use of low intensity laser irradiation in the treatment of thrombophlebitic complications during subclavian vein catheterization. Anesteziol Reanimatol. 1993; (6): 66-68.

Shore S E, Vass Z, Wyss N L,Altschuler R A. Trigeminal ganglion innervates the auditory brainstem. J Comparative Neurology 2000; 419: 271-285.

Shuvalova I N, Klimenko I T, Zhukova L P et al. [The effect of low-intensity laser radiation in the infrared and red ranges on arterial pressure regulation in patients with borderline hypertension]. Lik Sprava .1998; (7): 141-143.

Shuvalova I N et al. [The effect of low-intensity laser radiation in the infrared and red ranges on arterial pres-sure regulation in patients with borderline hypertension]. Likarska Sprava. 1998; (7): 141-143.

Siebert W et al. What is the efficacy of "soft" and "mid" lasers in therapy of tendinopathies? A double blind studie. Arch Ortop and Traum Surg. 1987; 106: 358-363.

Silva Junior A N, Pinheiro A, Oliveira M G et al. Computerized morphometric assessment of the effect of low-level laser therapy on bone repair: an experimental animal study. J Clin Laser Med Surg. 2002; 20 (2): 83-87.

Simunovic Z, Simunovic K. Status after multiple teeth extractions treatment with low level laser therapy: A randomised clinical study with control group. Lasers in Surgery and Medicine. 2001; Suppl 13: 11.

Simunovic Z, Trobonjaca T, Trobonjaca Z. Treatment of medial and lateral epicondylitis - tennis and golfer's elbow with low level laser therapy: a multicenter double blind, placebo-controlled clinical study on 324 patients. - J Clin Laser Med & Surg. 1998; 16 (3): 145-151.

Simunovic Z, Trobonjaca T. Comparison between low level laser therapy and visible incoherent polarised light in the treatment of lateral epicondylitis - tennis elbow. A pilot clinical study on 20 patients. Lasers in Surgery and Medicine. 2001; Suppl 13: 9.

Simunovic Z, Trobonjaca T. Low level laser therapy in the treatment of osteoarthrosis of joints of the upper extremity: a multicenter, double blind, placebo controlled clinical study of 154 patients. Lasers in Surg Med. Suppl 12, 2000: 7

Thorsen H. [Low energy laser treatment-effect in localized fibromyalgia in the neck and shoulder regions.] Ugeskrift for Laeger. 1991; 17; 153 (25):1801-1804. (in Danish).

Thwee T, Kato J , Hashimoto M et al. Pulp reaction after pulpotomy with He-Ne laser irradiation. In: Abstract handbook. Vol 4. Internat Soc Laser in Dentistry. 1994. Denics Pacific Ltd, Hong Kong. HeNe laser in combination with calcium hydroxide created dentin-like calcified layer after pulpotomy in Wistar rats.

Timirgalef M J et al. [Laser therapy of the inflammatory diseases of the accessory nasal sinuses]. Vestn Otorin. 1985; 3: 56-60.

Tiukhin N S et al. Laser therapy in patients with inflammatory pleural exudates. Problemy Tuberkuleza. 1997; 4: 38-40. (in Russian)

Tolle R. Psychotherapy of depressive disorders: on the theoretical background and its clinical relevance. Ner-venarzt. 1997; 68 (7): 602-605.

Toscani A, Bombelli G. [Laser therapy in post-extraction alveolitis]. Dent Cadmos. 1987; 55 (9): 73-74. (In Italian)

Toya S, Motegi M, Inomata K, Ohshiro T. Report on a computer-randomized double blind clinical trial to determine the effectiveness of the GaAlAs (830 nm) diode laser for pain attenuation in selected pain. Laser Therapy 1994; 6 (3): 143-148.

Trelles M et al. Bone Fracture Consolidates Faster With Low-Power Laser. Lasers in Surgery and Medicine. 1987; 7: 36-45.

Trelles M A, Rigau J, Soto P et al. Infrared Diode Laser in Low Reactive-Level Laser Therapy (laser therapy) for Knee Osteoarthroses. Laser Therapy. 1991; 3 (4): 149-154.

Trelles M, Mayayo E, Miro L, Rigau J, Baudin G, Calderhead G. The action of low reactive level laser therapy (laser therapy) on mast cells. Laser Therapy. 1989; 1: 27-30.

Trelles M, Mayayo E. Mast cells are implicated in low power laser effect on tissue. A preliminary study. Lasers in Medical Science. 1992; 7: 73-.

Trelles M A, Rotinen S. He/Ne laser treatment of hemorrhoids. Acupuncture & Electro-Therapeutics Research. 1983; 8 (3-4): 289-95.

Tsai CL et al. Effect of CO2 laser on healing of cultured meniscus. Lasers in Surgery and Medicine.1997; 20 (2): 172-178.

Tsai J-C, Kao M-C. The Biological Effects of Incident Low Power Density Laser Irradiation on Cultivated Rat Glial and Glioma Cells. Laser Therapy. 1989; 1 (4): 191-202.

Tsang D, Yew D T, Hui BS. Further studies on the effect of low-dose laser irradiation on cultured retinal pigment cells of the chick. Acta Anat (Basel) 1986; 125 (1):10-13.

Tsuchiya K et al. Diode laser irradiation selectively diminishes slow component of axonal volleys to dorsal roots from the saphenous nerve in the rat. Neuroscience Letters. 1993; 161: 65-68. Also: Tsuchiya K, Kawatani M, Takeshige C, et al.Laser irradiation abates neuronal responses to nociceptive stimulation of rat-paw skin.Brain Res Bull. 1994; 34 (4): 369-374

Tsurko V V, Muldiyarov PY, Sigidin YA. Laser therapy of rheumatoid arthritis. A clinical and morphological study. Terap Arkh. 1983; 55: 97-102. (in Russian).

Tsushima T et al. Effects of two-point linear polarised near-infrared irradiation in difficult temporomandibular joint disorders. Proc. 2nd Congress World Assn for Laser Therapy, Kansas City, September 1998; p. 29-30.

Tulebaev R K et al. Indicators of the activity of the immune system during laser therapy of vasomotor rhinitis. Vestn. Otorinolaringol. 19989; 1: 46-49. (in Russian)

Tunér J, Hode L. It's all in the parameters: a critical analysis of some well-known negative studies on low-level laser therapy. J Clin Laser Med Surg. 1998; 16 (5): 245-248.

Tunér J, Hode L. Are all the negative studies really negative? Laser Therapy. 1998; 10 (4): 165-174.

Tunér J. 100 positive double-blind studies: enough or too little? Proc. SPIE. 1999; Vol. 4166: 226-232.

Tunér J. The Cochrane analyses - can they be improved? Laser Therapy. 1999; 11 (3): 138-143.

Uchida K et al. Treatment of chronic prostatitis and prostatodynia with low reactive laser. Laser Therapy. (ILTA Okinawa Congr Abstr Issue) 1990; 2 (1): 36.

Ueda Y, Shimizu N. Pulse irradiation of low-power laser stimulates bone nodule formation. Journal of Oral Science. 2001; 43 (1): 55-560.

Ulrich M et al. Influence of laser light (830 nm) on the growth kinetics of rat rhabdomyosarcomas. University of Hamburg, Department of Accident Surgery. Part of M.D. thesis

Umeda Y et al. Blood pressure controlled by low reactive level diode laser therapy (laser therapy). Laser Therapy. 1990; 2 (2): 59-.

Umetov M A. Effects of laser therapy on psychophysiological parameters and arterial blood pressure in drivers with hypertension. Med Tr Prom Ekol. 1996; 8: 10-12. (in Russian)

Urazalin Zh B et al. Laser therapy in the combined treatment of mandibular fractures. Stomatologiia. 1983; 62: 34-.

Utsunomiya T A histopathological study of the effects of low-power laser irradiation on wound healing of exposed dental pulp tissues in dogs, with special reference to lectins and collagens. J Endod. 1998; 24 (3): 187-193.

Vacca R A et al. Activation of mitochondrial DNA replication by He-He laser irradiation. Biochem Biophys Res Commun. 1993; 195 (2): 704-709.

Valiente-Zaldivar C et al. Laserterapía en la neuralgía trigeminal. Informa preliminar. Rev Cubana de Estomat. 1990; 2 (22): 166-171.

Valiente-Zaldivar C et al. Lasers en estomatología. Rev Cubana de Estomat. 1989: 26: 336-343.

Velizhanina I A, Gapon L I, Shabalina M S et al. [Efficiency of low-intensity laser radiation in essential hypertension]. Klinicheskaia Meditsina (Mosk). 2001; 79 (1): 41-44.

van Breugel H et al. Low energy HeNe laser irradiation effects proliferation and laminin production of rat Schwann cells in vitro. Lasers in Surgery and Medicine. 1991;Suppl 3:10.

van Breugel H. et al. Power Density and Exposure Time of HeNe Laser Irradiation Are More Important Than Total Energy Dose in Photo-Biomodulation of Human Fibroblasts in Vitro. Lasers in Surgery and Medicine. 1992; 12: 528.

van den Brande P. Effect of HeNe - IR laser on cutaneous microcirculation in vascular patients. Proc. Lasertherapy III, Vrije Universiteit Brussel, October 1987.

van der Veen P, Lievens P. Low level laser therapy (laser therapy): The influence on the proliferation of fibroblasts and the influence of the regeneration process of lymphatic, muscular and cartilage tissue. In: Simunovic, Z (ed), Lasers in Medicine and Dentistry. Basic science and an up-to-date clinical application of low energy laser therapy. 2000: 187-217.

van der Ven P et al. The influence of IR-laser on the proliferation of fibroblasts: an in-vitro study. Proc. 2nd Congress World Assn for Laser Therapy, Kansas City, Sept 1998; p. 120-122.

van Dieten H E et al. Systematic review of the cost effectiveness of prophylactic treatments in the prevention of gastropathy in patients with rheumatoid arthritis or osteoarthritis taking non-steroidal anti-inflammatory drugs. Ann Rheum Dis. 2000; 59 (10): 753-759.

van Rensburg S D, Wiltshire W A. The effect of soft laser irradiation on fluoride release of two fluoride-containing orthodontic bonding materials. J Dent Assoc S Afr. 1994; 49 (3): 127-131.

Vasilotta A. I.R. laser: a new therapy in rhino-sino-nasal bronchial syndrome with asthmatic component. Proc X. Internat Congr Soc Lasers in Surgery and Medicine, Bangkok 1993, p. 161.

Vasseljen O et al. Low Level Laser versus placebo in the treatment of tennis elbow. Scand J Rehab Med. 1992; 24: 37-42. Also in Physiotherapy. 1992; 5: 329-334.

Vecchio P et al. A double-blind study of the effectiveness of low level laser treatment of rotator cuff tendinitis. Br J Rheum. 1993; 32: 740-742.

Vélez-González M et al. Activation of the subcutanus absorbtion of drugs previous laser irradiation. Proc. Ninth Congress of the International Society for Laser Surgery and Medicine, Anaheim, California, USA: 2-6 November 1991.

Vélez-Gonzáles M A. Absorción subcutaneo del salicilato de dietilamina tras la irradiación laser. Boletín CDL. 1987; 4 (12): 4-8.

Vélez-Gonzalez M et al. Treatment of relapse in Herpes Simplex on labial & facial areas and of primary herpes simplex on genital areas and "area pudenda" with low power laser (HeNe) or Acyclovir administred orally. Proc SPIE. 1995; Vol 2630: 43-50.

Velizhanina I A et al. [The laser therapy of hypertension patients in the initial stages.] Voprosy Kuror Fizioter Lecheb Fiziches Kult. 1998; 1: 9-11.

Verbruggen L A et al. Low-power laser therapy in chronic rheumatic diseases: Western and Soviet experiences. Phys Med Rehab. 1991; 1: 101.

Verdote-Robertson R, Munchua M M, Reddon J R. The use of low intensity laser therapy (LILT) for the treatment of open wounds in psychogeriatric patients: A pilot study. Physical and Occupational Therapy in Geriatrics. 2000, 18 (2): 1-19.

Verplanken M. Stimulation of wound healing after tooth extraction using low intensity laser therapy. Revue Belge de Medecine Dentaire. 1987; 42: 134-138.

Villaplana L A, Sarti M A, Trelles M A et al. Changes in albino rat testicle interstitial cells after pituitary stimulation in vivo with HeNe laser. Laser Therapy. 1995; 7 (1): 19-22.

Vizi E, Mester E, Tisza S, Mester A. Acetylcholine releasing effect of laser irradiation on Auerbach's plexus in guinea-pig ileum. J. Neural Transmission. 1977; 40: 305.

von Ahlften U et al. Erfahrungen bei der Behandlung aphtöser und herpetiformer Mundschleimhauterkrankungen mit einem neuen Infrarotlaser. Die Quintessenz. 1987; 5: 927.

Voronin I et al. [The use of laser therapy for restoring the fertilizing capacity of the ejaculate in men with chronic genital inflammation.] Vopr Kurortol Fizioter Lech Fiz Kult. 1994; 2: 24-26.

Vulliez C et al. Éffet du Laser Infra Rouge a Diode sur le Tissue Conjuctif. Innov. Tech Biol. Med. 1990; 11(1): 143-.

Wafa F et al. A clinical study of laser therapy in fixed posthodontic pain control after tooth preparation to receive a crown.. 1990; 2 (2): 83-88.

Wahl G, Bastianer S. Soft laser in postoperative care in dentoalveolar treatment. ZWR. 1991; 100 (8): 512-515.

Wakabayashi H et al. Effect of Irradiation by Semiconductor Laser on Responses Evoked in Trigeminal Caudal Neurons by Tooth Pulp Stimulation. Lasers in Surgery and Medicine. 1993; 13: 605-.

Wakabayashi H et al. Treatment of dentine hypersensitivity by GaAlAs soft laser irradiation. J Dent Research. 1988; 67: 182.

Walker J B, Swartzwelder H S, Bondy S C. Suppression of Hippocampal Epileptiform Activity In Vitro After Laser Exposure. Laser Therapy. 1989; 1 (1): 19-22.

Walker J B et al. Laser therapy for pain of rheumatoid arthritis. Lasers in Surgery and Medicine.1986; 6: 171-.

Walker J B et al. Laser Therapy for pain of trigeminal neuralgia. Pain 1987; 29: 585-.

Walker J B et al. Laser Therapy for pain of Rheumatoid Arthritis. The Clinical Journal of Pain. 1987; 3 (53): 54-59.

Walker J B. Relief from Chronic Pain by Low Power Laser Irradiation. Neuroscience Letters. 1983; 43: 339-344.

Walker J B. Temporary suppression of clonus in humans by brief photo-stimulation. Brain Research. 1985; 340: 109-113.

Walsh D et al. The effect of low intensity laser irradiation upon conduction and skin temperature in the superficial radial nerve. Double blind placebo controlled investigation using experimental ischaemic pain. Proc. Second Meeting of the International Laser Therapy Association, London Sept 1992.

Walsh D, Baxter D, Allen J. Lack of effect of pulsed low-intensity infrared (820) nm laser irradiation on nerve conduction in the human superficial radial nerve. Lasers in Surg Med. 2000; 26: 485-490.

Walsh L J. The use of lasers in implantology: an overview. J Oral Implantol. 1992; 18: 335-340.

Walter Wintsch, Switzerland, personal communication

Wang F, Wang Z. Observation on clinical effect of 70 cases of acute otitis media treated by He-Ne laser radiation on acupoints. Chin J Acupunct Moxibustion. 1991; 4 (1): 30-33.

Wang L-S, Kameya T, Yamada H. A Review of Clinical Applications of Low Level Laser Therapy in Veterinary Medicine. Laser Therapy. 1989; 1 (4): 183-190.

Wang Ya Zhu Jing et al. Vascular low level laser irradiation therapy in treatment of brain injury. Acta Laser Biol Sinica. 1999; 8 (2).

Wasserman I, Rabau M Y, Shoshan S. Collagen metabolism in lowpower CO2 laser welded intesitinal anastomosis in rats. Proc Ninth Congress of the International Society for Laser Surgery and Medicine, Anaheim, Cal., 2-6 November 1991.

Watanabe H, Ishikawa I, Susuki M et al. Clinical assessment of the Erbium:YAG laser for soft tissue surgery and scaling. J Clin Laser Med Surg. 1996; 14 (2): 67-75.

Waylonis G W et al. Chronic myofascial pain: management by low-output helium-neon laser therapy. Arch Phys Med Rehab. 1988; 69: 1017-.

Webb C et al. Stimulatory effect of 660 nm low level laser energy on hypertrophic scar-derived fibroblasts. Possible mechanisms for increase in cell count. Lasers in Surgery and Medicine. 1998; 22: 294.

Webb C, Dyson M, Lewis W H. Stimulatory effect of 660 nm low level laser energy on hypertrophic scar-derived fibroblasts: possible mechanisms for increase in cell counts. .Lasers in Surgery and Medicine. 1998; 22 (5): 294-301.

Wedel H, Calero L, Walger M et al. Soft-laser/Ginkgo therapy in chronic tinnitus. A placebo-controlled study. Adv Otorhinolaryngol.1995; 49: 105-108

Wedlock P, Shephard R A, Little C, McBurney F. Analgesic effects of cranial laser treatment in two rat nociception models. Physiol Behav. 1999; 59 (3): 445-448.

Weintraub M I. Noninvasie laser neurolysis in carpal tunnel syndrome. Muscle Nerve. 1997; 20 (8): 1029-1031.

Weiss N, Oron U. Enhancement of muscle regeneration in the rat gastrocnemius muscle by low energy laser irradiation. Anat Embryol. 1992; 186: 497-503

Wetterberg L et al. Light therapy of depression. Läkartidningen. 1991; Jan 30; 88 (5): 310-312. (in Swedish)

Wetterberg L. Light and biological rhythms. J Intern Med. 1994; 235 (1): 5-19.

Wetterberg L. Light therapy of depression; basal and clinical aspects. Pharmacol Toxicol 1992; 71, Suppl 1: 96-106.

Wetterberg L. Lighting. Nonvisual effects. Scand J Work Environ Health. 1990; 16 Suppl 1: 26-28.

Wetterberg L. Melatonin and affective disorders. Ciba Found Symp. 1985; 117: 253-65

Wetterberg L. The importance of light for health and well-being. Läkartidningen. 1991; 30; 88 (5): 295-296. (in Swedish)

Wetterberg L. The significance of lighting for health and wellbeing. Nord Med. 1991; 106 (3): 90-91. (in Swedish)

Wetterberg L. Light and biological rhythms. Läkartidningen. 1992; 89 (37): 2915-2918. (in Swedish)

Wikner J, Andersson DE, Wetterberg L, Röjdmark S. Impaired melatonin secretion in patients with Wernicke-Korsakoff syndrome. J Intern Med. 1995; 237 (6): 571-575.

Wilden L, Dindinger D. Treatment of chronic diseases in the inner ear with low level laser therapy (laser therapy): pilot project. Laser Therapy. 1996; 8 (2): 209-212.

Wilden L, Ellerbrock D. Verbesserung der Hörkapazität durch Low-Level-Laser-Licht (LLLL). [Amelioration of the hearing capacity by low-level-laser-light (LLL)]. Lasermedizin. 1999; 14: 129-138.

Wilden L. The effect of low level laser light on innear ear diseases. In: Low Level Laser Therapy, Clinical Practice and Scientific Background. Jan Tunér and Lars Hode. Prima Books in Sweden AB (1999). ISBN 91-630-7616-0.

Wilden L, Karthein R. Import of radiation phenomena of electrons and therapeutic low-level laser in regard to the mitochondrial energy transfer. J Clin Med Surg. 1998; 16 (3): 159-165.

Williams R, Havoonjian H, Isagholian K, Menaker G, Moy R. A clinical study of hair removal using the long-pulsed ruby laser. Dermatol Surg. 1998; 24 (8): 837-42.

Wilson M et al. Bacteria in supragingival plaque samples can be killed by low-power laser light in the presence of a photosensitizer. J Appl Bacteriol 1995; 78 (5): 569-74 .

Wilson M, Pratten A. Lethal photosensitisation of Staphylococcus aureus in vitro: effect of growth phase, serum, and pre-irradiation time. Lasers Med Surg. 1995; 16 (3): 272-276.

Winther A, Laserklinikken, Copenhagen, Denmark. 1997. Personal communication.

Wirz-Justice A. Beginning to see the light. Arch Gen Psychiatry. 1998; 55 (10): 861-862. Review.

Witt U, Felix C. Selektive photo-Biochemotherapie in der Kombination Laser und Ginkgo-Pflanzenextrakt nach der Methode Witt. Neue Möglichkeiten bei Innerohrstörungen. (1989). Unpublished material.

Wollman Y et al. Low power laser irradiation enhances migration and neurite sprouting of cultured rat embryonal brain cells. Neurol Res. 1996; 18 (5); 467-470.

Wong E et al. Successful management of female office workers with "repetitive stress injury" or "carpal tunnel syndrome" by a new treatment modality - application of low level laser. Int J Clin Pharmacol Ther. 1995; 33 (4): 208-211.

Wong E et al. Efficiacy of Low Power Laser Therapy in the Pain Relief of Migraine Headaches. Proc Ninth Congress Soc Laser Surgery and Medicine, Anaheim, California, USA: 2-6 November 1991.

Wong E, Lee G, Mason D T. Temporal headaches and associated symptoms related to the styloid process and its attachments. Annn Acad Med Singapore. 1995; 24: 124-128.

Wong F. Laser treatment for headaches of neurogenic and neuromuscular origin. Lasers in Surgery and Medicine. Suppl 12, 2000: 13.

Wu J, Sanchez de la Pena S, Hallberg F et al. Chronosynergistic effects of lighting schedule-shift and cefodizime on plasmacy-toma growth and host survival time. Chronobiologia. 1988; 15 (1-2) : 105-128.

Wu XB. 100 cases of facial paralysis treated with He-Ne laser irradiation on acupoints. J Tradit Chin Med 1990; 10 (4) :300-301.

Wu Wen-hsien, Ponnudurai R, Katz J et al. Failure to confirm report of light-evoked response of peripheral nerve to low power helium-neon laser light stimulus. Brain Research. 1987; 407-408.

Xiaoa X, Donga J, Chua X et al. A single photon emission computed tomography of the therapy of intravascular low intensity laser irradiation on blood for brain infarction. Laser Therapy. 2001; 13: 110-113.

Xijing Wu et al. Observations on the effect of HeNe laser acupoint radiation in chronic pelvic inflammation. J Trad Chin Med. 1983; 7 (4): 263-265.

Xu Yong-Qing et al. Experimental study of the effects of helium-neon laser radiation on repair of injured ten-don. Proc. SPIE.1993; Vol 1616: 598-604. (International Conference on Photodynamic Therapy and Laser Medicine)

Yaakobi T et al. Promotion of bone repair in the cortical bone of the tibia in rats by low energy laser (He-Ne) irradiation. Calcif Tissue Int. 1996; 59 (4): 297-300.

Yaakobi T, Oron U. Enhancement of bone repair in the rat tibia by low energy laser irradiation. Laser Therapy. 1996; 8 (1):19. (Abstract).

Yaakov N, Ben-Haim S, Oron U. Low level laser irradiation reduces interstitial scarring in the isoproternol-induced hypertrohpic rat heart. Laser Therapy. 1999; 11 (4): 190-197.

Yaakov N, Bdolah A, Wollberg Z et al. Recovery from Sarafotoxin-b induced cardiopathological effects in mice following low energy laser irradiation. Basic Research Cardiology. 2000; 95: 385-389.

Yamada H, Kameya T, Abe N, Miyahara K. Low Level Laser Therapy in Horses. Laser Therapy. 1989; 1 (2): 31-36.

Yamada H, Ogawa H. Comparative study of 60 mW diode laser therapy and 150 mW diode laser therapy in the treatment of postherpetic neutralgia. Laser Therapy. 1995; 7 (2): 71-74.

Yamada H, Yamanaka Y, Orihara H et al. Preliminary clinical study comparing the effect of low level laser therapy (laser therapy) and corticosteroid therapy in the treatment of facial palsy. Laser Therapy. 1995; 7 (4): 157-162.

Yamada K. Biological effects of low power laser irradiation on clonal osteoblastic cells (MC3T3-E1). Nippon Seikeigeka Gakkai Zasshi. 1991; 65 (9): 787-799.

Yamada K. Effect of low power laser irradiation on osteoblastic cell growth. Surgical and Medical Lasers. 1989; 2-3 (2): 67. (abstract)

Yamaguchi M et al. Clinical study on the treatment of hypersensitive dentine by GaAlAs laser diode using the double blind test. Aichi Gakuin Daigaku Shigakkai Shi - Aichi-Gakuin Journal of Dental Science 1990; 28(2): 703-707. (In Japanese)

Yamamoto H et al. Pain clinic. 1987; 8: 43-48. (In Japanese).

Yamamoto J.et al. Effect of long-term aerobic exercise on helium-neon-laser-induced thrombogenesis in rat mesenteric arterioles and platelet aggregation. Haemostasis. 1993; 23 (3): 129-134.

Yamamoto Y et al. Effect of low-power laser irradiation on procollagen synthesis in human fibroblasts. J Clin Laser Med Surg. 1996; 14 (3): 129-132.

Yamaya M, Shiroto C, Kobayashi Mechanistic approach to GaAlAs diode laser effects on production of reactive oxygen species from human neutrophils as a model for therapeutic modality at cellular level. Laser Therapy. 1993; 5 (3): 111-116.

Yan Li, Timon Cheng-Yi Liu, Rui Duan. Effects of some anaesthetics on wound healing: laser biomodulation mechanisms. Lasers in Surgery and Medicine. 2001; Suppl 13: 9. Lasers in Surgery and Medicine. 2001; Suppl 13: 9.

Yarita T et al. Effect of low power laser on gingival microcirculation. Proc. X Internat Congress Int Soc Laser Surgery and Medicine, Bangkok 1993, p 235.

Yasuda, Kubota J, Ohshiro T. The effects of diode laser low reactive-level laser therapy (laser therapy) on musculocutaneous flaps. Laser Therapy. 1993; 5 (4): 159-163.

Yew D T et al. Low dose laser and the developing retina. A histochemical and scanning electronmicroscopic study. Acta Morphol Neerl Scand. 1982; 20: 57-63.

Yew D T et al. Responses of astrocytes in culture after low dose laser irradiation. Scand Microscopy. 1990; 4: 151-159.

Yilmaz S, Kuru B, Kuru L et al. Effect of galium arsenide diode laser on human periodontal disease: A microbiological and clinical study. Lasers Surg Med. 2002; 30 (1): 60-66

Yo-Chen Zhou. Practical Applications of Non-contact laser therapy in Various Fields. In: Low Level Laser Therapy. A Practical Introduction, Eds. Ohshiro & Calderhead. John Wiley & Sons. 1988: 71.

Yonaga T, Kimura Y, Matsumoto K. Treatment of cervical dentin hypersensitivity by various methods using pulsed Nd:YAG laser. Journal of Clinical Laser Medicine and Surgery. 1999; 17 (5): 205-210.

Yoo C, Lee W K, Kemmotsu O. Efficacy of polarized light therapy for musculoskeletal pain. Laser Therapy. 1993; 5 (4): 153-157.

Yoshida K, Kato M, Ishida S, Arao M, Fukaya M. The management of the facial palsy patients using lower power output laser irradiation. 4th International Congress on Lasers in Dentistry, Singapore, 1994: 39.

Yoshida T et al. Pain reduction effect of soft laser in orthodontic therapy. Proc. Annual Meeting Jpn Orthodont Soc. 1992: 69.

Young JM, Altschuler BR. Laser holography in dentistry. J Prosthet Dent. 1977; 38 (2): 216-225.

Yu H S et al. Low energy helium-neon laser irradiation stimulates interleukin-1 alpha and interleukin-8 release from cultured human keratinocytes. J Invest Dermatol. 1996; 107 (4): 593-596.

Yu W et al. Effects of photostimulation on wound healing in diabetic mice. Lasers in Surgery and Medicine. 1997; 20 (1): 56-63.

Yu W et al. Improvement of host response to sepsis by photobiomodulation. Lasers in Surg Med. 1997; 21: 262-268.

Yu W et al. The effect of laser irradiation on the release of bFGF from 3T3 fibroblasts. Photochem Photobiol. 1994; 59 (2): 167-170.

Yu W, Naim JO, McGowan M, Ippolito K, Lanzafame RJ. Photomodulation of oxidative metabolism and electron chain enzymes in rat liver mitochondria. Photochem Photobiol 1997; (6):866-871.

Yu, I. Low Power Laser Therapy for carpal tunnel syndrome.Proc X Internat Congress Int Soc Laser Surg Med, Bangkok 1993, p. 197

Zalesskiy V N, Belousova I A, Frolov G V. Laser-acupuncture reduces cigarette smoking: a preliminary report. Acupunct Electrother Res. 1983 ;8 (3-4): 297-302.

Zarkovic J et al. Use of HeNe laser for treatment of soft tissue trauma: evaluation by Gallium-67 citrate scanning. J Orthop and Sports Physical Therapy. 1986; 8 (2): 93-96.

Zhang D, Gao Q. Treatment of facial paralysis with laser and acupuncture; report of 76 cases. Int J Clin Acupunct 1993; 4 (3): 327-329.

Zhang D, Zhou Y, Xiao B, Li G. The effect of postoperative irradiation with low incident levels of CO2 laser irradiation on skin flap survival and the possible mechanisms. Laser Therapy. 1992; 4 (2): 75-80.

Zheng H, Qin J, Xin H, Xin S: The activation action of low level Helium Neon laser radiation on macrophages in the mouse model. Laser Therapy. 1992; 4 (2): 55-58.

Zhong X et al. Correlation between endogenous opiate-like peptides and serotonin in laseracupuncture analgesia. Am J Acupunct. 1989; 17: 39-43.

Zhou Y C. An Advanced Clinical Trial with Laser Acupuncture Anaesthesia for Minor Operations in the Oro-maxillofacial Region. Lasers in Surgery and Medicine. 1984; 4: 297-.

Zhou Y C. Effect of HeNe laser irradiation of acupoint on analgesia and met-enkephalin contents in different regions in the rat. Laser Journal. 1986; 7: 41-. (in Chinese with English abstract.)

Zhou, Chuannong; Song, Xuyan; Deng, Jinsheng; Liang, Junlin; Zhang, Hua; Huang, Wenjia; Liu, Tao; Ha, Xian-Wen Photodynamic effect of copper-vapor pumped-dye laser, HeNe laser, and noncoherent red light to the liver in normal mice. Proc. SPIE.1993; Vol 1616: 239-245. (International Conference on Photodynamic Therapy and Laser Medicine, Jun-Heng Li; Ed.)

Zhu Q, Yu W, Yang X et al. Photoirradiation improved functional preservation of the isolated rat heart. Lasers in Surgery and Medicine. 1997; 20: 332-339.

Zubkova S T. [The use of helium-neon laser radiation in the treatment of trophic disorders in patients with diabetes mellitus]. Klin Khir. 1992; 3: 47-49. (in Russian with English abstract)

14.3 Abbreviations

Abbreviations used in this book are explained but not everywhere you meet them in the text. The following is a list of some of these abbreviations.

ASA	Acetylsalicylic Acid
ATP	Adenosine Triphosphate
BMP	Bone Morphogenetic Protein
CL	Chemiluminescence
CO_2	Carbon Dioxide
CTS	Carpal Tunnel Syndrome
CW	Continuous Wave
DNA	Deoxyribonucleic Acid
ED	Energy Density
EDL	Emitted Defocused Laser-Light
EMG	Electromyogram
ENT	Ear-Nose-Throat
Er:YAG	Erbium Yttrium-Aluminium-Garnet
FCS	Fetal Calf Serum
FDA	Food and Drug Administration
GaAlAs	Gallium Aluminium Arsenide
GaAs	Gallium Arsenide
Gy	Gray
HeNe	Helium Neon
Ho:YAG	Holmium Yttrium-Aluminium-Garnet
HSV	Herpes Simplex Virus
InGaAlP	Indium Gallium Aluminium Phosphide

IR	Infra Red
IRB	Institutional Review Board
KTP	Potassium (Kalium) Titanyle Phosphide
LED	Light Emitting Diode
MRI	Magnetic Resonance Imaging
Nd:YAG	Neodymium Yttrium-Aluminium-Garnet
NMRI	Nuclear Magnetic Resonance Imaging
NO	Nitric Oxide
NSAID	Non-Steriodal Anti-Inflammatory Drug
OA	Osteoarthritis
PD	Power Density
PDT	Photodynamic Therapy
PGE	Prostaglandine E
PHN	Postherpetic Neuralgia
RA	Rheumatic Arthritis
RNA	Ribonucleic Acid
ROM	Range Of Movement
SEM	Sweep Electron Microscopy
SOD	Super Oxide Dismutase
SPIE	The International Society for Optical Engineering
TBO	Tolouidine Blue
TMD	Temporo Mandibular Disorders
TMJ	Temporomandibular joint
TMR	Transmyocardial Revascularisation
VAS	Visual Analogue Scale
YAG	Yttrium Aluminium Garnet

Alphabetic index

A

Absorption 4, 25, 28, 38
Acetylcholine 357
Achilles 175, 177
Acne 31, 36, 100, 116
ACTH 168, 336
Acute calculous pyelonephritis 89
Acyclovir 148, 149
Adhesion 82, 163, 177
Alexandrite 20, 26, 27, 39
Allergy 4, 116
Alveolitis 85, 166, 204, 221
Anaesthesia 33, 84, 204
Anaesthetics 85, 204, 205
Angiogenesis 134, 225, 405
Angular cheilitis 220
Ankle sprain 175, 408
Ankylosing spondylarthritis 124
Aphthae 33, 36, 205, 206, 221, 222
Argon 19, 26, 27, 37, 39
Arndt-Schulz law 320
Asthma 117
ATP 97, 151, 185, 357, 361
Average power output 17

B

Bacteria 67, 102, 130, 149, 208, 209
Bechterew 118, 124
Bell's paralysis 160
Biostimulation 26, 27, 30, 37, 38, 40, 43, 61, 72, 98, 110, 112
Bleeding 85, 206, 207
Blink reflex 22, 24
Blood flow 79, 91, 105, 106, 153, 154, 162, 190, 196, 207, 214, 226
Blood pressure 125
Bone regeneration 100, 126, 130, 211
Bright Light Phototherapy 345
Bürger's disease 141

Burns 194
Bursitis 121, 143, 176

C

Calcium ion balance 65
Cancer 4, 33, 39, 97, 102, 205
Candida albicans 79
Canker sore 205
Carbon dioxide laser (acupuncture) 85, 87
Carbon dioxide laser (surgical) 28
Carbon dioxide laser (therapeutic) 98
Cardiac conditions 134
Caries 207, 234
Caries detection 235
Carpal tunnel 111, 135
Cartilage 118, 120, 121, 127, 129
Case reports 198, 235
Cellulites 199
Cerebral palsy 136
C-fibre 156, 356
Chemiluminescence 69, 96, 106
Chromophore 65, 162, 351, 352
Chronic pain 78, 139, 168, 174, 336, 356
Circulatory encephalopathy 89
Cluster probe 407
Coagulation 85, 193, 211, 225
Cochrane 139, 412
Collagen 63, 65, 74, 97, 99, 100, 106
Collimation 19, 92, 339, 345
Combination probe 319
Composite curing 235
Contraindications 285
Copper vapour laser 37
Corticosteroid 143, 160
C-reactive protein 213
Cross-over study 86, 142, 196
Crural ulcer 137, 335
Cumulative effect 80, 81, 168
Cytotoxin 205, 288

D

de Quervain's disease 142
Delayed onset muscle soreness 174
Dentitio dificilis 170, 209
Depolarisation 157, 357
Depression 88, 139, 334, 345
Diabetes 289
Divergence 22, 24, 92, 297, 318, 404
DNA 65, 97, 121, 127, 133, 134, 192, 214, 218
Dosage 69, 70, 73, 176, 179
Double blind studies 380, 388, 391
Dressings 194
Dry socket 204
Duodenal ulcer 141
Duty cycle 16, 17, 18, 40, 371
Dye laser 26, 37, 39, 194

E

Eczema 116
Electromagnetic radiation 2, 3, 4
Endodontics 210
Endorphin 168, 336, 356
Epicondylitis 98, 141, 177
Epilepsy 279, 286, 376
Epithelium down-growth 32, 225
Er:YAG 26, 198
Er:YAG (dental) 204, 205
Er:YAG (surgical) 33, 35
ErCr:YSGG 36
Excimer laser 19, 27, 39, 126
Extraction 85, 129, 211
Eye hazard 318

F

Fibrin network 162, 207
Fibroblast 32, 65, 70, 74, 80, 96, 100, 120, 121, 133, 158, 191, 195, 205, 212-214, 227
Fibromyalgia 121, 143, 236
Flap operation 32, 100, 225, 227
Fluorescence 39, 235, 351, 353, 363

Fracture 127, 219
Frenectomy 35, 36
Frequency 2, 16
Frequency doubled Nd:YAG 37

G

GaAlInP laser 41
GaAs laser 42
GAlAs laser 41
Genital 31, 147, 188
Gingivectomy 32, 215
Gingivitis 213
Glossitis 219
Goggles (protective) 19, 25, 42, 164
Gynaecology 31, 145

H

Haemangioma 29, 32, 37, 94
Haemoglobin 95, 162, 207, 345, 359
Haemorrhoids 147
Hair laser 199
Headache 86, 146, 182
Heat sensation 40, 42, 54, 65, 91, 105, 200, 352
HeNe laser 40, 49
Herpes simplex 34
Hologram 38, 235
Hyperaemia 208
Hyperplasia 32, 36, 234
Hyperreflexic bladder 145
Hypersensitive dentine 215

I

Immune system 65, 88, 89, 91, 102, 130, 149
Impacted wisdom teeth 212
Implantology 218
Incoherent polarised light 142, 334, 338
Infected wounds 193
Infertility 145, 186
Inflammation 78, 82, 95, 108, 120, 143, 151, 163, 165, 172, 176, 177, 187, 188, 195

Inhibition 74, 96, 97
Inner ear 94, 151, 178
Interleukin 118, 192, 222, 231
Intraligamental anaesthesia 205, 224
Ischemia 84, 141, 405
Ischemic heart conditions 89, 135, 420

J

Jaw fracture 219
Joule 69, 70, 71

K

Keloid 31, 100, 248
Keratinocyte 96, 192, 274, 349, 406
Keratoconjunctivitis 49, 165
Krypton laser 44, 148, 192
KTP 26, 37

L

Laryngitis 151
Laser acupuncture 78, 84, 86, 105
Laser cytofluorometry 364
Laser Doppler Velocimeter 363
Laser microscopy 364
Laser speckle flowmetry 153
Laser spectroscopy 364
Lasing effects in tissue 354
LED 6, 46, 51, 57, 79, 226, 235, 293, 298, 300, 319, 334, 335, 336, 340, 341, 351
Leukoplakia 219, 236
Lichen 29, 151
Lingua geographica 219
Lip fissure 220
Lip wounds 220
Liver 194
Low back pain 43, 152, 176
Lumbago 99
Lumbar disc herniation 152
Luminescence 353
Lung abscess 89, 420

Lymph nodes 83, 91, 209, 224
Lymphatic system 66, 162, 163, 164, 190
Lymphocytes 97, 102, 120, 149, 150, 151, 184, 187, 359

M

Macrophage 354, 359
Mastitis 146, 194, 279
Ménière 178
Menstrual pain 145
Meta analysis 109, 125, 167, 191, 195, 382, 414
Microcirculation 88, 89, 141, 152, 154, 173
Migraine 146
Mononucleated cell 155
Moxa 84, 87
Mucocele 32
Mucositis 82, 130, 132
Muscle regeneration 155
Myofibroblast 65, 226
Myoses 53, 230
Myotube 131, 155, 156

N

Naloxone 167, 356
Nausea 84, 220
Nd:YAG (dental) 33
Nd:YAG (surgical) 33
Nd:YAG (therapeutic) 100
Nephritis 89, 420
Nerve conduction 156
Nerve regeneration 68

O

Oedema 85, 88, 135, 163, 188, 195
OPH gestosis 89
Ophthalmic problems 164
Opioid 336
Optical field 3
Oral surgery 221
Orthodontics 222

Osteoarthritis 118, 123
Osteoblast 126, 128
Osteoclast 126, 223
Osteocyte 126

P

Pacemaker 286
Paediatric patients 133, 224
Pain 166
Pain reaction 103
Paraesthesia 100, 136, 159, 161, 221
Parameters 68
PDT 26, 150, 225, 337, 343, 354, 363
Peak pulse power 17, 58, 95
Penetration depth 17, 28, 39, 41, 42, 43, 68, 69, 83, 92, 94, 95
Periodontics 34, 225
Periostitis 174, 237
PGE1 120
PGE2 .... 118, 120, 123, 215
Phantom pain 169
Pharyngitis 100
Photo dynamic therapy 234, 337
Photobiomodulation .... VI, 67
Photon energy 2, 10, 235, 343, 354, 355, 362
Photosensitivity 158
Pituitary gland 67, 167
Plantar fasciitis 170
Plaque (dental) 209, 214, 215
Plaque (viral) 148
Pneumonia 89, 420
Polarisation 15, 294, 334, 337, 350, 358
Porphyrin 65, 293, 350, 351, 355, 357
Postherpetic neuralgia 55, 148, 168, 196, 197
Prostaglandin 120, 222, 256, 259, 273
Prostatitis 186, 188, 420
Prosthetics 228
Proximal priority 142, 175
Psoriasis 98
Psoriatic arthritis 118, 121
Pulp capping 210
Pulse frequency 2, 17, 42, 50, 72, 78, 96, 167, 172, 185, 278, 295, 296, 301

Pulse train 37, 42, 372

Q

Q-switched 11, 39

R

Radiation risks 3
Ranula 32
Raynaud's disease 105, 153, 197
Retention cyst 32
Rheumatoid arthritis 100, 105, 121, 414
Risks and side effects 101
RNA 65, 121, 127, 192, 215, 218, 286
Root canal 26, 32, 35, 36, 127, 210
Ruby laser 8, 27

S

Salivary glands 171
Scanner 43, 48, 117, 137, 371
Scattering 315, 321, 334, 341, 343, 344, 351
Schizophrenia 89, 420
Schlatter 287
Schwann cell 157
Sciatic nerve 157, 158, 159, 160, 167
Secondary dentine 100, 210, 211, 229
Semiconductor laser 26, 39, 40
Serotonin 168, 345, 346, 347, 348, 354
Shingles 49, 196
Shoulder tendinitis 112, 143, 337
Sialoadenitis 172
Side effects 101
Singlet oxygen 65, 82, 354, 357
Sinuitis 172
Sjögren's syndrome 171
Sluder 155, 420
Soft laser 46
Somatosensory tinnitus 181, 182
Speckle Interferometry 363
Speckles 13, 14, 294, 339, 340, 341, 350

Spectrum 2, 5, 7
Sperm 185, 186
Spinal cord 88, 158, 162, 173
Sports injuries 68, 174
Stellate ganglion 104, 161, 168, 197
Steroid 112, 143, 230, 231
Strain injuries 175
Stye 25, 165
Superpulse 17, 28, 42, 43, 77, 92
Suppression 66, 131, 135, 157
Swimmers Ear 180
Synovia 104, 118, 121, 123, 124, 231
Systemic effect 65, 66, 67, 95, 140, 190, 322, 344, 374, 391, 400, 405

T

Tattoo 26, 31, 37, 38, 39
Temporo-mandibular disorders 181, 230
Tendinitis 109, 112, 143, 176, 177
Tennis elbow 88, 176, 338
Tensile strength 66, 106, 225, 226
Terminology VI
Therapeutic window 100, 323, 336
Thermography 85, 105, 123, 140, 153, 170
Thrombophlebitis 185
Thyroid gland 133, 151, 286
Tissue condition 95
TMD 181, 230, 233, 234
Tonsillitis 183
Tooth bleaching 235
Tourette's syndrome 89, 420
Treatment dose 70
Treatment interval 74, 80
Treatment technique 68, 83, 329
Trigeminal neuralgia 79, 100, 184
Trigger point 77, 84, 87
Trismus 85, 163, 222, 230
Tuberculosis 44, 66

U

Urology 185

Uveitis 165

V

Vaginitis 146
Vasoconstriction 206
Vasodilatation 86, 105, 206
Venous ulcer 137
Vertigo 178, 230, 238
Veterinary 59, 278, 363
Virus 28, 96, 98, 102, 147, 149, 157

W

Warts 188
Wavelength 2, 3
Wound healing 189
Wrinkles 31, 36, 37, 198, 334

X

Xerostomia 172
X-ray 3, 4, 82, 104, 129, 156

Y

Yttrium 33, 36

Z

Zoster 38, 80, 88, 147, 196

About the authors

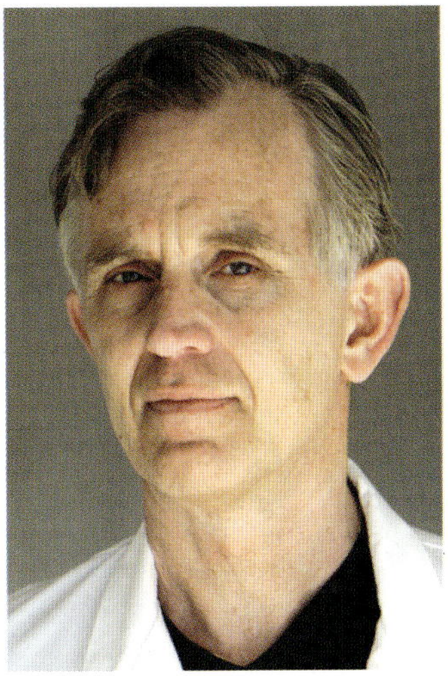

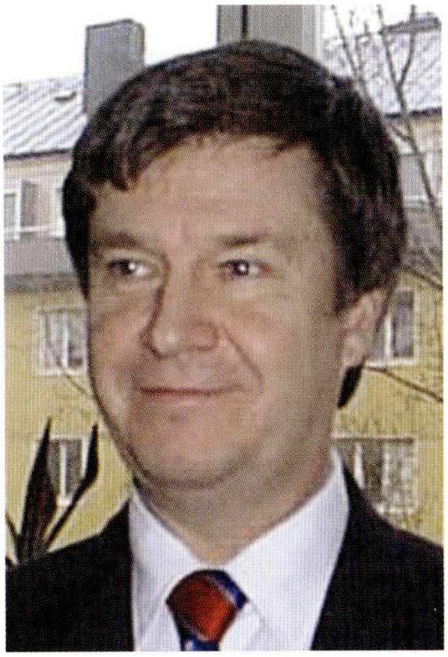

Jan Tunér is a dentist in private practise, working with lasers since 1986. He is a board member of the World Association for Laser Therapy.

Lars Hode is a physicist, specialised in medical laser applications and working with laser therapy since 1985. He is the president and founder of the Swedish Laser-Medical Society.